Recent Advancements in Brain Injury Medicine

Recent Advancements in Brain Injury Medicine

Editor: Emily Miller

AMERICAN
MEDICAL PUBLISHERS
www.americanmedicalpublishers.com

AMERICAN
MEDICAL PUBLISHERS
www.americanmedicalpublishers.com

Cataloging-in-Publication Data

Recent advancements in brain injury medicine / edited by Emily Miller.
p. cm.
Includes bibliographical references and index.
ISBN 979-8-88740-420-2
1. Brain--Wounds and injuries. 2. Brain damage. 3. Brain--Wounds and injuries--Treatment.
4. Brain damage--Treatment. 5. Brain--Wounds and injuries--Patients--Rehabilitation.
6. Brain--Wounds and injuries--Patients--Care. I. Miller, Emily.
RD594 .R43 2023
617.481--dc23

American Medical Publishers,
41 Flatbush Avenue,
1st Floor, New York,
NY 11217, USA

ISBN 979-8-88740-420-2 (Hardback)

Contents

Preface

The disorders which affect the brain and which are caused by an injury are treated within the field of brain injury medicine. It encompasses medical, physical, cognitive, sensory, and behavioral disorders. Acute injury refers to any severe injury that happens suddenly or spontaneously. Sudden injury to the brain is known as acute brain injury or traumatic brain injury (TBI). Alternatively, the death or degeneration of brain cells is known as neurotrauma or brain damage. Several internal and external events can cause brain damage. The severity of acute brain injury is estimated by determining how the normal brain function has been affected, the duration of loss of consciousness, the period of apnea (cessation of breathing), and the time it takes for the self-righting reflex to recover. An inflammatory response to TBI within the brain or spinal cord is known as neuroinflammation. It is caused by generation of cytokines, chemokines, reactive oxygen species (ROS), and secondary messengers. Neurodegeneration refers to the progressive atrophy (a condition in which a body portion, cell, organ, or other tissue shrinks in size) and loss of neuronal functions which is usually observed in neurodegenerative disorders like Alzheimer's and Parkinson's. The book aims to shed light on some of the unexplored aspects of brain injury. It will provide comprehensive knowledge with respect to the recent advancements in brain injury medicine.

The information contained in this book is the result of intensive hard work done by researchers in this field. All due efforts have been made to make this book serve as a complete guiding source for students and researchers. The topics in this book have been comprehensively explained to help readers understand the growing trends in the field.

I would like to thank the entire group of writers who made sincere efforts in this book and my family who supported me in my efforts of working on this book. I take this opportunity to thank all those who have been a guiding force throughout my life.

Editor

1

Molecular magnetic resonance imaging of brain–immune interactions

Maxime Gauberti, Axel Montagne, Aurélien Quenault and Denis Vivien*

Inserm, Inserm UMR-S U919, Serine Proteases and Pathophysiology of the Neurovascular Unit, Université de Caen Basse-Normandie – GIP Cyceron, Caen, France

Correspondence:
Denis Vivien, Inserm, Inserm UMR-S U919, Serine Proteases and Pathophysiology of the Neurovascular Unit, Université de Caen Basse-Normandie – GIP Cyceron, Boulevard Henri Becquerel, BP5229, 14074 Caen, France
e-mail: vivien@cyceron.fr

Although the blood–brain barrier (BBB) was thought to protect the brain from the effects of the immune system, immune cells can nevertheless migrate from the blood to the brain, either as a cause or as a consequence of central nervous system (CNS) diseases, thus contributing to their evolution and outcome. Accordingly, as the interface between the CNS and the peripheral immune system, the BBB is critical during neuroinflammatory processes. In particular, endothelial cells are involved in the brain response to systemic or local inflammatory stimuli by regulating the cellular movement between the circulation and the brain parenchyma. While neuropathological conditions differ in etiology and in the way in which the inflammatory response is mounted and resolved, cellular mechanisms of neuroinflammation are probably similar. Accordingly, neuroinflammation is a hallmark and a decisive player of many CNS diseases. Thus, molecular magnetic resonance imaging (MRI) of inflammatory processes is a central theme of research in several neurological disorders focusing on a set of molecules expressed by endothelial cells, such as adhesion molecules (VCAM-1, ICAM-1, P-selectin, E-selectin, ...), which emerge as therapeutic targets and biomarkers for neurological diseases. In this review, we will present the most recent advances in the field of preclinical molecular MRI. Moreover, we will discuss the possible translation of molecular MRI to the clinical setting with a particular emphasis on myeloperoxidase imaging, autologous cell tracking, and targeted iron oxide particles (USPIO, MPIO).

Keywords: inflammation, stroke, Alzheimer, multiple sclerosis, hemorrhage, lymphocytes, microparticles, antibody

INTRODUCTION

Brain–immune interactions play a central role in acute neurological disorders including ischemic stroke, intracranial hemorrhage and traumatic brain injury (Wang and Dore, 2007; Iadecola and Anrather, 2011; Woodcock and Morganti-Kossmann, 2013). Given the proven and putative clinical benefits of modulating brain–immune interactions, non-invasive methods aimed at imaging the molecular players involved in these processes have been the subject of numerous studies. The most promising approaches to visualize brain–immune interactions are magnetic resonance imaging (MRI), positron emission tomography (PET), single photon emission computed tomography (SPECT), and optical imaging (in preclinical studies). Only molecular MRI combines fast acquisition time, wide clinical availability and acceptable safety profile for repeated scanning. However, molecular MRI lacks sensitivity compared to PET or SPECT. Notably, recent developments in the field of MRI contrast agent dramatically improved MRI sensitivity and allowed, for the first time, reliable imaging of the proteins involved in brain immune interactions with high spatial and temporal resolutions.

Brain–immune interactions occur all over the time course of acute neurological diseases. Upon injury, endothelial cells of the cerebrovasculature become activated and release the content of their Weibel-Palade bodies. This leads to P-selectin exposure on their surface and subsequent adhesion of neutrophils through P-selectin – P-selectin Glycoprotein Ligand-1 (PSGL-1) interactions (Ley et al., 2007). In parallel, in the brain parenchyma, an early phase of microglial activation is followed by a local inflammatory response (including microgliosis, astrogliosis, and cytokines/chemokines secretion) which sustains the activation state of brain endothelial cells. Expression of E-selectin, intercellular adhesion molecule-1 (ICAM-1), and vascular cell adhesion molecule-1 (VCAM-1) on the luminal endothelial surface allows adhesion and subsequent diapedesis of systemic immune cells inside the brain parenchyma. These infiltrated cells further enhance the inflammatory reaction in order to fight potential pathogens and clear cellular debris. To this aim, they secrete numerous cytokines/chemokines, proteolytic enzymes, and peroxydases (including myeloperoxidase, MPO). Neuroinflammation is also deemed necessary for the post-injury reparation phase that can last for weeks after the initial brain insult (Kyritsis et al., 2012; Tobin et al., 2014). This phase involves neurogenesis, dendritogenesis, oligodendrogenesis, axon sprouting, and matrix remodeling to restore tissue integrity (Peruzzotti-Jametti et al., 2014). All these mechanisms are common to acute brain injuries (including ischemia, hemorrhage, and trauma), neuroinflammatory (including multiple sclerosis) and neurodegenerative disorders (Schwartz et al., 2013). However, discrepancies exist in terms of kinetic, localization, and intensity of the inflammatory responses.

Improvement in our general knowledge of the brain–immune interactions taking place during acute neurological disorders revealed new potential therapeutic targets. Nevertheless, the successes and failures of immunomodulatory treatments for acute brain injury remind us that precise characterization of the interplay between leukocytes, endothelial adhesion molecules, glial, and neuronal cells is mandatory for efficient design of therapeutic strategies targeting brain–immune interactions. For instance, Natalizumab, a monoclonal antibody targeting the interaction between very late antigen 4 (VLA-4) and VCAM-1, has been successfully developed as a treatment for multiple sclerosis (Miller et al., 2003). In contrast, Enlimomab, a monoclonal antibody targeting neutrophils diapedesis by ICAM-1 blockade, has failed in phase III trials involving ischemic stroke patients (Enlimomab Acute Stroke Trial, 2001), despite preclinical evidence of its potent neuroprotective effects (Matsuo et al., 1994; Connolly et al., 1996). In fact, contrary to what initially thought, a recent study demonstrated that neutrophils do not reach the brain parenchyma after stroke in humans (Enzmann et al., 2013). Moreover, it becomes now clearer that one size does not fit all: variability in individual inflammatory response following acute brain injury suggests that modulation of brain–immune interaction may prove beneficial in some individuals but not in others. Considering that blockade of leukocytes subsets may also be associated with impaired host defense against pathogens, adequate selection of patients should be performed before administration of immunomodulatory drugs.

In this context, molecular MRI appears highly promising to select patient candidates for immunomodulatory treatments, monitor treatment efficiency, and more generally improve our knowledge on brain–immune interactions in human patients. The purpose of this review is to present recent advances in the field of molecular MRI of brain–immune interactions. After presentation of the theoretical bases of molecular MRI and of the brain-specific issues of this non-invasive method, we will present recent studies relevant to brain–immune interactions after acute cerebral injury with a particular focus on MPO imaging, autologous cell tracking, unlabeled ultrasmall superparamagnetic particles of iron oxide (USPIOs), targeted USPIOs, and targeted microsized particles of iron oxide (MPIOs; **Figure 1**).

BASIS OF MOLECULAR MAGNETIC RESONANCE IMAGING

Magnetic resonance imaging signal is generated by the magnetization of the hydrogen nuclei (protons) from biological tissues. Basically, two different classes of MRI contrast agents are available: T1 contrast agents increase the signal on T1-weighted images by shortening the spin-lattice relaxation time (T1 constant). T2 and T2* contrast agents decrease the signal on T2- and T2*-weighted images by both shortening the spin–spin relaxation time (T2 constant) and dephasing adjacent protons (by modification of their precession angular velocity). Therefore, depending on the contrast material injected, a molecular target can be revealed by an increase (paramagnetic T1 contrast agent, mainly Gadolinium-based) or a decrease (superparamagnetic T2 or T2* contrast agent, mainly iron-oxide-based) in the MRI signal (**Figure 2**). New methods of molecular MRI have been recently developed [such as chemical exchange saturation transfer (CEST), positive contrast imaging or MRI of non-hydrogen nuclei] but they still present a

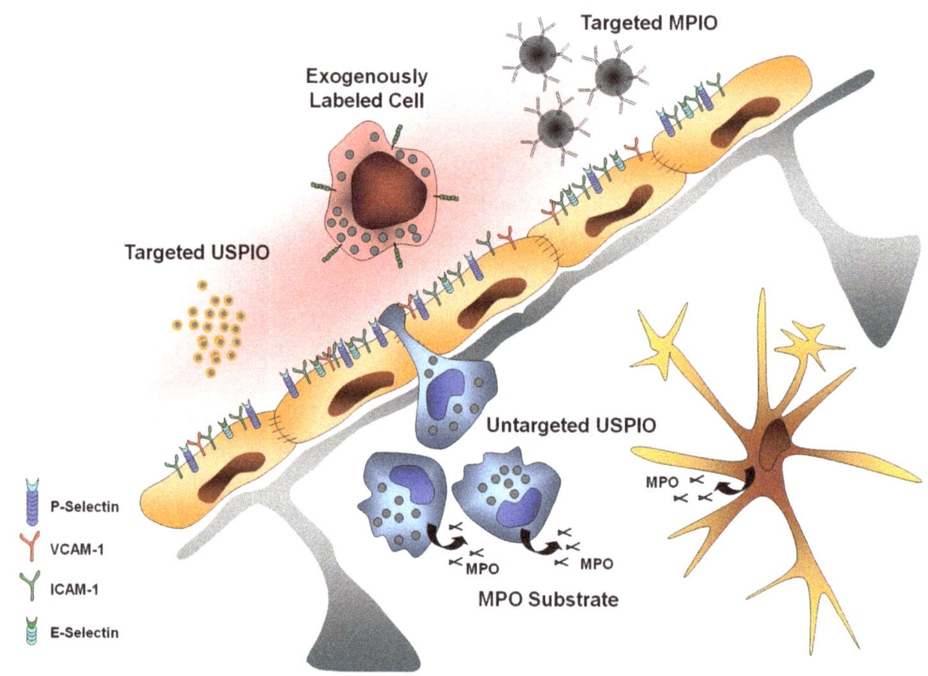

FIGURE 1 | Main targets of molecular imaging. USPIO, ultrasmall particles of iron oxide; MPIO, microsized particles of iron oxide; MPO, myeloperoxidase; VCAM-1, vascular cell adhesion molecule-1; ICAM-1, intercellular adhesion molecule-1.

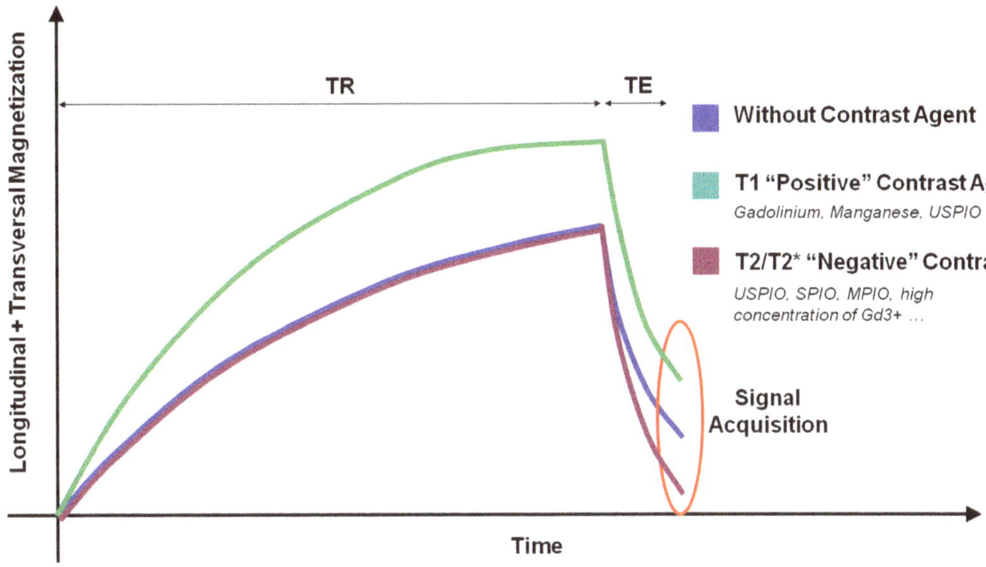

FIGURE 2 | Schematic representation of the effects of different contrast agents on water magnetization in biological samples. TR, repetition time; TE, Echo Time.

limited sensitivity compared to more conventional methods. Their development remains however of great interest since such contrast agents could allow imaging multiple targets simultaneously (Woods et al., 2006).

Independently of the contrast agent, the general concept of molecular MRI is to target a contrastophore (either Gadolinium- or Iron-oxide-based) to a protein of interest using a targeting moiety (pharmacophore). This targeting moiety can be either a specific ligand (such as a protein, an antibody or a specifically designed peptide) or a substrate of an enzyme which can accumulate in the regions where its corresponding enzyme is overexpressed/active. For instance, VCAM-1 imaging can be performed using microparticles of iron oxide (MPIO, the contrastophore) coupled to monoclonal antibodies targeting VCAM-1 (the pharmacophore). After intravenous injection, this agent binds to endothelial VCAM-1 and induces T2* effects leading to decreased signal on T2*-weighted images (i.e., signal voids) in regions presenting activated endothelial cells (McAteer et al., 2007).

The concentration of contrast material is one of the most important limits of molecular MRI. Indeed, whereas PET can detect β^+ emitting atoms at picomolar concentration, MRI using classical Gadolinium-based contrast agent (GBCA) presents a sensitivity in the micromolar range. To overcome this limitation, contrast agent carrying large payload of gadolinium or iron oxide have been developed, including paramagnetic liposomes and iron oxide particles (**Figure 3**). In this regard, MPIOs (1–4 μm in diameter) are particularly interesting since even a single particle can be detected by high-field MRI at high resolution (Montagne et al., 2012). After binding to its target, targeted MPIOs induce dephasing of the surrounding protons, leading to strong and large T2* effects, up to 50 times larger than the original particle size (~50 μm; Shapiro et al., 2006). At equal concentrations of iron, MPIOs induce much stronger T2* effects than USPIOs (10–50 nm; Montagne et al., 2012). This new generation of contrastophores is therefore especially efficient for the detection of targets present at low concentration on the surface of brain endothelial cells.

The use of high resolution and strongly T2*-weighted images to improve MRI sensitivity may also favor endogenous contrasts and false positive detection of iron oxide particles. In particular, hemorrhages and blood oxygen level dependent (BOLD) effects induce signal voids on T2*-weighted images which are comparable to MPIO-induced signal void and could therefore lead to false positive results. To overcome this, we demonstrated in a recent study in mice that a short preparation time (30 min) of normobaric hyperoxia can be sufficient to transform deoxyhemoglobin (paramagnetic) into oxyhemoglobin (diamagnetic) by increasing the tissular concentration of O_2 (Gaberel et al., 2013). Thus, the susceptibility effect of endogenous blood is blunted, allowing observing changes in signal intensity that are specific to the contrast agent injected. Importantly, this preparation period of hyperoxia did not impair behavioral testing in mice presenting intracranial hemorrhages suggesting that this strategy is safe. Further studies should look at the effect of normobaric hyperoxia on T2*-weighted images in larger animals and humans.

BRAIN SPECIFIC ISSUES IN MOLECULAR IMAGING

The presence of the BBB represents a challenge for molecular imaging of the brain. Indeed, to reach parenchymal targets, contrast agents should be able to cross the BBB. To date, there is no contrast agent able to cross the BBB in sufficiently large quantities to induce significant changes in MRI signal. Therefore molecular imaging of the brain is limited to endothelial proteins (such as VCAM-1, ICAM-1, E-selectin, and P-selectin), to diseases with compromised BBB (such as stroke, multiple sclerosis or severe

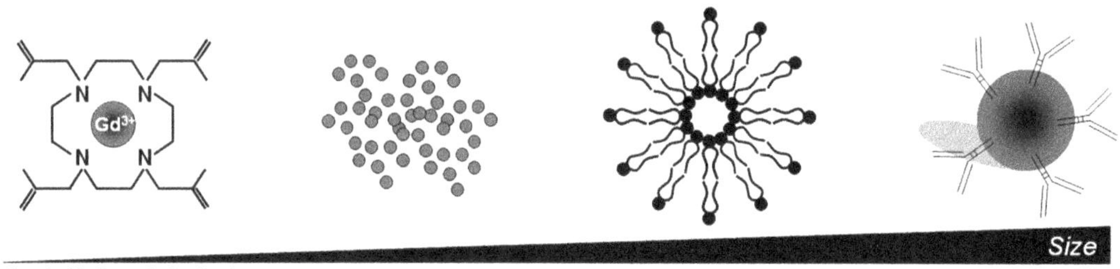

	Gadolinium labeled contrast agent	USPIO	Loaded-Liposomes	MPIO
Diameter	1 – 7 nm	10-50 nm	80-300 nm	1000 - 4000 nm
T1 Effect	+++	+	+++ or ~0	~0
T2 Effect	+/-	+	+	+
T2* Effect	+/-	+	+ or +++	+++

FIGURE 3 | Main characteristics of the most widely used contrastophores.

traumatic brain injury) and to cells capable of crossing the BBB (such as monocytes). The purpose of this paragraph is to present the main issues related to each imaging targets that should be kept in mind when performing molecular MRI of brain–immune interactions.

Endothelial proteins are targets easily accessible to large contrast-carrying particles and have been accordingly successfully imaged using different contrast agents (from small GBCA to large iron oxide particles). The first issue related to imaging of endothelial targets is the requirement of a high affinity of the pharmacophore for its target because of the force exerted by the blood flow. These shear forces promote detachment of the contrast agent from the endothelial wall and thus limit the time window for imaging (von Zur Muhlen et al., 2008). Moreover, since MRI should be performed after complete washout of the contrast agent from the blood, a short half-life of the contrast agent is required to allow imaging before its detachment from the endothelium. Therefore, for efficient detection of endothelial targets, the contrast agent should combine a high affinity for its target and a short half-life. Importantly, to avoid false positive findings, the molecular weight of the contrast agent should be large enough to prevent passive extravasation across the BBB. Of note, once in the brain parenchyma, low molecular weight compounds are able to spread throughout the brain thanks to the glymphatic system (Gaberel et al., 2014).

Issues related to imaging of intraparenchymal targets in conditions of injured BBB are numerous. First, the molecular weight of the contrast agent should be low to maximize its passive extravasation through the BBB. The drawback is that this limits the quantity of contrast material carried by contrast agent molecules. In fact, only GBCA have been used for this purpose. Second, the specificity of this method is limited: even in the absence of the molecular target, the contrast agent accumulates in an unspecific manner in the brain regions with BBB leakage. Activatable contrast agents such as bis-5HT-DTPA(Gd) (a substrate for MPO) might partially overcome this limitation (Breckwoldt et al., 2008). Enzyme processing induces oligomerization and protein binding of the contrast agent leading to accumulation and increased T1 effect. Indeed, the T1 effect of paramagnetic contrast agents increases in parallel with the molecular weight due to limitation of motion of the Gadolinium atom. Therefore processed contrast agent molecules induce more important changes in signal intensity, allowing reduction of the injected dose and thus reducing unspecific signals. Nevertheless, interpretation of changes in signal intensity after contrast agent injection is difficult since it depends both on the importance of the BBB leakiness and on the concentration of the molecular target. Accordingly, post-contrast images would be similar in a condition of severe BBB impairment without MPO secretion and in a condition of mild BBB impairment with MPO secretion. This lack of specificity remains one of the main limitations of molecular MRI of parenchymal targets, even using activatable contrast agents.

Imaging of leukocyte diapedesis is the third strategy developed for molecular MRI of the brain. Accumulation of leucocytes (especially blood-derived monocytes/macrophages) in the brain is a specific feature of neuroinflammation and then represents an attractive target for molecular imaging. However, this is a relatively delayed event after injury and requires a delay between injection of the contrast agent and imaging in order to allow its uptake and accumulation of leukocytes within the parenchyma. The prototypic contrast agents used to label leukocytes are unlabeled ultrasmall particles of iron oxide (USPIO; Corot et al., 2004). These small-sized iron-oxide-based contrast agents are internalized by circulating monocytes after intravenous injection. USPIOs-labeled monocytes are then detected by MRI once they have accumulated in the inflamed region of the brain. The delay between injection and imaging is usually long, about 24 h, limiting the interest of such contrast agents in the acute phases.

Moreover, the relative amount of contrast agent eventually reaching the parenchyma is directly dependent on the number of monocytes entering the brain, thus limiting the sensitivity of the method. The other limitation is the possibility of false positive findings in case of BBB leakage, since USPIO readily crosses the BBB after stroke as well as in active plaques of multiple sclerosis for instance (Desestret et al., 2009). The different contrast appearances and the influence of the BBB status are illustrated on **Figure 4**.

In the next paragraphs, we will present the main studies reporting the use of molecular MRI for studying brain–immune interactions after acute cerebral injury (**Table 1**).

MYELOPEROXIDASE IMAGING

Myeloperoxidase is an abundant enzyme expressed by activated inflammatory cells of the myeloid lineage (Bradley et al., 1982), especially macrophages, monocytes, and neutrophils. MPO can induce endothelial dysfunction and increased inflammation due to upregulation of inducible nitric oxide synthase and carbamylation of lipoproteins. Indeed, MPO interacts with hydrogen peroxide to generate highly reactive species, such as OCl^-, $O_2{}^-$, $ONOO^-$ that can covalently modify lipids, causing further local tissue damage and perpetuating the inflammatory cascade (Klinke et al., 2011). MPO-generated free radicals induce apoptosis and nitro-tyrosination of proteins (Heinecke, 2002). Therefore, MPO is included in a complex cascade of inflammatory events involving different types of cells and molecules. Accordingly, molecular imaging of MPO could help detecting areas of brain inflammation (endogenous microglia and infiltrated macrophages/neutrophils) in several CNS disorders.

The idea to non-invasively "image" inflammation by targeting MPO expression/activity had first been investigated by Chen et al. (2004), in a key article in which the authors synthesized and tested a series of activatable paramagnetic MR contrast agents. After several developments, the same team selected a candidate, called bis-5HT-DTPA(Gd) (Querol et al., 2005, 2006).

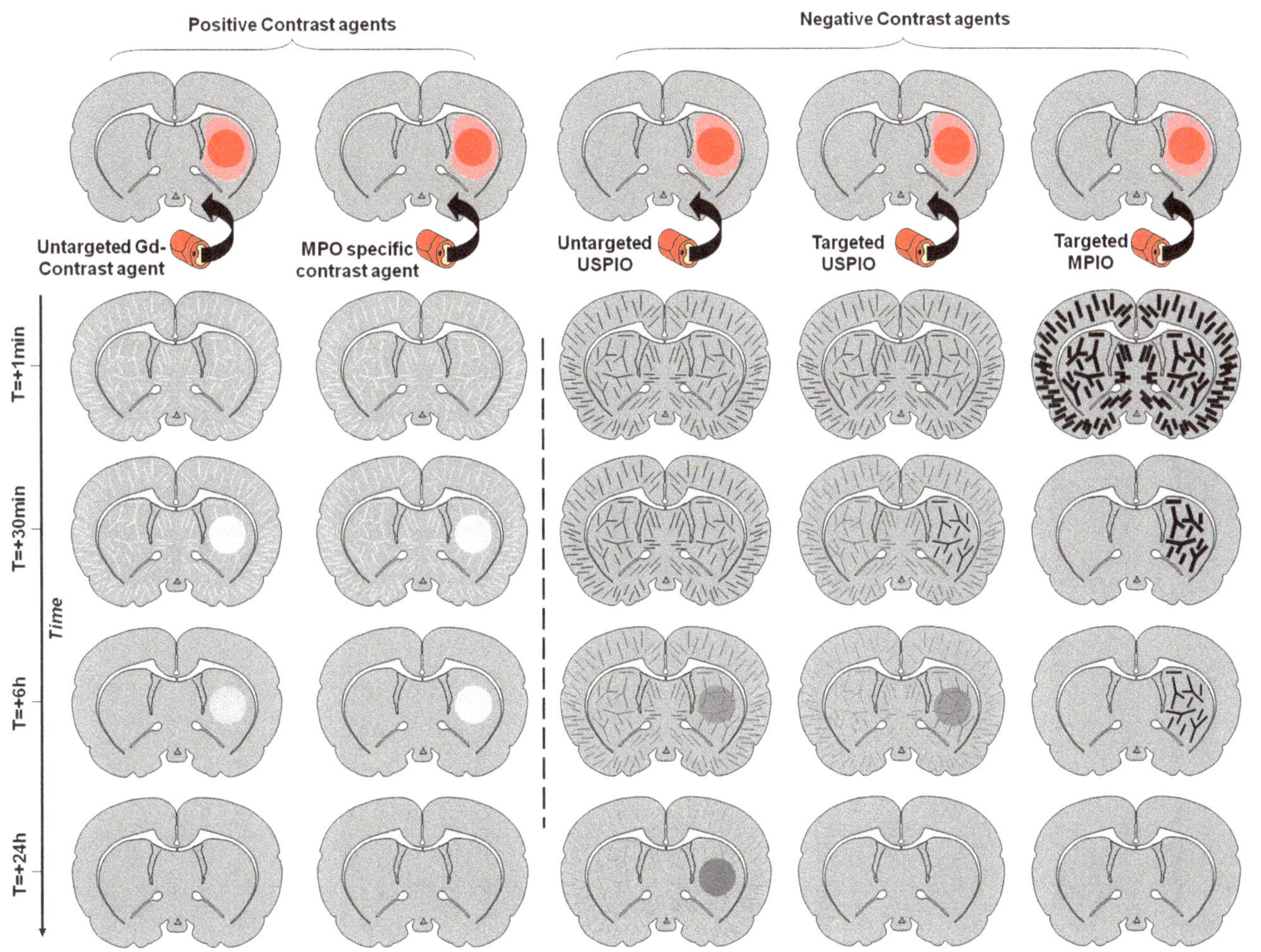

FIGURE 4 | Schematic representation of the effect of different contrast agents on brain MRI of a rodent with inflammation in the right striatum. The inflammatory region with impaired BBB is represented in dark red, whereas the inflammatory region without BBB impairment is in light red. Time-dependent signal changes after contrast agent injection are represented vertically. In contrast to the signal changes induced by targeted MPIOs which are independent of the BBB status, the contrast enhancement induced by other contrast agents is not inflammation specific and strongly depends on the permeability of the BBB.

Table 1 | List of all studies reporting *in vivo* molecular MRI of brain immune interactions in the last 15 years.

Target	Contrast carrying particle	Targeting moeity	Species	Experimental model	Reference
Macrophages	USPIO (Sinerem) diameter: 35 nm	Untargeted	Male Wistar rats	Ischemic Stroke: transient MCAo (60 min) by intraluminal filament	Farr et al. (2011)
Macrophages	USPIO (Sinerem) diameter: 35 nm	Untargeted	Male Lewis rats	EAE model: induction by 20mg of guinea pig myelin basic protein	Oude Engberink et al. (2010)
Macrophages	USPIO G 534-70 (ferumoxtran,Sinerem) diameter: 35 nm	Untargeted	Male Wistar rats	Ischemic Stroke: photo-sensitive dye rose induced a ischemic lesion in the right sensorimotor cortex	Saleh et al. (2004b)
Macrophages	USPIO AMI-227 (Sinerem) diameter: 40 nm	Untargeted	Male Fischer rats	Ischemic Stroke: transient MCAo (30 min) by intraluminal filament	Rausch et al. (2002)
Macrophages	Anionic iron oxide nanoparticles (AMNP)	Untargeted	Sprague-Dawley rats	Ischemic Stroke: transient MCAO (60 min) intraluminal filament	Riou et al. (2013)
Macrophages	USPIO AMI-227 (Sinerem) diameter: 40 nm	Untargeted	Female Lewis rats	EAE model: induction with xenogenic CNS proteins (guinea pig spinal cord).	Rausch et al. (2004)
Macrophages	VSOP (VSOP-R1) diameter: 7 nm	Untargeted	Female SJL/J mice	EAE model: induction 200μg of PLP (proteolipid protein)	Millward et al. (2013)
Macrophages	SPIO (Feridex) diameter: 60 μm	Untargeted	Male C57BL/6J mice	Traumatic Brain Injury model: induced by a controlled cortical injury.	Mills et al. (2012)
Macrophages	USPIO AMI-227 (Sinerem) diameter: 40 nm	Untargeted	Rat	Ischemic Stroke: cortical ischemic lesion (Rose Bengal)	Schroeter et al. (2004)
Macrophages	USPIO AMI-227 (Sinerem) diameter: 40 nm	Untargeted	Male Lewis rats	EAE model: induction with xenogenic CNS proteins (guinea pig spinal cord).	Rausch et al. (2003)
Macrophages	USPIO AMI-227 (Sinerem) diameter: 40 nm	Untargeted	Male Fischer rats	Ischemic Stroke: permanent MCAO by electrocoagulation	Rausch et al. (2001)
Macrophages	USPIO AMI-227 (Sinerem) diameter: 40 nm	Untargeted	Female Lewis rats	EAE model: induction with xenogenic CNS proteins (guinea pig spinal cord).	Dousset et al. (1999b)
Macrophages	SPIO (Resovist) diameter: 40 nm	Untargeted	Female rats	EAE model: induction with human MOG	Ladewig et al. (2009)
Macrophages	MPIO diameter: 0.9 μm	Untargeted	Male C57BL/6J mice	TBI model: induced by a controlled cortical injury.	Foley et al. (2009)
Macrophages	USPIO AMI-227 (Sinerem) diameter: 40nm	Untargeted	Male Swiss mice	Ischemic Stroke: permanent MCAO	Desestret et al. (2009)
Macrophages	USPIO AMI-227 (Sinerem) diameter: 40 nm	Untargeted	Female Lewis rats	EAE model: induction with myelin basic protein (MBP)	Baeten et al. (2008)

(Continued)

Table 1 | Continued

Target	Contrast carrying particle	Targeting moeity	Species	Experimental model	Reference
Macrophages	USPIO (Sinerem) diameter: 40 nm and SPIO (Endorem) diameter: 120 nm	Untargeted	Male Lewis rats	Ischemic Stroke: photo-sensitive dye rose induced a cortical ischemic lesion	Oude Engberink et al. (2008)
Macrophages	USPIO Ferumoxtran-10 (Sinerem) diameter: 35 nm	Untargeted	Male Swiss mice	Ischemic Stroke: permanent MCAO by electrocoagulation	Wiart et al. (2007)
Macrophages	USPIO AMI-227 (Sinerem) diameter: 40 nm	Untargeted	Female DA rats	EAE model: induction with xenogenic CNS proteins (guinea pig spinal cord).	Brochet et al. (2006)
Macrophages	USPIO AMI-227 (Sinerem) diameter: 40 nm	Untargeted	Female Lewis rats	EAE model: induction with xenogenic CNS proteins (guinea pig spinal cord).	Dousset et al. (1999a)
Macrophages	USPIO AMI-227 (Sinerem) diameter: 40 nm	Untargeted	Female Lewis rat	EAE model: induction with xenogenic CNS proteins (guinea pig spinal cord).	Berger et al. (2006)
Macrophages	USPIO 7228 diameter: 30 nm	Untargeted	Male Lewis rats	EAE model: induction with myelin basic protein (MBP)	Floris et al. (2004)
Macrophages	SPIO Feridex diameter: 40 nm	Untargeted	Male SHR/NCrl rats	Ischemic Stroke: transient MCAo (30 min) by intraluminal filament	Henning et al. (2009)
Macrophages	USPIO AMI-227 (Sinerem) diameter: 40 nm	Untargeted	Human	Stroke	Saleh et al. (2007)
Macrophages	USPIO SHU555C diameter: 25 nm	Untargeted	Human	Multiple sclerosis	Vellinga et al. (2008))
Macrophages	USPIO SHU555C diameter: 25 nm	Untargeted	Female DA rats	EAE model: induction with rat MOG	Chin et al. (2009)
Macrophages	USPIO SHU555C diameter: 25 nm	Untargeted	Human	Multiple sclerosis	Vellinga et al. (2009)
Macrophages	SPIO (Resovist) diameter: 40 nm	Untargeted	Male Wistar rats	Ischemic Stroke: cortical ischemic lesion (Rose Bengal)	Kleinschnitz et al. (2003)
Macrophages	SPIO (Resovist) diameter: 40 nm	Untargeted	Male rats	Ischemic Stroke: transient MCAo (60 min) by intraluminal filament	Kim et al. (2008)
Macrophages	USPIO AMI-227 (Sinerem) diameter: 40 nm	Untargeted	Human	Stroke	Nighoghossian et al. (2007)
Macrophages	SPIO (Resovist) diameter: 40 nm	Untargeted	Female DA rats	EAE model: induction with human MOG	Ladewig et al. (2009)
Macrophages	SPIO (Resovist) diameter: 40 nm	Untargeted	Male Sprague Dawley rats	Peripheral and central nerve injury: left sciatic and optic nerves were crushed	Bendszus and Stoll (2003)
Macrophages	USPIO AMI-227 (Sinerem) diameter: 40 nm	Untargeted	Human	Multiple sclerosis	Dousset et al. (2006)
Macrophages	USPIO (ferumoxtran-10) diameter 30 nm	Untargeted	Human	Multiple sclerosis	Manninger et al. (2005)
Macrophages	USPIO (Sinerem) diameter: 30 nm	Untargeted	Human	Severe internal carotid artery (ICA) stenosis	Trivedi et al. (2006)

(Continued)

Table 1 | Continued

Target	Contrast carrying particle	Targeting moeity	Species	Experimental model	Reference
Macrophages	USPIO AMI-227 (Sinerem) diameter: 40 nm	Untargeted	Human	Socioeconomic deprivation in elderly stroke/transient ischaemic attack and control medical patients	Cho et al. (2007)
Macrophages	USPIO AMI-227 (Sinerem) diameter: 40 nm	Untargeted	Male C57Bl/6J mice	Ischemic Stroke: Transient Middle Cerebral Artery Occlusion by clip (30 or 60 mins)	Denes et al. (2007)
Macrophages	monocrystalline iron oxide nanocolloid diameter: 4 nm	Untargeted	Male hypertensive rats	Ischemic Stroke: occlusion of the right middle cerebral artery by homologous blood clot	Dijkhuizen et al. (2002)
Macrophages	USPIO (Sinerem) diameter: 18 nm	Untargeted	Human	Stroke	Kooi et al. (2003)
Macrophages	USPIO	Untargeted	Sprague–Dawley rats	Ischemic Stroke: transient MCAO intraluminal filament	Yang et al. (2013)
Macrophages	SPIO (Resovist) diameter: 40 nm	Untargeted	Male pigs	hemorrhage model: sonication to open the BBB transcranially	Liu et al. (2011)
Mononuclear cells	VSOP C200 diameter: 62 nm	Spleen-derived MNCs	129/SV mice or C57/B6-GFP	Ischemic Stroke: transient MCAo (30 or 60 min) by intraluminal filament	Stroh et al. (2006)
T cells	SPIO (Ferumoxides) diameter: 120 nm	T-Cell isolated lymph node cells	Female SJL mice	EAE model: induction of PLP (proteolipid protein)	Anderson et al. (2004))
CD4+ T cells	USPIO (MACS) diameter: 30 nm	Antibodies against CD4+ T cells	Sprague–Dawley rats	ALS model: expressing mutated (G93A) human SOD-1	Machtoub et al. (2011)
CD4+ T cells	USPIO (MACS) diameter: 30 nm	Antibodies against CD4+	Female Wistar rats	Ischemic Stroke: global cerebral ischemia reversible by cardiac arrest	Sekeljic et al. (2012)
ICAM-1	MPIO (ProMag) diameter: 2 μm	Monoclonal antibody targeting ICAM-1 (YN1/1.7.4)	Female C57BL/6J mice	EAE model: induction with MOG	Blezer et al. (2014)
ICAM-1	Paramagnetic polymerized liposomes diameter: 200 nm	Monoclonal antibody targeting ICAM-1	SJL/J mice	EAE model: induction of PLP (proteolipid protein)	Sipkins et al. (2000)
ICAM-1	MPIO (ProMag) diameter: 1.05 μm	Monoclonal antibody targeting ICAM-1 (YN1/1.7.4)	Male C57Bl/6 mice	Ischemic Stroke: transient MCAO (30 min) by intraluminal filament	Deddens et al. (2013)
ICAM-1	SPIO diameter: 120 nm	Antibody targeting ICAM-1 (BD Biosciences)	Female Lewis rats	EAE model: induction with xenogenic CNS proteins (guinea pig spinal cord)	Schneider et al. (2009)
VCAM-1	MPIO (MyOne) diameter: 1.08 μm	Monoclonal antibody targeting VCAM-1 (clone A429)	Male C57Bl/6 mice	Ischemic Stroke: Permanent (electrocoagulation, FeCl3) and transient MCAO (Thrombin, Mechanical); Hemorrhage model: striatal injection of collagenase type VII and exogenous blood	Gauberti et al. (2013)

(Continued)

Table 1 | Continued

Target	Contrast carrying particle	Targeting moeity	Species	Experimental model	Reference
VCAM-1	MPIO (myOne) diameter: 1.08 μm	Monoclonal antibody targeting VCAM-1 (clone M/K2)	Male C57Bl/6 mice	Ischemic Stroke: transient MCAO (30 min) intraluminal filament	Hoyte et al. (2010)
VCAM-1	MPIO (myOne) diameter: 1.08 μm	Monoclonal antibody targeting VCAM-1 (clone M/K2)	Female SJL mice (8–12 wk old, 25 g; Harlan, Bicester, UK)	EAE model: induction of PLP (proteolipid protein)	Serres et al. (2011)
VCAM-1	USPIO (P03007) diameter: 26 nm	Monoclonal antibody targeting VCAM-1 (MCA 2297)	Male Swiss albino mice	Ischemic Stroke: transient MCAO (60 min) intraluminal filament	Fréchou et al. (2013)
VCAM-1	MPIO (myOne) diameter: 1.08 μm	Monoclonal antibody targeting VCAM-1 (clone M/K2)	Female adult Biozzi antibody high (ABH) mice	CR-EAE model: induction of mouse spinal cord homogenate	Mardiguian et al. (2013)
VCAM-1	MPIO (myOne) diameter: 1.08 μm	Monoclonal antibody targeting VCAM-1 (clone A429)	Male C57BL6/J mice	Alzheimer's disease model: APP/PS1 mice Vascular dementia: Unilateral common carotid artery ligature EAE model: induction with MOG (rMOG 1-125)	Montagne et al. (2012)
P-selectin	SPIO (MNP-NH2) diameter: 50 nm	Sialyl Lewis X (sLeX)	Male C57/BL 6 mice	Ischemic Stroke: transient MCAO intraluminal filament	Jin et al. (2009)
Selectin (P-E)	GD-DTPA (Magnevist). Gd-DTPA-B(sLeX)	Sialyl Lewis X (sLeX)	Male C57 mice	Ischemic Stroke: transient MCAO (30 min) intraluminal filament	Barber et al. (2004)
E-selectin	USPIO	Heptapeptide for E-selectin targeting (IELLQAR)	Female Sprague–Dawley rats	TBI model: fluid percussion	Chapon et al. (2009)
PECAM-1	MPIO (ProMag) diameter: 1.05 μm	Monoclonal antibody targeting PECAM-1	Male C57Bl/6 mice	Ischemic Stroke: transient MCAO (30 min) intraluminal filament	Deddens et al. (2013)
Myeloperoxidase (MPO)	bis-5HT-DTPA(Gd)	bis-5HT-DTPA(Gd)	Female SJL mice	Venous stenosis model: ligation of the right and left jugular veins EAE model: induction of PLP (proteolipid protein)	Atkinson et al. (2012)
MPO	DTPA(Gd)	bis-5HT	Female SJL mice	EAE model: induction of PLP (proteolipid protein)	Forghani et al. (2012))
MPO	DTPA(Gd)	bis-5HT	Male New Zealand rabbits	Aneurysm model: induction by Elastase	DəLeo et al. (2009)
MPO	DTPA(Gd)	bis-5HT	Male C57/mice	Ischemic Stroke: transient MCAO (30 min) by intraluminal filament	Breckwoldt et al. (2008)
MPO	DTPA(Gd)	bis-5HT	Female SJL mice	EAE model: induction of PLP (proteolipid protein)	Chen et al. (2008)

Basically, a specific substrate of MPO (5-hydroxytryptamide) is associated with a Gadolinium-based contrastophore which is responsible for the paramagnetic effect. In the presence of MPO, the 5-hydroxytryptamide moiety of bis-5HT-DTPA(Gd) is oxidized and radicalized by hydrogen peroxide. The radicalized bis-5HT-DTPA(Gd) molecule can react with another radicalized bis-5HT-DTPA(Gd) molecule to form a polymer of up to five subunits leading to an amplification of the enzymatic reaction. In mice, the activated agent can also bind to proteins within inflammatory sites, trapping the agent, further increasing its molecular weight, and increasing the signal intensity on T1-weighted MRI (Chen et al., 2006). Converted products are locally retained, so that pharmacokinetics properties are improved: prolonged enhancement can be detected for up to 60 min at sites of increased MPO activity. The specificity of Bis-5HT-DTPA(Gd) was demonstrated using a substrate not specific for MPO (di-tyrosine), a pharmacological inhibitor of MPO (ABAH) or MPO knockout mice. In conclusion, bis-5HT-DTPA(Gd) appeared as a biocompatible agent with good sensitivity and specificity. Accordingly, this agent has been tested in several pathological contexts.

In experimental autoimmune encephalomyelitis (EAE) induced with synthetic proteolipid protein, a model of multiple sclerosis, MPO imaging has been tested for its ability to detect active plaques before clinical symptoms appearance in mice. The authors found that bis-5HT-DTPA allows detection of MPO, as a surrogate marker of the appearance and size of active plaques, and was correlated to clinical grading (Chen et al., 2008). In the same model of multiple sclerosis, another group used MPO imaging as an objective evidence of the therapeutic efficiency of an inhibitor (ABAH) of MPO. Bis-5HT-DTPA-based signals on imaging were smaller and matched with less demyelination and reduced severity of symptoms (Forghani et al., 2012). A study proposed that multiple sclerosis could be due to chronic cerebrospinal venous insufficiency (CCVI). However, bis-5HT-DTPA imaging performed in EAE mice subjected to ligature of the jugular vein to induce CCVI invalidated this hypothesis. Indeed, the authors did not observe any effect of CCVI on the correlation between MPO activity and neuroinflammation, demyelination, or clinical signs (Atkinson et al., 2012). Whether these negative results could be explained by the low sensitivity of this imaging method to detect subtle inflammatory changes remains, however, unclear.

Bis-5HT-DTPA has also been used in a model of transient focal stroke (transient mechanical vascular occlusion model during 30 min). In this study, MPO imaging correlated with infarct size, and the authors hypothesized that MPO imaging could be used to select and stratify patients for clinical trials of therapies targeting inflammation (Breckwoldt et al., 2008). In an experimental model of common carotid artery aneurysm induced by elastase, MPO imaging was shown to be valuable to identify unstable aneurysms, at risk of subsequent rupture (DeLeo et al., 2009).

Myeloperoxidase imaging has thus proven relevant to diagnose, predict, or evaluate therapeutic efficiencies in several models of CNS disorders. However, as already mentioned, it is widely recognized that these MRI techniques have limitations because contrast enhancement reflects breakdown of the BBB with leakage of paramagnetic chelates rather than active inflammation, and the two may not always correspond. Another potential limitation is that MPO imaging does not discriminate between MPO secreted from resident microglia, infiltrated macrophages or neutrophils.

Finally, the activated MPO sensor is cleared from the brain within 6 h after administration; the protein-bound, activated MPO agents are likely digested and released by proteases that are present at sites of inflammation (Querol et al., 2006).

Therefore, enzymatic imaging targeting MPO points to an interesting technology for non-invasive confirmation of active inflammatory lesions in brain disease. This could potentially not only improve disease diagnosis and treatment assessment in the clinical setting, but may also lead to a better evaluation of drug development and clinical trials of new therapies. This method is, however, impaired by its lack of specificity due to passive extravasation and accumulation of the unprocessed contrast agent, which contributes significantly to MRI signal changes.

IMMUNE CELL TRACKING

Administration of exogenously labeled cells and subsequent tracking by non-invasive imaging has encountered numerous successes in molecular imaging of brain immune interactions. Unlike *in vivo* labeling of circulating cells using untargeted USPIO, this method has the advantage of a higher specificity since the contrast agent particles are clustered inside immune cells and are thus less susceptible to reach the brain in an unspecific manner (such as passive extravasation through a leaky BBB). Moreover, it allows direct imaging of brain–immune interactions as a whole, taking into account all the processes involved in the regulation of endothelial binding and blood to brain diapedesis of autologous cells. The basis of this method is to harvest autologous cells (most frequently leukocytes) and to label them with a high payload of contrast agent without impairing their ability to reach the CNS. Several labeling methods have been performed, based either on phagocytic uptake of contrast agent particles or on direct transfection of the cells with iron particles or Gadolinium using permeating agents.

One of the first studies investigating the use of systemically injected autologous labeled cells for molecular imaging demonstrated that rat bone marrow stromal cells were able to invade a photochemically induced brain lesion 7 days after intravenous injection (Jendelová et al., 2004). Later, Stroh et al. (2006) labeled spleen-derived mononuclear cells (MNCs) with very small superparamagnetic iron-oxide particles and transfused them into recipient mice subjected to transient ischemic stroke (filament model). Areas of signal hypointensities started to appear 24–48 h after intravenous injection of MNCs and corresponded to grafting of the cells in the ischemic lesion.

A similar method has been used by Anderson et al. (2004) in a mouse model of EAE by adoptive transfer of encephalitogenic T cells. They labeled endosomes from murine T-cells *ex vivo* using polylysine and ferumoxide and injected the labeled cells intraperitoneally in recipient mice. The authors were able to detect both *ex vivo* and *in vivo* the labeled cells in the lumbar spinal cord of EAE mice after the onset of clinical signs. Interestingly, the primary location of the encephalitogenic T-cells revealed by molecular MRI in this study was later confirmed by Arima et al. (2012), who demonstrated that autoreactive T cells access the CNS via the fifth lumbar spinal cord. Other immune-related cell-types can be labeled and subsequently imaged using the same labeling strategy, such as bone marrow-derived cells (Anderson et al., 2005).

Besides these proof-of-concept studies, molecular imaging of exogenously labeled cells allows to easily investigate the mechanisms driving the interactions between circulating cells and the brain endothelium. For instance, Gorelik et al. (2012) demonstrated in rats that iron oxide labeled glial-precursor cells can be targeted to the brain by the virtue of the interaction between circulating cell expressed VLA-4 and endothelial VCAM-1. Using MRI, they compared the efficiency of brain delivery of VLA-4 transfected and control glial precursor cells with or without VCAM-1 overexpression in the brain induced *in situ* by lipopolysaccharide injection. They found that brain delivery was dramatically enhanced when the injected cells and the brain expressed VLA-4 and VCAM-1, respectively. This kind of clever experiment can be performed using various types of circulating cells to improve our knowledge of brain–immune interactions.

The main limitation of this method is its reduced applicability for diagnostic purposes in humans. Although radiolabeling of autologous cells has been used successfully for imaging inflammation using SPECT and PET (Pulli and Chen, 2014), the limited sensitivity of MRI requires high payload of contrast agent per cell and a large amount of cells to be reinjected to achieve reliable imaging. Moreover, labeled cells might lose their iron oxide particles or die leading to false negative results. Another limitation is the effects of the labeling procedure including cell collection, purification, iron-oxide particles engulfment, and reinjection which can all influence the phenotype of the cells. To make this procedure faster and overcome some of its drawbacks, endogenous labeling of the monocyte/macrophage lineage using USPIOs has been developed.

UNLABELED USPIO

Unlabeled USPIOs are virus-sized molecules with a very long blood clearance time (over 24 h). Iron oxide agents have greater contrast sensitivity compared to GBCA, generating signal voids on MRI, due to shortening of T2 and T2* relaxation times. A large range of sizes exist, from nano- to micron-sized iron oxide particles. USPIOs are among the most famous MR contrast agents, with a range in size from 10–50 nm, and should be differentiated from the larger SPIOs and MPIOs with diameters about 50–300 nm and 0.9–5 μm, respectively. Iron oxide particles are based on magnetite (Fe_3O_4), and are usually encased in polysaccharide, synthetic polymers, or monomer coatings (Thorek et al., 2006; Laurent et al., 2008). The utility of these particles as MRI contrast agents has been studied for more than two decades and the list of available agents is still expanding.

Ultrasmall superparamagnetic particles of iron oxides are readily internalized by phagocytic cells such as the Kupffer cell of the liver, circulating monocytes/macrophages and mononuclear T cells, as well as reactive astrocytes, microglia, and dendritic cells within the CNS. The USPIOs are cleared from the circulation primarily by the reticulo-endothelial system (Bourrinet et al., 2006); these properties (i.e., degree of cellular uptake and rate of clearance) are dependent on size, coating, and method of delivery.

The USPIOs ferumoxytol (Feraheme®, *AMAG Pharmaceuticals Inc*) was initially approved for iron-replacement therapy in patients with chronic renal failure. However, ferumoxytol has also been investigated in humans for various CNS imaging applications (Neuwelt et al., 2007), as well as ferumoxtran-10 (Manninger et al., 2005; Saleh et al., 2007) and SHU 555 C (Vellinga et al., 2008) to name a few. Ferumoxytol, in particular, is attractive as an MRI contrast agent because it is approved for use in humans and it is safe in patients with chronic kidney disease. It can be given as a bolus for first-pass perfusion imaging and at a later time point (e.g., 24 h) ferumoxytol accumulation is obvious in regions of BBB dysfunction that may be related to inflammation from any cause.

Several groups have shown that molecular imaging is an important new diagnostic tool for studying *in vivo* cellular and molecular biology across a wide range of disciplines, especially regarding inflammatory processes and associated immune cells, in both humans and animal models. Such applications may be relevant for earlier disease detection, more precise prognosis, personalized treatment strategies, monitoring of treatment efficiency and finally to improved our understanding of how cells behave and interact in their microenvironment *in vivo* (Thorek et al., 2006).

The most common strategy for cellular MRI of neuroinflammation involves tagging of circulating monocytes by systemic injection of iron oxide nanoparticles. In 2001, Rausch and coworkers first developed this approach in a stroke model in rats, where a single dose of USPIOs (Sinerem®, *AMAG Pharmaceuticals Inc*) was injected intravenously 5 h post-onset (Rausch et al., 2001). An accumulation of USPIOs was shown in the periphery of the lesion 24 h post-injection. At day 7, the USPIOs signal was still present and spread out within the lesion area, spatially correlating with areas displaying activated macrophages. Several groups have used a similar protocol to assess the spatiotemporal profile of monocyte infiltration in various stroke models in rodents (Kleinschnitz et al., 2003; Saleh et al., 2004b; Wiart et al., 2007; Kim et al., 2008). These studies raise an interesting technical point related to the USPIOs uptake by circulating white blood cells and, therefore, the USPIOs blood half-life. It has been shown that phagocytic cellular uptake of iron oxide increases with particle size (Daldrup-Link et al., 2003; Matuszewski et al., 2005). With a hydrodynamic diameter of 10 to 50 nm, USPIOs are less efficiently phagocytosed than SPIOs with sizes of 50–300 nm. The maximum intracellular iron oxide concentration of *in vitro*-labeled, isolated human macrophages is 50 pg iron/cell for the SPIOs ferucarbotran (Resovist®, *Bayer Schering Pharma AG*) whereas for USPIOs SHU 555 C (Supravist®, *Bayer Schering Pharma AG*), it is below 8 pg iron/cell (Metz et al., 2004). Besides the particle size of the iron oxide, phagocytic uptake is also dependent on nanoparticle surface properties (e.g., neutral versus charged). Numerous studies employed neutrally charged dextran-coated USPIOs (e.g., Sinerem®) with a long blood half-life compared to larger ferumoxides, such as dextran- (Endorem®in Europe, Feridex®in the USA) or anionic-carboxydextran- (Resovist®) coated SPIOs (Weissleder et al., 1989; Rausch et al., 2002; Briley-Saebo et al., 2006). Thus, the USPIOs extended blood half-life is assumed to promote the uptake by circulating cells. Furthermore, pharmacological strategies, using the protamine sulfate peptide, may be also used to enhance USPIOs uptake, as reported *in vitro* (Arbab et al., 2004) and *in vivo* in rats (Wu et al., 2007).

Although internalization of contrast agents in activated macrophages and its correlation with MRI contrast have been reported in different studies, there is still debate on the specificity of the observed MRI contrast. For instance, some studies suggested that USPIOs-induced contrast could be non-specific, i.e., due to a passive diffusion of iron particles through the BBB (Kleinschnitz et al., 2003; Saleh et al., 2004a; Denes et al., 2007; Nighoghossian et al., 2007; Saleh et al., 2007). The passive diffusion is patently increased because of a disrupted BBB in a context of stroke (Dijkhuizen et al., 2002). To distinguish between USPIOs passive diffusion in the brain parenchyma and inflammation, USPIOs-based MRI have been combined with Gadolinium-enhanced MRI to correlate USPIOs accumulation and BBB integrity, both in animal models and in humans (Kleinschnitz et al., 2003; Saleh et al., 2004a, 2007; Denes et al., 2007; Nighoghossian et al., 2007). As an alternative to the approach of labeling within the bloodstream, blood cells may also be extracted, labeled *in vitro* and then reinjected as presented above (exogenously labeled cells). This would avoid non-specific free iron particles leakage over the BBB and/or entrapment in the vasculature (Stroh et al., 2006; Oude Engberink et al., 2008). One of the latest unlabeled USPIO is P904 (Guerbet), for which phase I clinical trial has been initiated, demonstrating a significantly higher uptake by macrophages because of their pegylated coating compared to dextran-coated USPIOs (Yancy et al., 2005; Sigovan et al., 2009).

Despite the technical issues described above, this cellular MRI approach has given encouraging results to pursue further investigations. Non-targeted USPIOs may also be interesting in the field of atherosclerosis (including intracranial atherosclerosis), as suggested by experimental *in vivo* studies in hyperlipidemic rabbits (Ruehm et al., 2001; Briley-Saebo et al., 2008) and in humans (Kooi et al., 2003; Trivedi et al., 2006). These groups have shown non-targeted USPIOs accumulation in atherosclerotic plaques rich in macrophages, both in animals and humans. Additionally, USPIOs were shown to localize to atherosclerotic plaques-containing macrophages in apolipoprotein E knockout mice (Morris et al., 2008). Using the same transgenic model, a p38 MAP kinase inhibitor has been shown to decrease USPIOs uptake by atherosclerotic plaques, which correlated with a reduction in macrophage activity by histology.

TARGETED USPIO

To counteract potential problems related to untargeted-USPIOs, targeted-nanoparticles of iron oxide have been developed to image neuroinflammation. VCAM-1 which promotes monocytes recruitment to the vascular wall and subsequent lesion development, is a promising marker for molecular imaging of cerebrovascular inflammation in several CNS disorders, since it is not constitutively expressed in normal vessels but is rapidly up-regulated on activated vascular endothelial cells (Davies et al., 1993; Cybulsky et al., 2001). On this basis, several generations of VCAM-1 targeted (using monoclonal antibodies or peptides generated by phage display) iron oxide nanoparticles conjugated with fluorescent molecules (Cy5.5) have been produced and applied in mouse models of acute inflammation and atherosclerosis (Kelly et al., 2005; Tsourkas et al., 2005; Nahrendorf et al., 2006). Molecular imaging of endothelial activation has been performed using USPIO labeled with a specifically designed targeting moiety consisting in a small peptide which triggers internalization of the USPIO by activated endothelial cells (Kelly et al., 2005). This amplification strategy allowed efficient intravital microscopic detection of the particles but this method lacked sensitivity for reliable *in vivo* imaging. Moreover, USPIOs conjugated to a VCAM-1 specific cyclic peptide (P03011 or R832, Guerbet) have recently been developed for *in vivo* detection of inflamed vessels in early and advanced atherosclerotic plaques by ultra-high field strength MRI (Burtea et al., 2012; Michalska et al., 2012), as well as in an ischemic stroke model in mice (Fréchou et al., 2013). Again, the sensitivity and specificity of VCAM-1 imaging using these USPIO-based strategies remained limited.

Among the different target of labeled USPIOs, E-selectin has been extensively studied in peripheral inflammation in mice (ear inflammation, muscle inflammation ...; Reynolds et al., 2006). Selectins have also been investigated as target for MR molecular imaging of inflammation owing to their role in recruiting immune cells (i.e., leukocytes) to the vascular wall. Platelet-selectin (P-selectin), for example, is involved in early events of the inflammatory pathway, which make them an ideal target for early diagnosis of vascular inflammation. In addition, its baseline expression is near zero, which enables subtle changes to be detected in the vascular wall. E-selectin targeting is usually achieved using a Sialyl-Lewis X targeting moiety (USPIO-sLeX; Radermacher et al., 2009). But other USPIOs have been developed with peptidic (Chapon et al., 2009) or F(ab') – based targeting moieties (Reynolds et al., 2006, Radiology). A study reported the use of E-selectin targeted USPIOs to detect endothelial activation in a mouse model of traumatic brain injury (Chapon et al., 2009). However, the sensitivity achieved using this agent is limited and does not allow reliable detection of brain E-selectin. A similar approach with P-selectin as a target has been developed and tested in an ischemic stroke model in mice (Jin et al., 2009), but presents the same limit as E-selectin.

While targeted USPIO-based molecular imaging remains an active field of investigation, targeted-USPIOs may have potential for toxicity, the sensitivity remains low even when amplification strategies are used and the specificity is impaired in condition of BBB leakage because of passive USPIOs extravasation. In addition, the long clearance time of USPIOs delays imaging until several hours after administration, which is not ideal for clinical use. For all these reasons, the feasibility of reliable *in vivo* molecular MRI using targeted USPIOs remains elusive.

TARGETED MPIOs

Micro-sized particles of iron oxide have singular properties for endothelial cell-specific molecular imaging. First, their micron size range allows endovascular specificity unlike USPIOs agents which are susceptible to passive diffusion within the brain parenchyma, passive accumulation in atherosclerotic plaques or even non-specific macrophage uptake. Second, MPIOs convey a large payload of iron oxide (usually 0.1–1.6 pg Iron/MPIO particle), which is an order of magnitude larger than USPIOs contrast agents, resulting in strong hypointense contrast effects that may extend up to 50 times the physical diameter of the particle. This phenomenon, known as "blooming effect," provides high sensitivity *in vivo* MRI detection, using only a small number of MPIO particles (Shapiro et al., 2005, 2006; Heyn et al., 2006). Third, MPIOs have very short blood half-life of 50–100 s (Ye et al., 2008; Yang et al., 2010), allowing imaging immediately after injection (Montagne et al., 2012; Gaberel et al., 2013; Gauberti et al., 2013). Finally, MPIOs are readily functionalized by covalent conjugation of ligands (monoclonal antibodies or their immunospecific fragments F(ab), single chain antibodies or peptides derived from phage display) to functional groups (amine, carboxyl acid or *p*-toluene sulphydryl (tosyl)) on the MPIOs surface.

Limitations of these agents for CNS imaging are related to their non-biodegradable coat and their potential iron toxicity. Indeed, MPIOs' coated-sheath includes inert polymers giving them a non-biodegradable nature. Micro-sized particles may therefore accumulate in the reticulo-endothelial system (McAteer et al., 2007, 2008). To overcome this problem, more related to a clinical use, development of biodegradable MPIOs is currently in process, and some have already been developed (Nkansah et al., 2011). Although commercially available MPIOs did not show any side effects in cultured hepatocytes in terms of iron homeostasis and cell survival (Raschzok et al., 2011), these particles might have a potential long-term toxicity in humans due to the iron. Furthermore, the dose of iron used in most of experimental studies using MPIOs is around 4 mg iron/kg (McAteer et al., 2007), which is higher than the dose used in clinical practice to visualize tumors with USPIOs (2.6 mg iron/kg; Will et al., 2006). In addition, although their large size improves the specificity of MPIO-based molecular MRI, they are not able to enter the brain parenchyma and their targets are therefore limited to proteins expressed by the endothelium such as cell adhesion molecules.

Microsized particles of iron oxides have been applied for imaging of inflammation in many experimental studies, including various animal models of CNS disorders. Due to its properties mentioned earlier, VCAM-1 is an interesting biomarker in the field of molecular imaging and has been thoroughly studied over the last years. For instance, MPIOs targeting VCAM-1 has been studied in mouse models of acute cerebral inflammation (McAteer et al., 2007, 2012), chronic cerebral hypoperfusion (Montagne et al., 2012), atherosclerosis (McAteer et al., 2008), strokes (Hoyte et al., 2010; Gauberti et al., 2013), myocardial ischemia (Grieve et al., 2013; von Elverfeldt et al., 2014), Alzheimer's disease (Montagne et al., 2012), multiple sclerosis (Serres et al., 2011; Montagne et al., 2012), and even in normal aging and systemic challenges related to risk factors of CNS disorders (e.g., peripheral inflammation, ethanol consumption, and hyperglycemia; Montagne et al., 2012).

Our group developed MPIOs conjugated to monoclonal VCAM-1 antibodies (MPIOs-αVCAM-1) and used them for non-invasive and high-sensitive *in vivo* detection of cerebrovascular inflammation in pre-clinical models in mice (Montagne et al., 2012). They provide higher sensitivity than previously reported methods and molecular contrast agents (McAteer et al., 2007), and are able to detect changes at a time that is otherwise undetectable using conventional MRI. Using an antibody anti-VCAM-1 carefully preselected by histology and a small dose of MPIOs (e.g., 1 mg iron/kg), we reported a dramatically higher sensitivity to assess cerebrovascular cell activation compared to previously published studies (**Figure 5**). In a model of acute inflammation in mice receiving a microinjection of pro-inflammatory cytokine tumor necrosis factor (TNF) into the right striatum, while the left striatum was not injected and served as internal control, we reported that *in vivo* T2*-weighted MRI reveals a potent hypointense contrast effect in the TNF injected hemisphere after MPIOs-αVCAM-1 injection 24 h post-onset. No contrast effects were seen in the non-injected hemisphere or in animals injected with control MPIOs-IgG. Similarly, although pre-contrast MRI images failed to reveal the ongoing pathology, contrast-enhanced MRI using MPIOs-αVCAM-1 revealed hypoperfusion-triggered CNS injury in vascular dementia, unmasked amyloid-induced cerebrovascular activation in Alzheimer's disease and allowed monitoring of disease activity during EAE (Montagne et al., 2012).

Other vascular biomarkers (mostly cell adhesion molecules) have been studied over the last few years as potential targets for MR molecular imaging of inflammation. ICAM-1, unlike VCAM-1, is constitutively expressed in endothelial cells. ICAM-1 is nevertheless up-regulated during an inflammatory response. Deddens et al. (2013) studied ICAM-1 up-regulation after stroke in mice using a similar approach based on MPIOs coupled to anti-ICAM-1 antibodies. Using the same custom contrast agent, this group also showed ICAM-1 overexpression during EAE, providing an early tracer of disease activity (Blezer et al., 2014). McAteer et al. (2012) constructed dual antibody-conjugated MPIOs, targeting both VCAM-1 and P-selectin (50:50 ratio). They did not show further enhance contrast effects compared to single VCAM-1 antibody-conjugated MPIOs in a model of acute inflammation in mice (McAteer et al., 2012). Endothelial-Selectin (E-selectin) has also been investigated *in vitro* using similar dual antibody-conjugated MPIOs, targeting both VCAM-1 and E-selectin (Jefferson et al., 2011).

Microsized particles of iron oxides are well-tolerated in mice, with no short-term ill effects. Clearance experiments showed that MPIOs are sequestered by the liver and spleen 24 h after injection, with no evidence of adverse effects such as tissue infarction, inflammation, or hemorrhage. The MPIOs used so far in experimental studies are non-biodegradable, due to their inert coat. However, the basic iron contrast mechanism is potentially transferable to humans with suitable adaptation of the surface coat.

Their size similar to circulating platelets, their short blood half-life and the exceptionally potent T2* MRI contrast effects of targeted MPIOs, together with advancement of biocompatible MPIOs, provide translational imaging opportunities for improved diagnosis and treatment of endovascular inflammation in various CNS disorders. However, extensive toxicological profiling and synthesis of sterile, clinical-grade targeted MPIOs according to good manufacturing practice will be required before clinical translation is feasible.

LAST AND FUTURE DEVELOPMENTS

To date, molecular MRI studies consisted primarily on proof-of-concept studies reporting the feasibility to image a particular

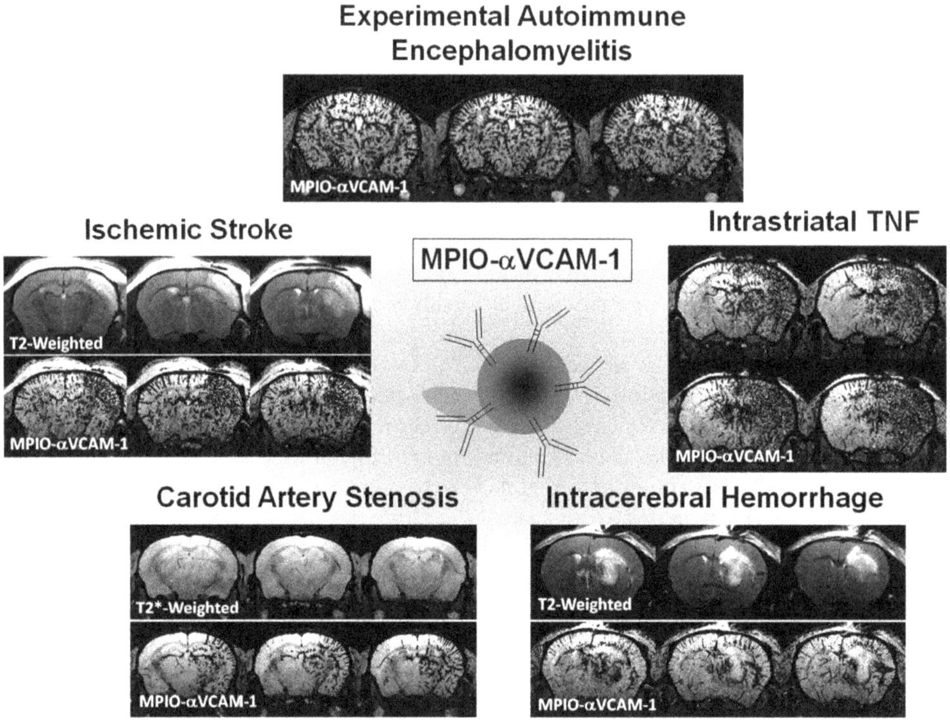

FIGURE 5 | Example of ultrasensitive molecular MRI of brain inflammation using optimized MPIO-αVCAM-1. All the images presented were acquired 20 min after MPIO-αVCAM-1 injection as described by Montagne et al. (2012) and Gauberti et al. (2013). Experimental autoimmune encephalomyelitis was induced by Myelin oligodendrocyte glycoprotein (MOG) in C57BL6J mice. The T2*-weighted image presented is from a mouse with a clinical score of 3. Intrastriatal injection of TNF (1 μg) was performed 24 h before imaging. Intracerebral hemorrhage was induced by intrastriatal collagenase. Carotid artery stenosis was performed by ligation of the right common carotid artery. Ischemic stroke was induced by intra-arterial administration of thrombin.

target. Very few studies used molecular MRI as a tool to investigate brain–immune interactions. Reasons for this are numerous including the lack of reliability of the imaging procedures with the already mentioned false negative (mainly due to a lack of sensitivity of most molecular MRI procedures) and false positive results (due to passive extravasation through an altered BBB, endogenous contrast induced by microhemorrhages or iron accumulation, inadequate post-processing analyses...). In particular, most of the MRI contrast agents are described in unique studies and no confirmatory results in other models or by other groups are presented. Altogether, these drawbacks limited the confidence of the molecular imaging community in molecular MRI and finally raised doubts about its feasibility. Of note, the recent use of MPIO-based contrast agents dramatically improved the reliability of molecular MRI and the latest studies were able to provide new insights into brain immune interactions.

For instance, numerous studies investigated the impact and timing of leukocyte diapedesis after ischemic stroke. However, the spatiotemporal modulation of the expression of adhesion molecules by the brain endothelium after ischemic onset was unknown. Using MPIOs-αVCAM-1 in mice, we demonstrated that stroke induced overexpression of VCAM-1 (involved in monocyte and T-Cell diapedesis) not only in the ischemic lesion, but also in intact brain regions (Gauberti et al., 2013). In particular, VCAM-1 overexpression was very strong in the close periphery of the lesion. Using longitudinal imaging, we were able to demonstrate that this overexpression was sustained for 5 days after permanent ischemia (by electrocoagulation or permanent thrombosis of the middle cerebral artery) but much quicker after transient ischemia (Gauberti et al., 2014; Le Behot et al., 2014). Interestingly, when VCAM-1 overexpression is sustained, the corresponding inflammatory region is recruited by the ischemic core in a delayed fashion. Since this secondary lesion growth can be blocked by anti-inflammatory treatments (such as celecoxib or high-dose statins) and by analogy with the ischemic penumbra, we proposed the concept of inflammatory penumbra to describe this peri-lesional area overexpressing VCAM-1 (**Figure 6**). This pathophysiological concept is supported by other studies demonstrating the critical role of VCAM-1 dependent T-cells diapedesis in delayed lesion growth after ischemic stroke (Liesz et al., 2011). In our study, the ability to simultaneously and longitudinally observe VCAM-1 expression and ischemic lesion development offered by molecular MRI was critical to determine the fate of the inflammatory penumbra. In a clinical setting, such imaging strategy may help to discriminate patients who will experience malignant stroke characterized by an exacerbated inflammation (Vivien et al., 2011). Experimental studies on the impact of peripheral inflammation on brain–immune interactions also benefited from molecular MRI. It is for instance

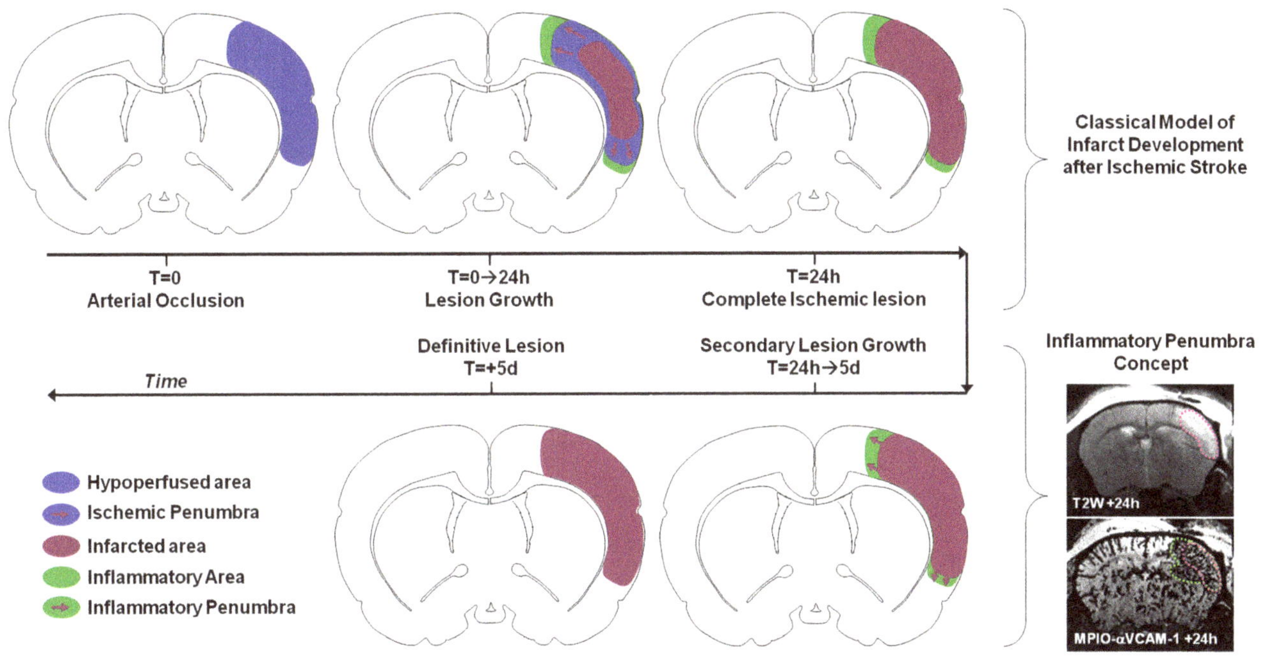

FIGURE 6 | Schematic representation of the inflammatory penumbra concept after ischemic stroke as revealed by MPIO-αVCAM-1 enhanced MRI. VCAM-1 overexpression is sustained and particularly significant in the peri-infarct area after ischemic stroke. From 24 h to 5 days post-stroke onset this inflammatory penumbra is recruited by the ischemic core. Interestingly, anti-inflammatory treatments block this secondary infarct expansion. In this context, the presence of an inflammatory penumbra 24 h after stroke onset revealed by molecular MRI of VCAM-1 may be used as a selection criteria for anti-inflammatory treatment in stroke patients.

possible to reveal the impact of sepsis, acute hyperglycemia, acute ethanol intoxication, or aging on brain endothelium expression of VCAM-1 using MPIO-based molecular MRI in mice (Montagne et al., 2012). The exceptional sensitivity of the method and its ease of use offer new avenues of investigations in the field of neuroinflammation.

Given the huge improvement in sensitivity and specificity of molecular imaging of inflammation offered by MPIO-based molecular MRI, efforts are ongoing to adapt this method for clinical imaging. Indeed, currently used MPIOs are not biodegradable, especially because of their poly-urethane coating. Therefore, the development of biodegradable and biocompatible MPIOs is mandatory for further development of this imaging technology. For instance, the production of multimeric magnetite particles forming large MPIO-like particles which are biodegradable has been described (Nkansah et al., 2011). Another active subject is the impact of MPIO binding on endothelium physiology. Indeed, several studies demonstrated outside-in signaling after binding of leukocytes on ICAM-1 expressing endothelial cells. ICAM-1 clustering due to leukocyte binding triggers intra-cellular calcium release and subsequent activation of RhoA and the formation of actin stress filaments (Jefferson et al., 2013). Concerning VCAM-1, a recent *in vitro* study demonstrated that MPIOs labeled with VCAM-1 targeting antibodies do not promote endothelial inflammation, in contrast to monocytes (Jefferson et al., 2013). However, this potential side effect of targeted MPIOs should be tested for all endothelial targets before clinical investigations. The risk of immunization of the receiver of targeted MPIOs preparation must also be studied and potentially counteracted using non-immunogenic targeting moieties.

Besides toxicity issues, translation of MPIO-based molecular MRI from bench to bedside will require the demonstration of the feasibility to detect MPIOs using magnet at clinical field strength and using standard coils. Indeed, the sensitivity of MPIO detection depends both on the field strength (higher field strength would produce larger susceptibility effect of the MPIOs) and on the spatial resolution of the MRI acquisition. This last parameter would be crucial to optimize for clinical translation since the resolution achieved in preclinical study is below 80 μm (isotropic) and allows single MPIO imaging whereas the highest resolution of 3D T2*-weighted images on clinical magnet is around 500 μm. This lower resolution, because of partial volume effects, will lower the sensitivity of the MRI acquisition to detect MPIOs. To overcome this issue, longer acquisition times to increase the signal to noise ratio and strengthen the T2*-weighting will be necessary and could limit the clinical availability of this method. Interestingly, a whole brain 3D T2*-weighted image with an isotropic resolution of 500 μm can be acquired using a 7 Tesla clinical magnet in 6 min with a high signal to noise ratio using echo planar imaging (Zwanenburg et al., 2011). Such imaging method with a clinically compatible acquisition time would be particularly well suited for MPIO-based molecular MRI and argue toward the feasibility of sensitive and timely molecular MRI in humans. Studies in large animals such as non-human primates are awaited to demonstrate the feasibility of MPIO-based imaging in humans.

CONCLUSION

While several years ago the feasibility of rapid and reliable molecular imaging of brain–immune interactions using MRI was elusive, the mini-revolution represented by the development of MPIO-based contrast agent has changed this view. Although molecular MRI using targeted MPIOs still remains restricted to preclinical imaging, studies aiming at closing the translational gap are ongoing. Once available, such contrast agents will undoubtedly help to improve our knowledge on the brain–immune interactions taking place in the human brain after acute neurological injury. Besides, they will represent potent tools to select patient for anti-inflammatory treatment and subsequently monitor the therapeutic response. Nevertheless, molecular MRI using targeted MPIOs is limited to imaging of endothelial targets and does not allow long term investigation of the fate of leukocyte once in the brain parenchyma. To this aim, exogenous labeling of autologous cells and subsequent cell tracking using MRI remains the method of choice. These two imaging strategies (i.e., targeted MPIOs and MRI cell tracking) appear today as the most promising technologies to non-invasively study immune cells trafficking in both preclinical and clinical studies. These tools will help to determine whether molecular MRI of brain–immune interactions can improve the management of patients presenting acute brain injury.

REFERENCES

Anderson, S. A., Glod, J., Arbab, A. S., Noel, M., Ashari, P., Fine, H. A., et al. (2005). Noninvasive MR imaging of magnetically labeled stem cells to directly identify neovasculature in a glioma model. *Blood* 105, 420–425. doi: 10.1182/blood-2004-06-2222

Anderson, S. A., Shukaliak-Quandt, J., Jordan, E. K., Arbab, A. S., Martin, R., Mcfarland, H., et al. (2004). Magnetic resonance imaging of labeled T-cells in a mouse model of multiple sclerosis. *Ann. Neurol.* 55, 654–659. doi: 10.1002/ana.20066

Arbab, A. S., Yocum, G. T., Kalish, H., Jordan, E. K., Anderson, S. A., Khakoo, A. Y., et al. (2004). Efficient magnetic cell labeling with protamine sulfate complexed to ferumoxides for cellular MRI. *Blood* 104, 1217–1223. doi: 10.1182/blood-2004-02-0655

Arima, Y., Harada, M., Kamimura, D., Park, J.-H., Kawano, F., Yull, F. E., et al. (2012). Regional neural activation defines a gateway for autoreactive T cells to cross the blood-brain barrier. *Cell* 148, 447–457. doi: 10.1016/j.cell.2012.01.022

Atkinson, W., Forghani, R., Wojtkiewicz, G. R., Pulli, B., Iwamoto, Y., Ueno, T., et al. (2012). Ligation of the jugular veins does not result in brain inflammation or demyelination in mice. *PLoS ONE* 7:e33671. doi: 10.1371/journal.pone.0033671

Baeten, K., Hendriks, J. J., Hellings, N., Theunissen, E., Vanderlocht, J., Ryck, L. D., et al. (2008). Visualisation of the kinetics of macrophage infiltration during experimental autoimmune encephalomyelitis by magnetic resonance imaging. *J. Neuroimmunol.* 195, 1–6. doi: 10.1016/j.jneuroim.2007.11.008

Barber, P. A., Foniok, T., Kirk, D., Buchan, A. M., Laurent, S., Boutry, S., et al. (2004). MR molecular imaging of early endothelial activation in focal ischemia. *Ann. Neurol.* 56, 116–120. doi: 10.1002/ana.20162

Bendszus, M., and Stoll, G. (2003). Caught in the act: in vivo mapping of macrophage infiltration in nerve injury by magnetic resonance imaging. *J. Neurosci.* 23, 10892–10896.

Berger, C., Hiestand, P., Kindler-Baumann, D., Rudin, M., and Rausch, M. (2006). Analysis of lesion development during acute inflammation and remission in a rat model of experimental autoimmune encephalomyelitis by visualization of macrophage infiltration, demyelination and blood-brain barrier damage. *NMR Biomed.* 19, 101–107. doi: 10.1002/nbm.1007

Blezer, E. L. A., Deddens, L. H., Kooij, G., Drexhage, J., Van Der Pol, S. M. A., Reijerkerk, A., et al. (2014). In vivo MR imaging of intercellular adhesion molecule-1 expression in an animal model of multiple sclerosis. *Contrast Media Mol. Imaging.* doi: 10.1002/cmmi.1602 [Epub ahead of print].

Bourrinet, P., Bengele, H. H., Bonnemain, B., Dencausse, A., Idee, J.-M., Jacobs, P. M., et al. (2006). Preclinical safety and pharmacokinetic profile of ferumoxtran-10, an ultrasmall superparamagnetic iron oxide magnetic resonance contrast agent. *Invest. Radiol.* 41, 313–324. doi: 10.1097/01.rli.0000197669.80475.dd

Bradley, P. P., Christensen, R. D., and Rothstein, G. (1982). Cellular and extracellular myeloperoxidase in pyogenic inflammation. *Blood* 60, 618–622.

Breckwoldt, M. O., Chen, J. W., Stangenberg, L., Aikawa, E., Rodriguez, E., Qiu, S., et al. (2008). Tracking the inflammatory response in stroke in vivo by sensing the enzyme myeloperoxidase. *Proc. Natl. Acad. Sci. U.S.A.* 105, 18584–18589. doi: 10.1073/pnas.0803945105

Briley-Saebo, K. C., Johansson, L. O., Hustvedt, S. O., Haldorsen, A. G., Bjørnerud, A., Fayad, Z. A., et al. (2006). Clearance of iron oxide particles in rat liver: effect of hydrated particle size and coating material on liver metabolism. *Invest. Radiol.* 41, 560–571. doi: 10.1097/01.rli.0000221321.90261.09

Briley-Saebo, K. C., Mani, V., Hyafil, F., Cornily, J.-C., and Fayad, Z. A. (2008). Fractionated feridex and positive contrast: in vivo MR imaging of atherosclerosis. *Magn. Reson. Med.* 59, 721–730. doi: 10.1002/mrm.21541

Brochet, B., Deloire, M. S., Touil, T., Anne, O., Caille, J. M., Dousset, V., et al. (2006). Early macrophage MRI of inflammatory lesions predicts lesion severity and disease development in relapsing EAE. *Neuroimage* 32, 266–274. doi: 10.1016/j.neuroimage.2006.03.028

Burtea, C., Ballet, S., Laurent, S., Rousseaux, O., Dencausse, A., Gonzalez, W., et al. (2012). Development of a magnetic resonance imaging protocol for the characterization of atherosclerotic plaque by using vascular cell adhesion molecule-1 and apoptosis-targeted ultrasmall superparamagnetic iron oxide derivatives. *Arterioscler. Thromb. Vasc. Biol.* 32, e36–e48. doi: 10.1161/atvbaha.112.245415

Chapon, C., Franconi, F., Lacoeuille, F., Hindré, F., Saulnier, P., Benoit, J.-P., et al. (2009). Imaging E-selectin expression following traumatic brain injury in the rat using a targeted USPIO contrast agent. *MAGMA* 22, 167–174. doi: 10.1007/s10334-008-0161-z

Chen, J. W., Breckwoldt, M. O., Aikawa, E., Chiang, G., and Weissleder, R. (2008). Myeloperoxidase-targeted imaging of active inflammatory lesions in murine experimental autoimmune encephalomyelitis. *Brain* 131, 1123–1133. doi: 10.1093/brain/awn004

Chen, J. W., Pham, W., Weissleder, R., and Bogdanov, A. (2004). Human myeloperoxidase: a potential target for molecular MR imaging in atherosclerosis. *Magn. Reson. Med.* 52, 1021–1028. doi: 10.1002/mrm.20270

Chen, J. W., Querol Sans, M., Bogdanov, A., and Weissleder, R. (2006). Imaging of myeloperoxidase in mice by using novel amplifiable paramagnetic substrates. *Radiology* 240, 473–481. doi: 10.1148/radiol.2402050994

Chin, C. L., Pai, M., Bousquet, P. F., Schwartz, A. J., O'connor, E. M., Nelson, C. M., et al. (2009). Distinct spatiotemporal pattern of CNS lesions revealed by USPIO-enhanced MRI in MOG-induced EAE rats implicates the involvement of spino-olivocerebellar pathways. *J. Neuroimmunol.* 211, 49–55. doi: 10.1016/j.jneuroim.2009.03.012

Cho, T.-H., Nighoghossian, N., Wiart, M., Desestret, V., Cakmak, S., Berthezène, Y., et al. (2007). USPIO-enhanced MRI of neuroinflammation at the sub-acute stage of ischemic stroke: preliminary data. *Cerebrovasc. Dis.* 24, 544–546. doi: 10.1159/000111222

Connolly, E. S. Jr., Winfree, C. J., Springer, T. A., Naka, Y., Liao, H., et al. (1996). Cerebral protection in homozygous null ICAM-1 mice after middle cerebral artery occlusion. Role of neutrophil adhesion in the pathogenesis of stroke. *J. Clin. Invest.* 97, 209–216. doi: 10.1172/JCI118392

Corot, C., Petry, K. G., Trivedi, R., Saleh, A., Jonkmanns, C., Le Bas, J. F., et al. (2004). Macrophage imaging in central nervous system and in carotid atherosclerotic plaque using ultrasmall superparamagnetic iron oxide in magnetic resonance imaging. *Invest. Radiol.* 39, 619–625. doi: 10.1097/01.rli.0000135980.08491.33

Cybulsky, M. I., Iiyama, K., Li, H., Zhu, S., Chen, M., Iiyama, M., et al. (2001). A major role for VCAM-1, but not ICAM-1, in early atherosclerosis. *J. Clin. Invest.* 107, 1255–1262. doi: 10.1172/jci11871

Daldrup-Link, H. E., Rudelius, M., Oostendorp, R. A. J., Settles, M., Piontek, G., Metz, S., et al. (2003). Targeting of hematopoietic progenitor cells with MR contrast agents. *Radiology* 228, 760–767. doi: 10.1148/radiol.2283020322

Davies, M. J., Gordon, J. L., Gearing, A. J., Pigott, R., Woolf, N., Katz, D., et al. (1993). The expression of the adhesion molecules ICAM-1, VCAM-1, PECAM, and E-selectin in human atherosclerosis. *J. Pathol.* 171, 223–229. doi: 10.1002/path.1711710311

Deddens, L. H., Van Tilborg, G. A. F., Van Der Toorn, A., Van Der Marel, K., Paulis, L. E. M., Van Bloois, L., et al. (2013). MRI of ICAM-1 upregulation after stroke: the importance of choosing the appropriate target-specific particulate contrast agent. *Mol. Imaging Biol.* 15, 411–422. doi: 10.1007/s11307-013-0617-z

DeLeo, M. J., Gounis, M. J., Hong, B., Ford, J. C., Wakhloo, A. K., and Bogdanov, A. A. (2009). Carotid artery brain aneurysm model: in vivo molecular enzyme-specific MR imaging of active inflammation in a pilot study. *Radiology* 252, 696–703. doi: 10.1148/radiol.2523081426

Denes, A., Vidyasagar, R., Feng, J., Narvainen, J., Mccoll, B. W., Kauppinen, R. A., et al. (2007). Proliferating resident microglia after focal cerebral ischaemia in mice. *J. Cereb. Blood Flow Metab.* 27, 1941–1953. doi: 10.1038/sj.jcbfm.9600495

Desestret, V., Brisset, J. C., Moucharrafie, S., Devillard, E., Nataf, S., Honnorat, J., et al. (2009). Early-stage investigations of ultrasmall superparamagnetic iron oxide-induced signal change after permanent middle cerebral artery occlusion in mice. *Stroke* 40, 1834–1841. doi: 10.1161/strokeaha.108.531269

Dijkhuizen, R. M., Asahi, M., Wu, O., Rosen, B. R., and Lo, E. H. (2002). Rapid breakdown of microvascular barriers and subsequent hemorrhagic transformation after delayed recombinant tissue plasminogen activator treatment in a rat embolic stroke model. *Stroke* 33, 2100–2104. doi: 10.1161/01.STR.0000023534.37670.F7

Dousset, V., Ballarino, L., Delalande, C., Coussemacq, M., Canioni, P., Petry, K. G., et al. (1999a). Comparison of ultrasmall particles of iron oxide (USPIO)-enhanced T2-weighted, conventional T2-weighted, and gadolinium-enhanced T1-weighted MR images in rats with experimental autoimmune encephalomyelitis. *AJNR Am. J. Neuroradiol.* 20, 223–227.

Dousset, V., Delalande, C., Ballarino, L., Quesson, B., Seilhan, D., Coussemacq, M., et al. (1999b). In vivo macrophage activity imaging in the central nervous system detected by magnetic resonance. *Magn. Reson. Med.* 41, 329–333. doi: 10.1002/(SICI)1522-2594(199902)41:2<329::AID-MRM17>3.0.CO;2-Z

Dousset, V., Brochet, B., Deloire, M. S., Lagoarde, L., Barroso, B., Caille, J. M., et al. (2006). MR imaging of relapsing multiple sclerosis patients using ultra-small-particle iron oxide and compared with gadolinium. *AJNR Am. J. Neuroradiol.* 27, 1000–1005.

Enlimomab Acute Stroke Trial, I. (2001). Use of anti-ICAM-1 therapy in ischemic stroke: results of the Enlimomab Acute Stroke Trial. *Neurology* 57, 1428–1434. doi: 10.1212/WNL.57.8.1428

Enzmann, G., Mysiorek, C., Gorina, R., Cheng, Y.-J., Ghavampour, S., Hannocks, M.-J., et al. (2013). The neurovascular unit as a selective barrier to polymorphonuclear granulocyte (PMN) infiltration into the brain after ischemic injury. *Acta Neuropathol.* 125, 395–412. doi: 10.1007/s00401-012-1076–1073

Farr, T. D., Seehafer, J. U., Nelles, M., and Hoehn, M. (2011). Challenges towards MR imaging of the peripheral inflammatory response in the subacute and chronic stages of transient focal ischemia. *NMR Biomed.* 24, 35–45. doi: 10.1002/nbm.1553

Floris, S., Blezer, E. L., Schreibelt, G., Dopp, E., Van Der Pol, S. M., Schadee-Eestermans, I. L., et al. (2004). Blood-brain barrier permeability and monocyte infiltration in experimental allergic encephalomyelitis: a quantitative MRI study. *Brain* 127, 616–627. doi: 10.1093/brain/awh068

Foley, L. M., Hitchens, T. K., Ho, C., Janesko-Feldman, K. L., Melick, J. A., Bayir, H., et al. (2009). Magnetic resonance imaging assessment of macrophage accumulation in mouse brain after experimental traumatic brain injury. *J. Neurotrauma* 26, 1509–1519. doi: 10.1089/neu.2008.0747

Forghani, R., Wojtkiewicz, G. R., Zhang, Y., Seeburg, D., Bautz, B. R. M., Pulli, B., et al. (2012). Demyelinating diseases: myeloperoxidase as an imaging biomarker and therapeutic target. *Radiology* 263, 451–460. doi: 10.1148/radiol.12111593

Fréchou, M., Beray-Berthat, V., Raynaud, J.-S., Mériaux, S., Gombert, F., Lancelot, E., et al. (2013). Detection of vascular cell adhesion molecule-1 expression with USPIO-enhanced molecular MRI in a mouse model of cerebral ischemia. *Contrast Media Mol. Imaging* 8, 157–164. doi: 10.1002/cmmi.1512

Gaberel, T., Gakuba, C., Goulay, R., Martinez De Lizarrondo, S., Hanouz, J. L., Emery, E., et al. (2014). Impaired glymphatic perfusion after strokes revealed by contrast-enhanced MRI: a new target for fibrinolysis? *Stroke* 45, 3092–3096. doi: 10.1161/STROKEAHA.114.006617

Gaberel, T., Gakuba, C., Hebert, M., Montagne, A., Agin, V., Rubio, M., et al. (2013). Intracerebral hematomas disappear on T2*-weighted images during normobaric oxygen therapy. *Stroke.* 44, 3482–3489. doi: 10.1161/STROKEAHA.113.002045

Gauberti, M., Martinez De Lizarrondo, S., Orset, C., and Vivien, D. (2014). Lack of secondary microthrombosis after thrombin-induced stroke in mice and non-human primates. *J. Thromb. Haemost.* 12, 409–414. doi: 10.1111/jth.12487

Gauberti, M., Montagne, A., Marcos-Contreras, O. A., Le Béhot, A., Maubert, E., and Vivien, D. (2013). Ultra-sensitive molecular MRI of vascular cell adhesion molecule-1 reveals a dynamic inflammatory penumbra after strokes. *Stroke* 44, 1988–1996. doi: 10.1161/strokeaha.111.000544

Gorelik, M., Orukari, I., Wang, J., Galpoththawela, S., Kim, H., Levy, M., et al. (2012). Use of MR cell tracking to evaluate targeting of glial precursor cells to inflammatory tissue by exploiting the very late antigen-4 docking receptor. *Radiology* 265, 175–185. doi: 10.1148/radiol.12112212

Grieve, S. M., Lønborg, J., Mazhar, J., Tan, T. C., Ho, E., Liu, C.-C., et al. (2013). Cardiac magnetic resonance imaging of rapid VCAM-1 up-regulation in myocardial ischemia-reperfusion injury. *Eur. Biophys. J.* 42, 61–70. doi: 10.1007/s00249-012-0857-x

Heinecke, J. W. (2002). Tyrosyl radical production by myeloperoxidase: a phagocyte pathway for lipid peroxidation and dityrosine cross-linking of proteins. *Toxicology* 177, 11–22. doi: 10.1016/S0300-483X(02)00192-0

Henning, E. C., Ruetzler, C. A., Gaudinski, M. R., Hu, T. C., Latour, L. L., Hallenbeck, J. M., et al. (2009). Feridex preloading permits tracking of CNS-resident macrophages after transient middle cerebral artery occlusion. *J. Cereb. Blood Flow Metab.* 29, 1229–1239. doi: 10.1038/jcbfm.2009.48

Heyn, C., Ronald, J. A., Mackenzie, L. T., Macdonald, I. C., Chambers, A. F., Rutt, B. K., et al. (2006). In vivo magnetic resonance imaging of single cells in mouse brain with optical validation. *Magn. Reson. Med.* 55, 23–29. doi: 10.1002/mrm.20747

Hoyte, L. C., Brooks, K. J., Nagel, S., Akhtar, A., Chen, R., Mardiguian, S., et al. (2010). Molecular magnetic resonance imaging of acute vascular cell adhesion molecule-1 expression in a mouse model of cerebral ischemia. *J. Cereb. Blood Flow Metab.* 30, 1178–1187. doi: 10.1038/jcbfm.2009.287

Iadecola, C., and Anrather, J. (2011). The immunology of stroke: from mechanisms to translation. *Nat. Med.* 17, 796–808. doi: 10.1038/nm.2399

Jefferson, A., Ruparelia, N., and Choudhury, R. P. (2013). Exogenous microparticles of iron oxide bind to activated endothelial cells but, unlike monocytes, do not trigger an endothelial response. *Theranostics* 3, 428–436. doi: 10.7150/thno.5895

Jefferson, A., Wijesurendra, R. S., Mcateer, M. A., Digby, J. E., Douglas, G., Bannister, T., et al. (2011). Molecular imaging with optical coherence tomography using ligand-conjugated microparticles that detect activated endothelial cells: rational design through target quantification. *Atherosclerosis* 219, 579–587. doi: 10.1016/j.atherosclerosis.2011.07.127

Jendelová, P., Herynek, V., Urdzíková, L., Glogarová, K., Kroupová, J., Andersson, B., et al. (2004). Magnetic resonance tracking of transplanted bone marrow and embryonic stem cells labeled by iron oxide nanoparticles in rat brain and spinal cord. *J. Neurosci. Res.* 76, 232–243. doi: 10.1002/jnr.20041

Jin, A. Y., Tuor, U. I., Rushforth, D., Filfil, R., Kaur, J., Ni, F., et al. (2009). Magnetic resonance molecular imaging of post-stroke neuroinflammation with a P-selectin targeted iron oxide nanoparticle. *Contrast Media Mol. Imaging* 4, 305–311. doi: 10.1002/cmmi.292

Kelly, K. A., Allport, J. R., Tsourkas, A., Shinde-Patil, V. R., Josephson, L., and Weissleder, R. (2005). Detection of vascular adhesion molecule-1 expression using a novel multimodal nanoparticle. *Circ. Res.* 96, 327–336. doi: 10.1161/01.RES.0000155722.17881.dd

Kim, J., Kim, D. I., Lee, S.-K., Kim, D. J., Lee, J. E., and Ahn, S. K. (2008). Imaging of the inflammatory response in reperfusion injury after transient cerebral ischemia in rats: correlation of superparamagnetic iron oxide-enhanced magnetic resonance imaging with histopathology. *Acta Radiol.* 49, 580–588. doi: 10.1080/02841850802020484

Kleinschnitz, C., Bendszus, M., Frank, M., Solymosi, L., Toyka, K. V., and Stoll, G. (2003). In vivo monitoring of macrophage infiltration in experimental ischemic brain lesions by magnetic resonance imaging. *J. Cereb. Blood Flow Metab.* 23, 1356–1361. doi: 10.1097/01.wcb.0000090505.76664.db

Klinke, A., Nussbaum, C., Kubala, L., Friedrichs, K., Rudolph, T. K., Rudolph, V., et al. (2011). Myeloperoxidase attracts neutrophils by physical forces. *Blood* 117, 1350–1358. doi: 10.1182/blood-2010-05-284513

Kooi, M. E., Cappendijk, V. C., Cleutjens, K. B. J. M., Kessels, A. G. H., Kitslaar, P. J. E. H. M., Borgers, M., et al. (2003). Accumulation of ultrasmall superparamagnetic particles of iron oxide in human atherosclerotic plaques can be detected by in vivo magnetic resonance imaging. *Circulation* 107, 2453–2458. doi: 10.1161/01.cir.0000068315.98705.cc

Kyritsis, N., Kizil, C., Zocher, S., Kroehne, V., Kaslin, J., Freudenreich, D., et al. (2012). Acute inflammation initiates the regenerative response in the adult zebrafish brain. *Science* 338, 1353–1356. doi: 10.1126/science.1228773

Ladewig, G., Jestaedt, L., Misselwitz, B., Solymosi, L., Toyka, K., Bendszus, M., et al. (2009). Spatial diversity of blood-brain barrier alteration and macrophage invasion in experimental autoimmune encephalomyelitis: a comparative MRI study. *Exp. Neurol.* 220, 207–211. doi: 10.1016/j.expneurol.2009.08.027

Laurent, S., Forge, D., Port, M., Roch, A., Robic, C., Vander Elst, L., et al. (2008). Magnetic iron oxide nanoparticles: synthesis, stabilization, vectorization, physicochemical characterizations, and biological applications. *Chem. Rev.* 108, 2064–2110. doi: 10.1021/cr068445e

Le Behot, A., Gauberti, M., Martinez De Lizarrondo, S., Montagne, A., Lemarchand, E., Repesse, Y., et al. (2014). GpIbalpha-VWF blockade restores vessel patency by dissolving platelet aggregates formed under very high shear rate in mice. *Blood* 123, 3354–3363. doi: 10.1182/blood-2013-12-543074

Ley, K., Laudanna, C., Cybulsky, M. I., and Nourshargh, S. (2007). Getting to the site of inflammation: the leukocyte adhesion cascade updated. *Nat. Rev. Immunol.* 7, 678–689. doi: 10.1038/nri2156

Liesz, A., Zhou, W., Mracsko, E., Karcher, S., Bauer, H., Schwarting, S., et al. (2011). Inhibition of lymphocyte trafficking shields the brain against deleterious neuroinflammation after stroke. *Brain* 134, 704–720. doi: 10.1093/brain/awr008

Liu, H. L., Chen, P. Y., Yang, H. W., Wu, J. S., Tseng, I. C., Ma, Y. J., et al. (2011). In vivo MR quantification of superparamagnetic iron oxide nanoparticle leakage during low-frequency-ultrasound-induced blood-brain barrier opening in swine. *J. Magn. Reson. Imaging* 34, 1313–1324. doi: 10.1002/jmri.22697

Machtoub, L., Bataveljic, D., and Andjus, P. R. (2011). Molecular imaging of brain lipid environment of lymphocytes in amyotrophic lateral sclerosis using magnetic resonance imaging and SECARS microscopy. *Physiol. Res.* 60(Suppl. 1), S121–S127.

Manninger, S. P., Muldoon, L. L., Nesbit, G., Murillo, T., Jacobs, P. M., and Neuwelt, E. A. (2005). An exploratory study of ferumoxtran-10 nanoparticles as a blood-brain barrier imaging agent targeting phagocytic cells in CNS inflammatory lesions. *AJNR Am. J. Neuroradiol.* 26, 2290–2300.

Mardiguian, S., Serres, S., Ladds, E., Campbell, S. J., Wilainam, P., Mcfadyen, C., et al. (2013). Anti-IL-17A treatment reduces clinical score and VCAM-1 expression detected by in vivo magnetic resonance imaging in chronic relapsing EAE ABH mice. *Am. J. Pathol.* 182, 2071–2081. doi: 10.1016/j.ajpath.2013.02.029

Matsuo, Y., Onodera, H., Shiga, Y., Shozuhara, H., Ninomiya, M., Kihara, T., et al. (1994). Role of cell adhesion molecules in brain injury after transient middle cerebral artery occlusion in the rat. *Brain Res.* 656, 344–352. doi: 10.1016/0006-8993(94)91478-8

Matuszewski, L., Persigehl, T., Wall, A., Schwindt, W., Tombach, B., Fobker, M., et al. (2005). Cell tagging with clinically approved iron oxides: feasibility and effect of lipofection, particle size, and surface coating on labeling efficiency. *Radiology* 235, 155–161. doi: 10.1148/radiol.2351040094

McAteer, M. A., Mankia, K., Ruparelia, N., Jefferson, A., Nugent, H. B., Stork, L. A., et al. (2012). A leukocyte-mimetic magnetic resonance imaging contrast agent homes rapidly to activated endothelium and tracks with atherosclerotic lesion macrophage content. *Arterioscler. Thromb. Vasc. Biol.* 32, 1427–1435. doi: 10.1161/ATVBAHA.111.241844

McAteer, M. A., Schneider, J. E., Ali, Z. A., Warrick, N., Bursill, C. A., Von Zur Muhlen, C., et al. (2008). Magnetic resonance imaging of endothelial adhesion molecules in mouse atherosclerosis using dual-targeted microparticles of iron oxide. *Arterioscler. Thromb. Vasc. Biol.* 28, 77–83. doi: 10.1161/ATVBAHA.107.145466

McAteer, M. A., Sibson, N. R., Von Zur Muhlen, C., Schneider, J. E., Lowe, A. S., Warrick, N., et al. (2007). In vivo magnetic resonance imaging of acute brain inflammation using microparticles of iron oxide. *Nat. Med.* 13, 1253–1258. doi: 10.1038/nm1631

Metz, S., Bonaterra, G., Rudelius, M., Settles, M., Rummeny, E. J., and Daldrup-Link, H. E. (2004). Capacity of human monocytes to phagocytose approved iron oxide MR contrast agents in vitro. *Eur. Radiol.* 14, 1851–1858. doi: 10.1007/s00330-004-2405-2402

Michalska, M., Machtoub, L., Manthey, H. D., Bauer, E., Herold, V., Krohne, G., et al. (2012). Visualization of vascular inflammation in the atherosclerotic mouse by ultrasmall superparamagnetic iron oxide vascular cell adhesion molecule-1-specific nanoparticles. *Arterioscler. Thromb. Vasc. Biol.* 32, 2350–2357. doi: 10.1161/atvbaha.112.255224

Miller, D. H., Khan, O. A., Sheremata, W. A., Blumhardt, L. D., Rice, G. P., Libonati, M. A., et al. (2003). A controlled trial of natalizumab for relapsing multiple sclerosis. *N. Engl. J. Med.* 348, 15–23. doi: 10.1056/NEJMoa020696

Mills, P. H., Hitchens, T. K., Foley, L. M., Link, T., Ye, Q., Weiss, C. R., et al. (2012). Automated detection and characterization of SPIO-labeled cells and capsules using magnetic field perturbations. *Magn. Reson. Med.* 67, 278–289. doi: 10.1002/mrm.22998

Millward, J. M., Schnorr, J., Taupitz, M., Wagner, S., Wuerfel, J. T., and Infante-Duarte, C. (2013). Iron oxide magnetic nanoparticles highlight early involvement of the choroid plexus in central nervous system inflammation. *ASN Neuro* 5, e00110. doi: 10.1042/an20120081

Montagne, A., Gauberti, M., Macrez, R., Jullienne, A., Briens, A., Raynaud, J.-S., et al. (2012). Ultra-sensitive molecular MRI of cerebrovascular cell activation enables early detection of chronic central nervous system disorders. *Neuroimage* 63, 760–770. doi: 10.1016/j.neuroimage.2012.07.018

Morris, J. B., Olzinski, A. R., Bernard, R. E., Aravindhan, K., Mirabile, R. C., Boyce, R., et al. (2008). p38 MAPK inhibition reduces aortic ultrasmall superparamagnetic iron oxide uptake in a mouse model of atherosclerosis: MRI assessment. *Arterioscler. Thromb. Vasc. Biol.* 28, 265–271. doi: 10.1161/atvbaha.107.151175

Nahrendorf, M., Jaffer, F. A., Kelly, K. A., Sosnovik, D. E., Aikawa, E., Libby, P., et al. (2006). Noninvasive vascular cell adhesion molecule-1 imaging identifies inflammatory activation of cells in atherosclerosis. *Circulation* 114, 1504–1511. doi: 10.1161/circulationaha.106.646380

Neuwelt, E. A., Várallyay, C. G., Manninger, S., Solymosi, D., Haluska, M., Hunt, M. A., et al. (2007). The potential of ferumoxytol nanoparticle magnetic resonance imaging, perfusion, and angiography in central nervous system malignancy: a pilot study. *Neurosurgery* 60, 601–611; discussion 611-602. doi: 10.1227/01.neu.0000255350.71700.37

Nighoghossian, N., Wiart, M., Cakmak, S., Berthezène, Y., Derex, L., Cho, T.-H., et al. (2007). Inflammatory response after ischemic stroke: a USPIO-enhanced MRI study in patients. *Stroke* 38, 303–307. doi: 10.1161/01.STR.0000254548.30258.f2

Nkansah, M. K., Thakral, D., and Shapiro, E. M. (2011). Magnetic poly(lactide-co-glycolide) and cellulose particles for MRI-based cell tracking. *Magn. Reson. Med.* 65, 1776–1785. doi: 10.1002/mrm.22765

Oude Engberink, R. D., Blezer, E. L., Dijkstra, C. D., Van Der Pol, S. M., Van Der Toorn, A., and De Vries, H. E. (2010). Dynamics and fate of USPIO in the central nervous system in experimental autoimmune encephalomyelitis. *NMR Biomed.* 23, 1087–1096. doi: 10.1002/nbm.1536

Oude Engberink, R. D., Blezer, E. L., Hoff, E. I., Van Der Pol, S. M., Van Der Toorn, A., Dijkhuizen, R. M., et al. (2008). MRI of monocyte infiltration in an animal model of neuroinflammation using SPIO-labeled monocytes or free USPIO. *J. Cereb. Blood Flow Metab.* 28, 841–851. doi: 10.1038/sj.jcbfm.9600580

Peruzzotti-Jametti, L., Donega, M., Giusto, E., Mallucci, G., Marchetti, B., and Pluchino, S. (2014). The role of the immune system in central nervous system plasticity after acute injury. *Neuroscience* doi: 10.1016/j.neuroscience.2014.04.036 [Epub ahead of print].

Pulli, B., and Chen, J. (2014). Imaging neuroinflammation–from bench to bedside. *J. Clin. Cell. Immunol.* 5, 2.

Querol, M., Chen, J. W., and Bogdanov, A. A. (2006). A paramagnetic contrast agent with myeloperoxidase-sensing properties. *Org. Biomol. Chem.* 4, 1887–1895. doi: 10.1039/b601540a

Querol, M., Chen, J. W., Weissleder, R., and Bogdanov, A. (2005). DTPA-bisamide-based MR sensor agents for peroxidase imaging. *Org. Lett.* 7, 1719–1722. doi: 10.1021/ol050208v

Radermacher, K. A., Beghein, N., Boutry, S., Laurent, S., Vander Elst, L., Muller, R. N., et al. (2009). In vivo detection of inflammation using pegylated iron oxide particles targeted at E-selectin: a multimodal approach using MR imaging and EPR spectroscopy. *Invest. Radiol.* 44, 398–404. doi: 10.1097/RLI.0b013e3181a49639

Raschzok, N., Muecke, D. A., Adonopoulou, M. K., Billecke, N., Werner, W., Kammer, N. N., et al. (2011). In vitro evaluation of magnetic resonance imaging contrast agents for labeling human liver cells: implications for clinical translation. *Mol. Imaging Biol.* 13, 613–622. doi: 10.1007/s11307-010-0405-y

Rausch, M., Baumann, D., Neubacher, U., and Rudin, M. (2002). In-vivo visualization of phagocytotic cells in rat brains after transient ischemia by USPIO. *NMR Biomed.* 15, 278–283. doi: 10.1002/nbm.770

Rausch, M., Hiestand, P., Baumann, D., Cannet, C., and Rudin, M. (2003). MRI-based monitoring of inflammation and tissue damage in acute and chronic relapsing EAE. *Magn. Reson. Med.* 50, 309–314. doi: 10.1002/mrm.10541

Rausch, M., Hiestand, P., Foster, C. A., Baumann, D. R., Cannet, C., and Rudin, M. (2004). Predictability of FTY720 efficacy in experimental autoimmune encephalomyelitis by in vivo macrophage tracking: clinical implications for ultrasmall superparamagnetic iron oxide-enhanced magnetic resonance imaging. *J. Magn. Reson. Imaging* 20, 16–24. doi: 10.1002/jmri.20057

Rausch, M., Sauter, A., Fröhlich, J., Neubacher, U., Radü, E. W., and Rudin, M. (2001). Dynamic patterns of USPIO enhancement can be observed in macrophages after ischemic brain damage. *Magn. Reson. Med.* 46, 1018–1022. doi: 10.1002/mrm.1290

Reynolds, P. R., Larkman, D. J., Haskard, D. O., Hajnal, J. V., Kennea, N. L., George, A. J. T., et al. (2006). Detection of vascular expression of E-selectin in vivo with MR imaging. *Radiology* 241, 469–476. doi: 10.1148/radiol.2412050490

Riou, A., Chauveau, F., Cho, T. H., Marinescu, M., Nataf, S., Nighoghossian, N., et al. (2013). MRI assessment of the intra-carotid route for macrophage delivery after transient cerebral ischemia. *NMR Biomed.* 26, 115–123. doi: 10.1002/nbm.2826

Ruehm, S. G., Corot, C., Vogt, P., Kolb, S., and Debatin, J. F. (2001). Magnetic resonance imaging of atherosclerotic plaque with ultrasmall superparamagnetic particles of iron oxide in hyperlipidemic rabbits. *Circulation* 103, 415–422. doi: 10.1161/01.CIR.103.3.415

Saleh, A., Schroeter, M., Jonkmanns, C., Hartung, H.-P., Mödder, U., and Jander, S. (2004a). In vivo MRI of brain inflammation in human ischaemic stroke. *Brain* 127, 1670–1677. doi: 10.1093/brain/awh191

Saleh, A., Wiedermann, D., Schroeter, M., Jonkmanns, C., Jander, S., and Hoehn, M. (2004b). Central nervous system inflammatory response after cerebral infarction as detected by magnetic resonance imaging. *NMR Biomed.* 17, 163–169. doi: 10.1002/nbm.881

Saleh, A., Schroeter, M., Ringelstein, A., Hartung, H.-P., Siebler, M., Mödder, U., et al. (2007). Iron oxide particle-enhanced MRI suggests variability of brain inflammation at early stages after ischemic stroke. *Stroke* 38, 2733–2737. doi: 10.1161/strokeaha.107.481788

Schneider, C., Schuetz, G., and Zollner, T. M. (2009). Acute neuroinflammation in Lewis rats - a model for acute multiple sclerosis relapses. *J. Neuroimmunol.* 213, 84–90. doi: 10.1016/j.jneuroim.2009.05.015

Schroeter, M., Saleh, A., Wiedermann, D., Hoehn, M., and Jander, S. (2004). Histochemical detection of ultrasmall superparamagnetic iron oxide (USPIO) contrast medium uptake in experimental brain ischemia. *Magn. Reson. Med.* 52, 403–406. doi: 10.1002/mrm.20142

Schwartz, M., Kipnis, J., Rivest, S., and Prat, A. (2013). How do immune cells support and shape the brain in health, disease, and aging? *J. Neurosci.* 33, 17587–17596. doi: 10.1523/JNEUROSCI.3241-13.2013

Sekeljic, V., Bataveljic, D., Stamenkovic, S., Ulamek, M., Jablonski, M., Radenovic, L., et al. (2012). Cellular markers of neuroinflammation and neurogenesis after ischemic brain injury in the long-term survival rat model. *Brain Struct. Funct.* 217, 411–420. doi: 10.1007/s00429-011-0336–337

Serres, S., Mardiguian, S., Campbell, S. J., Mcateer, M. A., Akhtar, A., Krapitchev, A., et al. (2011). VCAM-1-targeted magnetic resonance imaging reveals subclinical disease in a mouse model of multiple sclerosis. *FASEB J.* 25, 4415–4422. doi: 10.1096/fj.11–183772

Shapiro, E. M., Sharer, K., Skrtic, S., and Koretsky, A. P. (2006). In vivo detection of single cells by MRI. *Magn. Reson. Med.* 55, 242–249. doi: 10.1002/mrm.20718

Shapiro, E. M., Skrtic, S., and Koretsky, A. P. (2005). Sizing it up: cellular MRI using micron-sized iron oxide particles. *Magn. Reson. Med.* 53, 329–338. doi: 10.1002/mrm.20342

Sigovan, M., Boussel, L., Sulaiman, A., Sappey-Marinier, D., Alsaid, H., Desbleds-Mansard, C., et al. (2009). Rapid-clearance iron nanoparticles for inflammation imaging of atherosclerotic plaque: initial experience in animal model. *Radiology* 252, 401–409. doi: 10.1148/radiol.2522081484

Sipkins, D. A., Gijbels, K., Tropper, F. D., Bednarski, M., Li, K. C., and Steinman, L. (2000). ICAM-1 expression in autoimmune encephalitis visualized using magnetic resonance imaging. *J. Neuroimmunol.* 104, 1–9. doi: 10.1016/S0165-5728(99)00248-9

Stroh, A., Zimmer, C., Werner, N., Gertz, K., Weir, K., Kronenberg, G., et al. (2006). Tracking of systemically administered mononuclear cells in the ischemic brain by high-field magnetic resonance imaging. *Neuroimage* 33, 886–897. doi: 10.1016/j.neuroimage.2006.07.009

Thorek, D. L. J., Chen, A. K., Czupryna, J., and Tsourkas, A. (2006). Superparamagnetic iron oxide nanoparticle probes for molecular imaging. *Ann. Biomed. Eng.* 34, 23–38. doi: 10.1007/s10439-005-9002–9007

Tobin, M. K., Bonds, J. A., Minshall, R. D., Pelligrino, D. A., Testai, F. D., and Lazarov, O. (2014). Neurogenesis and inflammation after ischemic stroke: what is known and where we go from here. *J. Cereb. Blood Flow Metab. 34, 1573–1584.* doi: 10.1038/jcbfm.2014.130

Trivedi, R. A., Mallawarachi, C., U-King-Im, J.-M., Graves, M. J., Horsley, J., Goddard, M. J., et al. (2006). Identifying inflamed carotid plaques using in vivo USPIO-enhanced MR imaging to label plaque macrophages. *Arterioscler. Thromb. Vasc. Biol.* 26, 1601–1606. doi: 10.1161/01.ATV.0000222920.59760.df

Tsourkas, A., Shinde-Patil, V. R., Kelly, K. A., Patel, P., Wolley, A., Allport, J. R., et al. (2005). In vivo imaging of activated endothelium using an anti-VCAM-1 magnetooptical probe. *Bioconjug. Chem.* 16, 576–581. doi: 10.1021/bc050002e

Vellinga, M. M., Geurts, J. J., Rostrup, E., Uitdehaag, B. M., Polman, C. H., Barkhof, F., et al. (2009). Clinical correlations of brain lesion distribution in multiple sclerosis. *J. Magn. Reson. Imaging* 29, 768–773. doi: 10.1002/jmri.21679

Vellinga, M. M., Oude Engberink, R. D., Seewann, A., Pouwels, P. J. W., Wattjes, M. P., Van Der Pol, S. M. A., et al. (2008). Pluriformity of inflammation in multiple sclerosis shown by ultra-small iron oxide particle enhancement. *Brain* 131, 800–807. doi: 10.1093/brain/awn009

Vivien, D., Gauberti, M., Montagne, A., Defer, G., and Touze, E. (2011). Impact of tissue plasminogen activator on the neurovascular unit: from clinical data to experimental evidence. *J. Cereb. Blood Flow Metab.* 31, 2119–2134. doi: 10.1038/jcbfm.2011.127

von Elverfeldt, D., Maier, A., Duerschmied, D., Braig, M., Witsch, T., Wang, X., et al. (2014). Dual contrast molecular imaging allows noninvasive characterization of myocardial ischemia/reperfusion injury after coronary vessel occlusion in mice by MRI. *Circulation* 130, 676–687. doi: 10.1161/circulationaha.113.008157

von Zur Muhlen, C., Von Elverfeldt, D., Choudhury, R. P., Ender, J., Ahrens, I., Schwarz, M., et al. (2008). Functionalized magnetic resonance contrast agent selectively binds to glycoprotein IIb/IIIa on activated human platelets under flow conditions and is detectable at clinically relevant field strengths. *Mol. Imaging* 7, 59–67.

Wang, J., and Dore, S. (2007). Inflammation after intracerebral hemorrhage. *J. Cereb. Blood Flow Metab.* 27, 894–908. doi: 10.1038/sj.jcbfm.9600403

Weissleder, R., Stark, D. D., Engelstad, B. L., Bacon, B. R., Compton, C. C., White, D. L., et al. (1989). Superparamagnetic iron oxide: pharmacokinetics and toxicity. *AJR Am. J. Roentgenol.* 152, 167–173. doi: 10.2214/ajr.152.1.167

Wiart, M., Davoust, N., Pialat, J.-B., Desestret, V., Moucharrafie, S., Moucharaffie, S., et al. (2007). MRI monitoring of neuroinflammation in mouse focal ischemia. *Stroke* 38, 131–137. doi: 10.1161/01.str.0000252159.05702.00

Will, O., Purkayastha, S., Chan, C., Athanasiou, T., Darzi, A. W., Gedroyc, W., et al. (2006). Diagnostic precision of nanoparticle-enhanced MRI for lymph-node metastases: a meta-analysis. *Lancet Oncol.* 7, 52–60. doi: 10.1016/s1470-2045(05)70537–70534

Woodcock, T., and Morganti-Kossmann, M. C. (2013). The role of markers of inflammation in traumatic brain injury. *Front. Neurol.* 4:18. doi: 10.3389/fneur.2013.00018

Woods, M., Woessner, D. E., and Sherry, A. D. (2006). Paramagnetic lanthanide complexes as PARACEST agents for medical imaging. *Chem. Soc. Rev.* 35, 500–511. doi: 10.1039/b509907m

Wu, Y. J., Muldoon, L. L., Varallyay, C., Markwardt, S., Jones, R. E., and Neuwelt, E. A. (2007). In vivo leukocyte labeling with intravenous ferumoxides/protamine sulfate complex and in vitro characterization for cellular magnetic resonance imaging. *Am. J. Physiol. Cell Physiol.* 293, C1698–C1708. doi: 10.1152/ajpcell.00215.2007

Yancy, A. D., Olzinski, A. R., Hu, T. C.-C., Lenhard, S. C., Aravindhan, K., Gruver, S. M., et al. (2005). Differential uptake of ferumoxtran-10 and ferumoxytol, ultrasmall superparamagnetic iron oxide contrast agents in rabbit: critical determinants of atherosclerotic plaque labeling. *J. Magn. Reson. Imaging* 21, 432–442. doi: 10.1002/jmri.20283

Yang, Y. M., Feng, X. Y., Yin Le, K., Li, C. C., Li, A. N., Jia, J., et al. (2013). In vivo USPIO-enhanced MR signal characteristics of secondary degeneration in the ipsilateral substantia nigra after middle cerebral artery occlusion at 3T. *J. Neuroradiol.* 40, 198–203. doi: 10.1016/j.neurad.2012.11.002

Yang, Y., Yang, Y., Yanasak, N., Schumacher, A., and Hu, T. C.-C. (2010). Temporal and noninvasive monitoring of inflammatory-cell infiltration to myocardial infarction sites using micrometer-sized iron oxide particles. *Magn. Reson. Med.* 63, 33–40. doi: 10.1002/mrm.22175

Ye, Q., Wu, Y. L., Foley, L. M., Hitchens, T. K., Eytan, D. F., Shirwan, H., et al. (2008). Longitudinal tracking of recipient macrophages in a rat chronic cardiac allograft rejection model with noninvasive magnetic resonance imaging using micrometer-sized paramagnetic iron oxide particles. *Circulation* 118, 149–156. doi: 10.1161/circulationaha.107.746354

Zwanenburg, J. J. M., Versluis, M. J., Luijten, P. R., and Petridou, N. (2011). Fast high resolution whole brain T2* weighted imaging using echo planar imaging at 7T. *Neuroimage* 56, 1902–1907. doi: 10.1016/j.neuroimage.2011.03.046

2

Contributions of the immune system to the pathophysiology of traumatic brain injury – evidence by intravital microscopy

Susanne M. Schwarzmaier[1,2] and Nikolaus Plesnila[2,3] *

[1] Department of Anesthesiology, University of Munich Medical Center, Munich, Germany
[2] Institute for Stroke and Dementia Research (ISD), University of Munich Medical Center, Munich, Germany
[3] Munich Cluster of Systems Neurology, Munich, Germany

***Correspondence:**
Nikolaus Plesnila, Institute for Stroke and Dementia Research (ISD), University of Munich Medical Center, Max-Lebsche Platz 30, 81377 Munich, Germany
e-mail: nikolaus.plesnila@med.uni-muenchen.de

Traumatic brain injury (TBI) results in immediate brain damage that is caused by the mechanical impact and is non-reversible. This initiates a cascade of delayed processes which cause additional—secondary—brain damage. Among these secondary mechanisms, the inflammatory response is believed to play an important role, mediating actions that can have both protective and detrimental effects on the progression of secondary brain damage. Histological data generated extensive information; however, this is only a snapshot of processes that are, in fact, very dynamic. In contrast, *in vivo* microscopy provides detailed insight into the temporal and spatial patterns of cellular dynamics. In this review, we aim to summarize data which was generated by *in vivo* microscopy, specifically investigating the immune response following brain trauma, and its potential effects on secondary brain damage.

Keywords: brain trauma, secondary brain damage, inflammation, leukocytes, microglia, innate immune answer, *in vivo* imaging, intravital microscopy

TRAUMATIC BRAIN INJURY

Traumatic brain injury (TBI) remains one of the major causes of death and severe disability in industrialized countries (Bruns and Hauser, 2003; Tagliaferri et al., 2006). It results in immediate primary damage that is caused by the mechanical impact and is non-reversible. This primary contusion initiates a cascade of secondary processes on a cellular, subcellular, and molecular level which cause additional—secondary—brain damage (Kontos et al., 1981; Baethmann et al., 1988; Allan and Rothwell, 2001; Sahuquillo et al., 2001; Bramlett and Dietrich, 2004; Nortje and Menon, 2004; Werner and Engelhard, 2007; Harhangi et al., 2008; Maas et al., 2008; Greve and Zink, 2009; Shlosberg et al., 2010): Both vasogenic and cytotoxic brain edema, generated by a disruption of the blood brain barrier (BBB) or swelling of astrocytes, respectively, lead to a raise in intracranial pressure (ICP; Unterberg et al., 2004). This results in reduced cerebral blood flow (CBF) and finally ischemia (Bouma et al., 1992; Golding et al., 1999). CBF is also impaired by alterations in the cerebral microcirculation, e.g., microthrombus formation, the generation of leukocyte/platelet aggregates, and the interaction of leukocytes with the cerebral endothelium (Schwarzmaier et al., 2010, 2013). Inflammatory processes result in the production of NO and free radicals, and the release of chemokines and cytokines which worsen BBB disruption and tissue damage and maintain the inflammatory reaction. Further damage is mediated by apoptotic and necrotic processes in neurons, glia cells, and endothelial cells. While the contusion volume, i.e., the area of irreversible neuronal cell death, reaches its peak already in the first 24–48 h as demonstrated in animal models (Kochanek et al., 1995; Zweckberger et al., 2003, 2006; Engel et al., 2008; Turtzo et al., 2014), ongoing processes orchestrating both inflammatory and recovery-related mechanisms may influence functional outcome and recovery over the following days, weeks and months (Kontos et al., 1981; Allan and Rothwell, 2001; Sahuquillo et al., 2001; Bramlett and Dietrich, 2004; Nortje and Menon, 2004; Unterberg et al., 2004; Werner and Engelhard, 2007; Harhangi et al., 2008; Maas et al., 2008; Greve and Zink, 2009; Shlosberg et al., 2010).

Most data on the pathophysiology of secondary brain damage has been generated in various animal models of TBI. The two most frequently used models mimic the two main features of TBI, i.e., cortical contusion (Controlled Cortical Impact, CCI), and diffuse axon damage (fluid percussion injury, FPI). However, so far none of the available models simultaneously mimics all features of TBI—e.g., additional vessel injury or systemic hypoxia (Lighthall et al., 1989; Finnie and Blumbergs, 2002; Morales et al., 2005; Morganti-Kossmann et al., 2010).

INFLAMMATION

TBI causes tissue damage and, consequently, induces an acute as well as a chronic inflammatory reaction, including the innate and the adaptive immune system. Both protective and detrimental aspects for the progression of secondary brain damage have been associated to different aspects of the immune response, depending e.g., on the (immune) cell type, the intensity of activation, and on the temporal and spatial relation of the immune response in relation to the initial brain injury (Whalen et al., 1999a; Allan and Rothwell, 2001; Morganti-Kossmann et al., 2001, 2002; Konsman et al., 2007; Rivest, 2009; Loane and Byrnes, 2010; Prinz et al., 2011; de Rivero Vaccari et al., 2014; Peruzzotti-Jametti et al., 2014). In this review we will mainly focus on *in vivo* microscopy studies investigating the pathophysiology of TBI. To be able to put the findings after TBI in the right context, we also included some particularly relevant studies on spinal cord injury (SCI) and cerebral ischemia in our review.

IN VIVO IMAGING

The main difficulty in determining the effects of inflammatory cells on secondary brain damage following TBI lies in the nature of the employed methods: histological data provide extensive information on spatial distribution of immune cells as well as their state of activation; however, these data will always remain only a snapshot of processes that are, in fact, very dynamic. In contrast, *in vivo* imaging, and more specifically *in vivo* microscopy, provides detailed insight into the temporal and spatial patterns of cellular and sometimes subcellular dynamics in the living brain. The two main *in vivo* imaging techniques used in animal research are epi-fluorescence and multiphoton microscopy (Denk et al., 1990; Helmchen and Denk, 2005; Shaner et al., 2005; Misgeld and Kerschensteiner, 2006; Xu et al., 2007; Holtmaat et al., 2013). For epi-fluorescence microscopy, fluorophores are excited by light and emit a fluorescent signal which is detected by a CCD camera at high speed. Main shortcomings of this technique are phototoxic tissue damage caused by high excitation energy, and the acquisition of only superficial fluorescent signals, thereby allowing only imaging in two dimensions. Multiphoton microscopy overcomes these problems by an elegant method: two—or more—photons sent consecutively by a laser arrive in the focal point of the objective at almost the same time. Their combined energy results in emission of only one photon with higher energy, i.e., longer wavelength. This phenomenon—the 2-photon effect—results in emission of fluorescence only in the focal point of the objective, and in improved tissue penetration. The consequence is a greatly improved signal to noise ratio which allows imaging of photons deriving deep from brain tissue without the necessity to use high intensity excitation energy which may damage the tissue of interest.

In contrast to histological techniques, *in vivo* imaging needs to (a) stain the cells of interest in the living animal, (b) use surgical techniques to expose the area of interest; and (c) keep animals under anesthesia for several hours. These interventions may interfere with the evolving immune response after TBI. For example, leukocytes were mostly imaged following *in vivo* staining, e.g., with Rhodamine 6G (Villringer et al., 1991), while microglia were studied in most cases in mice expressing CX3CR1-GFP (Jung et al., 2000). For superficial imaging, an open cranial window preparation was employed (Wahl et al., 1985). In contrast, for multiphoton microscopy either the skull was thinned (Frostig et al., 1990), or a bone flap and the underlying dura mater were removed and a cover glass was implanted (Levasseur et al., 1975; Kienast et al., 2010); a procedure already activating microglia and influencing dendritic spine turnover (Xu et al., 2007). The maintenance of sufficient anesthesia and of physiological parameters like body temperature, mean arterial blood pressure (MABP), and arteriolar blood gases (i.e., pH, pO_2 and pCO_2, electrolytes, etc.) both during surgery and the time of *in vivo* imaging is another important aspect. These parameters can significantly affect (patho-) physiological processes; consequently, their continuous monitoring and maintenance throughout *in vivo* imaging is important. While the body temperature is controlled and maintained in most *in vivo* imaging experiments discussed in this review, only very few studies provide information on MABP or blood gases (Härtl et al., 1997a,b; Utagawa et al., 2008; Schwarzmaier et al., 2010, 2013), or heart rate and oxygen saturation (Masuda et al., 2011). Since experiments including the preparation of a cranial window and/or imaging can last up to several hours—and the animal is under anesthesia for an equally long period of time—it is important that the ventilation of the animals is sufficient and adjustable to the individual animal. However, only few studies report that the animals were intubated (Masuda et al., 2011) or intubated and ventilated (Härtl et al., 1997a,b; Utagawa et al., 2008; Schwarzmaier et al., 2010, 2013; Herz et al., 2011). Accordingly, these points need to be critically taken into consideration when interpreting data obtained by *in vivo* imaging.

CEREBRAL INFLAMMATORY RESPONSE—RESIDENT CELLS

Microglia are the resident macrophages in the brain (Stoll and Jander, 1999; Soulet and Rivest, 2008; Ransohoff and Cardona, 2010; Kettenmann et al., 2011). Under physiological conditions, they have a ramified shape with small cell bodies and long processes which continuously scan their environment (Davalos et al., 2005; Nimmerjahn et al., 2005), monitoring synapses and responding to their functional state (Wake et al., 2009). Upon activation, microglia change both functionally and morphologically into their activated forms which are referred to as "M1" or "M2". M1 is considered to be the pro-inflammatory state, associated with actions such as phagocytosis, the presentation of antigens, and the production of reactive oxygen species (ROS) and NO. By contrast, microglia with the activation state M2, which is sometimes subdivided further into "acquired deactivation" and "alternative activation", are responsible for effects such as the fine tuning of inflammation, the recruitment of regulatory T-cells, and for scavenging of debris. They are also associated with the promotion of tissue remodeling or repair, and with angiogenesis (Stoll and Jander, 1999; Colton, 2009; Loane and Byrnes, 2010; Ransohoff and Cardona, 2010; David and Kroner, 2011; Kettenmann et al., 2011). Accordingly, microglia are believed to play both a beneficial and a detrimental role after brain injury, depending—among other factors such as age—both on the injury type, and the time investigated, i.e., the acute or the chronic inflammatory response (Block et al., 2007; Glezer et al., 2007; Rivest, 2009; Loane and Byrnes, 2010; Kettenmann et al., 2011; Nayak et al., 2012; Hernandez-Ontiveros et al., 2013; Peruzzotti-Jametti et al., 2014).

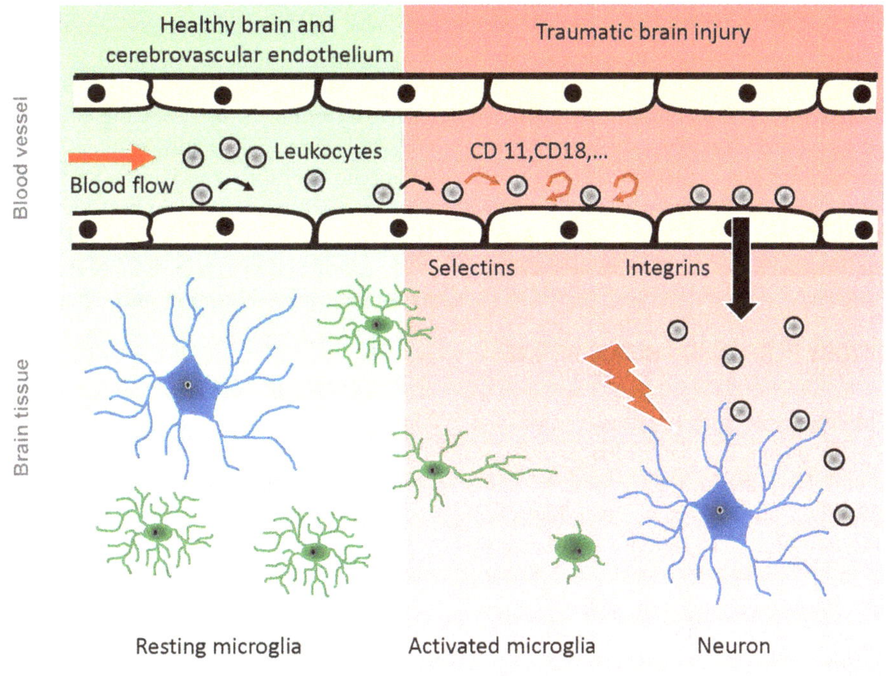

FIGURE 1 | Scheme of pathophysiological reactions of leukocytes and microglia after traumatic brain injury as demonstrated by *in vivo* experiments. Under physiological conditions (green background), leukocytes pass the cerebral microcirculation in undisturbed blood flow, while some of them occasionally role on the endothelium. Microglia have a ramified shape and continuously scan the brain parenchyma with their processes. Following TBI (red background), the intravascular leukocytes start rolling and adhering to the endothelium, mediated by selectins and integrins respectively. Finally, they migrate into the damaged tissue. Microglia become activated by brain trauma, extend their processes towards the site of injury, and finally migrate towards the injury, taking up an amoeboid shape.

Following brain injury, microglia extend their processes towards the damaged area as shown *in vivo* after laser or microelectrode injury (Davalos et al., 2005), or *ex vivo* on organotropic hippocampal slice cultures following MCAo (Neumann et al., 2008; **Figure 1**). Microglia morphologically become more amoeboid and finally migrate towards the site of injury (Kim and Dustin, 2006). These changes in morphology and/or migration resulted in encapsulation of the damaged area (Davalos et al., 2005; Kim and Dustin, 2006), or in engulfment of invading neutrophils (Neumann et al., 2008). The laser injury was performed by high laser power delivered to a dedicated area of interest for a certain time, and the microelectrode injury was induced with a glass electrode which was inserted into the cortex by a micromanipulator (Davalos et al., 2005). Both laser injury and microelectrode injury result in a very small, focal brain damage. Consequently, these techniques provide excellent models for studying very subtle alterations of cells or even subcellular processes in a well-defined area. While these studies generate valuable information on microglia and their functions, they do not mimic clinical brain injury. The dynamics of a TBI, however, can cause a much stronger and more complex damage—depending on injury severity and mechanism—which might affect or activate the resident immune cells quite differently.

Considering that TBI may also lead to cerebral ischemia, the reaction of microglia to ischemic events *in vivo* might also be helpful for a better understanding of the function of microglia after brain trauma. Severely decreased CBF initiated microglial de-ramification—i.e., activation—in different models of cerebral ischemia, while a moderate decrease or an increase in CBF had no visible effect on microglia and their processes (Masuda et al., 2011). Following ischemia, microglia seem to influence the fate of synapses in ischemic areas (Wake et al., 2009). The authors conclude that microglia detect the functional state of synapses and play a role in remodeling neuronal circuits. In both studies several different models of cerebral ischemia were investigated, such as photo-thrombotic stroke and global ischemia. CBF in the region of interest was assessed and directly compared and matched with alterations observed in microglia. Another study on cortical microhemorrhages induced by laser injury showed a local, inflammatory response including activated microglia, however this was limited to an area in close proximity around the lesion (Rosidi et al., 2011).

In contrast to their acute response, the chronic activation of microglia seems to mediate mainly detrimental effects, e.g., via (inadequate) release of cytotoxic chemokines, neurotoxic effects of receptor activation/upregulation (e.g., Toll-like receptors (TLRs)), or ROS production, as reviewed in detail by others (Stoll and Jander, 1999; Block et al., 2007; Rivest, 2009; Loane and Byrnes, 2010; Kettenmann et al., 2011; Giunta et al., 2012; Mannix and Whalen, 2012; Hernandez-Ontiveros et al., 2013).

In data obtained from histological sections *ex vivo*, different properties of acute and chronic activation post trauma were revealed. Microglia displayed mostly a classical activation (M1) or acquired deactivation at seven and up to 28 days after FPI, but no alternative activation (Cao et al., 2012). In line with that, M2 induced by CCI peaked already at day 3–5 post injury (Turtzo et al., 2014). Inhibition of microglia activation 1 month after CCI in mice resulted in less lesion progression at 3 months post injury as assessed by MRI (Byrnes et al., 2012). Unfortunately, so far, little information is available on the chronic activation of microglia following TBI *in vivo*.

SYSTEMIC INFLAMMATORY RESPONSE—BLOOD BORNE LEUKOCYTES

The contributions of the systemic inflammatory response to secondary brain damage following TBI have been investigated intensively (Kochanek and Hallenbeck, 1992; Rothlein, 1997; Ransohoff and Tani, 1998; Johnson-Léger et al., 2000; Ransohoff et al., 2003; Callahan and Ransohoff, 2004; Imhof and Aurrand-Lions, 2004; van Buul and Hordijk, 2004; David and Kroner, 2011). Within the first hours following TBI, leukocytes and leukocyte-platelet aggregates begin to roll on and adhere to the cerebrovascular endothelium (Härtl et al., 1997b; Schwarzmaier et al., 2010, 2013; **Figure 1**). These studies were performed using clinically relevant trauma models such as FPI and CCI, which mimic not all, but the main features induced by TBI (Lighthall et al., 1989; Finnie and Blumbergs, 2002; Morales et al., 2005; Morganti-Kossmann et al., 2010). Similar leukocyte-endothelium interactions (LEI) have been demonstrated in models of cerebral ischemia (Kataoka et al., 2004) and SAH (Ishikawa et al., 2009). In a model of liver inflammation, LEI was shown to activate cerebral microglia and alter neuronal excitability (D'Mello et al., 2013). For the development of secondary brain damage after TBI, however, rolling and adherence of leukocytes to the cerebral endothelium may have a limited pathophysiological relevance. *In vivo* data showed that BBB breakdown was not associated to LEI following FPI (Härtl et al., 1997a,b), which was confirmed by *ex vivo* data (Whalen et al., 1998, 1999b). Inhibition of leukocyte adherence to the endothelium did not have any effect on secondary lesion progression after CCI (Schwarzmaier et al., 2013). Following laser injury, leukocytes were not recruited into the injury focus but to perivascular spaces in close proximity to the injury as shown *in vivo*; however, this happened not before day one after injury (Kim and Dustin, 2006). There is, however, one study reporting a correlation between leukocyte adherence and vascular leakage 36 h following CCI *in vivo* (Pascual et al., 2013). In this study, however, the craniotomy for the CCI was not resealed, a procedure well known to prevent secondary brain injury after TBI (Zweckberger et al., 2003, 2006). In this setup, post trauma edema formation will not increase ICP and microcirculatory alterations are likely to differ significantly compared to a trauma model where the bone flap is resealed and intracranial hypertension is allowed to build up. These differences of pathophysiological processes with and without intracranial hypertension might well explain the differences in the observed effects of LEI.

While leukocyte rolling and adherence can be monitored by IVM, studying the migration into the affected tissue is technically demanding and has therefore been studied mostly *ex vivo*. Neutrophil depletion has been demonstrated to reduce secondary brain damage, but the effect only became significant at 2 weeks after CCI (Kenne et al., 2012). Another study investigating the effect of an antibody directed against a subunit of the CD11d/CD18 integrin on leukocytes reports a positive effect on lesion volume already 3 days after FPI (Utagawa et al., 2008). In a study conducted by our own laboratory, leukocytes were shown to migrate into the tissue only after secondary brain damage had already occurred (Schwarzmaier et al., 2013), findings in accordance with histological data published by others (Mathew et al., 1994; Holmin et al., 1995; Soares et al., 1995; Holmin and Mathiesen, 1999).

More conclusive *in vivo* data on the role of microglia vs. peripheral immune cells after SCI were presented by Evans et al. (2014). In this study, different chimeras of transgenic mice were generated in order to image either resident microglia or blood borne monocytes/macrophages and their respective contribution to the progression of the injury *in vivo*. The authors show that it is in fact blood-derived macrophages which facilitate secondary axon dieback, and not resident microglia. Invasion of blood borne monocytes/macrophages into the CNS was dependent on microglial TLR4 (Zhou et al., 2006). Accordingly, microglia do not only directly influence secondary brain damage, but also indirectly by recruiting blood borne immune cells.

ADAPTIVE IMMUNE RESPONSE

To date, the adaptive immune response to TBI and its contributions to secondary brain damage has not been investigated intensively. There are, however, reports indicating both a neuroprotective and a detrimental role of the adaptive immune system in the pathophysiology following SCI or in chronic neuronal diseases, which have been reviewed in detail by others (Ankeny and Popovich, 2009; Schwartz et al., 2013; Rodrigues et al., 2014; Walsh et al., 2014). Histological data suggest that adaptive immune cells migrate into the damaged tissue only after secondary brain damage has occurred (Holmin et al., 1995, 1998; Soares et al., 1995; Schwarzmaier et al., 2013).

One study investigating the behavior of T-cells in health and autoimmunity *in vivo* showed that naïve T-cells did not migrate into the healthy CNS, while they partly migrated into inflamed brain tissue after Experimental Autoimmune Encephalomyelitis (EAE) *in vivo*. In their paper, the authors show that the migratory capacity of T-cells depends more on the activation status rather than the phenotype or antigen specificity (Herz et al., 2011).

SUMMARY/OUTLOOK

TBI induces an inflammatory reaction which includes both the innate and the adaptive immune system. This inflammatory response can be roughly divided into an acute phase lasting hours to days, and a chronic phase lasting for weeks to months or even years. Upon TBI, microglia shift to different forms of activation, which have both detrimental and beneficial effects on secondary brain damage. By and large, the acute phase of microglia activation seems to provide various protective and beneficial mechanisms, reaching from phagocytosis to recovery and repair, while a chronic response is mainly associated with negative effects on the CNS. Following focal brain injury, data obtained *in vivo* demonstrate that microglia extend their processes towards the damaged area, change morphologically into a more amoeboid shape, and finally migrate towards the site of injury. This can result in the encapsulation of the damaged area or in the engulfment of invading leukocytes. While these observations were reported following laser injury or microelectrode injury, *in vivo* experiments on microglia activation in a clinically more relevant TBI model such as CCI or FPI are still missing. Additionally, no *in vivo* data is available on chronic microglia activation.

The systemic part of the inflammatory response following TBI has been studied intensively. It includes blood borne leukocytes which interact with the cerebrovascular endothelium and finally migrate into the damaged tissue. While this might influence outcome in other diseases, such as the early stage after a stroke, it does not seem to be of great importance for the mechanisms involved in secondary contusion expansion following TBI. However, a chronic response could worsen functional outcome and recovery.

Therapeutic alterations of the innate immune system might be promising not only in models of chronic inflammation, but also in TBI, specifically in view of the different forms of microglia activation after acute brain injury. Further studies are needed in order to investigate therapeutic options targeting inflammation, and to fully elucidate microglia activation *in vivo* following clinically relevant models of TBI.

AUTHOR CONTRIBUTIONS

Susanne M. Schwarzmaier: Review of the literature and writing the manuscript. Nikolaus Plesnila: Review of the literature and revision of the manuscript. Both authors approve the final version of the manuscript and are accountable for all aspects of the work.

ACKNOWLEDGMENTS

The authors would like to thank Joe Guerin for editing the manuscript.

REFERENCES

Allan, S. M., and Rothwell, N. J. (2001). Cytokines and acute neurodegeneration. *Nat. Rev. Neurosci.* 2, 734–744. doi: 10.1038/35094583

Ankeny, D. P., and Popovich, P. G. (2009). Mechanisms and implications of adaptive immune responses after traumatic spinal cord injury. *Neuroscience* 158, 1112–1121. doi: 10.1016/j.neuroscience.2008.07.001

Baethmann, A., Maier-Hauff, K., Kempski, O., Unterberg, A., Wahl, M., and Schurer, L. (1988). Mediators of brain edema and secondary brain damage. *Crit. Care Med.* 16, 972–978. doi: 10.1097/00003246-198810000-00008

Block, M. L., Zecca, L., and Hong, J. S. (2007). Microglia-mediated neurotoxicity: uncovering the molecular mechanisms. *Nat. Rev. Neurosci.* 8, 57–69. doi: 10.1038/nrn2038

Bouma, G. J., Muizelaar, J. P., Stringer, W. A., Choi, S. C., Fatouros, P., and Young, H. F. (1992). Ultra-early evaluation of regional cerebral blood flow in severely head-injured patients using xenon-enhanced computerized tomography. *J. Neurosurg.* 77, 360–368. doi: 10.3171/jns.1992.77.3.0360

Bramlett, H. M., and Dietrich, W. D. (2004). Pathophysiology of cerebral ischemia and brain trauma: similarities and differences. *J. Cereb. Blood Flow Metab.* 24, 133–150. doi: 10.1097/01.wcb.0000111614.19196.04

Bruns, J. Jr., and Hauser, W. A. (2003). The epidemiology of traumatic brain injury: a review. *Epilepsia* 44(Suppl. 10), 2–10. doi: 10.1046/j.1528-1157.44.s10.3.x

Byrnes, K. R., Loane, D. J., Stoica, B. A., Zhang, J., and Faden, A. I. (2012). Delayed mGluR5 activation limits neuroinflammation and neurodegeneration after traumatic brain injury. *J. Neuroinflammation* 9:43. doi: 10.1186/1742-2094-9-43

Callahan, M. K., and Ransohoff, R. M. (2004). Analysis of leukocyte extravasation across the blood-brain barrier: conceptual and technical aspects. *Curr. Allergy Asthma Rep.* 4, 65–73. doi: 10.1007/s11882-004-0046-9

Cao, T., Thomas, T. C., Ziebell, J. M., Pauly, J. R., and Lifshitz, J. (2012). Morphological and genetic activation of microglia after diffuse traumatic brain injury in the rat. *Neuroscience* 225, 65–75. doi: 10.1016/j.neuroscience.2012.08.058

Colton, C. A. (2009). Heterogeneity of microglial activation in the innate immune response in the brain. *J. Neuroimmune Pharmacol.* 4, 399–418. doi: 10.1007/s11481-009-9164-4

Davalos, D., Grutzendler, J., Yang, G., Kim, J. V., Zuo, Y., Jung, S., et al. (2005). ATP mediates rapid microglial response to local brain injury in vivo. *Nat. Neurosci.* 8, 752–758. doi: 10.1038/nn1472

David, S., and Kroner, A. (2011). Repertoire of microglial and macrophage responses after spinal cord injury. *Nat. Rev. Neurosci.* 12, 388–399. doi: 10.1038/nrn3053

Denk, W., Strickler, J. H., and Webb, W. W. (1990). Two-photon laser scanning fluorescence microscopy. *Science* 248, 73–76. doi: 10.1126/science.2321027

de Rivero Vaccari, J. P., Dietrich, W. D., and Keane, R. W. (2014). Activation and regulation of cellular inflammasomes: gaps in our knowledge for central nervous system injury. *J. Cereb. Blood Flow Metab.* 34, 369–375. doi: 10.1038/jcbfm.2013.227

D'Mello, C., Riazi, K., Le, T., Stevens, K. M., Wang, A., Mckay, D. M., et al. (2013). P-selectin-mediated monocyte-cerebral endothelium adhesive interactions link peripheral organ inflammation to sickness behaviors. *J. Neurosci.* 33, 14878–14888. doi: 10.1523/jneurosci.1329-13.2013

Engel, D. C., Mies, G., Terpolilli, N. A., Trabold, R., Loch, A., De Zeeuw, C. I., et al. (2008). Changes of cerebral blood flow during the secondary expansion of a cortical contusion assessed by 14C-iodoantipyrine autoradiography in mice using a non-invasive protocol. *J. Neurotrauma* 25, 739–753. doi: 10.1089/neu.2007.0480

Evans, T. A., Barkauskas, D. S., Myers, J. T., Hare, E. G., You, J. Q., Ransohoff, R. M., et al. (2014). High-resolution intravital imaging reveals that blood-derived macrophages but not resident microglia facilitate secondary axonal dieback in traumatic spinal cord injury. *Exp. Neurol.* 254, 109–120. doi: 10.1016/j.expneurol.2014.01.013

Finnie, J. W., and Blumbergs, P. C. (2002). Traumatic brain injury. *Vet. Pathol.* 39, 679–689.

Frostig, R. D., Lieke, E. E., Ts'o, D. Y., and Grinvald, A. (1990). Cortical functional architecture and local coupling between neuronal activity and the microcirculation revealed by in vivo high-resolution optical imaging of intrinsic signals. *Proc. Natl. Acad. Sci. U S A* 87, 6082–6086. doi: 10.1073/pnas.87.16.6082

Giunta, B., Obregon, D., Velisetty, R., Sanberg, P. R., Borlongan, C. V., and Tan, J. (2012). The immunology of traumatic brain injury: a prime target for Alzheimer's disease prevention. *J. Neuroinflammation* 9:185. doi: 10.1186/1742-2094-9-185

Glezer, I., Simard, A. R., and Rivest, S. (2007). Neuroprotective role of the innate immune system by microglia. *Neuroscience* 147, 867–883. doi: 10.1016/j.neuroscience.2007.02.055

Golding, E. M., Robertson, C. S., and Bryan, R. M. Jr. (1999). The consequences of traumatic brain injury on cerebral blood flow and autoregulation: a review. *Clin. Exp. Hypertens.* 21, 299–332. doi: 10.3109/10641969909068668

Greve, M. W., and Zink, B. J. (2009). Pathophysiology of traumatic brain injury. *Mt. Sinai J. Med.* 76, 97–104. doi: 10.1002/msj.20104

Harhangi, B. S., Kompanje, E. J., Leebeek, F. W., and Maas, A. I. (2008). Coagulation disorders after traumatic brain injury. *Acta Neurochir. (Wien)* 150, 165–175. doi: 10.1007/s00701-007-1475-8

Härtl, R., Medary, M., Ruge, M., Arfors, K. E., and Ghajar, J. (1997a). Blood-brain barrier breakdown occurs early after traumatic brain injury and is not related to white blood cell adherence. *Acta Neurochir. Suppl.* 70, 240–242. doi: 10.1007/978-3-7091-6837-0_74

Härtl, R., Medary, M. B., Ruge, M., Arfors, K. E., and Ghajar, J. (1997b). Early white blood cell dynamics after traumatic brain injury: effects on the cerebral microcirculation. *J. Cereb. Blood Flow Metab.* 17, 1210–1220. doi: 10.1097/00004647-199711000-00010

Helmchen, F., and Denk, W. (2005). Deep tissue two-photon microscopy. *Nat. Methods* 2, 932–940. doi: 10.1038/nmeth818

Hernandez-Ontiveros, D. G., Tajiri, N., Acosta, S., Giunta, B., Tan, J., and Borlongan, C. V. (2013). Microglia activation as a biomarker for traumatic brain injury. *Front. Neurol.* 4:30. doi: 10.3389/fneur.2013.00030

Herz, J., Paterka, M., Niesner, R. A., Brandt, A. U., Siffrin, V., Leuenberger, T., et al. (2011). In vivo imaging of lymphocytes in the CNS reveals different behaviour of naive T cells in health and autoimmunity. *J. Neuroinflammation* 8:131. doi: 10.1186/1742-2094-8-131

Holmin, S., and Mathiesen, T. (1999). Long-term intracerebral inflammatory response after experimental focal brain injury in rat. *Neuroreport* 10, 1889–1891. doi: 10.1097/00001756-199906230-00017

Holmin, S., Mathiesen, T., Shetye, J., and Biberfeld, P. (1995). Intracerebral inflammatory response to experimental brain contusion. *Acta Neurochir. (Wien)* 132, 110–119. doi: 10.1007/bf01404857

Holmin, S., Söderlund, J., Biberfeld, P., and Mathiesen, T. (1998). Intracerebral inflammation after human brain contusion. *Neurosurgery* 42, 291–298. doi: 10.1097/00006123-199809000-00159

Holtmaat, A., Randall, J., and Cane, M. (2013). Optical imaging of structural and functional synaptic plasticity in vivo. *Eur. J. Pharmacol.* 719, 128–136. doi: 10.1016/j.ejphar.2013.07.020

Imhof, B. A., and Aurrand-Lions, M. (2004). Adhesion mechanisms regulating the migration of monocytes. *Nat. Rev. Immunol.* 4, 432–444. doi: 10.1038/nri1375

Ishikawa, M., Kusaka, G., Yamaguchi, N., Sekizuka, E., Nakadate, H., Minamitani, H., et al. (2009). Platelet and leukocyte adhesion in the microvasculature at the cerebral surface immediately after subarachnoid hemorrhage. *Neurosurgery* 64, 546–553. doi: 10.1227/01.neu.0000337579.05110.f4

Johnson-Léger, C., Aurrand-Lions, M., and Imhof, B. A. (2000). The parting of the endothelium: miracle, or simply a junctional affair? *J. Cell Sci.* 113(Pt. 6), 921–933.

Jung, S., Aliberti, J., Graemmel, P., Sunshine, M. J., Kreutzberg, G. W., Sher, A., et al. (2000). Analysis of fractalkine receptor CX(3)CR1 function by targeted deletion and green fluorescent protein reporter gene insertion. *Mol. Cell. Biol.* 20, 4106–4114. doi: 10.1128/mcb.20.11.4106-4114.2000

Kataoka, H., Kim, S. W., and Plesnila, N. (2004). Leukocyte-endothelium interactions during permanent focal cerebral ischemia in mice. *J. Cereb. Blood Flow Metab.* 24, 668–676. doi: 10.1097/01.wcb.0000117812.35136.5b

Kenne, E., Erlandsson, A., Lindbom, L., Hillered, L., and Clausen, F. (2012). Neutrophil depletion reduces edema formation and tissue loss following traumatic brain injury in mice. *J. Neuroinflammation* 9:17. doi: 10.1186/1742-2094-9-17

Kettenmann, H., Hanisch, U. K., Noda, M., and Verkhratsky, A. (2011). Physiology of microglia. *Physiol. Rev.* 91, 461–553. doi: 10.1152/physrev.00011.2010

Kienast, Y., von Baumgarten, L., Fuhrmann, M., Klinkert, W. E., Goldbrunner, R., Herms, J., et al. (2010). Real-time imaging reveals the single steps of brain metastasis formation. *Nat. Med.* 16, 116–122. doi: 10.1038/nm.2072

Kim, J. V., and Dustin, M. L. (2006). Innate response to focal necrotic injury inside the blood-brain barrier. *J. Immunol.* 177, 5269–5277. doi: 10.4049/jimmunol.177.8.5269

Kochanek, P. M., and Hallenbeck, J. M. (1992). Polymorphonuclear leukocytes and monocytes/macrophages in the pathogenesis of cerebral ischemia and stroke. *Stroke* 23, 1367–1379. doi: 10.1161/01.str.23.9.1367

Kochanek, P. M., Marion, D. W., Zhang, W., Schiding, J. K., White, M., Palmer, A. M., et al. (1995). Severe controlled cortical impact in rats: assessment of cerebral edema, blood flow and contusion volume. *J. Neurotrauma* 12, 1015–1025. doi: 10.1089/neu.1995.12.1015

Konsman, J. P., Drukarch, B., and Van Dam, A. M. (2007). (Peri)vascular production and action of pro-inflammatory cytokines in brain pathology. *Clin. Sci. (Lond.)* 112, 1–25. doi: 10.1042/cs20060043

Kontos, H. A., Wei, E. P., and Povlishock, J. T. (1981). Pathophysiology of vascular consequences of experimental concussive brain injury. *Trans. Am. Clin. Climatol. Assoc.* 92, 111–121.

Levasseur, J. E., Wei, E. P., Raper, A. J., Kontos, A. A., and Patterson, J. L. (1975). Detailed description of a cranial window technique for acute and chronic experiments. *Stroke* 6, 308–317. doi: 10.1161/01.str.6.3.308

Lighthall, J. W., Dixon, C. E., and Anderson, T. E. (1989). Experimental models of brain injury. *J. Neurotrauma* 6, 83–97. doi: 10.1089/neu.1989.6.83

Loane, D. J., and Byrnes, K. R. (2010). Role of microglia in neurotrauma. *Neurotherapeutics* 7, 366–377. doi: 10.1016/j.nurt.2010.07.002

Maas, A. I., Stocchetti, N., and Bullock, R. (2008). Moderate and severe traumatic brain injury in adults. *Lancet Neurol.* 7, 728–741. doi: 10.1016/s1474-4422(08)70164-9

Mannix, R. C., and Whalen, M. J. (2012). Traumatic brain injury, microglia and Beta amyloid. *Int. J. Alzheimers Dis.* 2012:608732. doi: 10.1155/2012/608732

Masuda, T., Croom, D., Hida, H., and Kirov, S. A. (2011). Capillary blood flow around microglial somata determines dynamics of microglial processes in ischemic conditions. *Glia* 59, 1744–1753. doi: 10.1002/glia.21220

Mathew, P., Graham, D. I., Bullock, R., Maxwell, W., Mcculloch, J., and Teasdale, G. (1994). Focal brain injury: histological evidence of delayed inflammatory response in a new rodent model of focal cortical injury. *Acta Neurochir. Suppl. (Wien)* 60, 428–430. doi: 10.1007/978-3-7091-9334-1_116

Misgeld, T., and Kerschensteiner, M. (2006). In vivo imaging of the diseased nervous system. *Nat. Rev. Neurosci.* 7, 449–463. doi: 10.1038/nrn1905

Morales, D. M., Marklund, N., Lebold, D., Thompson, H. J., Pitkanen, A., Maxwell, W. L., et al. (2005). Experimental models of traumatic brain injury: do we really need to build a better mousetrap? *Neuroscience* 136, 971–989. doi: 10.1016/j.neuroscience.2005.08.030

Morganti-Kossmann, M. C., Rancan, M., Otto, V. I., Stahel, P. F., and Kossmann, T. (2001). Role of cerebral inflammation after traumatic brain injury: a revisited concept. *Shock* 16, 165–177. doi: 10.1097/00024382-200116030-00001

Morganti-Kossmann, M. C., Rancan, M., Stahel, P. F., and Kossmann, T. (2002). Inflammatory response in acute traumatic brain injury: a double-edged sword. *Curr. Opin. Crit. Care* 8, 101–105. doi: 10.1097/00075198-200204000-00002

Morganti-Kossmann, M. C., Yan, E., and Bye, N. (2010). Animal models of traumatic brain injury: is there an optimal model to reproduce human brain injury in the laboratory? *Injury* 41(Suppl 1), S10–13. doi: 10.1016/j.injury.2010.03.032

Nayak, D., Zinselmeyer, B. H., Corps, K. N., and Mcgavern, D. B. (2012). In vivo dynamics of innate immune sentinels in the CNS. *Intravital* 1, 95–106. doi: 10.4161/intv.22823

Neumann, J., Sauerzweig, S., Ronicke, R., Gunzer, F., Dinkel, K., Ullrich, O., et al. (2008). Microglia cells protect neurons by direct engulfment of invading neutrophil granulocytes: a new mechanism of CNS immune privilege. *J. Neurosci.* 28, 5965–5975. doi: 10.1523/jneurosci.0060-08.2008

Nimmerjahn, A., Kirchhoff, F., and Helmchen, F. (2005). Resting microglial cells are highly dynamic surveillants of brain parenchyma in vivo. *Science* 308, 1314–1318. doi: 10.1126/science.1110647

Nortje, J., and Menon, D. K. (2004). Traumatic brain injury: physiology, mechanisms, and outcome. *Curr. Opin. Neurol.* 17, 711–718. doi: 10.1097/00019052-200412000-00011

Pascual, J. L., Murcy, M. A., Li, S., Gong, W., Eisenstadt, R., Kumasaka, K., et al. (2013). Neuroprotective effects of progesterone in traumatic brain injury: blunted in vivo neutrophil activation at the blood-brain barrier. *Am. J. Surg.* 206, 840–845; discussion 845–846. doi: 10.1016/j.amjsurg.2013.07.016

Peruzzotti-Jametti, L., Donega, M., Giusto, E., Mallucci, G., Marchetti, B., and Pluchino, S. (2014). The role of the immune system in central nervous system plasticity after acute injury. *Neuroscience.* doi: 10.1016/j.neuroscience.2014.04.036. [Epub ahead of print].

Prinz, M., Priller, J., Sisodia, S. S., and Ransohoff, R. M. (2011). Heterogeneity of CNS myeloid cells and their roles in neurodegeneration. *Nat. Neurosci.* 14, 1227–1235. doi: 10.1038/nn.2923

Ransohoff, R. M., and Cardona, A. E. (2010). The myeloid cells of the central nervous system parenchyma. *Nature* 468, 253–262. doi: 10.1038/nature09615

Ransohoff, R. M., Kivisakk, P., and Kidd, G. (2003). Three or more routes for leukocyte migration into the central nervous system. *Nat. Rev. Immunol.* 3, 569–581. doi: 10.1038/nri1130

Ransohoff, R. M., and Tani, M. (1998). Do chemokines mediate leukocyte recruitment in post-traumatic CNS inflammation? *Trends Neurosci.* 21, 154–159. doi: 10.1016/s0166-2236(97)01198-3

Rivest, S. (2009). Regulation of innate immune responses in the brain. *Nat. Rev. Immunol.* 9, 429–439. doi: 10.1038/nri2565

Rodrigues, M. C., Sanberg, P. R., Cruz, L. E., and Garbuzova-Davis, S. (2014). The innate and adaptive immunological aspects in neurodegenerative diseases. *J. Neuroimmunol.* 269, 1–8. doi: 10.1016/j.jneuroim.2013.09.020

Rosidi, N. L., Zhou, J., Pattanaik, S., Wang, P., Jin, W., Brophy, M., et al. (2011). Cortical microhemorrhages cause local inflammation but do not trigger widespread dendrite degeneration. *PLoS One* 6:e26612. doi: 10.1371/journal.pone.0026612

Rothlein, R. (1997). Overview of leukocyte adhesion. *Neurology* 49, S3–S4. doi: 10.1212/wnl.49.5_suppl_4.s3

Sahuquillo, J., Poca, M. A., and Amoros, S. (2001). Current aspects of pathophysiology and cell dysfunction after severe head injury. *Curr. Pharm. Des.* 7, 1475–1503. doi: 10.2174/1381612013397311

Schwartz, M., Kipnis, J., Rivest, S., and Prat, A. (2013). How do immune cells support and shape the brain in health, disease and aging? *J. Neurosci.* 33, 17587–17596. doi: 10.1523/jneurosci.3241-13.2013

Schwarzmaier, S. M., Kim, S. W., Trabold, R., and Plesnila, N. (2010). Temporal profile of thrombogenesis in the cerebral microcirculation after traumatic brain injury in mice. *J. Neurotrauma* 27, 121–130. doi: 10.1089/neu.2009.1114

Schwarzmaier, S. M., Zimmermann, R., Mcgarry, N. B., Trabold, R., Kim, S. W., and Plesnila, N. (2013). In vivo temporal and spatial profile of leukocyte adhesion and migration after experimental traumatic brain injury in mice. *J. Neuroinflammation* 10:32. doi: 10.1186/1742-2094-10-32

Shaner, N. C., Steinbach, P. A., and Tsien, R. Y. (2005). A guide to choosing fluorescent proteins. *Nat. Methods* 2, 905–909. doi: 10.1038/nmeth819

Shlosberg, D., Benifla, M., Kaufer, D., and Friedman, A. (2010). Blood-brain barrier breakdown as a therapeutic target in traumatic brain injury. *Nat. Rev. Neurol.* 6, 393–403. doi: 10.1038/nrneurol.2010.74

Soares, H. D., Hicks, R. R., Smith, D., and Mcintosh, T. K. (1995). Inflammatory leukocytic recruitment and diffuse neuronal degeneration are separate pathological processes resulting from traumatic brain injury. *J. Neurosci.* 15, 8223–8233.

Soulet, D., and Rivest, S. (2008). Microglia. *Curr. Biol.* 18, R506–R508. doi: 10.1016/j.cub.2008.04.047

Stoll, G., and Jander, S. (1999). The role of microglia and macrophages in the pathophysiology of the CNS. *Prog. Neurobiol.* 58, 233–247. doi: 10.1016/s0301-0082(98)00083-5

Tagliaferri, F., Compagnone, C., Korsic, M., Servadei, F., and Kraus, J. (2006). A systematic review of brain injury epidemiology in Europe. *Acta Neurochir. (Wien)* 148, 255–268; discussion 268. doi: 10.1007/s00701-005-0651-y

Turtzo, L. C., Lescher, J., Janes, L., Dean, D. D., Budde, M. D., and Frank, J. A. (2014). Macrophagic and microglial responses after focal traumatic brain injury in the female rat. *J. Neuroinflammation* 11:82. doi: 10.1186/1742-2094-11-82

Unterberg, A. W., Stover, J., Kress, B., and Kiening, K. L. (2004). Edema and brain trauma. *Neuroscience* 129, 1021–1029. doi: 10.1016/j.neuroscience.2004.06.046

Utagawa, A., Bramlett, H. M., Daniels, L., Lotocki, G., Dekaban, G. A., Weaver, L. C., et al. (2008). Transient blockage of the CD11d/CD18 integrin reduces contusion volume and macrophage infiltration after traumatic brain injury in rats. *Brain Res.* 1207, 155–163. doi: 10.1016/j.brainres.2008.02.057

van Buul, J. D., and Hordijk, P. L. (2004). Signaling in leukocyte transendothelial migration. *Arterioscler. Thromb. Vasc. Biol.* 24, 824–833. doi: 10.1161/01.atv.0000122854.76267.5c

Villringer, A., Dirnagl, U., Them, A., Schürer, L., Krombach, F., and Einhäupl, K. M. (1991). Imaging of leukocytes within the rat brain cortex in vivo. *Microvasc. Res.* 42, 305–315. doi: 10.1016/0026-2862(91)90064-i

Wahl, M., Unterberg, A., and Baethmann, A. (1985). Intravital fluorescence microscopy for the study of blood-brain-barrier function. *Int. J. Microcirc. Clin. Exp.* 4, 3–18.

Wake, H., Moorhouse, A. J., Jinno, S., Kohsaka, S., and Nabekura, J. (2009). Resting microglia directly monitor the functional state of synapses in vivo and determine the fate of ischemic terminals. *J. Neurosci.* 29, 3974–3980. doi: 10.1523/jneurosci.4363-08.2009

Walsh, J. T., Watson, N., and Kipnis, J. (2014). T cells in the central nervous system: messengers of destruction or purveyors of protection? *Immunology* 141, 340–344. doi: 10.1111/imm.12187

Werner, C., and Engelhard, K. (2007). Pathophysiology of traumatic brain injury. *Br. J. Anaesth.* 99, 4–9. doi: 10.1093/bja/aem131

Whalen, M. J., Carlos, T. M., Clark, R. S., and Kochanek, P. M. (1999a). An acute inflammatory response to the use of granulocyte colony-stimulating factor to prevent infections in patients with brain injury: what about the brain? *Crit. Care Med.* 27, 1014–1018. doi: 10.1097/00003246-199905000-00049

Whalen, M. J., Carlos, T. M., Kochanek, P. M., Clark, R. S., Heineman, S., Schiding, J. K., et al. (1999b). Neutrophils do not mediate blood-brain barrier permeability early after controlled cortical impact in rats. *J. Neurotrauma* 16, 583–594. doi: 10.1089/neu.1999.16.583

Whalen, M. J., Carlos, T. M., Kochanek, P. M., and Heineman, S. (1998). Blood-brain barrier permeability, neutrophil accumulation and vascular adhesion molecule expression after controlled cortical impact in rats: a preliminary study. *Acta Neurochir. Suppl.* 71, 212–214. doi: 10.1007/978-3-7091-6475-4_61

Xu, H. T., Pan, F., Yang, G., and Gan, W. B. (2007). Choice of cranial window type for in vivo imaging affects dendritic spine turnover in the cortex. *Nat. Neurosci.* 10, 549–551. doi: 10.1038/nprot.2007.186

Zhou, H., Lapointe, B. M., Clark, S. R., Zbytnuik, L., and Kubes, P. (2006). A requirement for microglial TLR4 in leukocyte recruitment into brain in response to lipopolysaccharide. *J. Immunol.* 177, 8103–8110. doi: 10.4049/jimmunol.177.11.8103

Zweckberger, K., Erös, C., Zimmermann, R., Kim, S. W., Engel, D., and Plesnila, N. (2006). Effect of early and delayed decompressive craniectomy on secondary brain damage after controlled cortical impact in mice. *J. Neurotrauma* 23, 1083–1093. doi: 10.1089/neu.2006.23.1083

Zweckberger, K., Stoffel, M., Baethmann, A., and Plesnila, N. (2003). Effect of decompression craniotomy on increase of contusion volume and functional outcome after controlled cortical impact in mice. *J. Neurotrauma* 20, 1307–1314. doi: 10.1089/089771503322686102

3

Neuroinflammation after intracerebral hemorrhage

Eva Mracsko*[1] *and Roland Veltkamp*[1,2]

[1] *Department of Neurology, University Heidelberg, Heidelberg, Germany*
[2] *Division of Brain Sciences, Imperial College, London, UK*

Correspondence:
Roland Veltkamp, Department of Neurology, University Heidelberg, Im Neuenheimer Feld 400, 69120 Heidelberg, Germany
e-mail: Roland.Veltkamp@med.uni-heidelberg.de

Spontaneous intracerebral hemorrhage (ICH) is a particularly severe type of stroke for which no specific treatment has been established yet. Although preclinical models of ICH have substantial methodological limitations, important insight into the pathophysiology has been gained. Mounting evidence suggests an important contribution of inflammatory mechanisms to brain damage and potential repair. Neuroinflammation evoked by intracerebral blood involves the activation of resident microglia, the infiltration of systemic immune cells and the production of cytokines, chemokines, extracellular proteases and reactive oxygen species (ROS). Previous studies focused on innate immunity including microglia, monocytes and granulocytes. More recently, the role of adaptive immune cells has received increasing attention. Little is currently known about the interactions among different immune cell populations in the setting of ICH. Nevertheless, immunomodulatory strategies are already being explored in ICH. To improve the chances of translation from preclinical models to patients, a better characterization of the neuroinflammation in patients is desirable.

Keywords: stroke, intracerebral hemorrhage, neuroinflammation, innate immunity, adaptive immunity

INTRODUCTION

Intracerebral hemorrhages (ICH) account for 10–15% of all strokes (Qureshi et al., 2009). It is a particularly severe stroke subtype that is associated with a mortality rate of 30–50%. Moreover, 74% of the survivors remain functionally dependent 12 months after the ictus (van Asch et al., 2010). Currently, the overall incidence of ICH is 24.6 per 100,000 person per year (van Asch et al., 2010) but incidence is expected to have doubled by 2050 (Qureshi et al., 2001) due to aging and the spreading use of anticoagulants (Wang, 2010). Intracerebral hemorrhages is strongly associated with cerebral microvascular diseases (Xi et al., 2006). The most frequent underlying disorder is hypertensive microangiopathy which predominantly manifests in deep cerebral structures (basal ganglia, brain stem and cerebellum) (Fisher, 1971, 2003). In the elderly, cerebral amyloid angiopathy develops in cortical arteriolar and venular microvessels (Thanvi and Robinson, 2006). Intracerebral hemorrhages in association with the use of oral anticoagulants is increasingly frequently encountered. Hemorrhage originating from aneurysms or vascular malformations is less frequent (Qureshi et al., 2001). Risk factors for ICH include genetic variants of apolipoprotein E, ethnic differences and life style factors such as smoking and alcohol intake (O'Donnell et al., 2010). Several determinants of outcome have been clearly identified. Predictors of poor clinical outcome are the initial hematoma volume, hematoma expansion during the first day, location of the hematoma, extent of brain edema, age and neurological status on admission (Hanley, 2009; Mendelow et al., 2011; Kuramatsu et al., 2013). Although several of these factors are potentially modifiable, no effective medical or surgical therapy has been firmly established for acute ICH beyond treatment in dedicated stroke and critical care units (Steiner et al., 2006, 2014; Xi et al., 2006; Morgenstern et al., 2010; Keep et al., 2012). Current efforts in clinical trials focus on blood pressure control (Anderson et al., 2013), modified surgical approaches or hemostasis in selected patients (Mayer et al., 2008; Morgan et al., 2008; Newell et al., 2011; Ziai et al., 2014). Despite the lack of evidence from randomized clinical trials, specialized neurovascular centers offer medical and surgical therapies for selected patients but otherwise ICH therapy remains supportive within a framework of general critical care management (Kuramatsu et al., 2013).

The need for new therapeutic approaches for ICH has prompted a search for the molecular and cellular mechanisms that underlie early and delayed brain damage after ICH. Clearly, several research themes are shared with other acute and chronic degenerative brain disorders. However, the appearance of extracellular blood in the brain, that results in the release of the hemoglobin constituents heme and iron, triggers specific pathophysiological cascades or modifies the timing of other processes.

In particular, there is increasing evidence that inflammatory mechanisms participate in early and delayed phases after ICH. After reviewing some limitations of preclinical modeling of ICH, the present review will summarize the evidence supporting an essential role of inflammation to brain damage and potential repair after ICH.

PRECLINICAL MODELS OF ICH

Animal models of ICH have been established in many different species (for review see James et al., 2008). A major limitation of most models is that an invasive procedure is required to induce the hemorrhage that inadvertently implies a limited brain trauma. The most frequently used methods and species, respectively, are the intracerebral injection of autologous blood or bacterial collagenase in rodents (MacLellan et al., 2008, 2010). Although both models are suitable to induce hematomas of various sizes and location, the differences between these models may influence the pathomechanisms of ICH and the neurological outcome.

Injection of autologous blood (Bullock et al., 1984) creates a single large bleeding and allows studying the mechanisms of hemorrhage-induced neuronal damage. However, it fails to reproduce the aspect of continuing bleeding and hematoma expansion. Secondary hematoma enlargement occurs in about 1/3 of patients during the first day after ICH and is an important predictor of poor neurological outcome (Brott et al., 1997; Davis et al., 2006). In contrast, injection of bacterial collagenase (Rosenberg et al., 1990) dissolves the basal lamina of small cerebral blood vessels and results in continuous parenchymal bleeding for several hours (MacLellan et al., 2008). However, the vascular source of bleeding in the collagenase model differs from most human ICH in which bleeding is of penetrating arteriolar origin (Clark et al., 1998; Wang et al., 2003; Tang et al., 2004). Another disadvantage of this model is that higher doses of collagenase can induce direct neurotoxicity (Matsushita et al., 2000; Chu et al., 2004) which may complicate the interpretation of results with neuroprotective strategies.

The size of the hematoma, which determines outcome both in man (Broderick et al., 1993) and in rodents (MacLellan et al., 2006), can be varied in both ICH-models by changing the injected blood volume or collagenase dose. However, injection of a higher blood volume may produce difficulties by the injected blood spreading along the corpus callosum or flowing back through the needle insertion canal. These problems can be reduced by using the double injection method (Belayev et al., 2003), where a small amount of blood is allowed to clot and followed by the injection of the remaining blood volume. In comparison with the blood injection model where the tissue is split apart by the hematoma, collagenase induces a less dense hemorrhage which infiltrates the parenchyma (MacLellan et al., 2008) resulting in bigger hematoma volume in case of matched blood content between the two models (Mracsko et al., 2014).

In both models, macroscopic hematoma size decreases already during the first days after surgery (Mracsko et al., 2014), and the hematoma resolves completely in about 21 days (Zhao et al., 2007). In contrast, the resolution of the hematoma takes several weeks in patients and usually leaves a cavity in the brain with focal atrophy and ventricular enlargement (Dolinskas et al., 1977).

In conclusion, both ICH methods have their advantages and limitations. These differences should be carefully considered when choosing a model to address the outcome parameters of interest and when interpreting the findings.

DELETERIOUS MECHANICAL EFFECTS OF THE HEMATOMA

Primary brain injury after ICH is caused by the tissue disruption due to parenchymal blood accumulation and the mechanical damage associated with the mass effect (**Figure 1**). Besides treating increased intracranial pressure (Helbok et al., 2011), surgical interventions to remove the blood clot and release the pressure would appear a plausible approach in this phase (Gautschi and Schaller, 2013). In about one third of patients (Kazui et al., 1996; Brott et al., 1997), re-bleeding and the expansion of the hemorrhage within the first day after the ictus further exacerbates the mass effect and thus neurological damage. Preventing this complication by aggressive antihypertensive therapy or by administration of hemostatic factors may prevent secondary hematoma growth. (Sakamoto et al., 2013). However, evidence for clinical efficacy is limited. The concept of brain damage resulting from peri-hematomal ischemia induced by the increased intracranial pressure has not been confirmed in studies using positron emission tomography in patients (Zazulia et al., 2001). However, a recent magnetic resonance imaging (MRI) study found ischemic events in one third of ICH patients within 1 month after the ictus (Menon et al., 2012).

Immediately after ICH, peri-hematomal edema develops which increases intracranial pressure and contributes to the mass effect (Xi et al., 2006). Edema in ICH is associated with higher in-hospital mortality (Staykov et al., 2011). In animal models, edema peaks already 3–4 days after ICH-induction (Xi et al., 1998). In contrast, the edema expands in ICH patients until at least 10 days after the ictus (Staykov et al., 2011). In the first hours after ICH, edema is mainly formed by plasma egress due to the increased hydrostatic pressure and the damaged blood-brain barrier (BBB); edema also results from extruded serum during clot retraction (Wagner et al., 1996). Later on, thrombin production, erythrocyte lysis and the triggered inflammatory processes are responsible for edema formation (Xi et al., 2001a).

MECHANISMS OF SECONDARY BRAIN DAMAGE

Besides the mechanical tissue damage caused by the initial hematoma, injured brain cells and the extravasated components of the blood clot trigger a complex sequence of parallel and sequential deleterious mechanisms including inflammatory and oxidative stress pathways (Aronowski and Zhao, 2011; **Figure 1**).

Activation of hemostatic mechanisms is a physiological tissue response to hemorrhage to stop the bleeding. Thrombin is essential for the blood coagulation processes and gets activated within the first hour after ICH (Gong et al., 2008). Intracerebral injection of thrombin leads to early brain edema formation by direct opening of the BBB (Lee et al., 1997) and to neuronal damage at days 1 and 3 after ICH (Gong et al., 2008). High concentrations of thrombin induce neuronal damage *in vitro*, however, low concentrations are neuroprotective against various insults including ischemia or oxidative stress (Vaughan et al., 1995; Donovan et al., 1997; Striggow et al., 2000). Moreover, thrombin has an important role in brain recovery after intracerebral hemorrhage (Hua et al., 2009) possibly via the initiation of neurogenesis (Yang et al., 2008) and angiogenesis (Tarzami et al., 2006; Tsopanoglou and Maragoudakis, 2007). Therefore, the role of thrombin after ICH remains controversial (Xi et al., 2003, 2006; Keep et al., 2012).

The lysis of erythrocytes within the first days after ICH leads to the release of hemoglobin which is then converted by the heme

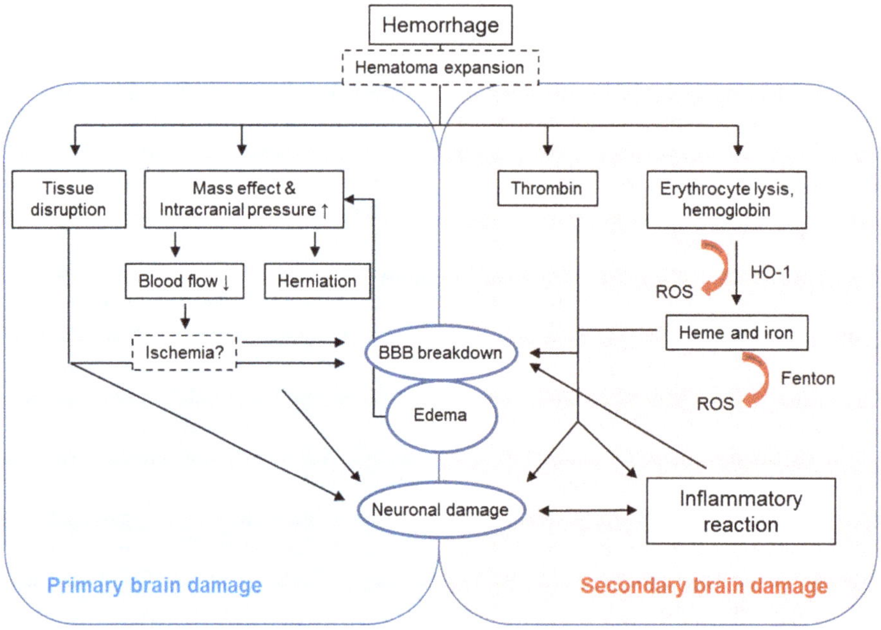

FIGURE 1 | Primary and secondary brain damage after intracerebral hemorrhage.

oxygenase-1 enzyme (HO-1) into neurotoxic components such as heme and iron which are major contributors to secondary brain injury (Wagner et al., 2003; Wu et al., 2003; Keep et al., 2012). Intracerebral injection of lyzed erythrocytes or hemoglobin and iron result in brain edema formation and neuronal damage (Xi et al., 1998; Huang et al., 2002). The proposed mechanism of heme- and iron-induced neurotoxicity is the induction of oxidative stress due to the activity of HO-1 (Koeppen et al., 2004; Wang and Doré, 2007a) and the iron-mediated free radical production via the Fenton-reaction (Wu et al., 2003, 2011; Clark et al., 2008).

The inflammatory reaction comprising both cellular and molecular components is a common response of the central nervous system (CNS) to various stimuli. Neuroinflammation after ICH involves the early activation of resident microglia, release of proinflammatory mediators and the influx of peripheral leukocytes and has major role in the pathophysiology of secondary brain damage (Wang and Doré, 2007b; Wang, 2010). Components of both innate and adaptive immune system take part of ICH-induced neuroinflammation. At present, the involvement of antigen specific immune processes remains unclear in both ischemic and hemorrhagic stroke (Iadecola and Anrather, 2011).

MICROGLIA/MACROPHAGES

The first activated innate immune cells are microglia which reside in the CNS. They continuously scan the extracellular brain environment and can be activated within minutes after tissue damage. Danger-associated molecular patterns including ATP, neurotransmitters, nucleic acids, heat shock proteins and high mobility group box 1 are released to the extracellular space from necrotic neurons after ICH (Ohnishi et al., 2011). These stimuli act on distinct microglia receptors including Toll-like receptors (TLRs) and the receptor of advanced glycosylation end-products (Taylor and Sansing, 2013). Several TLRs including TLR4 are involved in the neuroinflammatory processes after ICH (Fang et al., 2013). TLR4 is predominantly expressed in CD11b+ microglial cells and is upregulated early after ICH subsequently leading to the upregulation of proinflammatory genes via nuclear factor-κB (NF-κB) signaling (Teng et al., 2009; Lin et al., 2012). Besides danger signals originating from damaged neuronal cells, blood components such as thrombin, fibrin and heme can also trigger inflammatory processes through the TLR/NF-κB pathway (Loftspring et al., 2010; Lin et al., 2012; Wang et al., 2014). Hemoglobin triggers an inflammatory response via assembly of TLR2/TLR4 heterodimers (Wang et al., 2014). Experimental and clinical data suggest that TLR4 contributes to neuronal damage in ICH. TLR4 deficiency (Teng et al., 2009; Sansing et al., 2011b; Lin et al., 2012) or blockade (Wang et al., 2013) lowers brain water content (i.e., edema) and reduces neurological deficit. In patients, higher expression of TLR2 and TLR4 in monocytes on admission was independently associated with poor outcome (Rodríguez-Yáñez et al., 2012). Therefore, antagonization of the TLR4 signaling may represent a therapeutic target after ICH.

Besides TLRs, microglia can be activated by thrombin via the proteinase activated receptor-1 (PAR-1) and mitogen-activated protein kinase signaling pathways (Fujimoto et al., 2007; Ohnishi et al., 2007). This leads to increased production of tumor necrosis factor-α (TNF-α) and neuronal death (Ohnishi et al., 2010). Microglia endocytose erythrocyte remnants via scavenger receptors such as CD36, which initiates microglial activation (Aronowski and Zhao, 2011; Fang et al., 2014).

Upon stimulation, microglia cells will be rounded gaining an ameboid appearance and high phagocytic activity (Kreutzberg, 1996). They are difficult to distinguish from activated macrophages which express the same cellular surface markers including CD11b, Iba-1, isolectin B4 (Ginhoux et al., 2010). However, multi-parameter characterization by flow cytometry allows the definition of microglia population as $CD45^{low}$/CD11b+ cells (Campanella et al., 2002; D'Mello et al., 2009; Parney et al., 2009; Gabrusiewicz et al., 2011; Patel et al., 2013; Mracsko et al., 2014; Tang et al., 2014). Both macrophages and microglia can have either the classically activated M1 or the alternatively activated M2 phenotype (Kigerl et al., 2009; David and Kroner, 2011). M1 polarized microglia produce proinflammatory, largely deleterious cytokines such as TNF-α, interleukin-1β (IL-1β) or IL-6 and pro-oxidant enzymes such as inducible nitric oxide synthase (Liao et al., 2012; Kobayashi et al., 2013). In contrast, M2 polarized microglia have arginase activity, produce neurotrophic factors and IL-10. The M2 microglia phenotype has been associated with neuroprotective and regenerative effects after brain injury (Ponomarev et al., 2007). Due to this polarity, microglia/macrophage can exert controversial effects in brain diseases and injuries (Taylor and Sansing, 2013).

Microglial activation takes place in various neurological disorders including CNS and peripheral infections, neurodegenerative diseases, traumatic brain injury, ischemic and hemorrhagic stroke (Suzuki et al., 2011; Püntener et al., 2012; Hernandez-Ontiveros et al., 2013; Patel et al., 2013; Taylor and Sansing, 2013; Doens and Fernández, 2014). Besides the clearance of cell debris, microglia play also an important role in the phagocytosis of blood components released into the brain parenchyma (Aronowski and Zhao, 2011). In experimental ICH, microglial activation occurs as early as 1 h following collagenase injection (Wang and Doré, 2007a) and 4 h after autologous blood injection (Xue and Del Bigio, 2000). The number of activated microglia/macrophages peaks at 72 h and returns to normal level 3–4 weeks after ICH (Wang, 2010; Yabluchanskiy et al., 2010; Sansing et al., 2011b).

Upon various stimuli, microglia and brain macrophages produce proinflammatory cytokines including TNF-α and IL-1β (Wang and Doré, 2007b), chemokines (Matsushita et al., 2014) and reactive oxygen species (ROS; Yang et al., 2014a). Beyond the neurotoxic cytokines, chemokines such as CXCL2 produced by microglia (Shiratori et al., 2010) have chemotactic activity on neutrophils and thus exacerbate the inflammatory reaction (Tessier et al., 1997). Moreover, M1 polarized microglia create microglia-T cell crosstalk due to antigen presentation via MHCII expression (Starossom et al., 2012). Thus, microglia also enforce early neuroinflammation by recruiting and activating blood-derived leukocytes which may worsen ICH-induced neuronal damage.

On the other hand, microglia play a key role in hematoma resolution and therefore in the recovery phase after ICH. A more effective and faster clearance of intracerebral blood could limit the inflammatory processes that are triggered by blood constituents in the brain parenchyma (Zhao et al., 2007). Moreover, the chemokine receptor CX3CR1 is required for M2 polarization of microglia facilitating recovery after ICH (Taylor and Sansing, 2013).

The essential pathophysiological role of microglia/macrophages after ICH suggests a therapeutic potential. On the other hand, microglial functions are diverse and cannot be classified as either good or bad. Moreover, different microglial subsets may send opposing signals, and predominant functional effects may differ depending on timing after the event (cp ischemia; Lalancette-Hébert et al., 2007).

In experimental ICH, blockade of TLR4 reduced neuronal loss and edema formation and improved neurological function. The effects resulted from inhibition of downstream signaling mechanisms and the lower expression of proinflammatory cytokines (Wang et al., 2013). In another study, the TLR4 inhibitor TAK-242 upregulated CD36 scavenger receptor expression thereby promoting faster hematoma resolution and attenuating neurological deficit (Fang et al., 2014). Minocycline is a tetracycline-based molecule which can inhibit microglia activation (Tikka and Koistinaho, 2001). Minocyclin has been tested in numerous studies to moderate neuronal damage after ICH. Minocycline reduces thrombin-induced microglial TNF-α and IL-1β expression *in vitro* (Wu et al., 2009). In the same study, minocycline reduced brain edema 3 days after intracerebral blood injection, diminished neurological deficit and decreased brain atrophy 28 days following ICH (Wu et al., 2010). These effects were accompanied by reduced numbers of microglia/macrophages around the hematoma 5 days following ICH (Szymanska et al., 2006). Others found preserved microvessels along with reduced brain water content, and lower levels of TNF-α and matrix metalloproteinase-12 (MMP-12) in minocycline-treated rats (Wasserman and Schlichter, 2007). In these studies, the treatment was applied from up to 6 h after induction of ICH suggesting clinical relevance. As a consequence, a randomized,-single-blinded clinical trial of minocycline in ICH has been initiated (A Pilot Study of Minocycline in Intracerebral Hemorrhage Patients (MACH); NCT01805895). Further molecules targeting microglia activation and function have been recently tested after ICH. The mitogen-activated protein kinase inhibitor sesamin (Ohnishi et al., 2013), as well as sinomenine (Yang et al., 2014a) and curcumin (Yang et al., 2014c) with anti-inflammatory and anti-oxidant properties were neuroprotective in ICH. However, their distinct mechanisms of action require further investigation.

Hematoma resolution by microglia/macrophages has also been recognized as a therapeutic target after ICH. Peroxisome proliferator-activated receptor-γ agonist induced CD36-mediated clearance of erythrocytes by microglia *in vitro*. It promoted hematoma resolution, reduced neuronal loss and neurological deficit *in vivo* (Zhao et al., 2007, 2009). Therefore, besides blocking the acute detrimental effects of microglia activation, stimulating microglial phagocytosis and thus enhancing recovery may also have therapeutic potential.

BBB BREAKDOWN AND INVASION OF SYSTEMIC IMMUNE CELLS

The physical BBB is formed by capillary endothelial cells, which are connected via tight junctions resulting in very low permeability. Besides endothelial cells, perivascular cells such as pericytes and astrocytes and the extracellular matrix have an important regulatory role on BBB function. Increased permeability of the BBB can be caused by changes in the para- and transcellular routes or by disruption of the extracellular matrix (Keep et al., 2014; Knowland et al., 2014). In ischemic stroke, BBB dysfunction results from insufficient oxygen and glucose supply (Ronaldson and Davis, 2012). In contrast, the absence of ICH-induced ischemic damage (Zazulia et al., 2001) suggests that other mechanisms induce BBB hyperpermeability in ICH. Thrombin has been shown to induce BBB disruption via proteinase activated receptor-1 mediated mechanisms (Liu et al., 2010). Hemoglobin itself and its degradation products heme and iron also increase permeability of the BBB (Yang et al., 2013). Accordingly, the iron chelator deferoxamine (Nakamura et al., 2004; Okauchi et al., 2010) and HO inhibitors (Gong et al., 2006) reduce ICH-induced brain edema.

Matrix metalloproteinases belong to the group of endopeptidases just as other proteases like serine or cysteine proteases. They have important role in the remodeling of extracellular matrix but under inflammatory conditions activation of MMPs results in BBB dysfunction, increased capillary permeability and brain edema formation after ICH (Rosenberg and Navratil, 1997). Matrix metalloproteinases have been intensively studied in ICH in the last two decades and the available information on their role in ICH has been reviewed in detail (Wang and Doré, 2007b; Florczak-Rzepka et al., 2012). Although inhibition of MMPs may decrease ICH-induced brain injury, MMPs also have an important role in the regulation of neurogenesis, myelin function and axonal growth (Pepper, 2001; Kaczmarek et al., 2002; Cunningham et al., 2005). Therefore rather the modulation than long-term inhibition of MMPs may be considered for ICH treatment.

The strict regulation of the immune cell infiltration into the brain parenchyma through the immunological BBB plays an important role in the immune privilege of the CNS (Pachter et al., 2003). During neuroinflammatory processes, the expression of adhesion molecules on leukocytes and of their ligands on endothelial cells in postcapillary venules increases. As a consequence, leukocytes adhere to the wall of these venules. Infiltration through the BBB involves rolling, adhesion and transendothelial migration of leukocytes. Adhesion molecules that participate in this process are classified into three types: selectins, the superfamily of immunoglobulins and the integrins (Brea et al., 2009; Iadecola and Anrather, 2011). The expression of intracellular adhesion molecule-1 is upregulated already hours after ICH (Gong et al., 2000; Yang et al., 2011). The vascular adhesion protein-1 has been also shown to be upregulated after ICH, and its inhibitors reduced neutrophil invasion and brain damage (Ma et al., 2011).

The brain infiltrating leukocytes produce proinflammatory cytokines and MMPs leading to further disruption of the BBB (Xi et al., 2006; Wang and Doré, 2007b; Aronowski and Zhao, 2011). Therefore, peripheral leukocytes and the BBB are in tight reciprocal connection that makes it difficult to evaluate the effect of distinct compounds on BBB integrity. Essentially, any compound that influences the ICH-induced inflammatory reaction also affects BBB integrity and vica versa.

In experimental and clinical ICH blood-borne leukocytes invade the hemorrhagic brain (Lee et al., 1975; Del Bigio et al., 1996; Gong et al., 2000; Xue and Del Bigio, 2000; Mayne et al., 2001a; Peeling et al., 2001; Wang and Tsirka, 2005). In principle, leukocytes found in the brain after ICH could originate from the inflowing blood in the hematoma. Alternatively, systemic immune cells may actively migrate across the BBB to enter the brain (Xi et al., 2006). The origin of leukocytes located in the brain after ICH can be determined by using the leukocyte marker CD45.1 transgenic mice in blood injection models (Sansing et al., 2011b; Hammond et al., 2012; Mracsko et al., 2014). In this approach, blood from CD45.2 expressing wild type mice is injected into the brain of CD45.1 expressing mice or vice versa and brain located leukocytes are analyzed by flow cytometry for CD45.2 and CD45.1 expression. These studies agree that already 1 day after blood injection the majority of leukocytes isolated from the brain originates from the blood circulation rather than from the injected blood. A methodological limitation of this approach is that the traumatic injury caused by the insertion of the injection needle alone results in a relatively high number of infiltrating leukocyte in sham operated animals (Loftspring et al., 2009; Mracsko et al., 2014). Therefore, differences of injection techniques and even needles can result in discrepancies between different workgroups regarding infiltrating cell numbers.

MONOCYTES

Monocytes are produced by bone marrow from monoblasts and mature into different types of macrophages. In the CNS the renewal of the microglia cell population takes place by local expansion and, at lower rate, by replenishment by circulating monocytes (Ajami et al., 2007). As mentioned above, the distinction of infiltrating monocyte/macrophages from microglia is difficult due to the identical surface activation markers they express. To distinguish the roles and distributions of microglia and peripheral monocytes, several studies on cerebral ischemia used bone marrow chimeric mice generated by transplanting green fluorescent protein transgenic bone marrow into irradiated wild-type recipients (Schilling et al., 2003, 2005; Tanaka et al., 2003). So far the application of this approach in ICH is limited to one study (Hammond et al., 2014). Taking advantage of differential CD45 expression between microglia and monocyte/macrophages, flow cytometry studies have also differentiated infiltrating monocytes (Sansing et al., 2011a,b; Hammond et al., 2012; Mracsko et al., 2014). Monocytes invade already within 12 h after ICH outnumbering the neutrophil population (Hammond et al., 2012), and their number peaks by day 5 (Mracsko et al., 2014). Monocyte infiltration is reduced after neutrophil depletion (Sansing et al., 2011a) or in TLR4 deficiency (Sansing et al., 2011b). The monocyte chemoattractant protein-1 and its receptor CC chemokine receptor 2 (CCR2) are involved in the migration of monocytes into the hemorrhagic brain (Yao and Tsirka, 2012b). Monocyte chemoattractant protein-1 is elevated in the brain 24 h after experimental ICH (Chang et al., 2011; Ma et al., 2011) as well as in the serum of patients associated with poor functional outcome 7 days following ICH (Hammond et al., 2014). Accordingly, chimeric mice with wild type CNS and CCR2 deficiency exhibit attenuated motor dysfunction after ICH (Hammond et al., 2014). At the same time, CCR2+ inflammatory monocytes seem to be important regulators of hematoma clearance and functional recovery after ICH (Yao and Tsirka, 2012a).

GRANULOCYTES

Neutrophils are the leukocyte population that immigrates first into the brain after injury. In ICH, infiltrating neutrophils were found in and around the hematoma as early as 4 h after collagenase-induced ICH in mice (Wang and Tsirka, 2005). Their number peaks at 3–5 days after ICH (Gong et al., 2000; Xue and Del Bigio, 2000; Mracsko et al., 2014). Although the temporal pattern of neutrophil infiltration is similar in blood and collagenase injection models, higher neutrophil numbers are found after collagenase than after blood injection (Xue and Del Bigio, 2000; Mracsko et al., 2014). In experimental ICH, infiltrating neutrophils undergo apoptosis 2 days after entering the hematoma (Savill, 1997). Molecules released from dying leukocytes may further stimulate microglia/macrophages and exacerbate the neuroinflammatory process (Stern et al., 1996; Wang, 2010). Neutrophil accumulation in the blood vessels around the hematoma was observed already 6 h after the ictus (Wisniewski, 1961). In the peri-hematomal tissue obtained from ICH patients during craniotomy, neutrophil (and lymphocyte) infiltration further increased 12–24 h after ICH and correlated with the number of TUNEL positive cells (Guo et al., 2006). It should be noted however that in ischemic stroke histological techniques labeling components of the neurovascular unit showed that polymorphonuclear granulocytes were mainly located in the luminal surfaces or perivascular spaces of cerebral vessels and no granulocytes infiltrated the brain parenchyma (Enzmann et al., 2013). So far, no similar data are available for ICH.

Recent studies suggest an important role of activated microglia in neutrophil recruitment into the hemorrhagic brain. Heme-induced TLR4 activation on microglia increases CXCL2 production, which interacts with CXCR2 on the surface of neutrophils resulting in chemoattraction (Zarbock and Ley, 2009). Accordingly, TLR4-deficient mice show reduced neutrophil and monocyte infiltration 3 days after ICH (Sansing et al., 2011b).

Granulocytes appear to have mainly deleterious effects on the brain after ICH. Neutrophil depletion by intravenous injection of anti-polymorphonuclear neutrophil (anti-PMN) serum reduced BBB breakdown, axonal injury and neurological deficit (Moxon-Emre and Schlichter, 2011). After cerebral ischemia, anti-PMN therapy prevented endothelial dysfunction and thrombolysis-induced hemorrhagic transformation in another study (Gautier et al., 2009). As professional phagocytes, neutrophils use phagosomes containing digestive and oxidative compounds. During phagocytosis they produce an oxidative burst resulting in the release of ROSs via NADPH oxidase and myeloperoxidase (Hampton et al., 1998). Although these processes are needed for antimicrobial defence, high ROS levels due to microglial activation and neutrophil infiltration contribute to poor outcome after ICH (Nguyen et al., 2007; Han et al., 2008). The free radical scavenger edaravone decreases brain edema and neurological deficit after ICH (Nakamura et al., 2008). Other molecules with free radical trapping properties have been tested in ICH as reviewed earlier (Wang and Doré, 2007b) supporting the important role of ROS in secondary brain injury and their therapeutic potential after ICH.

Besides microglia/macrophages, the expression of the neurotoxic TNF-α has also been shown in neutrophils (Mayne et al., 2001b; Nguyen et al., 2007; Wasserman and Schlichter, 2007). Neutrophils may also recruit monocyte/macrophages amplifying inflammatory processes (Soehnlein and Lindbom, 2010). Accordingly, anti-PMN therapy decreased the number of infiltrating monocyte/macrophages around the hematoma and reduced glial scarring (Moxon-Emre and Schlichter, 2011).

CELLS OF THE ADAPTIVE IMMUNE SYSTEM

Mounting an antigen-specific immune response generally requires several (5–7) days. As cellular parts of the adaptive immune system, B cells participate in humoral immune responses, while T cells are involved in cellular immunity. T cells express either the CD4 or the CD8 cell surface marker determining their function: modulating immune responses or eliciting cytotoxicity.

Increasing evidence suggests an important role of adaptive immunity and particularly T lymphocytes in secondary brain damage after ischemia (Yilmaz et al., 2006; Iadecola and Anrather, 2011; Liesz et al., 2011; Chamorro et al., 2012). In contrast, little is known about the role of lymphocytes after experimental and clinical ICH. Lymphocytes were found in cerebrospinal fluid early (starting at 6 h) following human ICH (Lee et al., 1975). Lymphocytes were also detected in peri-hematomal brain tissue obtained during craniotomy of ICH patients (Guo et al., 2006). In contrast, most studies using animal models of ICH reported more delayed infiltration of T cells 48–96 h after ICH (Xue and Del Bigio, 2000, 2003; Loftspring et al., 2009). Using flow cytometry, we found that CD4+ T cells are the predominating brain infiltrating leukocyte population in mice already 1 day after ICH and their number peaked at day 5 (Mracsko et al., 2014). At the same time, infiltration of CD8+ T cell appears to be less prominent in ICH compared to cerebral ischemia (Schwab et al., 2001; Loftspring et al., 2009; Chaitanya et al., 2010; Mracsko et al., 2014).

An important unresolved question is whether T cell invasion and activation is antigen dependent both in cerebral ischemia and in ICH (Iadecola and Anrather, 2011). Along with other T cell populations, both proinflammatory γδT cells and immunosuppressive regulatory T cells (Treg) infiltrate the hemorrhagic brain (Gao et al., 2014). According to the neuroprotective role of Treg in cerebral ischemia (Liesz et al., 2009), Treg transfer also attenuated neurological deficit after ICH (Yang et al., 2014b). The pathophysiological role of B cells and natural killer cells after ICH has barely been studied to date. Their low rate of infiltration (Mracsko et al., 2014) suggests a minor role in ICH-induced brain injury.

Fingolimod is a modulator of the sphingosine 1-phosphate receptor 1 and has been approved for the treatment of the relapsing form of multiple sclerosis. Fingolimod downregulates the expression of sphingosine receptors on T cells thereby inhibiting their egress from lymphoid tissue (Chiba, 2005). Fingolimod reduced brain edema and improved neurological function after experimental ICH in one study (Rolland et al., 2011). Interestingly, it was recently tested in a Chinese clinical pilot study ($n = 23$ patients) where it decreased peri-hematomal edema and reduced neurological impairment compared with control individuals (Fu et al., 2014). A better understanding of the mechanism of activation and action of T cell population is needed.

HUMORAL INFLAMMATORY MEDIATORS

Nuclear factor-κB is a ubiquitous transcription factor that is a critical regulator of numerous responses including inflammation (Barnes, 1996) and pro-inflammatory genes such as TNF-α, IL-1β, nitric oxide synthase, HO-1 and intracellular adhesion molecule-1 (Barnes and Karin, 1997; Emsley and Tyrrell, 2002). Nuclear factor-κB has high sensitivity towards oxidative stress (Grilli and Memo, 1999) and gets immediately activated in the peri-hematomal brain tissue in both experimental (Hickenbottom et al., 1999; Wagner, 2007) and human ICH (Wang et al., 2011). Peroxisome proliferator-activated receptor-γ, a member of the nuclear hormone receptor superfamily has been shown to suppress NF-κB function leading to decreased inflammation and neuronal death, increased hematoma resolution and improved functional outcome after experimental ICH (Zhao et al., 2006). Information on the role of NF-κB in ICH has been reviewed elsewhere in detail (Aronowski and Hall, 2005; Wagner, 2007).

Cytokines can be divided into pro- and anti-inflammatory cytokines. Tumor necrosis factor-α is a pleiotropic cytokine which is mainly produced by microglia/macrophages (Lambertsen et al., 2005) and neutrophils (Mayne et al., 2001b). Tumor necrosis factor-α plays a central role in extending neuronal damage after CNS injury (Rodríguez-Yáñez and Castillo, 2008). Tumor necrosis factor-α knockout mice showed reduced ICH-induced brain edema compared to wild type mice (Hua et al., 2006). Treatment with TNF-α antibody after ICH attenuated microglia/macrophage activation, reduced cleaved caspase-3 and resulted in less brain edema and better neurological function (Mayne et al., 2001b; Lei et al., 2013). The IL-1 cytokine family contains an increasing number of members; the most important are IL-1α, IL-β and the natural receptor antagonist IL-Ra (Luheshi et al., 2009). In neuroinflammatory conditions, IL-1β is mostly produced by microglia/macrophages and is neurotoxic (Pearson et al., 1999; Vezzani et al., 1999). Overexpression of IL-1 receptor antagonist decreased thrombin-induced brain edema (Masada et al., 2001), BBB breakdown and neuronal loss (Greenhalgh et al., 2012). Both TNF-α and IL-1 are overexpressed as early as 2 h after experimental ICH (Xi et al., 2001b; Aronowski and Hall, 2005; Wagner et al., 2006).

Interferon-γ (IFN-γ) is one of the main effector molecule of T lymphocytes (Schroder et al., 2004) and T cells are the major source of IFN-γ in cerebral ischemia (Liesz et al., 2009). In contrast to the well-established expression pattern and role of IFN-γ in ischemic stroke (Yilmaz et al., 2006; Liesz et al., 2011), the role of this cytokine in ICH remains to be elucidated. Interferon-γ protein expression was increased at 72 h after ICH which was prevented by fingolimod treatment (Rolland et al., 2011).

Clinical studies on the role of cytokines in ICH are limited on serum measurements. Increased serum concentrations of IL-6 and IL-10 were found 24 h after ICH where IL-6 level correlated with blood volume and the mass effect of the hemorrhage (Dziedzic et al., 2002). In another study, elevated plasma levels of TNF-α and IL-6 12 and 24 h after the ictus correlated with peri-hematomal edema (Castillo et al., 2002). These reports support the deleterious effect of proinflammatory cytokines after ICH. Although cytokines may be promising therapeutic targets in ICH, to date no clinical trials examining the effect of cytokine antagonization have been conducted.

IMAGING OF NEUROINFLAMMATION

Due to the spatial and temporal complexity of the neuroinflammatory processes, anatomical and functional *in vivo* imaging techniques are increasingly recognized for diagnosis and follow-up in patient care. Furthermore, the fast development of these techniques already allows their implication for the understanding of neuroinflammatory mechanisms in the cellular and molecular level in experimental studies.

As microglia activation is an essential part of the neuroinflammatory response to cerebral injury and disease progression, it has become an important target for *in vivo* imaging of neuroinflammation. Upon activation, the microglial translocator protein (TSPO) is upregulated (Chauveau et al., 2008) and can be detected by radiolabeled ligands for positron-emission tomography (PET) or single-photon emission computed tomography (SPECT; Winkeler et al., 2010; Chauveau et al., 2011; Ciarmiello, 2011; Kiferle et al., 2011).

To investigate the mechanisms underlying the trafficking of systemic immune cells into the brain, contrast media targeting endothelial selectin, ICAM and VCAM have been developed. These include ^{125}I-labeled gold nanorods (GdNRs) and 64Cu-labeled nanoparticles conjugated with anti-ICAM-1 antibody (Rossin et al., 2008; Shao et al., 2011) or iron oxide microparticles conjugated with anti-VCAM antibody (McAteer et al., 2007; Hoyte et al., 2010) (for detailed review cp. Jacobs and Tavitian, 2012)). Infiltrating leukocytes can be labelled either *ex vivo* by incubation with a tracer or *in vivo* taking advantage of their phagocytic properties. For *ex vivo* labelling ^{111}In- or ^{99m}Tc-labeled compounds for SPECT or [^{18}F] fluorodeoxyglucose (FDG) for PET imaging have been developed (Wunder et al., 2009). *In vivo* labelling is performed using MRI agents including iron-oxide nanoparticles (Stuber et al., 2007), liposomes encapsulating monodisperse single core superparamagnetic iron-oxide particles (Soenen et al., 2010) or paramagnetic lanthanide-based agents (Castelli et al., 2009; Stoll and Bendszus, 2010).

The above detailed labeling methods are increasingly used in clinical and experimental studies to characterize inflammatory processes in neurologic disorders including cerebral ischemia, multiple sclerosis, Alzheimer's and Parkinson's disease (Jacobs and Tavitian, 2012). In contrast, *in vivo* neuroimaging has been barely used to investigate the ICH-induced inflammatory processes. In collagenase-induced ICH, enhanced MRI with microparticles of iron oxide targeted to VCAM-1 revealed the maximal VCAM-1 expression 24 h after ICH which returned to baseline 5 days following hemorrhage induction (Gauberti et al., 2013). However, so far we do not have neuroimaging data about tracking leukocytes infiltrating the hemorrhagic brain.

CONCLUSIONS

Inflammatory processes are increasingly recognized as important players in the pathophysiology of secondary brain damage after ICH. There is now solid information on the infiltration pattern of leukocytes in experimental ICH. The pathophysiological role of specific leukocyte populations is beginning to be better understood but little is known about the interactions among these immune cells. Because of the delayed nature of brain damage after ICH, adaptive immune cells may play an important role in the subacute and the regenerative phases after ICH. Translation of preclinical findings into the clinical setting is challenging because of limitations of current animal models of ICH. Moreover, the local and systemic neuroinflammatory response in ICH patients remains to be better characterized.

AUTHORS' CONTRIBUTIONS

All authors were involved in writing the review.

REFERENCES

Ajami, B., Bennett, J. L., Krieger, C., Tetzlaff, W., and Rossi, F. M. (2007). Local self-renewal can sustain CNS microglia maintenance and function throughout adult life. *Nat. Neurosci.* 10, 1538–1543. doi: 10.1038/nn2014

Anderson, C. S., Heeley, E., Huang, Y., Wang, J., Stapf, C., Delcourt, C., et al. (2013). Rapid blood-pressure lowering in patients with acute intracerebral hemorrhage. *N. Engl. J. Med.* 368, 2355–2365. doi: 10.1056/NEJMoa1214609

Aronowski, J., and Hall, C. E. (2005). New horizons for primary intracerebral hemorrhage treatment: experience from preclinical studies. *Neurol. Res.* 27, 268–279. doi: 10.1179/016164105x25225

Aronowski, J., and Zhao, X. (2011). Molecular pathophysiology of cerebral hemorrhage: secondary brain injury. *Stroke* 42, 1781–1786. doi: 10.1161/strokeaha.110.596718

Barnes, P. J. (1996). Is immunotherapy for asthma worthwhile? *N Engl J. Med.* 334, 531–532. doi: 10.1056/NEJM199602223340811

Barnes, P. J., and Karin, M. (1997). Nuclear factor-κB: a pivotal transcription factor in chronic inflammatory diseases. *N Engl J. Med.* 336, 1066–1071. doi: 10.1056/nejm199704103361506

Belayev, L., Saul, I., Curbelo, K., Busto, R., Belayev, A., Zhang, Y., et al. (2003). Experimental intracerebral hemorrhage in the mouse: histological, behavioral and hemodynamic characterization of a double-injection model. *Stroke* 34, 2221–2227. doi: 10.1161/01.str.0000088061.06656.1e

Brea, D., Sobrino, T., Ramos-Cabrer, P., and Castillo, J. (2009). Inflammatory and neuroimmunomodulatory changes in acute cerebral ischemia. *Cerebrovasc. Dis.* 27(Suppl. 1), 48–64. doi: 10.1159/000200441

Broderick, J. P., Brott, T. G., Duldner, J. E., Tomsick, T., and Huster, G. (1993). Volume of intracerebral hemorrhage. A powerful and easy-to-use predictor of 30-day mortality. *Stroke* 24, 987–993. doi: 10.1161/01.str.24.7.987

Brott, T., Broderick, J., Kothari, R., Barsan, W., Tomsick, T., Sauerbeck, L., et al. (1997). Early hemorrhage growth in patients with intracerebral hemorrhage. *Stroke* 28, 1–5. doi: 10.1161/01.str.28.1.1

Bullock, R., Mendelow, A. D., Teasdale, G. M., and Graham, D. I. (1984). Intracranial haemorrhage induced at arterial pressure in the rat. Part 1: description of technique, ICP changes and neuropathological findings. *Neurol. Res.* 6, 184–188.

Campanella, M., Sciorati, C., Tarozzo, G., and Beltramo, M. (2002). Flow cytometric analysis of inflammatory cells in ischemic rat brain. *Stroke* 33, 586–592. doi: 10.1161/hs0202.103399

Castelli, D. D., Terreno, E., Cabella, C., Chaabane, L., Lanzardo, S., Tei, L., et al. (2009). Evidence for in vivo macrophage mediated tumor uptake of paramagnetic/fluorescent liposomes. *NMR Biomed.* 22, 1084–1092. doi: 10.1002/nbm.1416

Castillo, J., Dávalos, A., Alvarez-Sabín, J., Pumar, J. M., Leira, R., Silva, Y., et al. (2002). Molecular signatures of brain injury after intracerebral hemorrhage. *Neurology* 58, 624–629. doi: 10.1212/wnl.58.4.624

Chaitanya, G. V., Schwaninger, M., Alexander, J. S., and Babu, P. P. (2010). Granzyme-b is involved in mediating post-ischemic neuronal death during focal cerebral ischemia in rat model. *Neuroscience* 165, 1203–1216. doi: 10.1016/j.neuroscience.2009.10.067

Chamorro, Á., Meisel, A., Planas, A. M., Urra, X., van de Beek, D., and Veltkamp, R. (2012). The immunology of acute stroke. *Nat. Rev. Neurol.* 8, 401–410. doi: 10.1038/nrneurol.2012.98

Chang, C. F., Chen, S. F., Lee, T. S., Lee, H. F., Chen, S. F., and Shyue, S. K. (2011). Caveolin-1 deletion reduces early brain injury after experimental intracerebral hemorrhage. *Am. J. Pathol.* 178, 1749–1761. doi: 10.1016/j.ajpath.2010.12.023

Chauveau, F., Boutin, H., Van Camp, N., Dollé, F., and Tavitian, B. (2008). Nuclear imaging of neuroinflammation: a comprehensive review of [C-11]PK11195 challengers. *Eur. J. Nucl. Med. Mol. Imaging* 35, 2304–2319. doi: 10.1007/s00259-008-0908-9

Chauveau, F., Boutin, H., Van Camp, N., Thominiaux, C., Hantraye, P., Rivron, L., et al. (2011). In vivo imaging of neuroinflammation in the rodent brain with [C-11]SSR180575, a novel indoleacetamide radioligand of the translocator protein (18 kDa). *Eur. J. Nucl. Med. Mol. Imaging* 38, 509–514. doi: 10.1007/s00259-010-1628-5

Chiba, K. (2005). FTY720, a new class of immunomodulator, inhibits lymphocyte egress from secondary lymphoid tissues and thymus by agonistic activity at sphingosine 1-phosphate receptors. *Pharmacol. Ther.* 108, 308–319. doi: 10.1016/j.pharmthera.2005.05.002

Chu, K., Jeong, S. W., Jung, K. H., Han, S. Y., Lee, S. T., Kim, M., et al. (2004). Celecoxib induces functional recovery after intracerebral hemorrhage with reduction of brain edema and perihematomal cell death. *J. Cereb. Blood Flow Metab.* 24, 926–933. doi: 10.1097/01.wcb.0000130866.25040.7d

Ciarmiello, A. (2011). Imaging of neuroinflammation. *Eur. J. Nucl. Med. Mol. Imaging* 38, 2198–2201. doi: 10.1007/s00259-011-1959-x

Clark, W., Gunion-Rinker, L., Lessov, N., and Hazel, K. (1998). Citicoline treatment for experimental intracerebral hemorrhage in mice. *Stroke* 29, 2136–2140. doi: 10.1161/01.str.29.10.2136

Clark, J. F., Loftspring, M., Wurster, W. L., Beiler, S., Beiler, C., Wagner, K. R., et al. (2008). Bilirubin oxidation products, oxidative stress and intracerebral hemorrhage. *Acta Neurochir. Suppl.* 105, 7–12. doi: 10.1007/978-3-211-094 69-3_2

Cunningham, L. A., Wetzel, M., and Rosenberg, G. A. (2005). Multiple roles for MMPs and TIMPs in cerebral ischemia. *Glia* 50, 329–339. doi: 10.1002/glia.20169

David, S., and Kroner, A. (2011). Repertoire of microglial and macrophage responses after spinal cord injury. *Nat. Rev. Neurosci.* 12, 388–399. doi: 10.1038/nrn3053

Davis, S. M., Broderick, J., Hennerici, M., Brun, N. C., Diringer, M. N., Mayer, S. A., et al. (2006). Hematoma growth is a determinant of mortality and poor outcome after intracerebral hemorrhage. *Neurology* 66, 1175–1181. doi: 10.1212/01.wnl.0000208408.98482.99

Del Bigio, M. R., Yan, H. J., Buist, R., and Peeling, J. (1996). Experimental intracerebral hemorrhage in rats. Magnetic resonance imaging and histopathological correlates. *Stroke* 27, 2312–2319; discussion 2319–2320. doi: 10.1161/01.str.27.12.2312

D'Mello, C., Le, T., and Swain, M. G. (2009). Cerebral microglia recruit monocytes into the brain in response to tumor necrosis factoralpha signaling during peripheral organ inflammation. *J. Neurosci.* 29, 2089–2102. doi: 10.1523/jneurosci.3567-08.2009

Doens, D., and Fernández, P. L. (2014). Microglia receptors and their implications in the response to amyloid β for Alzheimer's disease pathogenesis. *J. Neuroinflammation* 11:48. doi: 10.1186/1742-2094-11-48

Dolinskas, C. A., Bilaniuk, L. T., Zimmerman, R. A., Kuhl, D. E., and Alavi, A. (1977). Computed tomography of intracerebral hematomas. II. Radionuclide and transmission CT studies of the perihematoma region. *AJR Am. J. Roentgenol.* 129, 689–692. doi: 10.2214/ajr.129.4.689

Donovan, F. M., Pike, C. J., Cotman, C. W., and Cunningham, D. D. (1997). Thrombin induces apoptosis in cultured neurons and astrocytes via a pathway requiring tyrosine kinase and RhoA activities. *J. Neurosci.* 17, 5316–5326.

Dziedzic, T., Bartus, S., Klimkowicz, A., Motyl, M., Slowik, A., and Szczudlik, A. (2002). Intracerebral hemorrhage triggers interleukin-6 and interleukin-10 release in blood. *Stroke* 33, 2334–2335. doi: 10.1161/01.str.0000027211.73567.fa

Emsley, H. C., and Tyrrell, P. J. (2002). Inflammation and infection in clinical stroke. *J. Cereb. Blood Flow Metab.* 22, 1399–1419. doi: 10.1097/00004647-200212000-00001

Enzmann, G., Mysiorek, C., Gorina, R., Cheng, Y. J., Ghavampour, S., Hannocks, M. J., et al. (2013). The neurovascular unit as a selective barrier to polymorphonuclear granulocyte (PMN) infiltration into the brain after ischemic injury. *Acta Neuropathol.* 125, 395–412. doi: 10.1007/s00401-012-1076-3

Fang, H., Chen, J., Lin, S., Wang, P., Wang, Y., Xiong, X., et al. (2014). CD36-mediated hematoma absorption following intracerebral hemorrhage: negative regulation by TLR4 signaling. *J. Immunol.* 192, 5984–5992. doi: 10.4049/jimmunol.1400054

Fang, H., Wang, P. F., Zhou, Y., Wang, Y. C., and Yang, Q. W. (2013). Toll-like receptor 4 signaling in intracerebral hemorrhage-induced inflammation and injury. *J. Neuroinflammation* 10:27. doi: 10.1186/1742-2094-10-27

Fisher, C. M. (1971). Pathological observations in hypertensive cerebral hemorrhage. *J. Neuropathol. Exp. Neurol.* 30, 536–550. doi: 10.1097/00005072-197107000-00015

Fisher, C. M. (2003). Hypertensive cerebral hemorrhage. Demonstration of the source of bleeding. *J. Neuropathol. Exp. Neurol.* 62, 104–107.

Florczak-Rzepka, M., Grond-Ginsbach, C., Montaner, J., and Steiner, T. (2012). Matrix metalloproteinases in human spontaneous intracerebral hemorrhage: an update. *Cerebrovasc. Dis.* 34, 249–262. doi: 10.1159/000341686

Fu, Y., Hao, J., Zhang, N., Ren, L., Sun, N., Li, Y. J., et al. (2014). Fingolimod for the treatment of intracerebral hemorrhage: a 2-arm proof-of-concept study. *JAMA Neurol.* 71, 1092–1101. doi: 10.1001/jamaneurol.2014.1065

Fujimoto, S., Katsuki, H., Ohnishi, M., Takagi, M., Kume, T., and Akaike, A. (2007). Thrombin induces striatal neurotoxicity depending on mitogen-activated protein kinase pathways in vivo. *Neuroscience* 144, 694–701. doi: 10.1016/j.neuroscience.2006.09.049

Gabrusiewicz, K., Ellert-Miklaszewska, A., Lipko, M., Sielska, M., Frankowska, M., and Kaminska, B. (2011). Characteristics of the alternative phenotype of microglia/macrophages and its modulation in experimental gliomas. *PLoS One* 6:e23902. doi: 10.1371/journal.pone.0023902

Gao, L., Lu, Q., Huang, L. J., Ruan, L. H., Yang, J. J., Huang, W. L., et al. (2014). Transplanted neural stem cells modulate regulatory T, $\gamma\delta$ T cells and corresponding cytokines after intracerebral hemorrhage in rats. *Int. J. Mol. Sci.* 15, 4431–4441. doi: 10.3390/ijms15034431

Gauberti, M., Montagne, A., Marcos-Contreras, O. A., Le Béhot, A., Maubert, E., and Vivien, D. (2013). Ultra-sensitive molecular MRI of vascular cell adhesion molecule-1 reveals a dynamic inflammatory penumbra after strokes. *Stroke* 44, 1988–1996. doi: 10.1161/strokeaha.111.000544

Gautier, S., Ouk, T., Petrault, O., Caron, J., and Bordet, R. (2009). Neutrophils contribute to intracerebral haemorrhages after treatment with recombinant tissue plasminogen activator following cerebral ischaemia. *Br. J. Pharmacol.* 156, 673–679. doi: 10.1111/j.1476-5381.2009.00068.x

Gautschi, O. P., and Schaller, K. (2013). Surgery or conservative therapy for cerebral haemorrhage? *Lancet* 382, 377–378. doi: 10.1016/s0140-6736(13)61087-9

Ginhoux, F., Greter, M., Leboeuf, M., Nandi, S., See, P., Gokhan, S., et al. (2010). Fate mapping analysis reveals that adult microglia derive from primitive macrophages. *Science* 330, 841–845. doi: 10.1126/science.1194637

Gong, C., Hoff, J. T., and Keep, R. F. (2000). Acute inflammatory reaction following experimental intracerebral hemorrhage in rat. *Brain Res.* 871, 57–65. doi: 10.1016/s0006-8993(00)02427-6

Gong, Y., Tian, H., Xi, G., Keep, R. F., Hoff, J. T., and Hua, Y. (2006). Systemic zinc protoporphyrin administration reduces intracerebral hemorrhage-induced brain injury. *Acta Neurochir. Suppl.* 96, 232–236. doi: 10.1007/3-211-30714-1_50

Gong, Y., Xi, G., Hu, H., Gu, Y., Huang, F., Keep, R. F., et al. (2008). Increase in brain thrombin activity after experimental intracerebral hemorrhage. *Acta Neurochir. Suppl.* 105, 47–50. doi: 10.1007/978-3-211-09469-3_10

Greenhalgh, A. D., Brough, D., Robinson, E. M., Girard, S., Rothwell, N. J., and Allan, S. M. (2012). Interleukin-1 receptor antagonist is beneficial after subarachnoid haemorrhage in rat by blocking haem-driven inflammatory pathology. *Dis. Model Mech.* 5, 823–833. doi: 10.1242/dmm.008557

Grilli, M., and Memo, M. (1999). Possible role of NF-kappaB and p53 in the glutamate-induced pro-apoptotic neuronal pathway. *Cell Death Differ.* 6, 22–27. doi: 10.1038/sj.cdd.4400463

Guo, F. Q., Li, X. J., Chen, L. Y., Yang, H., Dai, H. Y., Wei, Y. S., et al. (2006). Study of relationship between inflammatory response and apoptosis in perihematoma region in patients with intracerebral hemorrhage. *Zhongguo Wei Zhong Bing Ji Jiu Yi Xue* 18, 290–293.

Hammond, M. D., Ai, Y., and Sansing, L. H. (2012). Gr1+ macrophages and dendritic cells dominate the inflammatory infiltrate 12 hours after experimental intracerebral hemorrhage. *Transl. Stroke Res.* 3, s125–s131. doi: 10.1007/s12975-012-0174-9

Hammond, M. D., Taylor, R. A., Mullen, M. T., Ai, Y., Aguila, H. L., Mack, M., et al. (2014). CCR2+ Ly6C(hi) inflammatory monocyte recruitment exacerbates acute disability following intracerebral hemorrhage. *J. Neurosci.* 34, 3901–3909. doi: 10.1523/jneurosci.4070-13.2014

Hampton, M. B., Kettle, A. J., and Winterbourn, C. C. (1998). Inside the neutrophil phagosome: oxidants, myeloperoxidase and bacterial killing. *Blood* 92, 3007–3017.

Han, N., Ding, S. J., Wu, T., and Zhu, Y. L. (2008). Correlation of free radical level and apoptosis after intracerebral hemorrhage in rats. *Neurosci. Bull.* 24, 351–358. doi: 10.1007/s12264-008-0711-4

Hanley, D. F. (2009). Intraventricular hemorrhage: severity factor and treatment target in spontaneous intracerebral hemorrhage. *Stroke* 40, 1533–1538. doi: 10.1161/strokeaha.108.535419

Helbok, R., Kurtz, P., Schmidt, J. M., Stuart, R. M., Fernandez, L., Malhotra, R., et al. (2011). Effect of mannitol on brain metabolism and tissue oxygenation in severe haemorrhagic stroke. *J. Neurol. Neurosurg. Psychiatry* 82, 378–383. doi: 10.1136/jnnp.2009.198754

Hernandez-Ontiveros, D. G., Tajiri, N., Acosta, S., Giunta, B., Tan, J., and Borlongan, C. V. (2013). Microglia activation as a biomarker for traumatic brain injury. *Front. Neurol.* 4:30. doi: 10.3389/fneur.2013.00030

Hickenbottom, S. L., Grotta, J. C., Strong, R., Denner, L. A., and Aronowski, J. (1999). Nuclear factor-kappaB and cell death after experimental intracerebral hemorrhage in rats. *Stroke* 30, 2472–2477; discussion 2477–2478. doi: 10.1161/01.str.30.11.2472

Hoyte, L. C., Brooks, K. J., Nagel, S., Akhtar, A., Chen, R. L., Mardiguian, S., et al. (2010). Molecular magnetic resonance imaging of acute vascular cell adhesion molecule-1 expression in a mouse model of cerebral ischemia. *J. Cereb. Blood Flow Metab.* 30, 1178–1187. doi: 10.1038/jcbfm.2009.287

Hua, Y., Keep, R. F., Gu, Y., and Xi, G. (2009). Thrombin and brain recovery after intracerebral hemorrhage. *Stroke* 40, S88–S89. doi: 10.1161/strokeaha.108.533281

Hua, Y., Wu, J., Keep, R. F., Nakamura, T., Hoff, J. T., and Xi, G. (2006). Tumor necrosis factor-alpha increases in the brain after intracerebral hemorrhage and thrombin stimulation. *Neurosurgery* 58, 542–550; discussion 542–550. doi: 10.1227/01.neu.0000197333.55473.ad

Huang, F. P., Xi, G., Keep, R. F., Hua, Y., Nemoianu, A., and Hoff, J. T. (2002). Brain edema after experimental intracerebral hemorrhage: role of hemoglobin degradation products. *J. Neurosurg.* 96, 287–293. doi: 10.3171/jns.2002.96.2.0287

Iadecola, C., and Anrather, J. (2011). The immunology of stroke: from mechanisms to translation. *Nat. Med.* 17, 796–808. doi: 10.1038/nm.2399

Jacobs, A. H., Tavitian, B., and INMiND consortium. (2012). Noninvasive molecular imaging of neuroinflammation. *J. Cereb. Blood Flow Metab.* 32, 1393–1415. doi: 10.1038/jcbfm.2012.53

James, M. L., Warner, D. S., and Laskowitz, D. T. (2008). Preclinical models of intracerebral hemorrhage: a translational perspective. *Neurocrit. Care* 9, 139–152. doi: 10.1007/s12028-007-9030-2

Kaczmarek, L., Lapinska-Dzwonek, J., and Szymczak, S. (2002). Matrix metalloproteinases in the adult brain physiology: a link between c-Fos, AP-1 and remodeling of neuronal connections? *EMBO J.* 21, 6643–6648. doi: 10.1093/emboj/cdf676

Kazui, S., Naritomi, H., Yamamoto, H., Sawada, T., and Yamaguchi, T. (1996). Enlargement of spontaneous intracerebral hemorrhage. Incidence and time course. *Stroke* 27, 1783–1787. doi: 10.1161/01.str.27.10.1783

Keep, R. F., Hua, Y., and Xi, G. (2012). Intracerebral haemorrhage: mechanisms of injury and therapeutic targets. *Lancet Neurol.* 11, 720–731. doi: 10.1016/s1474-4422(12)70104-7

Keep, R. F., Zhou, N., Xiang, J., Andjelkovic, A. V., Hua, Y., and Xi, G. (2014). Vascular disruption and blood-brain barrier dysfunction in intracerebral hemorrhage. *Fluids Barriers CNS* 11:18. doi: 10.1186/2045-8118-11-18

Kiferle, L., Politis, M., Muraro, P. A., and Piccini, P. (2011). Positron emission tomography imaging in multiple sclerosis-current status and future applications. *Eur. J. Neurol.* 18, 226–231. doi: 10.1111/j.1468-1331.2010.03154.x

Kigerl, K. A., Gensel, J. C., Ankeny, D. P., Alexander, J. K., Donnelly, D. J., and Popovich, P. G. (2009). Identification of two distinct macrophage subsets with divergent effects causing either neurotoxicity or regeneration in the injured mouse spinal cord. *J. Neurosci.* 29, 13435–13444. doi: 10.1523/JNEUROSCI.3257-09.2009

Knowland, D., Arac, A., Sekiguchi, K. J., Hsu, M., Lutz, S. E., Perrino, J., et al. (2014). Stepwise recruitment of transcellular and paracellular pathways underlies blood-brain barrier breakdown in stroke. *Neuron* 82, 603–617. doi: 10.1016/j.neuron.2014.03.003

Kobayashi, K., Imagama, S., Ohgomori, T., Hirano, K., Uchimura, K., Sakamoto, K., et al. (2013). Minocycline selectively inhibits M1 polarization of microglia. *Cell Death Dis.* 4:e525. doi: 10.1038/cddis.2013.54

Koeppen, A. H., Dickson, A. C., and Smith, J. (2004). Heme oxygenase in experimental intracerebral hemorrhage: the benefit of tin-mesoporphyrin. *J. Neuropathol. Exp. Neurol.* 63, 587–597.

Kreutzberg, G. W. (1996). Microglia: a sensor for pathological events in the CNS. *Trends Neurosci.* 19, 312–318. doi: 10.1016/0166-2236(96)10049-7

Kuramatsu, J. B., Huttner, H. B., and Schwab, S. (2013). Advances in the management of intracerebral hemorrhage. *J. Neural Transm.* 120(Suppl. 1), S35–S41. doi: 10.1007/s00702-013-1040-y

Lalancette-Hébert, M., Gowing, G., Simard, A., Weng, Y. C., and Kriz, J. (2007). Selective ablation of proliferating microglial cells exacerbates ischemic injury in the brain. *J. Neurosci.* 27, 2596–2605. doi: 10.1523/jneurosci.5360-06.2007

Lambertsen, K. L., Meldgaard, M., Ladeby, R., and Finsen, B. (2005). A quantitative study of microglial-macrophage synthesis of tumor necrosis factor during acute and late focal cerebral ischemia in mice. *J. Cereb. Blood Flow Metab.* 25, 119–135. doi: 10.1038/sj.jcbfm.9600014

Lee, M. C., Heaney, L. M., Jacobson, R. L., and Klassen, A. C. (1975). Cerebrospinal fluid in cerebral hemorrhage and infarction. *Stroke* 6, 638–641. doi: 10.1161/01.str.6.6.638

Lee, K. R., Kawai, N., Kim, S., Sagher, O., and Hoff, J. T. (1997). Mechanisms of edema formation after intracerebral hemorrhage: effects of thrombin on cerebral blood flow, blood-brain barrier permeability and cell survival in a rat model. *J. Neurosurg.* 86, 272–278. doi: 10.3171/jns.1997.86.2.0272

Lei, B., Dawson, H. N., Roulhac-Wilson, B., Wang, H., Laskowitz, D. T., and James, M. L. (2013). Tumor necrosis factor alpha antagonism improves neurological recovery in murine intracerebral hemorrhage. *J. Neuroinflammation* 10:103. doi: 10.1186/1742-2094-10-103

Liao, B., Zhao, W., Beers, D. R., Henkel, J. S., and Appel, S. H. (2012). Transformation from a neuroprotective to a neurotoxic microglial phenotype in a mouse model of ALS. *Exp. Neurol.* 237, 147–152. doi: 10.1016/j.expneurol.2012.06.011

Liesz, A., Suri-Payer, E., Veltkamp, C., Doerr, H., Sommer, C., Rivest, S., et al. (2009). Regulatory T cells are key cerebroprotective immunomodulators in acute experimental stroke. *Nat. Med.* 15, 192–199. doi: 10.1038/nm.1927

Liesz, A., Zhou, W., Mracskó, É., Karcher, S., Bauer, H., Schwarting, S., et al. (2011). Inhibition of lymphocyte trafficking shields the brain against deleterious neuroinflammation after stroke. *Brain* 134, 704–720. doi: 10.1093/brain/awr008

Lin, S., Yin, Q., Zhong, Q., Lv, F. L., Zhou, Y., Li, J. Q., et al. (2012). Heme activates TLR4-mediated inflammatory injury via MyD88/TRIF signaling pathway in intracerebral hemorrhage. *J. Neuroinflammation* 9:46. doi: 10.1186/1742-2094-9-46

Liu, D. Z., Ander, B. P., Xu, H., Shen, Y., Kaur, P., Deng, W., et al. (2010). Blood-brain barrier breakdown and repair by Src after thrombin-induced injury. *Ann. Neurol.* 67, 526–533. doi: 10.1002/ana.21924

Loftspring, M. C., Hansen, C., and Clark, J. F. (2010). A novel brain injury mechanism after intracerebral hemorrhage: the interaction between heme products and the immune system. *Med. Hypotheses* 74, 63–66. doi: 10.1016/j.mehy.2009.08.002

Loftspring, M. C., McDole, J., Lu, A., Clark, J. F., and Johnson, A. J. (2009). Intracerebral hemorrhage leads to infiltration of several leukocyte populations with concomitant pathophysiological changes. *J. Cereb. Blood Flow Metab.* 29, 137–143. doi: 10.1038/jcbfm.2008.114

Luheshi, N. M., Rothwell, N. J., and Brough, D. (2009). Dual functionality of interleukin-1 family cytokines: implications for anti-interleukin-1 therapy. *Br. J. Pharmacol.* 157, 1318–1329. doi: 10.1111/j.1476-5381.2009.00331.x

Ma, Q., Manaenko, A., Khatibi, N. H., Chen, W., Zhang, J. H., and Tang, J. (2011). Vascular adhesion protein-1 inhibition provides antiinflammatory protection after an intracerebral hemorrhagic stroke in mice. *J. Cereb. Blood Flow Metab.* 31, 881–893. doi: 10.1038/jcbfm.2010.167

MacLellan, C. L., Auriat, A. M., McGie, S. C., Yan, R. H., Huynh, H. D., De Butte, M. F., et al. (2006). Gauging recovery after hemorrhagic stroke in rats: implications for cytoprotection studies. *J. Cereb. Blood Flow Metab.* 26, 1031–1042. doi: 10.1038/sj.jcbfm.9600255

MacLellan, C. L., Silasi, G., Auriat, A. M., and Colbourne, F. (2010). Rodent models of intracerebral hemorrhage. *Stroke* 41, S95–S98. doi: 10.1161/strokeaha.110.594457

MacLellan, C. L., Silasi, G., Poon, C. C., Edmundson, C. L., Buist, R., Peeling, J., et al. (2008). Intracerebral hemorrhage models in rat: comparing collagenase to blood infusion. *J. Cereb. Blood Flow Metab.* 28, 516–525. doi: 10.1038/sj.jcbfm.9600548

Masada, T., Hua, Y., Xi, G., Yang, G. Y., Hoff, J. T., and Keep, R. F. (2001). Attenuation of intracerebral hemorrhage and thrombin-induced brain edema by overexpression of interleukin-1 receptor antagonist. *J. Neurosurg.* 95, 680–686. doi: 10.3171/jns.2001.95.4.0680

Matsushita, H., Hijioka, M., Ishibashi, H., Anan, J., Kurauchi, Y., Hisatsune, A., et al. (2014). Suppression of CXCL2 upregulation underlies the therapeutic effect of the retinoid Am80 on intracerebral hemorrhage in mice. *J. Neurosci. Res.* 92, 1024–1034. doi: 10.1002/jnr.23379

Matsushita, K., Meng, W., Wang, X., Asahi, M., Asahi, K., Moskowitz, M. A., et al. (2000). Evidence for apoptosis after intercerebral hemorrhage in rat striatum. *J. Cereb. Blood Flow Metab.* 20, 396–404. doi: 10.1097/00004647-200002000-00022

Mayer, S. A., Brun, N. C., Begtrup, K., Broderick, J., Davis, S., Diringer, M. N., et al. (2008). Efficacy and safety of recombinant activated factor VII for acute intracerebral hemorrhage. *N Engl J. Med.* 358, 2127–2137. doi: 10.1056/NEJMoa0707534

Mayne, M., Fotheringham, J., Yan, H. J., Power, C., Del Bigio, M. R., Peeling, J., et al. (2001a). Adenosine A2A receptor activation reduces proinflammatory events and decreases cell death following intracerebral hemorrhage. *Ann. Neurol.* 49, 727–735. doi: 10.1002/ana.1010

Mayne, M., Ni, W., Yan, H. J., Xue, M., Johnston, J. B., Del Bigio, M. R., et al. (2001b). Antisense oligodeoxynucleotide inhibition of tumor necrosis factor-alpha expression is neuroprotective after intracerebral hemorrhage. *Stroke* 32, 240–248. doi: 10.1161/01.str.32.1.240

McAteer, M. A., Sibson, N. R., von Zur Muhlen, C., Schneider, J. E., Lowe, A. S., Warrick, N., et al. (2007). In vivo magnetic resonance imaging of acute brain inflammation using microparticles of iron oxide. *Nat. Med.* 13, 1253–1258. doi: 10.1038/nm1631

Mendelow, A. D., Gregson, B. A., Mitchell, P. M., Murray, G. D., Rowan, E. N., and Gholkar, A. R. (2011). Surgical trial in lobar intracerebral haemorrhage (STICH II) protocol. *Trials* 12:124. doi: 10.1186/1745-6215-12-124

Menon, R. S., Burgess, R. E., Wing, J. J., Gibbons, M. C., Shara, N. M., Fernandez, S., et al. (2012). Predictors of highly prevalent brain ischemia in intracerebral hemorrhage. *Ann. Neurol.* 71, 199–205. doi: 10.1002/ana.22668

Morgan, T., Awad, I., Keyl, P., Lane, K., and Hanley, D. (2008). Preliminary report of the clot lysis evaluating accelerated resolution of intraventricular hemorrhage (CLEAR-IVH) clinical trial. *Acta Neurochir. Suppl.* 105, 217–220. doi: 10.1007/978-3-211-09469-3_41

Morgenstern, L. B., Hemphill, J. C. 3rd, Anderson, C., Becker, K., Broderick, J. P., Connolly, E. S. Jr., et al. (2010). Guidelines for the management of spontaneous intracerebral hemorrhage: a guideline for healthcare professionals from the American Heart Association/American Stroke Association. *Stroke* 41, 2108–2129. doi: 10.1161/STR.0b013e3181ec611b

Moxon-Emre, I., and Schlichter, L. C. (2011). Neutrophil depletion reduces blood-brain barrier breakdown, axon injury and inflammation after intracerebral hemorrhage. *J. Neuropathol. Exp. Neurol.* 70, 218–235. doi: 10.1097/nen.0b013e31820d94a5

Mracsko, E., Javidi, E., Na, S. Y., Kahn, A., Liesz, A., and Veltkamp, R. (2014). Leukocyte invasion of the brain after experimental intracerebral hemorrhage in mice. *Stroke* 45, 2107–2114. doi: 10.1161/strokeaha.114.005801

Nakamura, T., Keep, R. F., Hua, Y., Schallert, T., Hoff, J. T., and Xi, G. (2004). Deferoxamine-induced attenuation of brain edema and neurological deficits in a rat model of intracerebral hemorrhage. *J. Neurosurg.* 100, 672–678. doi: 10. 3171/jns.2004.100.4.0672

Nakamura, T., Kuroda, Y., Yamashita, S., Zhang, X., Miyamoto, O., Tamiya, T., et al. (2008). Edaravone attenuates brain edema and neurologic deficits in a rat model of acute intracerebral hemorrhage. *Stroke* 39, 463–469. doi: 10.1161/strokeaha. 107.486654

Newell, D. W., Shah, M. M., Wilcox, R., Hansmann, D. R., Melnychuk, E., Muschelli, J., et al. (2011). Minimally invasive evacuation of spontaneous intracerebral hemorrhage using sonothrombolysis. *J. Neurosurg.* 115, 592–601. doi: 10. 3171/2011.5.jns10505

Nguyen, H. X., O'barr, T. J., and Anderson, A. J. (2007). Polymorphonuclear leukocytes promote neurotoxicity through release of matrix metalloproteinases, reactive oxygen species and TNF-alpha. *J. Neurochem.* 102, 900–912. doi: 10. 1111/j.1471-4159.2007.04643.x

O'Donnell, M. J., Xavier, D., Liu, L., Zhang, H., Chin, S. L., Rao-Melacini, P., et al. (2010). Risk factors for ischaemic and intracerebral haemorrhagic stroke in 22 countries (the INTERSTROKE study): a case-control study. *Lancet* 376, 112–123. doi: 10.1016/s0140-6736(10)60834-3

Ohnishi, M., Katsuki, H., Fujimoto, S., Takagi, M., Kume, T., and Akaike, A. (2007). Involvement of thrombin and mitogen-activated protein kinase pathways in hemorrhagic brain injury. *Exp. Neurol.* 206, 43–52. doi: 10.1016/j.expneurol. 2007.03.030

Ohnishi, M., Katsuki, H., Fukutomi, C., Takahashi, M., Motomura, M., Fukunaga, M., et al. (2011). HMGB1 inhibitor glycyrrhizin attenuates intracerebral hemorrhage-induced injury in rats. *Neuropharmacology* 61, 975–980. doi: 10. 1016/j.neuropharm.2011.06.026

Ohnishi, M., Katsuki, H., Izumi, Y., Kume, T., Takada-Takatori, Y., and Akaike, A. (2010). Mitogen-activated protein kinases support survival of activated microglia that mediate thrombin-induced striatal injury in organotypic slice culture. *J. Neurosci. Res.* 88, 2155–2164. doi: 10.1002/jnr.22375

Ohnishi, M., Monda, A., Takemoto, R., Matsuoka, Y., Kitamura, C., Ohashi, K., et al. (2013). Sesamin suppresses activation of microglia and p44/42 MAPK pathway, which confers neuroprotection in rat intracerebral hemorrhage. *Neuroscience* 232C, 45–52. doi: 10.1016/j.neuroscience.2012.11.057

Okauchi, M., Hua, Y., Keep, R. F., Morgenstern, L. B., Schallert, T., and Xi, G. (2010). Deferoxamine treatment for intracerebral hemorrhage in aged rats: therapeutic time window and optimal duration. *Stroke* 41, 375–382. doi: 10. 1161/strokeaha.109.569830

Pachter, J. S., de Vries, H. E., and Fabry, Z. (2003). The blood-brain barrier and its role in immune privilege in the central nervous system. *J. Neuropathol. Exp. Neurol.* 62, 593–604.

Parney, I. F., Waldron, J. S., and Parsa, A. T. (2009). Flow cytometry and in vitro analysis of human glioma-associated macrophages. Laboratory investigation. *J. Neurosurg.* 110, 572–582. doi: 10.3171/2008.7.jns08475

Patel, A. R., Ritzel, R., McCullough, L. D., and Liu, F. (2013). Microglia and ischemic stroke: a double-edged sword. *Int. J. Physiol. Pathophysiol. Pharmacol.* 5, 73–90.

Pearson, V. L., Rothwell, N. J., and Toulmond, S. (1999). Excitotoxic brain damage in the rat induces interleukin-1beta protein in microglia and astrocytes: correlation with the progression of cell death. *Glia* 25, 311–323. doi: 10. 1002/(sici)1098-1136(19990215)25:4<311::aid-glia1>3.0.co;2-e

Peeling, J., Yan, H. J., Corbett, D., Xue, M., and Del Bigio, M. R. (2001). Effect of FK-506 on inflammation and behavioral outcome following intracerebral hemorrhage in rat. *Exp. Neurol.* 167, 341–347. doi: 10.1006/exnr.2000.7564

Pepper, M. S. (2001). Role of the matrix metalloproteinase and plasminogen activator-plasmin systems in angiogenesis. *Arterioscler. Thromb. Vasc. Biol.* 21, 1104–1117. doi: 10.1161/hq0701.093685

Ponomarev, E. D., Maresz, K., Tan, Y., and Dittel, B. N. (2007). CNS-derived interleukin-4 is essential for the regulation of autoimmune inflammation and induces a state of alternative activation in microglial cells. *J. Neurosci.* 27, 10714–10721. doi: 10.1523/jneurosci.1922-07.2007

Püntener, U., Booth, S. G., Perry, V. H., and Teeling, J. L. (2012). Long-term impact of systemic bacterial infection on the cerebral vasculature and microglia. *J. Neuroinflammation* 9:146. doi: 10.1186/1742-2094-9-146

Qureshi, A. I., Mendelow, A. D., and Hanley, D. F. (2009). Intracerebral haemorrhage. *Lancet* 373, 1632–1644. doi: 10.1016/S0140-6736(09)60371-8

Qureshi, A. I., Tuhrim, S., Broderick, J. P., Batjer, H. H., Hondo, H., and Hanley, D. F. (2001). Spontaneous intracerebral hemorrhage. *N Engl J. Med.* 344, 1450–1460. doi: 10.1056/NEJM200105103441907

Rodríguez-Yáñez, M., Brea, D., Arias, S., Blanco, M., Pumar, J. M., Castillo, J., et al. (2012). Increased expression of toll-like receptors 2 and 4 is associated with poor outcome in intracerebral hemorrhage. *J. Neuroimmunol.* 247, 75–80. doi: 10. 1016/j.jneuroim.2012.03.019

Rodríguez-Yáñez, M., and Castillo, J. (2008). Role of inflammatory markers in brain ischemia. *Curr. Opin. Neurol.* 21, 353–357. doi: 10.1097/wco. 0b013e3282ffafbf

Rolland, W. B. 2nd, Manaenko, A., Lekic, T., Hasegawa, Y., Ostrowski, R., Tang, J., et al. (2011). FTY720 is neuroprotective and improves functional outcomes after intracerebral hemorrhage in mice. *Acta Neurochir. Suppl.* 111, 213–217. doi: 10. 1007/978-3-7091-0693-8_36

Ronaldson, P. T., and Davis, T. P. (2012). Blood-brain barrier integrity and glial support: mechanisms that can be targeted for novel therapeutic approaches in stroke. *Curr. Pharm. Des.* 18, 3624–3644. doi: 10.2174/138161212802002625

Rosenberg, G. A., Mun-Bryce, S., Wesley, M., and Kornfeld, M. (1990). Collagenase-induced intracerebral hemorrhage in rats. *Stroke* 21, 801–807. doi: 10.1161/01. str.21.5.801

Rosenberg, G. A., and Navratil, M. (1997). Metalloproteinase inhibition blocks edema in intracerebral hemorrhage in the rat. *Neurology* 48, 921–926. doi: 10. 1212/wnl.48.4.921

Rossin, R., Muro, S., Welch, M. J., Muzykantov, V. R., and Schuster, D. P. (2008). In vivo imaging of Cu-64-labeled polymer nanoparticles targeted to the lung endothelium. *J. Nucl. Med.* 49, 103–111. doi: 10.2967/jnumed.107. 045302

Sakamoto, Y., Koga, M., Yamagami, H., Okuda, S., Okada, Y., Kimura, K., et al. (2013). Systolic blood pressure after intravenous antihypertensive treatment and clinical outcomes in hyperacute intracerebral hemorrhage: the stroke acute management with urgent risk-factor assessment and improvement-intracerebral hemorrhage study. *Stroke* 44, 1846–1851. doi: 10. 1161/STROKEAHA.113.001212

Sansing, L. H., Harris, T. H., Kasner, S. E., Hunter, C. A., and Kariko, K. (2011a). Neutrophil depletion diminishes monocyte infiltration and improves functional outcome after experimental intracerebral hemorrhage. *Acta Neurochir. Suppl.* 111, 173–178. doi: 10.1007/978-3-7091-0693-8_29

Sansing, L. H., Harris, T. H., Welsh, F. A., Kasner, S. E., Hunter, C. A., and Kariko, K. (2011b). Toll-like receptor 4 contributes to poor outcome after intracerebral hemorrhage. *Ann. Neurol.* 70, 646–656. doi: 10.1002/ana.22528

Savill, J. (1997). Apoptosis in resolution of inflammation. *J. Leukoc. Biol.* 61, 375–380.

Schilling, M., Besselmann, M., Leonhard, C., Mueller, M., Ringelstein, E. B., and Kiefer, R. (2003). Microglial activation precedes and predominates over macrophage infiltration in transient focal cerebral ischemia: a study in green fluorescent protein transgenic bone marrow chimeric mice. *Exp. Neurol.* 183, 25–33. doi: 10.1016/s0014-4886(03)00082-7

Schilling, M., Besselmann, M., Müller, M., Strecker, J. K., Ringelstein, E. B., and Kiefer, R. (2005). Predominant phagocytic activity of resident microglia over hematogenous macrophages following transient focal cerebral ischemia: an investigation using green fluorescent protein transgenic bone marrow chimeric mice. *Exp. Neurol.* 196, 290–297. doi: 10.1016/j.expneurol.2005. 08.004

Schroder, K., Hertzog, P. J., Ravasi, T., and Hume, D. A. (2004). Interferon-gamma: an overview of signals, mechanisms and functions. *J. Leukoc. Biol.* 75, 163–189. doi: 10.1189/jlb.0603252

Schwab, J. M., Nguyen, T. D., Meyermann, R., and Schluesener, H. J. (2001). Human focal cerebral infarctions induce differential lesional interleukin-16 (IL-16) expression confined to infiltrating granulocytes, CD8+ T-lymphocytes and activated microglia/macrophages. *J. Neuroimmunol.* 114, 232–241. doi: 10. 1016/s0165-5728(00)00433-1

Shao, X., Zhang, H. A., Rajian, J. R., Chamberland, D. L., Sherman, P. S., Quesada, C. A., et al. (2011). 125 I-labeled gold nanorods for targeted imaging of inflammation. *ACS Nano* 5, 8967–8973. doi: 10.1021/nn203138t

Shiratori, M., Tozaki-Saitoh, H., Yoshitake, M., Tsuda, M., and Inoue, K. (2010). P2X7 receptor activation induces CXCL2 production in microglia through

NFAT and PKC/MAPK pathways. *J. Neurochem.* 114, 810–819. doi: 10.1111/j.1471-4159.2010.06809.x

Soehnlein, O., and Lindbom, L. (2010). Phagocyte partnership during the onset and resolution of inflammation. *Nat. Rev. Immunol.* 10, 427–439. doi: 10.1038/nri2779

Soenen, S. J. H., Himmelreich, U., Nuytten, N., Pisanic, T. R. 2nd, Ferrari, A., and De Cuyper, M. (2010). Intracellular nanoparticle coating stability determines nanoparticle diagnostics efficacy and cell functionality. *Small* 6, 2136–2145. doi: 10.1002/smll.201000763

Starossom, S. C., Mascanfroni, I. D., Imitola, J., Cao, L., Raddassi, K., Hernandez, S. F., et al. (2012). Galectin-1 deactivates classically activated microglia and protects from inflammation-induced neurodegeneration. *Immunity* 37, 249–263. doi: 10.1016/j.immuni.2012.05.023

Staykov, D., Wagner, I., Volbers, B., Hauer, E. M., Doerfler, A., Schwab, S., et al. (2011). Natural course of perihemorrhagic edema after intracerebral hemorrhage. *Stroke* 42, 2625–2629. doi: 10.1161/strokeaha.111.618611

Steiner, T., Al-Shahi Salman, R., Beer, R., Christensen, H., Cordonnier, C., Csiba, L., et al. (2014). European Stroke Organisation (ESO) guidelines for the management of spontaneous intracerebral hemorrhage. *Int. J. Stroke* 9, 840–855. doi: 10.1111/ijs.12309

Steiner, T., Kaste, M., Forsting, M., Mendelow, D., Kwiecinski, H., Szikora, I., et al. (2006). Recommendations for the management of intracranial haemorrhage—part I: spontaneous intracerebral haemorrhage. The European stroke initiative writing committee and the writing committee for the EUSI executive committee. *Cerebrovasc. Dis.* 22, 294–316. doi: 10.1159/000094831

Stern, M., Savill, J., and Haslett, C. (1996). Human monocyte-derived macrophage phagocytosis of senescent eosinophils undergoing apoptosis. Mediation by alpha v beta 3/CD36/thrombospondin recognition mechanism and lack of phlogistic response. *Am. J. Pathol.* 149, 911–921.

Stoll, G., and Bendszus, M. (2010). New approaches to neuroimaging of central nervous system inflammation. *Curr. Opin. Neurol.* 23, 282–286. doi: 10.1097/wco.0b013e328337f4b5

Striggow, F., Riek, M., Breder, J., Henrich-Noack, P., Reymann, K. G., and Reiser, G. (2000). The protease thrombin is an endogenous mediator of hippocampal neuroprotection against ischemia at low concentrations but causes degeneration at high concentrations. *Proc. Natl. Acad. Sci. U S A* 97, 2264–2269. doi: 10.1073/pnas.040552897

Stuber, M., Gilson, W. D., Schär, M., Kedziorek, D. A., Hofmann, L. V., Shah, S., et al. (2007). Positive contrast visualization of iron oxide-labeled stem cells using inversion-recovery with ON-Resonant water suppression (IRON). *Magn. Reson. Med.* 58, 1072–1077. doi: 10.1002/mrm.21399

Suzuki, Y., Sa, Q., Gehman, M., and Ochiai, E. (2011). Interferon-gamma-and perforin-mediated immune responses for resistance against *Toxoplasma gondii* in the brain. *Expert Rev. Mol. Med.* 13:e31. doi: 10.1017/s1462399411002018

Szymanska, A., Biernaskie, J., Laidley, D., Granter-Button, S., and Corbett, D. (2006). Minocycline and intracerebral hemorrhage: influence of injury severity and delay to treatment. *Exp. Neurol.* 197, 189–196. doi: 10.1016/j.expneurol.2005.09.011

Tanaka, R., Komine-Kobayashi, M., Mochizuki, H., Yamada, M., Furuya, T., Migita, M., et al. (2003). Migration of enhanced green fluorescent protein expressing bone marrow-derived microglia/macrophage into the mouse brain following permanent focal ischemia. *Neuroscience* 117, 531–539. doi: 10.1016/s0306-4522(02)00954-5

Tang, Z., Gan, Y., Liu, Q., Yin, J. X., Shi, J., and Shi, F. D. (2014). CX3CR1 deficiency suppresses activation and neurotoxicity of microglia/macrophage in experimental ischemic stroke. *J. Neuroinflammation* 11:26. doi: 10.1186/1742-2094-11-26

Tang, J., Liu, J., Zhou, C., Alexander, J. S., Nanda, A., Granger, D. N., et al. (2004). Mmp-9 deficiency enhances collagenase-induced intracerebral hemorrhage and brain injury in mutant mice. *J. Cereb. Blood Flow Metab.* 24, 1133–1145. doi: 10.1097/01.wcb.0000135593.05952.de

Tarzami, S. T., Wang, G., Li, W., Green, L., and Singh, J. P. (2006). Thrombin and PAR-1 stimulate differentiation of bone marrow-derived endothelial progenitor cells. *J. Thromb. Haemost.* 4, 656–663. doi: 10.1111/j.1538-7836.2006.01788.x

Taylor, R. A., and Sansing, L. H. (2013). Microglial responses after ischemic stroke and intracerebral hemorrhage. *Clin. Dev. Immunol.* 2013:746068. doi: 10.1155/2013/746068

Teng, W., Wang, L., Xue, W., and Guan, C. (2009). Activation of TLR4-mediated NFkappaB signaling in hemorrhagic brain in rats. *Mediators Inflamm.* 2009:473276. doi: 10.1155/2009/473276

Tessier, P. A., Naccache, P. H., Clark-Lewis, I., Gladue, R. P., Neote, K. S., and Mccoll, S. R. (1997). Chemokine networks in vivo: involvement of C-X-C and C-C chemokines in neutrophil extravasation in vivo in response to TNF-alpha. *J. Immunol.* 159, 3595–3602.

Thanvi, B., and Robinson, T. (2006). Sporadic cerebral amyloid angiopathy—an important cause of cerebral haemorrhage in older people. *Age Ageing* 35, 565–571. doi: 10.1093/ageing/afl108

Tikka, T. M., and Koistinaho, J. E. (2001). Minocycline provides neuroprotection against N-methyl-D-aspartate neurotoxicity by inhibiting microglia. *J. Immunol.* 166, 7527–7533. doi: 10.4049/jimmunol.166.12.7527

Tsopanoglou, N. E., and Maragoudakis, M. E. (2007). Inhibition of angiogenesis by small-molecule antagonists of protease-activated receptor-1. *Semin. Thromb. Hemost.* 33, 680–687. doi: 10.1055/s-2007-991535

van Asch, C. J., Luitse, M. J., Rinkel, G. J., van der Tweel, I., Algra, A., and Klijn, C. J. (2010). Incidence, case fatality and functional outcome of intracerebral haemorrhage over time, according to age, sex and ethnic origin: a systematic review and meta-analysis. *Lancet Neurol.* 9, 167–176. doi: 10.1016/s1474-4422(09)70340-0

Vaughan, P. J., Pike, C. J., Cotman, C. W., and Cunningham, D. D. (1995). Thrombin receptor activation protects neurons and astrocytes from cell death produced by environmental insults. *J. Neurosci.* 15, 5389–5401.

Vezzani, A., Conti, M., De Luigi, A., Ravizza, T., Moneta, D., Marchesi, F., et al. (1999). Interleukin-1beta immunoreactivity and microglia are enhanced in the rat hippocampus by focal kainate application: functional evidence for enhancement of electrographic seizures. *J. Neurosci.* 19, 5054–5065.

Wagner, K. R. (2007). Modeling intracerebral hemorrhage: glutamate, nuclear factor-kappa B signaling and cytokines. *Stroke* 38, 753–758. doi: 10.1161/01.str.0000255033.02904.db

Wagner, K. R., Beiler, S., Beiler, C., Kirkman, J., Casey, K., Robinson, T., et al. (2006). Delayed profound local brain hypothermia markedly reduces interleukin-1beta gene expression and vasogenic edema development in a porcine model of intracerebral hemorrhage. *Acta Neurochir. Suppl.* 96, 177–182. doi: 10.1007/3-211-30714-1_39

Wagner, K. R., Sharp, F. R., Ardizzone, T. D., Lu, A., and Clark, J. F. (2003). Heme and iron metabolism: role in cerebral hemorrhage. *J. Cereb. Blood Flow Metab.* 23, 629–652. doi: 10.1097/01.wcb.0000073905.87928.6d

Wagner, K. R., Xi, G., Hua, Y., Kleinholz, M., de Courten-Myers, G. M., Myers, R. E., et al. (1996). Lobar intracerebral hemorrhage model in pigs: rapid edema development in perihematomal white matter. *Stroke* 27, 490–497. doi: 10.1161/01.str.27.3.490

Wang, J. (2010). Preclinical and clinical research on inflammation after intracerebral hemorrhage. *Prog. Neurobiol.* 92, 463–477. doi: 10.1016/j.pneurobio.2010.08.001

Wang, J., and Doré, S. (2007a). Heme oxygenase-1 exacerbates early brain injury after intracerebral haemorrhage. *Brain* 130, 1643–1652. doi: 10.1093/brain/awm095

Wang, J., and Doré, S. (2007b). Inflammation after intracerebral hemorrhage. *J. Cereb. Blood Flow Metab.* 27, 894–908.

Wang, J., Rogove, A. D., Tsirka, A. E., and Tsirka, S. E. (2003). Protective role of tuftsin fragment 1-3 in an animal model of intracerebral hemorrhage. *Ann. Neurol.* 54, 655–664. doi: 10.1002/ana.10750

Wang, J., and Tsirka, S. E. (2005). Neuroprotection by inhibition of matrix metalloproteinases in a mouse model of intracerebral haemorrhage. *Brain* 128, 1622–1633. doi: 10.1093/brain/awh489

Wang, Y. C., Wang, P. F., Fang, H., Chen, J., Xiong, X. Y., and Yang, Q. W. (2013). Toll-like receptor 4 antagonist attenuates intracerebral hemorrhage-induced brain injury. *Stroke* 44, 2545–2552. doi: 10.1161/STROKEAHA.113.001038

Wang, Y. X., Yan, A., Ma, Z. H., Wang, Z., Zhang, B., Ping, J. L., et al. (2011). Nuclear factor-kappaB and apoptosis in patients with intracerebral hemorrhage. *J. Clin. Neurosci.* 18, 1392–1395. doi: 10.1016/j.jocn.2010.11.039

Wang, Y. C., Zhou, Y., Fang, H., Lin, S., Wang, P. F., Xiong, R. P., et al. (2014). Toll-like receptor 2/4 heterodimer mediates inflammatory injury in intracerebral hemorrhage. *Ann. Neurol.* 75, 876–889. doi: 10.1002/ana.24159

Wasserman, J. K., and Schlichter, L. C. (2007). Minocycline protects the blood-brain barrier and reduces edema following intracerebral hemorrhage in the rat. *Exp. Neurol.* 207, 227–237. doi: 10.1016/j.expneurol.2007.06.025

Winkeler, A., Boisgard, R., Martin, A., and Tavitian, B. (2010). Radioisotopic imaging of neuroinflammation. *J. Nucl. Med.* 51, 1–4. doi: 10.2967/jnumed.109.065680

Wisniewski, H. (1961). The pathogenesis of some cases of cerebral hemorrhage (a morphologic study of thmargins of hemorrhagic foci and areas of the brain distant form the hemorrhage). *Acta Med. Pol.* 2, 379–390.

Wu, J., Hua, Y., Keep, R. F., Nakamura, T., Hoff, J. T., and Xi, G. (2003). Iron and iron-handling proteins in the brain after intracerebral hemorrhage. *Stroke* 34, 2964–2969. doi: 10.1161/01.str.0000103140.52838.45

Wu, H., Wu, T., Xu, X., Wang, J., and Wang, J. (2011). Iron toxicity in mice with collagenase-induced intracerebral hemorrhage. *J. Cereb. Blood Flow Metab.* 31, 1243–1250. doi: 10.1038/jcbfm.2010.209

Wu, J., Yang, S., Hua, Y., Liu, W., Keep, R. F., and Xi, G. (2010). Minocycline attenuates brain edema, brain atrophy and neurological deficits after intracerebral hemorrhage. *Acta Neurochir. Suppl.* 106, 147–150. doi: 10.1007/978-3-211-98811-4_26

Wu, J., Yang, S., Xi, G., Fu, G., Keep, R. F., and Hua, Y. (2009). Minocycline reduces intracerebral hemorrhage-induced brain injury. *Neurol. Res.* 31, 183–188. doi: 10.1179/174313209X385680

Wunder, A., Klohs, J., and Dirnagl, U. (2009). Non-invasive visualization of CNS inflammation with nuclear and optical imaging. *Neuroscience* 158, 1161–1173. doi: 10.1016/j.neuroscience.2008.10.005

Xi, G., Hua, Y., Bhasin, R. R., Ennis, S. R., Keep, R. F., and Hoff, J. T. (2001a). Mechanisms of edema formation after intracerebral hemorrhage: effects of extravasated red blood cells on blood flow and blood-brain barrier integrity. *Stroke* 32, 2932–2938. doi: 10.1161/hs1201.099820

Xi, G., Hua, Y., Keep, R. F., Younger, J. G., and Hoff, J. T. (2001b). Systemic complement depletion diminishes perihematomal brain edema in rats. *Stroke* 32, 162–167. doi: 10.1161/01.str.32.1.162

Xi, G., Keep, R. F., and Hoff, J. T. (1998). Erythrocytes and delayed brain edema formation following intracerebral hemorrhage in rats. *J. Neurosurg.* 89, 991–996. doi: 10.3171/jns.1998.89.6.0991

Xi, G., Keep, R. F., and Hoff, J. T. (2006). Mechanisms of brain injury after intracerebral haemorrhage. *Lancet Neurol.* 5, 53–63. doi: 10.1016/s1474-4422(05)70283-0

Xi, G., Reiser, G., and Keep, R. F. (2003). The role of thrombin and thrombin receptors in ischemic, hemorrhagic and traumatic brain injury: deleterious or protective? *J. Neurochem.* 84, 3–9. doi: 10.1046/j.1471-4159.2003.01268.x

Xue, M., and Del Bigio, M. R. (2000). Intracerebral injection of autologous whole blood in rats: time course of inflammation and cell death. *Neurosci. Lett.* 283, 230–232. doi: 10.1016/s0304-3940(00)00971-x

Xue, M., and Del Bigio, M. R. (2003). Comparison of brain cell death and inflammatory reaction in three models of intracerebral hemorrhage in adult rats. *J. Stroke Cerebrovasc. Dis.* 12, 152–159. doi: 10.1016/s1052-3057(03)00036-3

Yabluchanskiy, A., Sawle, P., Homer-Vanniasinkam, S., Green, C. J., and Motterlini, R. (2010). Relationship between leukocyte kinetics and behavioral tests changes in the inflammatory process of hemorrhagic stroke recovery. *Int. J. Neurosci.* 120, 765–773. doi: 10.3109/00207454.2010.523129

Yang, S., Chen, Y., Deng, X., Jiang, W., Li, B., Fu, Z., et al. (2013). Hemoglobin-induced nitric oxide synthase overexpression and nitric oxide production contribute to blood-brain barrier disruption in the rat. *J. Mol. Neurosci.* 51, 352–363. doi: 10.1007/s12031-013-9990-y

Yang, J. T., Lee, T. H., Lee, I. N., Chung, C. Y., Kuo, C. H., and Weng, H. H. (2011). Dexamethasone inhibits ICAM-1 and MMP-9 expression and reduces brain edema in intracerebral hemorrhagic rats. *Acta Neurochir. (Wien)* 153, 2197–2203. doi: 10.1007/s00701-011-1122-2

Yang, Z., Liu, Y., Yuan, F., Li, Z., Huang, S., Shen, H., et al. (2014a). Sinomenine inhibits microglia activation and attenuates brain injury in intracerebral hemorrhage. *Mol. Immunol.* 60, 109–114. doi: 10.1016/j.molimm.2014.03.005

Yang, S., Song, S., Hua, Y., Nakamura, T., Keep, R. F., and Xi, G. (2008). Effects of thrombin on neurogenesis after intracerebral hemorrhage. *Stroke* 39, 2079–2084. doi: 10.1161/STROKEAHA.107.508911

Yang, Z., Yu, A., Liu, Y., Shen, H., Lin, C., Lin, L., et al. (2014b). Regulatory T cells inhibit microglia activation and protect against inflammatory injury in intracerebral hemorrhage. *Int. Immunopharmacol.* 22, 522–525. doi: 10.1016/j.intimp.2014.06.037

Yang, Z., Zhao, T., Zou, Y., Zhang, J. H., and Feng, H. (2014c). Curcumin inhibits microglia inflammation and confers neuroprotection in intracerebral hemorrhage. *Immunol. Lett.* 160, 89–95. doi: 10.1016/j.imlet.2014.03.005

Yao, Y., and Tsirka, S. E. (2012a). The CCL2-CCR2 system affects the progression and clearance of intracerebral hemorrhage. *Glia* 60, 908–918. doi: 10.1002/glia.22323

Yao, Y., and Tsirka, S. E. (2012b). Chemokines and their receptors in intracerebral hemorrhage. *Transl. Stroke Res.* 3, 70–79. doi: 10.1007/s12975-012-0155-z

Yilmaz, G., Arumugam, T. V., Stokes, K. Y., and Granger, D. N. (2006). Role of T lymphocytes and interferon-gamma in ischemic stroke. *Circulation* 113, 2105–2112. doi: 10.1161/circulationaha.105.593046

Zarbock, A., and Ley, K. (2009). Neutrophil adhesion and activation under flow. *Microcirculation* 16, 31–42. doi: 10.1080/10739680802350104

Zazulia, A. R., Diringer, M. N., Videen, T. O., Adams, R. E., Yundt, K., Aiyagari, V., et al. (2001). Hypoperfusion without ischemia surrounding acute intracerebral hemorrhage. *J. Cereb. Blood Flow Metab.* 21, 804–810. doi: 10.1097/00004647-200107000-00005

Zhao, X., Grotta, J., Gonzales, N., and Aronowski, J. (2009). Hematoma resolution as a therapeutic target: the role of microglia/macrophages. *Stroke* 40, S92–S94. doi: 10.1161/STROKEAHA.108.533158

Zhao, X., Sun, G., Zhang, J., Strong, R., Song, W., Gonzales, N., et al. (2007). Hematoma resolution as a target for intracerebral hemorrhage treatment: role for peroxisome proliferator-activated receptor gamma in microglia/macrophages. *Ann. Neurol.* 61, 352–362. doi: 10.1002/ana.21097

Zhao, X., Zhang, Y., Strong, R., Grotta, J. C., and Aronowski, J. (2006). 15d-Prostaglandin J2 activates peroxisome proliferator-activated receptor-gamma, promotes expression of catalase and reduces inflammation, behavioral dysfunction and neuronal loss after intracerebral hemorrhage in rats. *J. Cereb. Blood Flow Metab.* 26, 811–820. doi: 10.1038/sj.jcbfm.9600233

Ziai, W. C., Tuhrim, S., Lane, K., McBee, N., Lees, K., Dawson, J., et al. (2014). A multicenter, randomized, double-blinded, placebo-controlled phase III study of clot lysis evaluation of accelerated resolution of intraventricular hemorrhage (CLEAR III). *Int. J. Stroke* 9, 536–542. doi: 10.1111/ijs.12097

4

Atypical "seizure-like" activity in cortical reverberating networks *in vitro* can be caused by LPS-induced inflammation: a multi-electrode array study from a hundred neurons

Francesca Gullo[1], Alida Amadeo[2], Giulia Donvito[1], Marzia Lecchi[1], Barbara Costa[1], Andrew Constanti[3] and Enzo Wanke[1]*

[1] Department of Biotechnologies and Biosciences, University of Milano-Bicocca, Milan, Italy
[2] Department of Biomolecular Sciences and Biotechnology, University of Milan, Milan, Italy
[3] UCL School of Pharmacy, University of London, London, UK

***Correspondence:**
Enzo Wanke, Department of Biotechnologies and Biosciences, University of Milano-Bicocca, Piazza della Scienza, 20129 Milan, Italy
e-mail: enzo.wanke@unimib.it

We show here that a mild sterile inflammation induced by the endotoxin lipopolysaccharide (LPS), in a neuron/astrocyte/microglial cortical network, modulates neuronal excitability and can initiate long-duration burst events resembling epileptiform seizures, a recognized feature of various central nervous neurodegenerative, neurological and acute systemic diseases associated with neuroinflammation. To study this action, we simultaneously analyzed the reverberating bursting activity of a hundred neurons by using *in vitro* multi-electrode array methods. ~5 h after LPS application, we observed a net increase in the average number of spikes elicited in engaged cells and within each burst, but no changes neither in spike waveforms nor in burst rate. This effect was characterized by a slow, twofold exponential increase of the burst duration and the appearance of rarely occurring long burst events that were never seen during control recordings. These changes and the time-course of microglia-released proinflammatory cytokine, tumor necrosis factor-alpha (TNF-α), were blocked by pre-treatment with 50 nM minocycline, an established anti-inflammatory agent which was inactive when applied alone. Assay experiments also revealed that application of 60 pM exogenous TNF-α after 12–15 h, produced non-washable changes of neuronal excitability, completely different from those induced by LPS, suggesting that TNF-α release alone was not responsible for our observed findings. Our results indicate that the link between neuroinflammation and hyperexcitability can be unveiled by studying the long-term activity of *in vitro* neuronal/astrocyte/microglial networks.

Keywords: sterile inflammation, LPS, burst activity, neocortical cultures, multi-electrode array, minocycline, TNF-α

INTRODUCTION

Since many years, the term "tripartite synapse" comprising of a presynaptic neuron, a postsynaptic neuron and an astrocyte, was proposed to summarize the evidence from many laboratories, that revealed the existence of bidirectional communication between neurons and astrocytes, especially at level of the synapse (for reviews see Perea et al., 2009). Also, microglial cells [the resident immune cells of the central nervous system (CNS)], play a critical role in neuropathology following brain injury (Perry et al., 2010; Krabbe et al., 2013). In activated microglial cells responding to the injury, migration and phagocytosis are promoted, and inflammatory mediators including nitric oxide (NO), inflammatory cytokines, such as interleukin-1 beta (IL-1β) and tumor necrosis factor-alpha (TNF-α) are released. Since both microglia and astrocytes are present and active in neuronal networks, it is still debated how complicated the cross-talk is between these three cell families (Kettenmann et al., 2013) and interesting mathematical models of this relationship have even been reported in a real-time artificial neuron-astrocyte network (Valenza et al., 2013). It is believed that spontaneous bursting in neuronal network assemblies is physiologically important especially during early development to ensure the reliability of synaptic transmission and information processing (O'Learly et al., 1994; Lisman, 1997; Catalano and Shatz, 1998; Komuro and Rakic, 1998; Garaschuk et al., 2000; Sanchez-Vives and McCormick, 2000; Corlew et al., 2004; Harris, 2005; Dupont et al., 2006).

The aim of the present study was to investigate the proinflammatory effects of low doses of the bacterial endotoxin lipopolysaccharide (LPS) on the spontaneous bursting activity of cortical network cultures derived from *ex vivo* neocortex and containing neurons, astrocytes and microglial cells. Contrary to the *in vivo* network counterpart that is governed by a sensory input and a up-and down-state behavior (see Chen et al., 2013), it is well known that cultured neuronal network activity is reverberating, and long-term data recording can be performed by using *in vitro* multi-site electrophysiology, fully established from many years (Keefer et al., 2001; Beggs and Plenz, 2003, 2004; Gramowski et al., 2004; Tateno et al., 2005; Eytan and Marom, 2006; Gullo et al., 2009, 2010, 2012).

Activity can be basically described by two interlaced time intervals called "burst" (with duration, BD) and "inter-burst interval"

(IBI), respectively. The former is characterized by short-lived (i.e., burst-like events, 1–5 s duration, with each neuron having its own duration) and synchronized synaptically mediated neuronal firing from ~85% of the engaged neurons, and the latter by silent periods of variable duration (7–100 s). Furthermore, by combining electrophysiological multi-electrode array (MEA) recording with fluorescence imaging of γ–aminobutyric acid (GABA)-containing neurons derived from mice expressing green fluorescent protein (GFP), we have previously described how it is possible to classify authentic inhibitory and excitatory cells within the network. Moreover, we showed that the metric which best recognized the firing mode of these different neurons was that defined by the Fano factor (FF; calculated from the ratio between spike-count variance and mean; for details see Becchetti et al., 2012). Thus, we concluded that this statistical analysis demonstrated that BDs of neurons designated as excitatory or inhibitory were qualitatively short or long, respectively.

In each MEA dish, we continuously recorded (over 10s of hours) from a hundred neurons (~2–3% of network neurons), the BD and excitability changes observed in the two identified clusters of neurons before and after LPS or other pharmacological manipulations. We found that besides a slow increase of excitability of both clusters after LPS, there was a surprising occurrence of atypical burst-like activity, characterized by rare but statistically significant long-duration events, never observed in control recordings before LPS application. Application of low concentrations of the anti-inflammatory agent minocycline (MC) before LPS was sufficient to occlude this hyperactivity. In conclusion, these novel results, obtained from *in vitro* neuronal/astrocyte/microglial networks, reinforce the important, but ultra-slow roles of proinflammatory cytokines (such as TNF-α, whose concentration was measured during LPS experiments) in modulating neuronal excitability as compared to their more well-known faster ionotropic and metabotropic synaptic counterparts. (Santello and Volterra, 2012; Béchade et al., 2013).

MATERIALS AND METHODS

CELL CULTURES

Primary cultures of cortical neurons were prepared as previously described (Gullo et al., 2009). Briefly, all of the cerebral cortex (excluding the hippocampus) was removed from decapitated post-natal mice (P1–P3), cut into 1 mm × 1 mm × 1 mm pieces, and digested by trypsin (0.15%) and DNAse (10 μg/ml) at 37°C for 20 min. After enzyme digestion, cells were mechanically dissociated by means of trituration, and plated at densities of 600–900 × 10^3 cells/ml on glass coverslips (for immunocytochemistry) or MEA Petri dishes pre-coated with polyethyleneimine 0.1% (wt/vol) and laminin 20 μg/ml (30 μm diameter ITO electrodes spaced 200 μm apart, Multichannels System, Germany). Each dish had a recording area of ~2 mm × ~2 mm, where on average ~7000 cells were present but only ~3000 were neurons. After 3 h incubation, the plating medium was replaced by neurobasal medium (NB) with B27 (Invitrogen, Italy), glutamine 1 mM and basic fibroblast growth factor (bFGF) 10 ng/ml, and the culture was maintained at 37°C in 5% CO_2. One-half of the medium volume was replaced every 3 days. The cultures in MEA dishes were covered with gas-permeable covers (MEA-MEM, Ala Scientific Instruments, Inc., USA) throughout the culture period [12–22 days-*in vitro* (DIV)].

CYTOCHEMICAL CHARACTERIZATION OF CORTICAL CELL CULTURES

To characterize the neuronal population in our cultures, we used monoclonal antibodies against microtubule-associated protein 2 (MAP2; 1:1000, Sigma) for neurons, gliofibrillar acid protein (GFAP; 1:500, Dako) for glial cells and the biotin-labeled tomato lectin, biotinylated *Lycopersicum esculentum* agglutinin (b-LEA, 1:500; Vector Inc.) for microglia (Saura, 2007). Controls were performed by omitting primary antibodies or b-LEA. In these cases, no labeling was observed. The cultured cortical cells of control and those treated with LPS (3 μg/ml for 7 h) were fixed at 13 DIV in 4% paraformaldehyde in 0.1M phosphate buffer (PB; pH 7.2) for 20 min, then washed and maintained in PB until cytochemical reactions.

IMMUNOFLUORESCENCE

After aldehyde quenching with 0.05M NH_4Cl and permeabilization with 0.1% Triton X-100, cells were preincubated with 1% bovine serum albumin (BSA) for 30 min. Successive incubation was performed for 48 h at 4°C in a mixture of anti-MAP2 and anti-GFAP primary antibodies and b-LEA in PBS/BSA 0.1%. This procedure was followed by incubation with a solution of PBS/BSA 0.1% containing the secondary antibodies DAM-Cy3 (polyclonal, anti-mouse IgG, made in donkey; 1:200 dilution; Cy3 fluorochrome; Jackson Immunoresearch Laboratories) and DAR-Cy5 (polyclonal, donkey anti-rabbit IgG conjugated to the indocarbocyanine Cy5, 1:200, Jackson Immunoresearch Laboratories) to reveal monoclonal and polyclonal antibodies, and Alexa-488-labeled streptavidin (1:200, Molecular Probes) for b-LEA lectin cytochemistry. After rinsing, samples were mounted on coverslips with PBS/glycerol and inspected with a TCS-NT (Leica Laserteknik GmbH) laser scanning confocal microscope, to visualize triple fluorescent labeling. The original emission color of fluorochrome conjugated to secondary antibody DAR-Cy5 has been set to blue to facilitate visual inspection of confocal images. All the thickness of cell cultures (about 12 μm) was acquired by digital superimposing of at least 10 serial optical sections.

LEA PEROXIDASE CYTOCHEMISTRY FOR MICROGLIAL CELLS COUNTING

Fixed cultures were pre-treated as previously reported for immunofluorescence, except for the additional H_2O_2 treatment (0.1% for 5 min) to block endogenous peroxidases. Overnight incubation at room temperature in a solution containing b-LEA in PBS/BSA 0.1% was followed by treatment with the avidin-biotinylated complex (ABC kit, Vector Inc., diluted 1:100) for 75 min and then with a freshly prepared solution (0.075%) of 3-3′-diaminobenzidine tetrahydrochloride (Sigma) and 0.002% H_2O_2. Finally, coverslips were dehydrated, cleared and mounted over clean slides. We selected four different cultures/coverslips per experimental set (controls/LPS-treated) from two animals. b-LEA positive (+) cells were counted in four non-overlapping random fields of the coverslips (340 × 250 μm). Image J software was used to count cells on acquired images. Statistical comparison was made using Student's t-test with $P < 0.05$ accepted as significantly different from control.

TNF-α CONCENTRATION MEASUREMENTS

In each MEA dish, small (150 μl) aliquots of the incubation medium were collected in control and during different times (30 min, 3, 6, 12, and 24 h) after the addition of LPS (3 μg/ml) or MC (50 nM) + LPS. Samples (50 μl) were analyzed in triplicate for murine TNFα with enzyme-linked immunosorbent assay (ELISA) kits (KCM3012, Invitrogen, Italy) accordingly to manufacture's instructions. The data were expressed as pg/ml following interpolation on the basis of a standard curve. As suggested by the manufacturer, the inter-assay and intra-assay variability were 3.5–4.3 and 2.6–8.2%, with a lower limit of detection <3 pg/ml. During the analysis we did not correct the data for the small change in the total incubation medium volume resulting from the aliquots removal. Data were analyzed using GraphPad 4.0 software employing Student t-test for group comparison. $P < 0.05$ was considered statistically significant.

MEA ELECTROPHYSIOLOGY

Drug application: general aspects

As previously described (Gullo et al., 2009), we report results obtained within a few hours after the MEA dish positioning into the incubator, which can thus be considered at the steady-state. The recording area in our MEA dishes was ~2 mm × ~2 mm, and in this area, the average number of neurons was in the order of ~5000, plus about the same number of astrocytes (see Figure 1 of supplementary material in Gullo et al., 2010 at http://journal.frontiersin.org/journal/10.3389/fncir.2010.00011/full) and the average space between cells was therefore relatively large. The drugs were kept as frozen stock solutions in distilled water (or DMSO < 0.1%) at −20°C, until diluted as appropriate with MEA culture medium before each experiment. All experiments were performed by adding the drugs in volumes that were always <1% of the total conditioned media volume bathing the neurons. When indicated, a washout was carried out with a solution pre-conditioned by the same network under control conditions. Murine TNF-α (T7539), thalidomide (THAL) and MC were purchased from Sigma, Italy. PPADS was kindly received from Prof. P. Illes, Rudolf-Boehm-Institut, Leipzig, Germany.

Recordings, waveform acquisition, and sorting

We used the same procedures previously described in Gullo et al. (2009, 2010). Briefly, analog signals sampled at 40 kHz were recorded at 36°C in CO_2-controlled incubators using MEA-1060BC or 1060INV pre-amplifiers (bandwidth 1–8000 Hz, Multichannel Systems, Germany) connected to a MEA Workstation (bandwidth 100–8000 Hz, Plexon Inc., USA). Data were sorted into timestamp files by the MEAWorkstation Sorter software (MEAWS, see details below) and cleaned of artifacts using the OFFLine Sorter program (Plexon Inc., USA). Next, during the PCA-based waveform sorting and for multi-unit electrodes, we applied one of the following procedures: (i) spike removal with a Mahalanobis threshold in the range 1.8–1.4; we concurrently checked that the P-value of multivariate ANOVA sorting quality statistics was <0.01 amongst the identified units; (ii) when the previous procedure led to excessive spike invalidation, we manually removed the spikes invading the adjacent unit ellipsoids (the latter method was very effective in decreasing the P-values, with only a limited number of erased spikes).

Neuronal cluster classification

The method of neuronal classification into excitatory or inhibitory is described in detail in Gullo et al. (2009, 2010) and Becchetti et al. (2012). For each identified unit and each burst, the following characteristics were computed in defined time segments: the autocorrelation function (ACF), the BD (see for recent details in Becchetti et al., 2012), the spike number (SN), the spike rate (SR), the intra-burst SR (IBSR), the IBIs and the FF (Baddeley et al., 1997). We classified the neurons on the basis of an unsupervised learning approach consisting of data reducing principal component analysis (PCA) based on FF as a feature (Becchetti et al., 2012), followed by the K-means clustering procedure. The large differences in these burst metrics was the basis for adopting FF as the best feature to clusterize neurons. As previously described (Becchetti et al., 2012), these procedures normally separated two statistically different clusters composed of numbers of excitatory (~60–90) and inhibitory (~15–25) neurons whose ratio always fitted the ratio present in the neocortex, i.e., from 4 to 5 (Gullo et al., 2010; Sahara et al., 2012).

Advanced burst classification into states and BD histograms

The global network burst structure was analyzed with standard techniques (see Ham et al., 2008) as well as procedures recently developed by us (Gullo et al., 2012). Briefly, we applied a running window of variable duration (10 ms to 1 s) in order to search for the start and end of the burst duration and collect all of the spikes which were precisely tagged to the engaged excitatory and inhibitory neurons already designated as previously explained above. In conclusion, for each spike, we knew exactly which neuron fired it, in which specific burst it was and how many other spikes were fired. This had the consequence that we could also compute for this neuron the average propensity for firing, namely, its "excitability" in terms of spikes per burst. Our new procedure consisted of performing a classification of all bursts into states (for simplicity here, we chose four), controlled by a PCA based on both BD and SN features. Accordingly, for each of these four states, we could obtain not only the total amounts of SN and the engaged neurons, but also their average time histogram spike number time histograms (SNTH) which specifically described the average time course of each burst from its start to its end (separately for excitatory and inhibitory neurons). Moreover, we computed also the cumulative distributions of BD (BD cum. probability). These last data were found not to be normally distributed (P-value < 0.0001, Shapiro-Wilk, Anderson-Darling, and Lilliefors tests by XLSTAT option Normality test, not shown).

Data analysis and statistical significance

All of the data are expressed as mean values ± SEM, with n indicating the number of experiments. For the non-normally distributed data, we used the non-parametric tests available from XLSTAT-Pro software (Addinsoft, USA). To compute statistical significance among BD cumulative distributions originating from different experiments in general, we preferred the non-parametric equivalent of the ANOVA (a test valid only for normally distributed data), i.e., the Kruskal-Wallis test, where the optional "multiple comparisons" method allowed us to identify various putative groups (we tested the Dunn and the Steel-Dwass-Critchlow-Fligner methods, with the Bonferroni correction). The data were analyzed and the figures prepared using OriginPro 7.0 software.

RESULTS

THE ACTIVITY PATTERN IN CONTROL (UNTREATED) AND IN LPS-TREATED NETWORKS

The simplest way to observe the reverberating burst activity of long-term cultured networks is to examine raster plots from multi-site recordings; these show the temporal sequence of action potential timestamps recorded simultaneously from ~2% of the total number of neurons attached on a square area of 2 mm × 2 mm forming the recorded network. Typical raster plots of a reverberating burst in control during 5 s of activity is shown in **Figure 1A**, where each line corresponds to one cell (the small vertical ticks are the spike timestamps) and the 65 upper and 27 lower lines belong to units classified as excitatory and inhibitory neurons respectively (Becchetti et al., 2012). **Figure 1B** shows the very different properties of an atypical burst recorded 6 h after the application of 3 μg/ml LPS in the same MEA dish (notice the change by a factor of ~6 on the time scale). While the burst duration (BD) in control (untreated) was around ~2–3 s, the application of LPS introduced a dramatic BD increase. Similar data were observed in 9 out of 10 different experiments. It can be seen that in 200 s windows, as shown in **Figure 1C**, in control before LPS, the duration of the spontaneous bursts (i.e., thickness of the vertical columns) was characterized by a distribution shifted toward short BDs. In contrast, in the presence of LPS (**Figure 1D**), the appearance of long atypical BD events increased significantly, suggesting an overall increase in neuronal excitability.

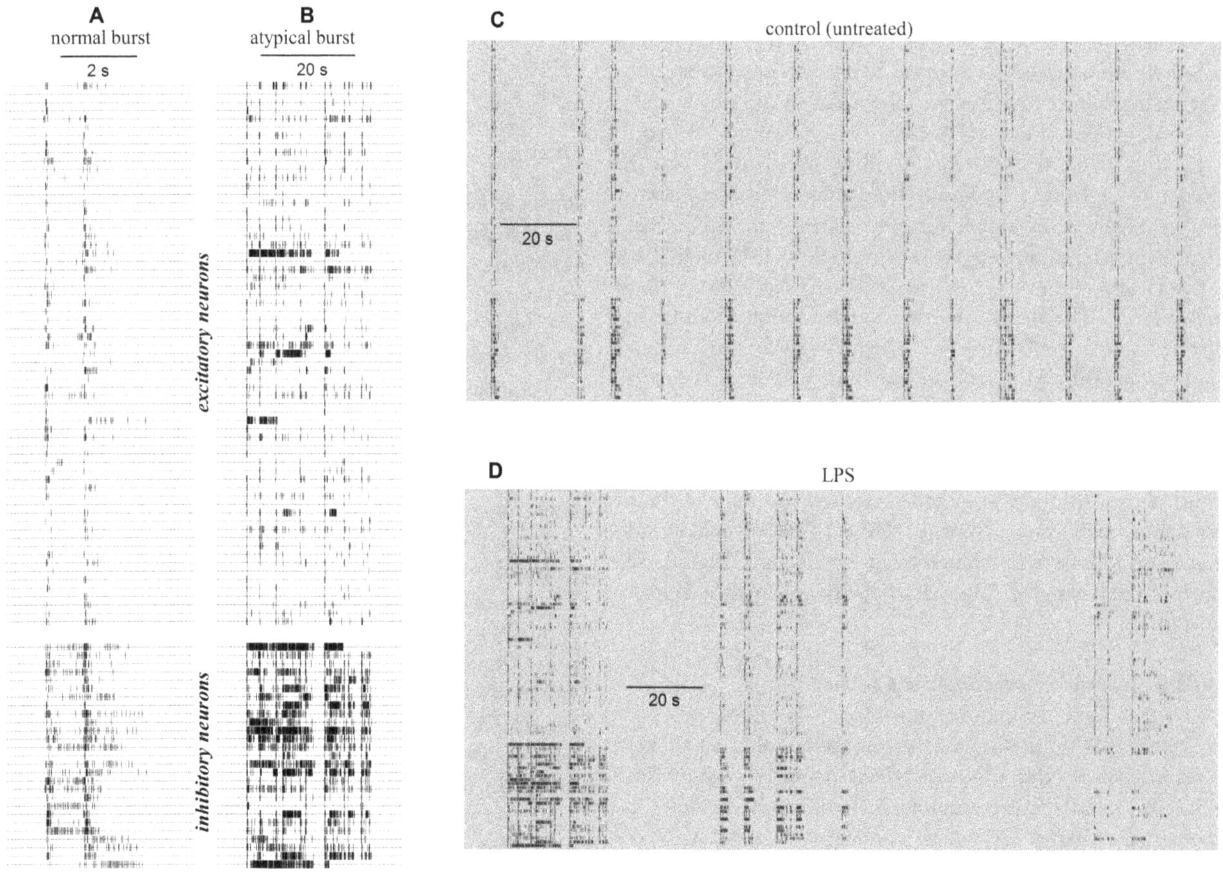

FIGURE 1 | Raster plots of exemplary normal and atypical reverberating bursts of the network activity recorded in a neocortical/astrocyte/microglial co-culture grown on an multi-electrode array (MEA) dish in control (CON) and 6 h after application of 3 μg/ml lipopolysaccharide (LPS). Data in **(A–D)** were recorded in control and in LPS, respectively. Small vertical ticks on horizontal lines are timestamps of spikes elicited by identified neurons as indicated. **(A)** Raster plot of a normal burst recorded in control before adding LPS. Note the time scale bar of 2 s. **(B)** Raster plot of an atypical burst recorded 6 h after adding LPS. Note the time scale bar of 20 s. **(C)** Plot of 13 similar normal bursts recorded in control during a time window of 200 s. **(D)** Plot of two atypical bursts recorded in LPS during 200 s (the first is shown in **Figure 1B**). The timestamps in **(C,D)** had the same pattern as in **(A,B)**, i.e., upper and lower ticks relate to identified excitatory and inhibitory cells, respectively.

To investigate the underlying properties of this activity, we performed a statistical analysis of the neuron type (excitatory or inhibitory, see Becchetti et al., 2012) and a classification of the durations of the acquired bursts (see Gullo et al., 2012). We found that, on average, the number of engaged neurons was not changing before and after LPS (not shown), but on the contrary, it was the number of elicited spikes (SN, in each burst) that was strongly increasing for both neuronal types (clusters). To quantify the heterogeneity of the BDs, we performed a classification procedure of all bursts into four states according to two features, namely, SN and BD. The assignment of each burst to one of the four states was performed automatically, and the states were significantly different according to our classification procedure (see Materials and Methods). During a typical whole experiment of 14 h, we computed the data in sequential time segments of 2 h in control (6 h) and after the LPS application (8 h). Each burst was characterized by how many spikes were elicited from burst onset up to its end; we then computed the temporal histogram of the SN (SNTH: Gullo et al., 2010, 2012) and plotted it by averaging all data in each 2 h time segment and among all the neurons belonging to the same cluster (see Materials and Methods). The SNTH data plots observed in control (untreated) and in LPS are shown in **Figures 2A,B**, respectively: for excitatory cluster: thin lines and open circles and for inhibitory cluster: thick lines and closed circles. During control, state 1 and 2 maximal BDs where in the range 2–3 s and for states 3 and 4 BDs were up to 6–7 s. In contrast, in LPS, the BDs were much longer: for states 1 and 2 BDs reached the range 5–11 s, but for states 3 and 4

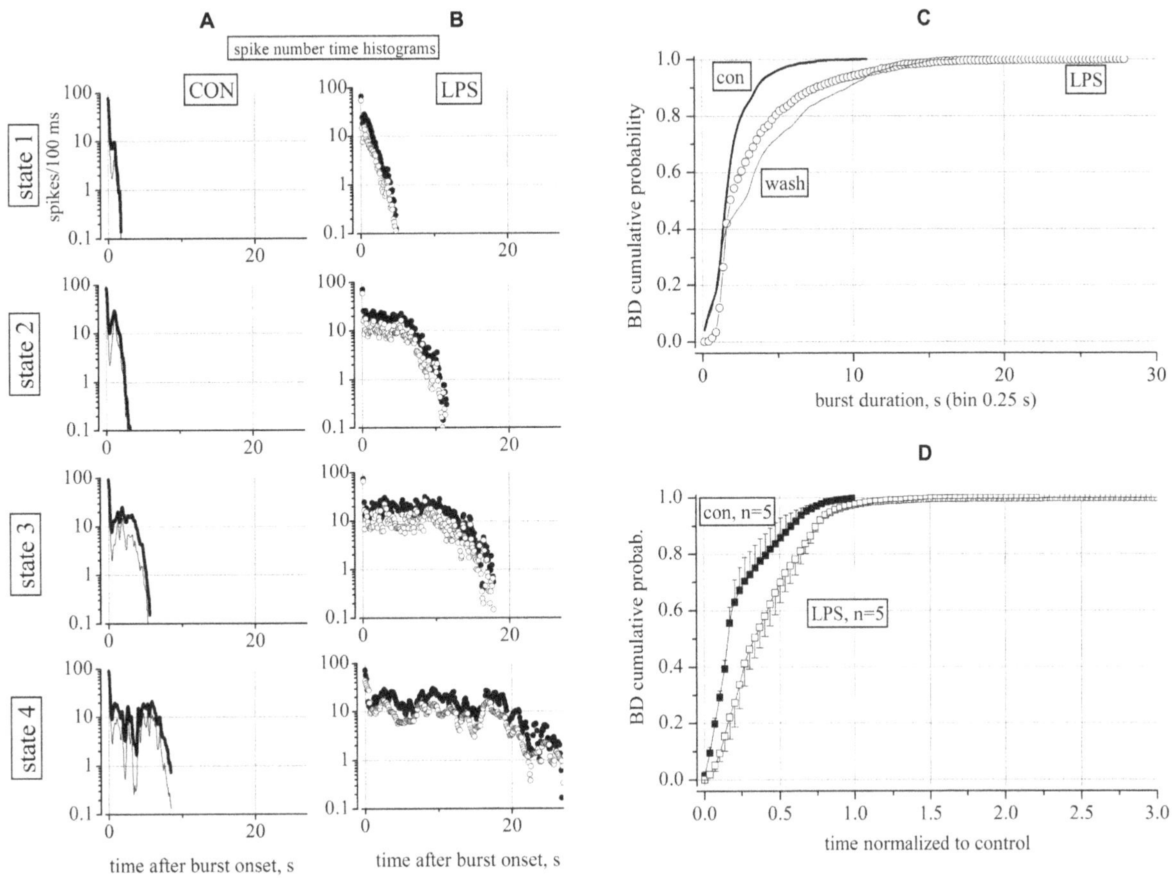

FIGURE 2 | Characterization of reverberating activity recorded in control and 4 h after application of 3 μg/ml LPS. Data (time segments of 2 h) in **(A,B)** show global firing properties during control (CON) and 4 h after application of LPS. **(A,B)** Plots of spike number time histograms (SNTH, spike number/0.1 s bin width: log-scale vs. time after burst onset in seconds) representing properties of bursts classified into four states from up to down. In control and in LPS (in parentheses) the number of events assigned to states 1, 2, 3, and 4 were: 122 (280), 255 (50), 66 (20), and 15 (6). LPS therefore strongly modified the pattern of the burst durations by favoring the large (>10 s) durations in 21% of the bursts as compared to control where all of the durations were below 10 s as shown in detail below in **Figure 3**. **(C)** Superimposed BD cumulative probability plots during control (5 h, thick line), 3 μg/ml LPS (6 h, open circles) and after washout (4 h, thin line). Data from an experiment with 65 excitatory and 26 inhibitory neurons (classified as described in Section "Materials and Methods") respectively. Number of analyzed bursts were 1208 in control, 1421 in LPS and 634 in washout respectively. The non-parametric Kruskal–Wallis statistical significance method gave, for the pairs con/LPS, LPS/wash and con/wash, the following results: $P < 0.0001$, $P < 0.029$, $P < 0.0001$, respectively. **(D)** Cumulative probability of BD averaged from 5 similar experiments done in different dishes after correctly normalizing the control part of each experiment for having a value of 1 and 60 equally spaced bins (error bars are ±SEM). Note that the LPS action on BD distribution was consistently different with respect to control; also for LPS data, after normalization, the time scale had a maximum value three times longer than for control data.

they were the longest from 18 up to 27 s (for details see Figure legend).

Taken together, these results suggest that LPS was able to barely modify the short burst states, but, in contrast, it largely increased the number of spikes of the long-lived atypical bursts compared to the control recording condition. This could indicate that the network (balanced in control and with burst ending on average after 6–7 s), was shifted toward a new steady-state characterized, in both neuronal clusters, by an increased excitability which favored a longer and atypical activity in bursts.

Although the SNTHs shown in **Figures 2A,B** clarified the temporal structure of the bursts in control conditions and in LPS, it was important to check that these results were complemented by an analysis independent from the burst classification method. To this aim, we used a standard cumulative probability analysis of BD as shown in **Figure 2C** for an exemplary experiment in which we could obtain also a tentative washout from LPS. These results were useful to better demonstrate the crucial effects of LPS: (1) in control at relatively long BDs, i.e., ~7 s, ~99% of bursts had BDs smaller than 7 s, (2) but in LPS, only 95% of the bursts had BDs <7 s and the rest of the bursts had longer BDs; (3) in LPS the short (<1 s) BD bursts practically disappeared, but, (4) on washout, the short bursts reappeared but the long ones did not disappeared, suggesting a non-completely washable effect of LPS. Since both the distribution of BD and its cumulative probability were not normal, a non-parametric Kruskal–Wallis statistical analysis (see Materials and Methods) was performed here and will be used in all of the following results. As indicated in the legend of **Figure 2**, this analysis suggests that the LPS data were highly significantly different ($P < 0.0001$) from both control untreated and washout, but control was different from washout with a $P < 0.029$, indicating a lingering action of LPS.

Since in each MEA dish, it was practically impossible to exactly control the precise composition and the amount of cells at div 0, each network started its activity and became mature at slightly different days. This implies also that each dish had different intrinsic properties such as the average values of BD, the IBIs, the total number of neurons and the ratio between the excitatory and inhibitory cells. These and other variables such as the density of astrocytes and microglia normally could in principle, produce different cumulative histograms. To average different experiments it was necessary to normalize the time scales of each LPS experiment to its control and then average data. From 5 independent and successful experiments, we plotted in **Figure 2D** the averaged control data ($n = 5$) of the control time segments (closed squares) and LPS segments (open squares) which proved to be significantly different ($P < 0.0001$). The averaged control "con" data had $P > 0.05$ with respect to each single control experiment, thus suggesting that they were not statistically different after normalization. The same was true for the LPS data.

On the whole, these results point out that the robust modifications in firing activity induced by LPS were long-lasting at least for 4–6 h during washout, although we observed only a weak recovery of short bursts. The data points of the LPS trace illustrate that novel bursts were also present in a BD range in which it was always impossible to capture such bursts during control. On the contrary, in the range from 0 to ~2 s the histograms were hardly different from each others.

LPS DID NOT AFFECT ACTION POTENTIAL WAVEFORM NEITHER IN EXCITATORY NOR IN INHIBITORY NEURONS

The results shown in **Figures 2A,B** suggested that the statistical analysis of the SNTHs in control and in LPS at a concentration of 3 μg/ml, differed dramatically for both neuronal clusters. The diversity was present not only in the BD that was much longer in LPS, but also in the mean SN of the inhibitory clusters, with respect to the excitatory clusters (values of closed symbols were always greater than those of open symbols). This consistent observation suggested to us to investigate in detail both the timing pattern of bursts and the waveforms of the action potentials in both types of clusters. To this aim, we compared the spike timing pattern and their waveforms acquired during control or 8 h after adding LPS, when the effects on excitability had become consistently established. In **Figure 3** we show how spike trains of classified neurons [excitatory (ex) inhibitory (inh)] looked during exemplary events in control and LPS. In a 35 s time-window, the two left (A) and right (D) raster plots (timestamps) show three brief bursts in control and one long burst (separated by a very short interval <3 s) in LPS, respectively. From two different electrodes, we identified two neurons classified as belonging to the excitatory (B,E) and inhibitory (C,F) clusters and we show how their spike trains (vertical lines) contributed differently to the global network burst. In the control windows, B and C, the spikes were rare or abundant according to the different modes of firing of excitatory and inhibitory cells, and the same pattern can also be followed in the companion windows E and F recorded in LPS. To investigate if the spike waveforms were changing from control to LPS, we superimposed the action potential waveforms relative to these bursts (see the insets in B,C and E,F); it is clearly evident that on average, they did not differ. Since no detectable changes were also observed at the level of IBI (the average time between bursts), a variable that is linked to the average probability of starting a burst, it is reasonable to assume that the average resting membrane potential of the engaged neurons was not dramatically affected by LPS, despite their increased propensity toward burst broadening. This observation suggests that the LPS-induced actions on excitability described above were quite subtle, perhaps originating from time-dependent alterations in the properties of voltage-gated ion channels responsible for maintaining the neuronal excitability (see Due et al., 2012); however, this would need to be confirmed in intracellular recording experiments from individual neurons.

THE TIME COURSE OF LPS ACTION

To further investigate the time-course of development of the LPS effects illustrated in **Figures 1** and **2** we re-analyzed some experiments by dividing the control and the LPS periods into shorter half-hour segments in order to check if during briefer periods of time, there were relevant fluctuations that were averaged out when longer segments were used. At the same time, a half-hour sampling had the advantage of verifying the exact time course of the changes introduced by LPS. This opened the possibility that some of the long bursts observed in control could be confounded or

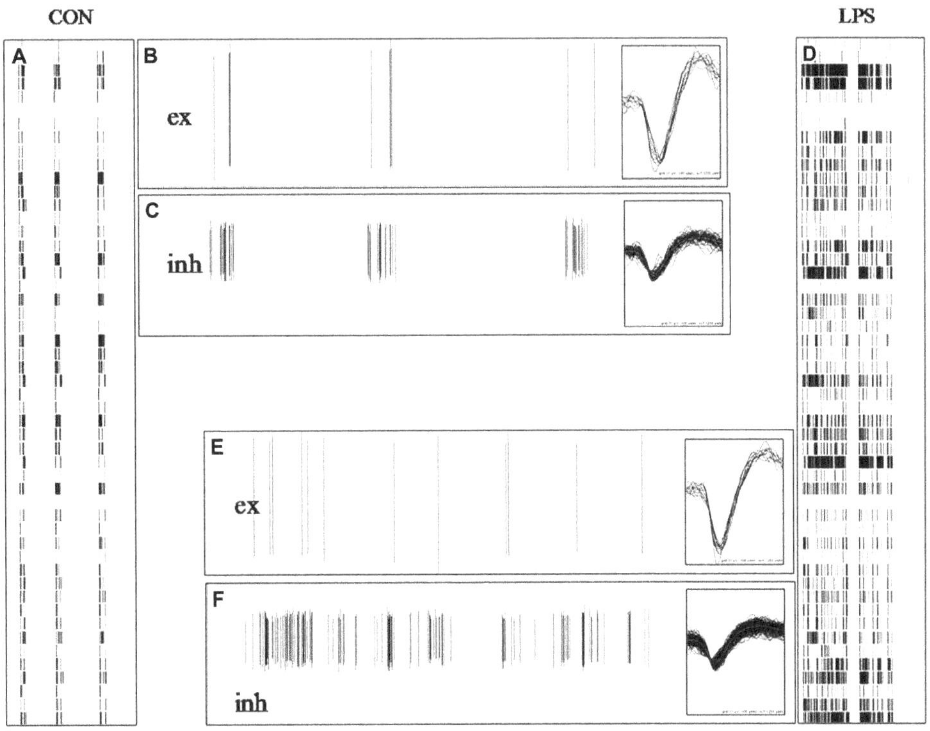

FIGURE 3 | Lipopolysaccharide did not affect action potential waveform neither in excitatory nor in inhibitory neurons. (A,D) 35 s-long windows in which are shown raster plots of timestamps of normal and atypical burst in control (CON) and 6 h after adding LPS (each point in a column contains data from one electrode). In **(A)** are present three brief bursts and in **(B)** one long burst in LPS (identified as one single up-state because the short; <3 s) inter-spike interval was well below the average IBI value of ~15 s. **(B,C,E,F)** 35 s-long windows showing plots of spike amplitude (vertical lines) vs. time in control and during LPS for identified excitatory **(B,E)** and inhibitory **(C,F)** neurons in two different electrodes. The number of identified excitatory and inhibitory cells was 69 and 24, respectively. The insets associated with **(B,C,E,F)** show the superimposed spikes recorded in the respective windows and their vertical and horizontal dimensions correspond to +62/−93 μV and 1.2 ms, respectively.

blurred with those observed during the LPS application. Furthermore, we wanted also to verify if briefer segments of control data could be considered statistically indistinguishable among themselves, and also to verify that the same concept was valid for the LPS-data when the action of the drug reached its final maximum steady-state level.

The BD data are shown as points in the time plot of **Figure 4A** where the tentative fitting to an analytical function describing drug onset time-course is shown by the red superimposed line. We found that the fitting of these data to an exponential relationship allowed us to suggest that the process really consists of a delayed exponential, namely $y = \exp - (t - \tau_0)/\tau_{LPS}$, where τ_0 and τ_{LPS} are the delay and LPS action time constants found to be ~1.5 and ~2.3 h, respectively. In conclusion, and taking into account the other successful experiments, we found that LPS, at a concentration of 3 μg/ml, was able to produce a considerable and significant increase in the BD duration in the neuronal cultures.

Given the fact that we never observed any significant change in the spike waveform in the presence of LPS (see **Figure 3**), we wanted to examine how these effects on BD could be interpreted at the level of neuronal excitability. Since in our experiments, we continuously sampled the same set of neurons, we could count the number of spikes elicited by each engaged cell during each burst. This analysis is shown at the same half-hour resolution in **Figure 4B** for the two clusters of neurons. The plot illustrates that excitatory and inhibitory cells behaved in a very different manner, the former class being much less active than the latter class, possibly indicating that they were under a strong "braking" influence from local inhibitory neurons as already shown in Gullo et al., 2010). A further interesting analysis is shown in **Figure 4C** where we normalized the previous data by the control values (averaged) to remove the different firing modes and this showed that despite their different background levels of activity, both clusters behaved similarly in the presence of LPS ($P > 0.05$, $n = 150$). We did not observe any other change in the activity properties like IBI, except for an obvious increase in mean SR of inhibitory and excitatory (in parenthesis) clusters which changed from 1.44 ± 0.08 ($n = 26$) [0.37 ± 0.03, ($n = 65$)] in control to 1.82 ± 0.15 ($n = 26$) [0.48 ± 0.06 ($n = 65$)] in LPS at the experiment end after 7 h. This finding suggests that the LPS action on the neuronal culture resembled a change of the working "set point" of the network activity as previously proposed to explain homeostatic plasticity (for a review see Turrigiano and Nelson, 2004).

To test the random BD changes observed during each half-hour segment, we did the complete study of the statistical significance of the BD data in this exemplary experiment whose behavior is illustrated in **Figures 4A–C** by using the Kruskal–Wallis test

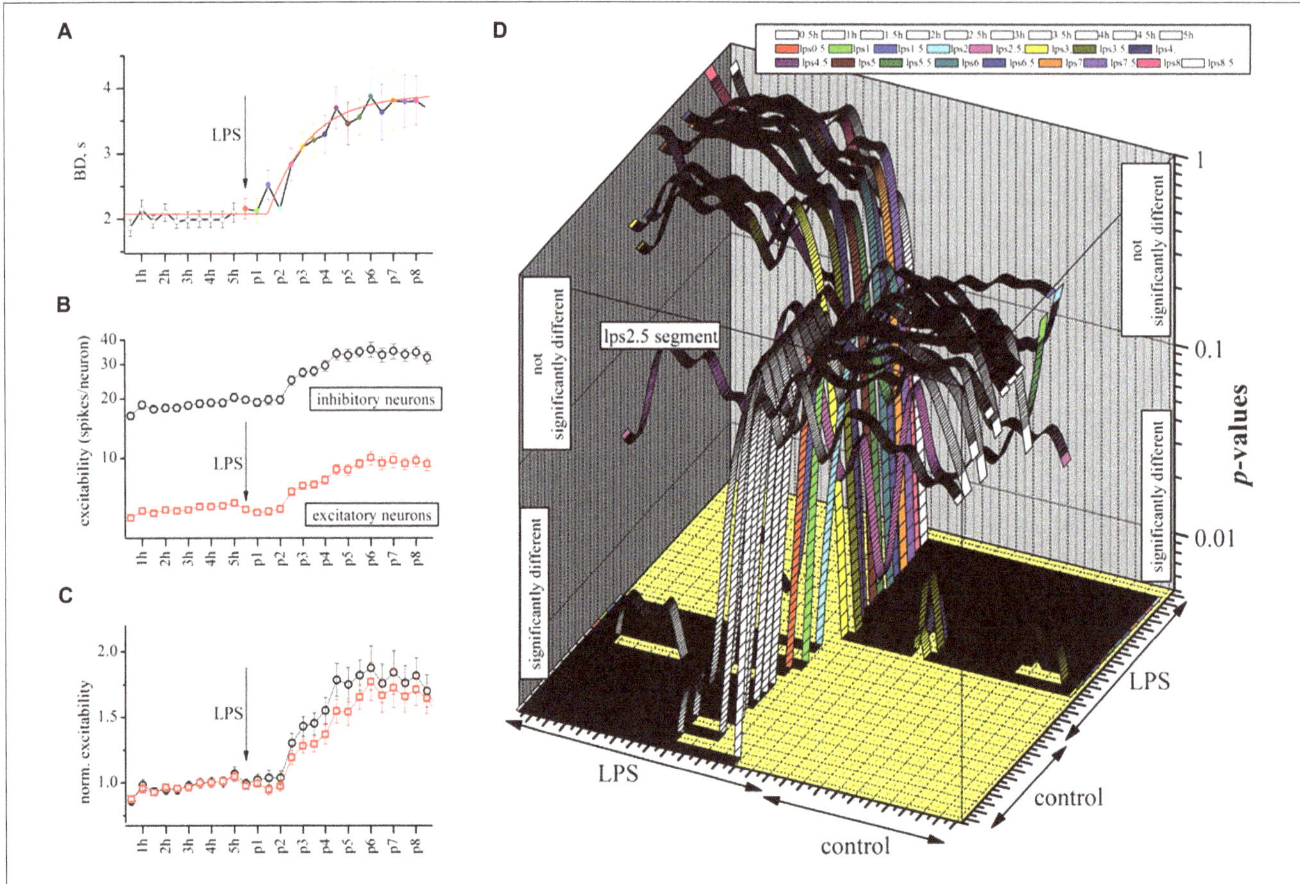

FIGURE 4 | The delayed excitatory action of LPS studied at a half-hour resolution by analyzing BD and engaged excitatory and inhibitory neuron excitability. (A) Plot of BD in an exemplary experiment where time was divided into half-hour segments (10 in control and 16 during LPS). The red line is the best fit to an exponential function of the following type: fit line $= 2.07 + 1.9^{*}[1 - \exp[-(x - \tau_d)/\tau_{LPS}]]$, where τ_d and τ_{LPS} are in seconds and represent the delay (5250 ± 970 s, $n = 13$) and the LPS onset time constant (8355 ± 2980 s, $n = 13$) which characterized the drug action, respectively. **(B)** For the same experiment, plot of excitability, defined as the average number of spikes elicited by engaged neurons in the same cluster in each up-state (red and black for excitatory and inhibitory cells). **(C)** For the same experiment, the data shown in **(C)** but normalized to the mean control data for each cluster (black and red symbols for inhibitory and excitatory neurons, respectively). Note the slow time course of excitability increase was similar in both neuron types. **(D)** 3D graph where each ribbon is the *P*-value of significance plotted vs. 27 time segments in the exemplary experiment of **(A–C)**. There are 27 such ribbons plotted in order to evaluate all of the 702 (but those significant were 351) multiple pairwise (those identical were omitted) comparisons to compute the statistical significance by the non-parametric Kruskal–Wallis test (Dunn analysis, Bonferroni correction). Each ribbon is for each 0.5 h segment (open ribbon for control, colored ribbons for LPS data). Control (before) and LPS regions (succeeding) are indicated. Since the vertical axis of the *P*-values is in the form of a log-scale whose middle point is 0.05, all the regions where ribbons are above or below 0.05 represent non significant or significant comparisons, respectively. The time segment "lps2.5" that is in between control and steady-state LPS segments resulted in a "strange" shape. The data show that during control and well after LPS application, the BD data are significantly similar; however, during the development of the LPS action, they slowly (after each half hour) changed consistently to the differences shown in **Figures 3A–C**.

(see Materials and Methods). To do so, we computed all of the *P*-values amongst all the sub-segments, both in control and during the action of LPS. In **Figure 4D**, these data are shown in a 3D graph where, on the z-axis, are plotted the *P*-values of the BD statistical analysis originating from the 27 time segments (0.5 h each) of this exemplary experiment (for a total of 351 comparisons, see legend). We found that all the segments in control (10, open symbols) and the first four LPS segments had highly similar properties, i.e., P-values $>>0.05$ before LPS and $<<0.05$ after LPS, suggesting that the BDs slowly shifted from the properties they had in control to a new stationary and significantly different longer mode. Conversely, when we examined the BD data in the LPS region, the behavior was symmetrical and opposite.

Lipopolysaccharide was not used at higher concentrations because it has been recently shown that at 10 μg/ml, other remarkable effects lead to apoptosis (Nimmervoll et al., 2012). Another 10 experiments performed at lower LPS concentrations of 1 μg/ml produced data that were either transient (3 out of 10) or subject to the intrinsic variability among different dishes (3 out of 10) and therefore were not sufficiently stable and trustable to be analyzed further. At a concentration of 0.3 μg/ml, only one experiment out of 5 was successful (not shown). The slowly developing LPS action described here is completely different from the fast action of any agonist or antagonist of voltage-gated ion channels or excitatory/inhibitory neurotransmitter receptors tested on MEA culture dishes (Gullo et al., 2009, 2010, 2012; Puia et al., 2012).

LPS EFFECTS CAN BE BLOCKED BY NANOMOLAR CONCENTRATIONS OF MINOCYCLINE

Minocycline, a semi-synthetic second generation tetracycline analog, has been extensively used therapeutically as an anti-inflammatory agent (for a recent review see Tikka et al., 2001; Filipovic and Zecevic, 2008; Henry et al., 2008; Garrido-Mesa et al., 2013) and also possesses neuroprotective and anticonvulsant properties (Beheshti Nasr et al., 2013; Dodd et al., 2013). Since our LPS experiments had a duration of 8–10 h, we decided to test MC at one of the lowest concentrations used by Tikka et al. (2001) in mixed spinal cord cultures, namely 50 nM. Since preliminary experiments at high concentrations of MC (3 μM) caused a persistent and irreversible strong *decrease* of neuronal activity (not shown), indicating an unwanted possibly toxic action, we wanted to control the MC putative intrinsic activity on our networks by performing some preliminary dose-response experiments as shown in **Figures 5B,C**.

We applied increasing concentrations of MC from 10 nM up to 3 μM to obtain a dose-response curve during short time segments (30, 20, and 10 min). In **Figures 5A–C** we plotted the BD cumulative histograms, the excitability and the IBI data recorded during a 6 h period which started with control (untreated) and finished with the washout. As shown in **Figures 5B,C**, the smallest concentration of 10 nM MC caused both a decrease of excitability and a smaller IBI which, taken together, resulted in a small (but non-significant) *increase* in global spiking rate (SR, not shown) which seems counter-intuitive.

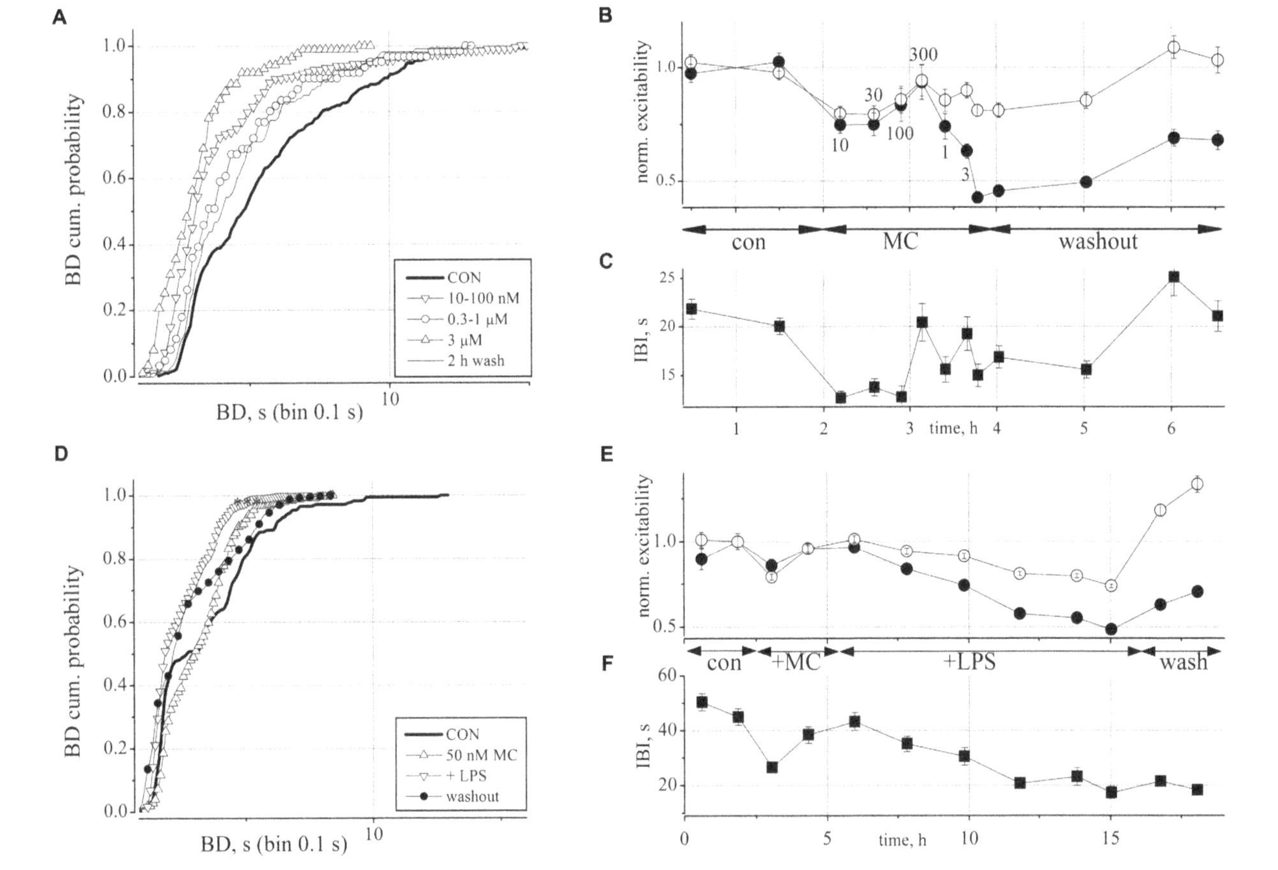

FIGURE 5 | Minocycline (MC) dose-response relationship and its antagonistic action toward the effects of LPS on neuronal excitability. (A) Plot of superimposed BD cumulative probability histograms in control (thick line), in 10–30–100 nM MC (inverted triangles), in 0.3–1 μM MC (circles), in 3 μM MC (upward triangles), and after 2 h of washout (thin line). Statistical significance was assessed on the cumulative probability data by Kruskal–Wallis method (*$P < 0.05$; ***$P < 0.0001$; $^{-}P > 0.05$) according to the following matrix-table that illustrates in a compact form the 10 P-values among all the possible combinations of the different probability curves (see **Table 1**). **(B)** Plot of the normalized excitability of identified excitatory/inhibitory neurons (open/closed symbols). Notice that the effects of the highest MC dose persisted for more than 1 h during washout. The small numbers near symbols indicate the increasing concentrations of MC. **(C)** Plot of IBI vs. time. Notice an early IBI decrease effect at the lowest MC dose. **(D)** Plot of superimposed BD cumulative probability histograms in control (thick line), in 50 nM MC (2 h, upward triangles), after adding 3 μg/ml LPS (10.5 h, inverted triangles), and after 2 h of washout (closed circles). This exemplary representative experiment is similar to other four experiments and shows that only small, i.e., <100 nM doses of MC produce small and transient (<1 h) and recoverable effects on the network activity. Number of analyzed bursts in control, +MC, +LPS and washout were 176, 250, 1300, and 405, respectively. Statistical significance was assessed on the cumulative probability data by Kruskal–Wallis method as follows: CON vs. MC $P < 0.001$; CON vs. LPS $P < 0.0001$; CON vs. WASH $P < 0.0001$; LPS vs. WASH, MC vs. WASH, LPS vs. MC $P > 0.05$. **(E)** Plot of the normalized excitability for identified excitatory (open circles) and inhibitory neurons (closed circles). **(F)** Plot of IBI vs. time.

Table 1 | The 10 *P*-values mentioned in the Figure 5A legend as Table 1.

	Con	10–100 nM	0.3–1 μM	3 μM
Con				
MC 10–100 nM	*			
MC 0.3–1 μM	*	–		
MC 3 μM	***	***	***	
2 h wash	*	–	–	***

This observation obviously suggests that in our cultured reverberating networks (and putatively in *in vivo* recordings during synchronized spontaneous activity or during sleep, see Discussion) the global activity is controlled by two distinct and functionally independent mechanisms: namely, burst activity (with BD duration) among neurons connected by glutamatergic and GABAergic synapses, with their different properties and therefore subject to different pathways leading to the burst onset and end and, in contrast, the IBIs characterized by quasi-silent periods in which all cells are temporarily hyperpolarized and recovering from the previous excessive firing activity (synaptic fatigue, slow voltage-gated ion channel inactivation, slow metabotropic neurotransmitter action, etc). Indeed, on average, SR (spike/s, a variable computed independently from BD and IBI definition) is proportional to excitability (spikes during the burst), but inversely proportional to IBI (because in IBI there are no spikes elicited). Thus, any excitability change with no IBI change leads obviously to the same SR change. On the contrary, if the excitability decrease is accompanied by a proportionally larger IBI decrease as shown in panel C, the effect on SR can result in a counter-intuitive increase (we show below in **Figures 6D–F** other counter-intuitive results). Since in the two clusters, SRs originate from different excitabilities of different numbers of neurons, we always found that in CNS networks, the average SR of the inhibitory cluster was higher than the SR of the excitatory neuron cluster (Gullo et al., 2010).

This effect persisted up to a concentration of 100 nM but recovered at 300 nM MC where both variables had the values seen in control. Since the successively higher concentrations of MC produced a further decrease in excitability and BD that was difficult to washout (see at the fifth hour), we interpreted the initial, but recoverable effects as a momentary disturbance that the network compensated by its own homeostasis. This was confirmed by the BD cumulative analysis of the data shown in **Figure 5A** (superimposed curves). In the plot, it is possible to follow the data in control (thick line) and the slow left-shift of the curves (symbols) during the increasing MC concentrations (see meaning of different symbols in the legend) and the final washout (thin line) which returned back toward the control curve.

In conclusion, we learned from these experiments that at very low concentrations, the putative early intrinsic action of MC should not interfere with other drugs working at a much slower rate. On the contrary, the specific inhibitory action of MC at higher concentrations on the excitability of inhibitory neurons and not on excitatory cells suggested that at these high concentrations the action was clearly not negligible. The fast but recoverable action of MC we observed will certainly need further investigation in the future.

In order to test whether the excitatory action of LPS could be blocked by MC, we pre-incubated the networks with 50 nM MC for 2 h, and then added LPS, in order to exclude the transient effects of MC mentioned above. The experiments were analyzed similarly to those shown in **Figures 2** and **3** and one exemplary test (out of 5) is illustrated in **Figures 5D–F**. We found that after pre-treatment with MC, LPS no longer produced rightward shifts of the BD probability to indicate significant BD increases ($n = 5$; cf. **Figures 2C,D**). This is shown in **Figure 5D** where, after a 4 h recording in control conditions, 50 nM MC was added and 2 h later, 3 μg/ml LPS was added on top. After 12 h, we washed out the dish for 3 further hours of recording. Although the BD probability plot of **Figure 5D** showed that control data (continuous thick line) were statistically different ($P < 0.0001$) from those obtained in MC (upward triangles), in LPS (inverted triangles) and in washout (thin line), all these last curves were positioned to the left of the control line, and this fact is the opposite of what we reported in **Figures 2C,D** for LPS alone. Moreover, these last three curves were not significantly different from control ($P > 0.05$, using the Kruskal–Wallis test). In **Figures 5E,F** are shown the details of excitability and IBI during an exemplary experiment lasting more than 18 h. The transient depressant effect of MC addition, seen in **Figures 5B,C** is barely visible in excitability, but clearly evident in IBI, which decreased from 45 ± 3.2 s to 26 ± 1.8 s (and SR that increased (excitatory cell in parenthesis) from 1.02 ± 0.15, ($n = 19$) [0.24 ± 0.025,($n = 60$)] Hz up to 1.38 ± 0.25 Hz, ($n = 19$) [0.30 ± 0.031, ($n = 60$)] not shown. The addition of LPS was followed over ~10 h, and a weak (~0.75 and ~0.5 for inhibitory and excitatory clusters, respectively) *decrease* in excitability and IBI (by a factor of ~0.5) can be observed before network washout where excitability recovered, but not IBI. Thus, in conclusion the average SR did not significantly change.

Minocycline, at the same concentration, was tested also in some dishes 7–8 h after the LPS application, but no consistent excitability decrease was evident, apart from the fast but transient negative jump already described above in **Figures 5E,F**. We thus conclude that MC at 50 nM was able to effectively inhibit the slow excitability increase produced by LPS, without significantly altering the other properties of the network activity.

EFFECTS OF CYTOKINE (TNF-α), PURINERGIC ANTAGONIST (PPADS), ANTICONVULSANT CARBAMAZEPINE (CBZ) AND NEUROPROTECTANT THALIDOMIDE

Brain inflammation is characterized by activation of CNS-resident microglia and astrocytes, and it is supposed that these cell types express, release and respond to cytokines (Allan et al., 2005). Indeed, it was suggested in 2002 that glial cells constitutively release the cytokine TNF-α (Beattie et al., 2002) and it was also shown that "synaptic scaling" was dependent on the same cytokine exogenously applied (Stellwagen and Malenka, 2006). On the contrary, it is now clear from transcriptome analysis of purified astrocytes, that this cytokine is only released from microglia (for a review see Béchade et al., 2013). Therefore, we did some tests and verification experiments to determine if our multi-site electrophysiology

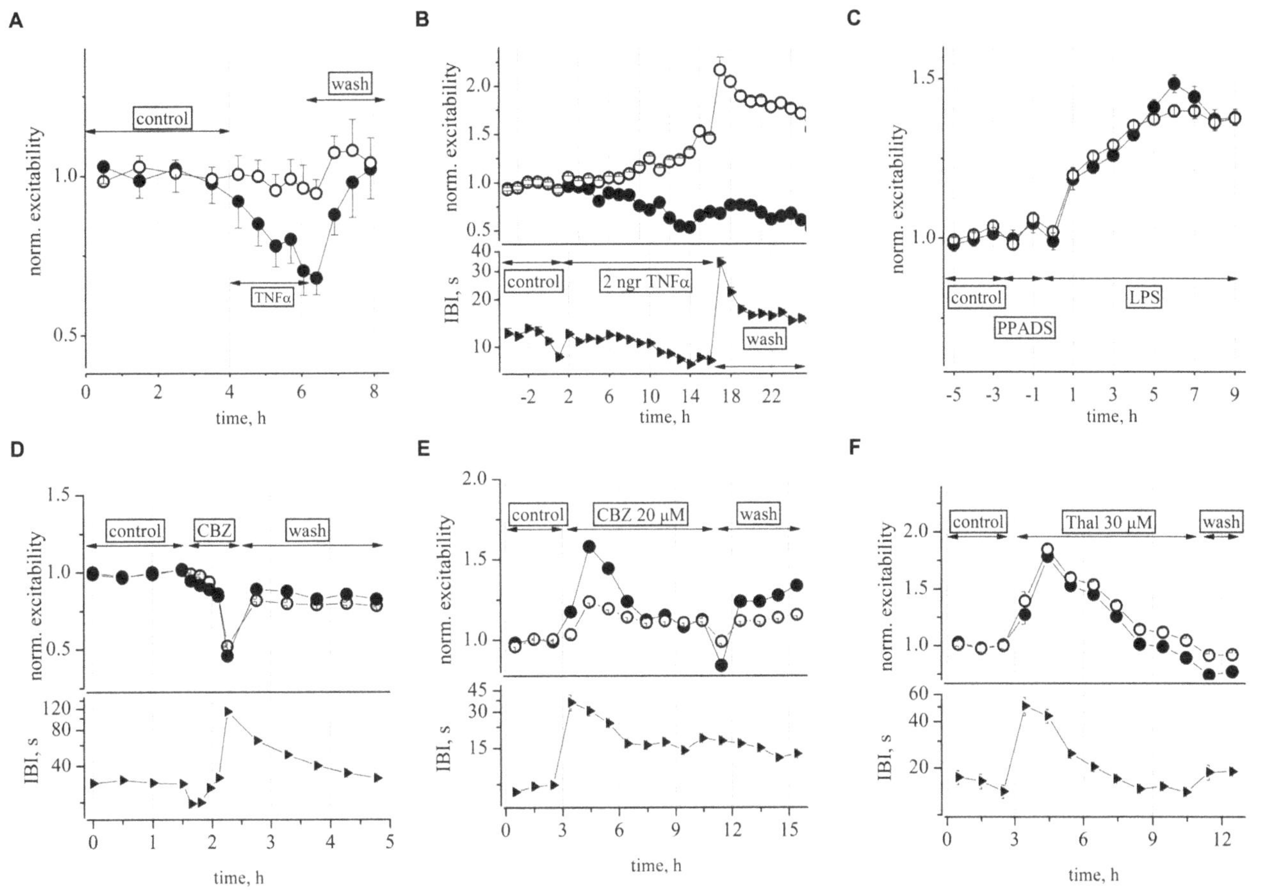

FIGURE 6 | Effects of TNF-α, PPADS, carbamazepine, and thalidomide on neuronal excitability. (A) Plot of normalized excitability (relative to control) in an exemplary dose-response 2 h experiment in which increasing concentrations of TNF-α from 10 to 300 pM [see arrows labeled TNF-α, 10 (15 min), 20 (15 min), 60 (25 min), 100 (25 min), 300 pM (15 min)] were applied to a culture while recording from a network of 95 excitatory and 19 inhibitory identified neurons, respectively. No effects were seen on IBI (not shown). **(B)** Plot of normalized excitability (upper) and IBI (lower) vs. time after addition of a single dose of TNF-α see line with arrows and the 60 pM TNF-α label. Notice the slow build-up of an unbalanced neuronal activity characterized by higher and lower excitability in both excitatory and inhibitory neuronal clusters, respectively. According to **(A)** experiment, we expected a small excitability decrease for inhibitory cells, but notice that here the averaging time is longer (3600 s for each symbol) than that of **(A)** (~900 s). Although it can be seen that ~3 h after washout, the excitability during the up-states resulted consistently changed, the network SR was not significantly altered. The mean IBI values during TNF-α were not significantly different from control (12.2 ± 0.2 vs. 15.4 ± 1 s, $n = 21$). A network of 70 excitatory and 21 inhibitory identified neurons were recorded, respectively. **(C)** Plot of normalized excitability in control, after the addition of PPADS (50 μM) and the subsequent co-addition of LPS at 3 μg/ml. Network of 86 and 17 excitatory and inhibitory identified neurons, respectively. Note that PPADS did not prevent the excitatory effect of LPS. **(D)** Plot of normalized excitability (upper) and IBI (lower) vs. time for increasing doses of CBZ (1, 3, 10, 30, and 100 μM) and the subsequent washout. Network of 91 excitatory and 37 inhibitory identified neurons, respectively. **(E)** Plot of excitability (upper) and IBI (lower) after the addition of a single dose of CBZ at 20 μM. Notice that the IBI change preceded and outlasted the excitability changes. Network of 99 and 47 excitatory and inhibitory identified neurons, respectively (see explanation in text). **(F)** Plot of excitability (upper) and IBI (lower) after the addition of thalidomide (THAL) at 30 μM. Notice again that the IBI change preceded the excitability change by ~1 h. Network of 121 and 27 excitatory and inhibitory identified neurons, respectively.

was able to detect a change in neuronal excitability in response to exogenously applied TNF-α.

Preliminary dose-response experiments suggested that 1 h-long exposures to TNF-α at concentrations in the picomolar range (from 10 to 300 pM, steps: 10, 20, 60, 100, 300), produced a net *decrease* of the inhibitory neuron excitability with no evident effects on excitatory cells as shown in **Figure 6A**. These data, obtained during brief successive dose-steps in a network free of any other drugs, suggest that the cytokine action was relatively fast and the effect of the highest concentration tested was completely washable after a few hours. No changes were present in the down-state duration, i.e., IBI ($n = 3$). On the contrary, in long-term experiments (2 h of control + 15 h in TNF-α + 8 h of recovery), a single application of a small TNF-α concentration (60 pM), produced a delayed and non-washable response characterized by a slow excitability increase in the excitatory neuronal cluster and a decrease in the inhibitory cluster. This is shown in **Figure 6B**, where the excitability data for excitatory and inhibitory neuronal clusters (upper) is shown together with the IBI change (lower). The washout was characterized by a partial 3 h-recovery, and in the further 5 h, the activity during the bursts remained substantially hyperexcitable because the excitatory neurons were more active, probably as a consequence of the lower excitability of inhibitory cells. TNF-α at this low dose, therefore partially mimicked the excitatory action of LPS but this was only apparent on the excitatory neuron clusters and prolonged atypical "seizure-like" burst episodes were not present.

It is now recognized that endogenous adenosine triphosphate (ATP) and ATP (purinergic) receptors play an important role in regulating microglial function, and in particular, the release of cytokines in the brain (Shieh et al., 2014). We therefore performed two experiments designed to investigate the putative role of purinergic receptors in our LPS-induced responses shown above (Pascual et al., 2012). Contrary to our expectation, as shown in **Figure 6C**, pre-conditioning the network with the non-selective P2X receptor antagonist PPADS (50 μM), did not prevent the LPS effects, suggesting that a modulatory effect of endogenous ATP on microglia was not involved.

Next, we were interested to examine the effects of other drugs as putative substitutes of MC as blockers of the LPS effects and tested the effects of the anticonvulsant drug carbamazepine (CBX) and of THAL, also a powerful anticonvulsant (Palencia et al., 2011) and anti-hyperalgesic (Cata et al., 2008). Both agents were tested first for their effects on neuronal excitability. A cumulative CBZ dose-response relation (1, 3, 10, 30, and 100 μM), performed in about 2 h, is shown in **Figure 6D** where a progressively *depressant* action on excitability is clearly evident up to the almost complete silencing of activity at 100 μM. On the contrary, when CBZ or THAL were applied on ultra-long time scales of more than 10 h, as a single dose of 20 and 30 μM, respectively, the actions were *excitatory* but only transient (about 2 h, decaying time constant about 2–3 h, see **Figures 6E,F**) and thereafter the network homeostatically recovered toward its quasi-normal equilibrium level of firing.

After the drug additions, the first effect was a strong and persistent IBI increase (by fourfold for more than 2 h), followed by a delayed hyperexcitability during the bursting activity. These early and late effects may be putatively explained as follows: (1) the initial fast action was probably caused by a generalized hyperpolarization of the resting membrane potential of neurons, with the consequence that fluctuations in their normal "baseline" activity could only rarely attain an amplitude exceeding action potential threshold (leading to the burst onset); (2) the delayed hyperexcitability (more pronounced in inhibitory cells in CBZ) persisted during firing sustained by the putative drug-induced effects on synaptic connectivity and/or ion channel properties. These results led us to conclude that: (1) CBZ concentrations as low as 20 μM (when briefly applied) did not apparently produce remarkable effects, but when applied at steady-state, they caused transient and non-washable long-term effects which were different in the two neuron clusters. In conclusion, the drug cannot be considered useful as a blocker of the very slow LPS effects; (2) likewise for THAL, the data in **Figure 6F** suggest considerations similar to those explained for CBZ: namely, that the drug was acting on time scales and pathways that competed with those activated by LPS, and thus any putative results obtained with it in combination would not clarify the LPS-induced effects in the same manner as shown for MC.

THE COEXISTENCE OF NEURONS, ASTROCYTES AND MICROGLIA AND THE LPS-INDUCED TNF-α RELEASE IN THE *EX VIVO* LONG-TERM CULTURED NEOCORTICAL NETWORKS

Finally, two different approaches were used to characterize the cortical cell cultures and to evaluate the microglial population in control and LPS-treated networks: immunofluorescence and tomato lectin cytochemistry methods. The identification of the MAP2-positive neuronal component (**Figures 7A,A'**) showed neurons distributed on the coverslips forming clusters with long dendritic processes. Numerous astroglial cells positive for GFAP (**Figures 7C,C'**) homogeneously surrounded this cortical neuronal network (**Figures 7D,D'**, merge). b-LEA+ microglial cells were scattered in the same fields (**Figures 7B,B'**). In control cultures (i.e., not LPS treated), both ramified resting and amoeboid/activated round microglial cells (Saura, 2007; Kettenmann et al., 2011) were observed (**Figure 7B**). In LPS-treated cultures, b-LEA+ microglial cells appeared more numerous than in control cultures, they showed a predominant round morphology and appeared concentrated in clusters (**Figure 7B'**). The total number of b-LEA+ cells in each examined culture was rather homogeneous both in control and in the LPS group. However, a significant difference was demonstrated by the statistical comparison of the two sets of samples, showing an increase of microglial population after LPS treatment in cell cultures. A quantitative statistical analysis, performed on non-overlapping fields ($n = 32$ for each control and LPS sample, see Materials and Methods), suggests that average microglial cell counts in control (650 cells) and in LPS-treated (852 cells) samples were 18.15 ± 0.98 and 23.75 ± 1.53, respectively (Student's t-test, $P < 0.01$, $n = 32$). Taken together, these results demonstrate that the cells cultured on MEAs include microglia, astrocytes and neurons and that LPS induces a functional increase in the microglial population as expected.

In order to test in our *ex vivo* neocortical networks, the functional state of microglia during the LPS-induced activity and under a MC-pretreatment, we decided to evaluate, by standard ELISA techniques (see Materials and Methods), the release of TNF-α, a cytokine that is universally considered as an index of microglia activation. Nakamura et al. (1999) originally showed that cultured microglia derived from neonatal rats, when stimulated by LPS concentrations as low as 1 μg/ml, release TNF-α with a 1 h lag time; later, interleukins were released and after ~6 h, NO. In primary retinal microglia cultures, similar effects of LPS were described and in addition, it was shown that MC pretreatment completely blocked the cytokine release (Wang et al., 2005).

To gain insight into the time-course of the LPS-induced cytokine release by microglia in our cultures, we collected from culture media, small aliquots before ($t = 0$) and after microglia activation. To perform the measurements, we used a total of 11 MEA dishes; six were treated with LPS alone, and five were pretreated with MC to check its inhibiting role. The results of our experiments are shown in **Figure 8** where the time-course of the TNF-α concentration is plotted vs. time (open symbols) and with MC pre-treatment (50 nM, 1 h: closed symbols). LPS induced a significant increase in mean TNF-α level at 3, 6, and 12 h (peak) post-LPS treatment, relative to control untreated conditions (where the TNF-α level was very small and at the limit of

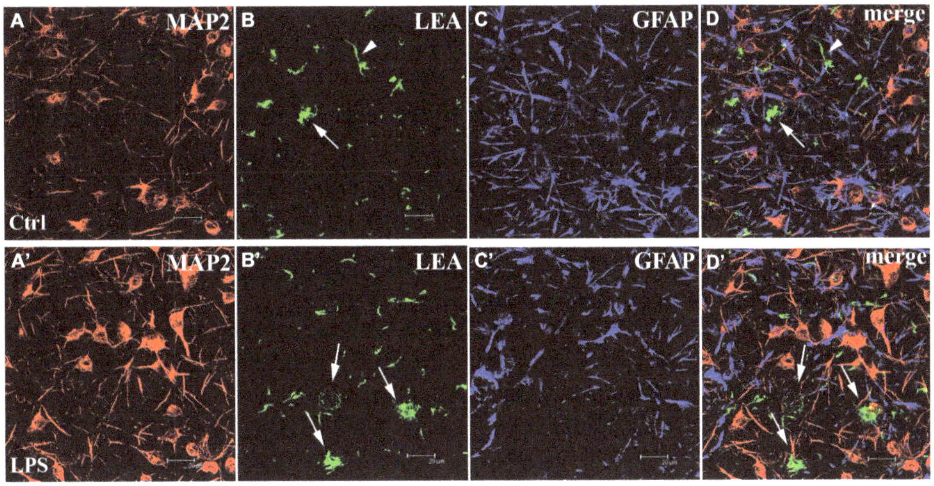

FIGURE 7 | The cortical networks are a mixture of neurons, astrocytes and microglia. (Upper panels) Untreated control (Ctrl) culture **(A–D)**. (Lower panels) LPS-treated (LPS) culture **(A′–D′)**. From left to right, confocal microscopical analysis of triple fluorescence staining for: (1) MAP2 (neuronal marker, red signal, **A,A′**), (2) b-LEA lectin cytochemistry (microglial marker, green signal, **B,B′**), (3) GFAP (astroglial marker, blue signal, **C,C′**), (4) **(D,D′)**: merged image of triple labeling. b-LEA lectin-positive (+) cells exhibited both ramified (arrowheads in **B**,**D**, merge) and round amoeboid morphology (arrows in **B,B′,D,D′**) and were sparsely interspersed among MAP2+ neurons and GFAP+ astrocytes. Amoeboid b-LEA lectin+ cells were more frequently observed after LPS treatment (compare **B,B′**) than in controls. Different cell populations in cortical cultures at DIV13. Note that the number of *neurons* in the different pictures was not related to the LPS action. Scale bars: 20 μm.

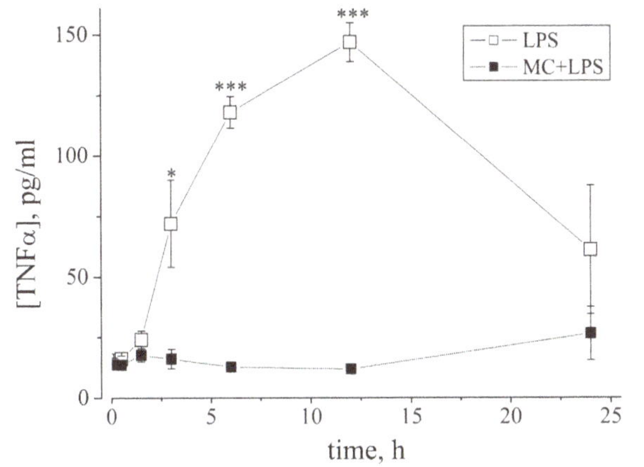

FIGURE 8 | The cytokine TNF-α is released from LPS-treated networks but not from MC-pre-treated networks. Graph shows the time-course of changes of TNF-α concentration (ordinate: expressed as pg/ml, see Materials and Methods) vs. time (abscissa: hours), measured from neuronal network culture media, induced by LPS (3 μg/ml) without (open squares) or with (closed squares) MC preconditioning (50 nM, 1 h). Aliquots were collected at different time points (30, 90 min, 3, 6, 12, and 24 h) and assayed with a TNF-α ELISA kit. As shown by asterisks, open square data for LPS alone (mean ± SEM, $n = 5$) were statistically different from data obtained after MC-preconditioning at 3 h with $*P < 0.015$, and at 6 and 12 h, with $***P < 0.0001$.

detection of the method). On the whole, these results indicate that quasi-simultaneously with the prolonged neuronal excitability changes described above, the TNF-α concentration also grew over a similar time-course with respect to control. In 1/6 LPS-experiments, the TNF-α concentration increase was not observed (not shown). Our results thus confirm the functional activation of microglia in our cultures and its LPS-synchronized and MC-sensitive link. It should however be noted, that the peak amplitude of the TNF-α level attained (corresponding to ~3 pM) is far from that necessary to produce the neuronal effects shown in **Figure 6B**, which were seen at 60 pM of exogenous TNF-α.

DISCUSSION

LPS INDUCES LONG-TERM ULTRA-SLOW CHANGES IN NETWORK EXCITABILITY

This study shows that the earlier steps of microglia-induced neuroinflammation induced by LPS can modulate network activity by producing a very slow change of the average firing properties of both excitatory and inhibitory neuronal clusters observed during burst events (without any apparent effect on burst rate), eventually leading to the appearance of abnormally long and atypical "seizure-like" activity in the network. Since the effect was occluded by the anti-inflammatory agent MC at nanomolar concentrations (shown to inhibit activation and proliferation of microglia, see Tikka et al., 2001), we suggest that the hyperexcitability effects are directly mediated by a complement of microglia-released factors (including TNF-α, as we have now demonstrated by ELISA assays; see below) released by LPS in our system, although the exact nature of all these factors and the mechanisms by which they subtly interact to alter cell-firing behavior are currently unclear. Nevertheless, we found that a purinergic antagonist was unable to occlude the LPS-induced effects, supporting a model probably not linked to astrocyte-mediated activity and release of endogenous ATP.

In our exogenous TNF-α-assay experiments in **Figure 6B**, using small non-saturating concentrations of TNF-α (60 pM), we did not reproduce the action of LPS, but instead, we found an un-washable ultra-slow dynamic effect of increasing/decreasing excitability of excitatory/inhibitory neurons, respectively. These data are in agreement with the *in vivo* inhibiting action of exogenous TNF-α injection on kainic acid-induced seizures in mice (Balosso et al., 2005), and with *in vitro* data obtained in rat hippocampal slices, with 100 nM applied TNF-α (Tancredi et al., 1992). The possible mechanisms underlying these TNF-α effects and the role of different MC preconditioning will be further investigated in future experiments.

Clearly, TNF-α *alone*, at the very low pM levels released by LPS in our cultures could not be responsible for the excitability changes we observed. However, it is worth noting that this cytokine has previously been shown to control basal synaptic functions such as plasticity (Stellwagen and Malenka, 2006), attributed to endogenous release by astrocytes, but these cells do not release this cytokine, which is only released by activated microglia (Lehnardt et al., 2002). Stellwagen et al. (2005), also studied the neuronal effects of applying TNF-α in hippocampal cultures and slices but used brief, 15 min, applications at 100 ng/ml (i.e., 2 nM, see the erratum to the Stellwagen et al., 2005 paper appeared in J. Neurosci. Jun 1; 25(22): 1 p following 5454) and demonstrated a differential regulation characterized by synaptic AMPA (α-amino-3-hydroxy-5-methyl-4-isoxazolepropionic acid)-type glutamate receptor (AMPAR) trafficking and $GABA_AR$ internalization, both by using immunocytochemistry techniques and miniature excitatory/inhibitory synaptic data. Similar applications of TNF-α (but only up to 300 pM), were also performed in our dose-response experiments shown in **Figure 6A** but we observed a dramatic *depression* in excitability of designated inhibitory neuron clusters that was completely reversed in <2 h. These effects resembled those obtained in our laboratory by enhancers of GABAergic neurotransmission such as neurosteroids or benzodiazepines (Puia et al., 2012), though whether a similar mechanism was involved at the level of $GABA_ARs$ remains to be determined.

MICROGLIA AND THE ROLE OF NEUROINFLAMMATION IN CNS DISEASES

Microglia are an integral part of CNS networks, forming the innate defensive system of the CNS and their pathological potential has been extensively investigated (Kettenmann et al., 2011). All CNS diseases involve microglia, which typically convert from the resting/surveillant cell type in the normal brain to an activated form specialized to operate within the diseased environment. In different pathologies, microglia acquire distinct functional states and during the disease progression, modify and change their activated phenotype. Activated microglia specifically interact with neurons and influence their survival either in a positive or in a negative direction. They can physically contact injured neurons and remove synapses, a process termed synaptic stripping (Kettenmann et al., 2013).

Conceptually, microglial cells can affect neural networks either through removal of cellular and subcellular elements (by phagocytosis) or through secreting factors with different properties: transmitter, trophic or neuroprotective. Thus, these factors, released in the activated state, are considered to be pathological signals and, as already mentioned in Introduction, include several types of cytokines, trophic factors, neurotransmitters (ATP and glutamate; Nakajima et al., 2007; Kettenmann et al., 2011; Viviani et al., 2014). On the other hand, studies in cell culture have indicated that microglial cells express a variety of receptors for neurotransmitters, neuropeptides, and neuromodulators and thus have also the capacity to sense neuronal activity (Pocock and Kettenmann, 2007).

Increasing evidence also supports the involvement of inflammatory and immune processes in the etiopathogenesis of seizures. Epilepsy is a disabling neurological disorder that in about 30% of affected individuals is refractory to pharmacological treatment (Perucca et al., 2007). Pharmacological and genetic studies in animal models have shown that specific inflammatory mediators such as cytokines, complement factors and prostaglandins substantially contribute to seizures and that interfering with these molecules or their receptors can reduce seizure frequency and severity (Vezzani et al., 2008).

Although there is substantial evidence that activated microglia can have negative effects in neurologic disease (Bamberger and Landreth, 2002), evidence also exists that under certain circumstances, microglia can be neuroprotective. Several groups have found that microglia express the glutamate uptake transporter, which may help microglia protect nerve cells during excitotoxic injury (Schwartz et al., 2003).

MECHANISM OF LPS ACTION

Small amounts of LPS from invading bacteria are one of the first signals detected by the body upon infection, and detection of LPS primes the immune system to mount a defense. Under some circumstances, the initial inflammatory response can become uncontrolled and ultimately lead to other deleterious effects including prolonged inflammation and cytokine release which is known to contribute to CNS dysfunction, chronic depressive disorders and neurodegenerative processes (Perry, 2004; Kettenmann, 2007). Although the CNS actions of pro-inflammatory cytokines have been implicated in "sickness behavior" that develops during the course of an infection (Cunningham et al., 2002), the mechanisms in the brain that trigger this adaptive behavioral response are not well understood. The Toll-like receptor 4 (TLR4) and its potent ligand LPS, represent one of the first and best characterized receptor/ligand systems (Gertig and Hanish, 2014). TLR4 receptors are expressed on microglia and not astrocytes (Lehnardt et al., 2002).

Systemic LPS acts on the CNS through several parallel pathways (Konsman et al., 2002) and given that TLR4 receptors are expressed in the brain (Chakravarty and Herkenham, 2005) and high LPS concentrations (100 μg/ml) lower the seizure threshold in rodents (Sayyah et al., 2003; Galic et al., 2008), its pathways have been investigated in some detail. Indeed, increasing evidence indicates that, in the absence of pathogens, TLR signaling can be activated also by molecules released by injured tissue (Bianchi and Manfredi, 2009) and among these is the high-mobility group box 1 protein (HMGB1), released by neurons and glia, that binds to TLR4 receptors (Scaffidi et al., 2002; Park et al., 2004; Maroso et al., 2010). Preliminary experiments done in our laboratory with increasing concentrations of HMGB1, produced slow actions similar to those reported here for LPS (Gullo et al., in preparation). Very recently, HMGB1 pulses have also been reported to enhance focal seizure generation in a brain slice preparation (Chiavegato et al., 2014).

The exact mechanism by which LPS activation of TLR4 signaling in our neuron system led to slow changes in excitability remain to be determined, although it is interesting to note that in a study of LPS action on dorsal root ganglion neurons recorded *in vitro*, a clear increase in cell excitability was observed, possibly through subtle changes in the density and gating of voltage-gated Na^+ channels involved in neuronal firing (Due et al., 2012). Moreover, also in acute hippocampal slices, 10 μg/ml LPS facilitated epileptiform activity (induced by Mg^{2+}-free ACSF + 4-AP) via enhanced excitatory synaptic transmission and release of TNF-α and IL-1β (Gao et al., 2014).

PREVIOUS LPS-INDUCED *IN VITRO* STUDIES IN BRAIN SLICES, ORGANOTYPIC AND DISSOCIATED CELL CULTURES

Depending on the LPS concentration used, the effects observed on single neurons or in brain slice activity can be either transient or sustained and can initiate irreversible changes like apoptosis. Moreover, the LPS-induced release of cytokines, chemokines and NO have been generally studied over several hours (Nakamura et al., 1999; Wang et al., 2005). The effects of LPS-induced microglial secretion of TNF-α and the consequent modulation of neurotransmission has also been studied in acute brain slices and in cultured cells as recently reported (Nimmervoll et al., 2012; Pascual et al., 2012). In H. J. Luhmann's laboratory, the experiments were both performed in organotypic and primary dissociated cells cultures by using an LPS concentration which caused rapid changes in spontaneous synaptic activity and caspase-3-dependent cell death in neurons, with no effects on astrocytes (Nimmervoll et al., 2012). Indeed, the LPS concentration used by these authors was more than three times higher (10 μg/ml) than our concentration and interestingly, their laboratory used the same multisite MEA recording dishes as ours. Unfortunately, in both brain slices and cultured neuron dishes, no spike sorting to find different units was performed. With respect to control, their results 1 h after the LPS treatment resulted in a significantly higher IBI between bursts ("oscillations") for slices and a "desynchronization" of the networks in dissociated neuronal cultures. On the whole, their results suggest that LPS concentrations of 10 μg/ml (higher than ours of 3 μg/ml) were able to produce after 2 h, large increases in TNF-α and macrophage inflammatory protein 2, but induced unwanted "toxic" effects, difficult to be compared with ours that were always recoverable on washout. Similar detrimental changes may also have occurred after chronic (7 day) exposure of organotypic hippocampal slices to LPS, which led to a persistent *decrease* in intrinsic neuronal excitability (Hellstrom et al., 2005).

Pascual et al. (2012) essentially carried out the same experiment in acute hippocampal brain slices as we did in dissociated neuron networks (with different techniques), for studying the LPS-induced excitability, by preconditioning networks with MC, and found exactly the same occlusion effect. Interestingly, they checked the TLR4 role in these experiments by also using TLR4 −/− KO mice and concluded that microglia are required for LPS to modulate neuronal activity. However, they observed only a transient (few minutes, but repeatable response) effect of LPS and ultra-slow effects were not studied as we did here. On the contrary, although we can exclude an important role for purinergic receptors during our experiments (see **Figure 6C**), they suggested that these receptors are "necessary" for the positive modulation of the synaptic mEPSC frequency (same purinergic receptor blocker at the same concentration). It is not easy to compare our and their experiments both on an electrophysiological and biological basis: we measured excitability of neurons and not mEPSCs, and in conclusion, we tested the functional outcome of the global synaptic bombardment in both neuronal clusters (simultaneously in many neurons), while they tested the miniature excitatory input and not the functional outcome, i.e., spikes in various principal neurons, not simultaneously. Interestingly, they also described an LPS-induced seizure-like activity, but only under facilitated conditions (0 external Mg^{2+} medium + block of $GABA_A$Rs with picrotoxin). In our experiments, LPS induced burst-like epileptiform events without background pharmacological intervention (see also Gao et al., 2014), most likely through the induced slow changes in overall network excitability.

On the whole, these data strongly suggest that the LPS-induced effects, seen in other laboratories in cell preparations containing viable microglia (releasing TNF-α) identified astrocytes and spiking neurons, have relatively large differences within themselves and with respect to our data. As reported, LPS concentrations at 1 μg/ml or below, strongly reduced successful experiments and statistical significance. On the contrary, the advantage of our *ex vivo* networks as compared to the other *in vitro* preparations, was the possibility to record: (1) stable excitable activity for hours in control, (2) follow long-term changes induced in LPS, and (3) during the action of picomolar TNF-α (as shown in **Figure 6A**); moreover, at the same time, we were able to test the effects of other drugs selective for different pathways, as shown in **Figure 6**).

EFFECTS OF MINOCYCLINE

Minocycline is a semi-synthetic, second-generation tetracycline antibiotic analog which effectively crosses the blood–brain barrier. It was first reported that MC had neuroprotective effects in animal models of ischemic injury (Yrjanheikki et al., 1998). It has been shown that this action of MC involves not only microglia but also T cells and their subsequent microglial activation (Giuliani et al., 2005); moreover, it attenuates the production of TNF-α in neuron/glia co-cultures (Lee et al., 2004). More recently, it was reported that MC promotes re-myelination in rat brain cultures (Defaux et al., 2011). These results suggest that MC attenuates microglial reactivity and favors re-myelination by enhancing the differentiation of oligodendrocytes. There are reports where MC has consistently been used in the 40–100 μM range, which is three orders of magnitude larger than the concentration used in our experiments (60 nM). We used the MC concentration reported by Tikka et al. (2001), which is one of the lowest reported in the literature, although in some papers, concentrations up to 60 μM were used in LPS-induced retinal microglia activation (Wang et al., 2005). MC was also tested for its effects on Na^+, K^+, and Ca^{2+} ion channels in hippocampal neurons, where it produced only weak inhibitory effects, but it has been suggested to reduce the release of glutamate with an EC_{50} of 60 μM.

Minocycline is an unusual type of tetracycline because its use is still increasing and has attracted many research areas of application, but it is no longer considered an antibiotic (see Garrido-Mesa et al., 2013). In addition to its own antimicrobacterial properties, MC has been reported to exert neuroprotective effects in various experimental models such as cerebral ischemia, traumatic brain injury, amyotrophic lateral sclerosis, Parkinson's disease, kainic acid treatment, Huntington' disease, and multiple sclerosis. Recently, the effect of MC in Alzheimer's disease has been also reported in mouse models at a concentration of 10 mg/kg/day and apparently it is not dangerous, but when given in Aβ-treated mice, the MC concentration that was necessary to improve latency times in behavioral tests had to be increased by five times (Choi et al., 2007). We also performed long-term experiments in our networks with MC at 2 μM and after a sudden 50% decrease of excitability, IBI slowly increased by the same amount producing a net marked SR decrease in the following 8 h, thus confirming that the network was substantially unrecoverable (not shown).

CONCLUSION

In conclusion, our study provides evidence that it is possible to characterize the network excitability and its response to the pro-inflammatory agent LPS in a standard culture of dissociated cortical neurons, astrocytes and microglia grown on a MEA recording environment. Our results show that this response can be prevented by pre-exposure of the network to a low dose of the anti-inflammatory drug MC. In view of the known involvement of neuroinflammatory components in a wide range of neurodegenerative, neurological, as well as psychiatric central nervous disorders, we would like to suggest that the use of anti-inflammatory agents like MC might be useful as adjuncts to conventional therapies in the management of these debilitating conditions. The fact that we can detect and analyze long-term effects on neuron activity during microglia activation also opens the possibility to study recently demonstrated roles of "resting" microglia, probably bi-directionally cross-talking with neurons in the developing CNS (Béchade et al., 2013; Kyungmin et al., 2013; Schafer et al., 2013; Sheridan and Murphy, 2013).

AUTHOR CONTRIBUTIONS

Enzo Wanke conceived and designed the research project. Francesca Gullo did all the MEA experiments on the dissociated cultures and performed the preliminary analysis of the data. Alida Amadeo did the immunohistochemistry analysis. Barbara Costa designed the TNF-α release experiments and Giulia Donvito performed the experiments. Marzia Lecchi, Andrew Constanti and Enzo Wanke wrote the manuscript.

ACKNOWLEDGMENTS

We thank Drs. Raimondo D'Ambrosio and Clifford L. Eastman, University of Washington, Seattle, WA, USA, for helpful discussions on a preliminary version of the manuscript. The authors also thank Dr. Marco Ferrari for help in microglial cytochemical analysis and immunofluorescence. Part of this work was carried out in CIMA, an advanced microscopy laboratory established by the State University of Milan. This study was supported by grants from the Italian Ministero dell'Università e della Ricerca Scientifica e Tecnologica (MURST-COFIN2007 – 2009), a Cariplo Foundation Grant "Functional regeneration of the mesocorticolimbic dopaminergic system as a model to study novel neuro reparative strategies" (2009–2012), and University of Milano-Bicocca, Grandi Attrezzature 2009 to Enzo Wanke.

REFERENCES

Allan, S. M., Tyrrell, P. J., and Rothwell, N. J. (2005). Interleukin-1 and neuronal injury. *Nat. Rev. Immunol.* 5, 629–640. doi: 10.1038/nri1664

Baddeley, R., Abbot, L. F., Booth, M. C., Sengpiel, F., Freeman, T., Wakeman, E. A., et al. (1997). Responses of neurons in primary and inferior temporal visual cortices to natural scenes. *Proc. Biol. Sci.* 264, 1775–1783. doi: 10.1098/rspb.1997.0246

Balosso, S., Ravizza, T., Perego, C., Peschon, J., Campbell, I. L., De Simoni, M. G., et al. (2005). Tumor necrosis factor-alpha inhibits seizures in mice via p75 receptors. *Ann. Neurol.* 57, 804–812. doi: 10.1002/ana.20480

Bamberger, M. E., and Landreth, G. E. (2002). Inflammation, apoptosis, and Alzheimer's disease. *Neuroscientist* 8, 276–283. doi: 10.1177/107385840200800301З

Beattie, E. C., Stellwagen, D., Morishita, W., Bresnahan, J. C., Ha, B. K., Zastrow, M. V., et al. (2002). Control of synaptic strength by glial TNFα. *Science* 295, 2282–2285. doi: 10.1126/science.1067859

Becchetti, A., Gullo, F., Bruno, G., Dossi, E., Lecchi, M., and Wanke, E. (2012). Exact distinction of excitatory and inhibitory neurons in neural networks: a study with GFP-GAD67 neurons optically and electrophysiologically recognized on multielectrode arrays. *Front. Neural Circuits* 6:63. doi: 10.3389/fncir.2012.00063

Béchade, C., Cantaut-Belarif, Y., and Bessis, A. (2013). Microglial control of neuronal activity. *Front. Cell. Neurosci.* 7:32. doi: 10.3389/fncel.2013.00032

Beggs, J. M., and Plenz, D. (2003). Neuronal avalanches in neocortical circuits. *J. Neurosci.* 23, 11167–11177.

Beggs, J. M., and Plenz, D. (2004). Neuronal avalanches are diverse and precise activity patterns that are stable for many hours in cortical slice cultures. *J. Neurosci.* 24, 5216–5229. doi: 10.1523/JNEUROSCI.0540-04.2004

Beheshti Nasr, S. M., Moghimi, A., Mohammad-Zadeh, M., Shamsizadeh, A., and Noorbakhsh, S. M. (2013). The effect of minocycline on seizures induced by amygdala kindling in rats. *Seizure* 22, 670–674. doi: 10.1016/j.seizure.2013.05.005

Bianchi, M. E., and Manfredi, A. A. (2009). Immunology. Dangers in and out. *Science* 323, 1683–1684. doi: 10.1126/science.1172794

Cata, J. P., Weng, H. R., and Dougherty, P. M. (2008). The effects of thalidomide and minocycline on taxol-induced hyperalgesia in rats. *Brain Res.* 1229, 100–110. doi: 10.1016/j.brainres.2008.07.001

Catalano, S. M., and Shatz, C. J. (1998). Activity-dependent cortical target selection by thalamic axons. *Science* 281, 559–562. doi: 10.1126/science.281.5376.559

Chakravarty, S., and Herkenham, M. (2005). Toll-like receptor 4 on nonhematopoietic cells sustains CNS inflammation during endotoxemia, independent of systemic cytokines. *J. Neurosci.* 25, 1788–1796. doi: 10.1523/JNEUROSCI.4268-04.2005

Chen, X., Rochefort, N. L., Sakmann, B., and Konnert, A. (2013). Reactivation of the same synapses during spontaneous up states and sensory stimuli. *Cell Rep.* 4, 31–39. doi: 10.1016/j.celrep.2013.05.042

Chiavegato, A., Zurolo, E., Losi, G., Aronica, E., and Carmignoto, G. (2014). The inflammatory molecules IL-1β and HMGB1 can rapidly enhance focal seizure generation in a brain slice model of temporal lobe epilepsy. *Front. Cell. Neurosci.* 8:155. doi: 10.3389/fncel.2014.00155

Choi, Y., Kim, H. S., Shin, K. Y., Kim, E. M., Kim, M., Kim, H. S., et al. (2007). Minocycline attenuates neuronal cell death and improves cognitive impairment in Alzheimer's disease models. *Neuropsychopharmacology* 32, 2393–2404. doi: 10.1038/sj.npp.1301377

Corlew, R., Bosma, M. M., and Moody, W. J. (2004). Spontaneous, synchronous electrical activity in neonatal mouse cortical neurones. *J. Physiol.* 560, 377–390. doi: 10.1113/jphysiol.2004.071621

Cunningham, C., Konsman, J. P., and Cartmell, T. (2002). Cytokines and the ageing brain. *Trends Neurosci.* 25, 546–547. doi: 10.1016/S0166-2236(02)02265-8

Defaux, A., Zurich, A. G., Honegger, P., and Monnet-Tschudi, F. (2011). Minocycline promotes remyelination in aggregating rat brain cell cultures after interferon-γ plus lipopolysaccharide-induced demyelination. *Neuroscience* 187, 84–92. doi: 10.1016/j.neuroscience.2011.04.053

Dodd, S., Maes, M., Anderson, G., Dean, O. M., Moylan, S., and Berk, M. (2013). Putative neuroprotective agents in neuropsychiatric disorders. *Prog. Neuropsychopharmacol. Biol. Psychiatry* 42, 135–145. doi: 10.1016/j.pnpbp.2012.11.007

Due, M. R., Piekarz, A. D., Wilson, N., Feldman, P., Ripsch, M. S., Chavez, S., et al. (2012). Neuroexcitatory effects of morphine-3-glucuronide are dependent on Toll-like receptor 4 signaling. *J. Neuroinflammation* 9, 200. doi: 10.1186/1742-2094-9-200

Dupont, E., Hanganu, I. L., Kilb, W., Hirsch, S., and Luhmann, H. J. (2006). Rapid development switch in the mechanisms driving early cortical columnar networks. *Nature* 435, 79–83. doi: 10.1038/nature04264

Eytan, D., and Marom, S. (2006). Dynamics and effective topology underlying sychronization in networks of cortical neurons. *J. Neurosci.* 26, 8465–8476. doi: 10.1523/JNEUROSCI.1627-06.2006

Filipovic, R., and Zecevic, N. (2008). Neuroprotective role of minocycline in co-cultures of human fetal neurons and microglia. *Exp. Neurol.* 211, 41–51. doi: 10.1016/j.expneurol.2007.12.024

Galic, M. A., Riazi, K., Heida, J. G., Mouihate, A., Fournier, N. M., Spencer, S. J., et al. (2008). Postnatal inflammation increases seizure susceptibility in adult rats. *J. Neurosci.* 28, 6904–6913. doi: 10.1523/JNEUROSCI.1901-08.2008

Gao, F., Liu, Z., Ren, W., and Jiang, W. (2014). Acute lipopolysaccharide exposure facilitates epileptic activity via enhanced excitatory transmission and neuronal excitability *in vitro*. *Neuropsychiatr. Dis. Treat.* 10, 1489–1495. doi: 10.2147/NDT.S65695

Garaschuk, O., Linn, J., Eilers, J., and Konnerth, A. (2000). Large-scale oscillatory calcium waves in the immature cortex. *Nat. Neurosci.* 3, 452–459. doi: 10.1038/74823

Garrido-Mesa, N., Zarzuelo, A., and Galvez, J. (2013). Minocycline: far beyond an antibiotic. *Br. J. Pharmacol.* 169, 337–352. doi: 10.1111/bph.12139

Gertig, U., and Hanish, U. K. (2014). Microglial diversity by responses and responders. *Front. Cell. Neurosci.* 8:101. doi: 10.3389/fncel.2014.00101

Giuliani, F., Hader, W., and Yong, V. W. (2005). Minocycline attenuates T cell and microglia activity to impair cytokine production in T cell-microglia interaction. *J. Leukoc. Biol.* 78, 135–143. doi: 10.1189/jlb.0804477

Gramowski, A., Jügelt, K., Weiss, D. G., and Gross, G. W. (2004). Substance identification by quantitative characterization of oscillatory activity in murine spinal cord networks on microelectrode arrays. *Eur. J. Neurosci.* 19, 2815–2825. doi: 10.1111/j.0953-816X.2004.03373.x

Gullo, F., Maffezzoli, A., Dossi, E., Lecchi, M., and Wanke, E. (2012). Classifying heterogeneity of spontaneous up-states: a method for revealing variations in firing probability, engaged neurons and Fano factor. *J. Neurosci. Methods* 203, 407–417. doi: 10.1016/j.jneumeth.2011.10.014

Gullo, F, Maffezzoli, A., Dossi, E., and Wanke, E. (2009). Short latency cross-and autocorrelation identify clusters of interacting neurons recorded from multi-electrode arrays. *J. Neurosci. Methods* 181, 186–198. doi: 10.1016/j.jneumeth.2009.05.003

Gullo, F., Mazzetti, S., Maffezzoli, A., Dossi, E., Lecchi, M., Amadeo, A., et al. (2010). Orchestration of "presto" and "largo" synchrony in up-down activity of cortical networks. *Front. Neural Circuits* 4:11. doi: 10.3389/fncir.2010.00011

Ham, M. I., Bettencourt, L. M., McDaniel, F. D., and Gross, G. W. (2008). Spontaneous coordinated activity in cultured networks: analysis of multiple ignition sites, primary circuits, and burst phase delay distributions. *J. Comput. Neurosci.* 24, 346–357. doi: 10.1007/s10827-007-0059-1

Harris, K. D. (2005). Neural signatures of cell assembly organization. *Nat. Rev. Neurosci.* 6, 399–407. doi: 10.1038/nrn1669

Hellstrom, I. C., Danik, M., Luheshi, G. N., and Williams, S. (2005). Chronic LPS exposure produces changes in intrinsic membrane properties and a sustained IL-beta-dependent increase in GABAergic inhibition in hippocampal CA1 pyramidal neurons. *Hippocampus* 15, 656–664. doi: 10.1002/hipo.20086

Henry, C. J., Huang Wynne, A., Hank, M., Himler, J., Bailey, M. T., Sheridan, J. F., et al. (2008). Minocycline attenuates lipopolysaccharide (LPS)-induced neuroinflammation, sickness behavior and anhedonia. *J. Neuroinflammation* 5, 15. doi: 10.1186/1742-2094-5-15

Keefer, E. W., Gramowsky, A., and Gross, G. W. (2001). NMDA receptor-dependent periodic oscillations in cultured spinal cord networks. *J. Neurophysiol.* 86, 3030–3042.

Kettenmann, H. (2007). Neuroscience: the brain's garbage men. *Nature* 446, 987–989. doi: 10.1038/nature05713

Kettenmann, H., Hanisch, U. K., Noda, M., and Verkhratsky, A. (2011). Physiology of microglia. *Physiol. Rev.* 91, 461–553. doi: 10.1152/physrev.00011.2010

Kettenmann, H., Kirchhoff, F., and Verkhratsky, A. (2013). Microglia: new roles for the synaptic stripper. *Neuron* 77, 10–18. doi: 10.1016/j.neuron.2012.12.023

Komuro, H., and Rakic, P. (1998). Orchestration of neuronal migration by activity of ion channels, neurotransmitter receptors, and intracellular ca2+ fluctuations. *J. Neurobiol.* 37, 110–130. doi: 10.1002/(SICI)1097-4695(199810)37:1<110::AID-NEU9>3.0.CO;2-C

Konsman, J. P., Parnet, P., and Dantzer, R. (2002). Cytokine-induced sickness behaviour: mechanisms and implications. *Trends Neurosci.* 25, 154–159. doi: 10.1016/S0166-2236(00)02088-9

Krabbe, G., Halle, A., Matyash, V., Rinnenthal, J. L., Eom, G. D., Bernhardt, U., et al. (2013). Functional impairment of microglia coincides with Beta-amyloid deposition in mice with Alzheimer-like pathology. *PLoS ONE* 8:e60921. doi: 10.1371/journal.pone.0060921

Kyungmin, J. I., Akgul, G., Wollmuth, L. P., and Tsirka, S. E. (2013). Microglia actively regulate the number of functional synapses. *PLoS ONE* 8:e56293. doi: 10.1371/journal.pone.0056293

Lee, S. M., Yune, T. Y., Kim, S. J., Kim, Y. C., Oh, Y. J., Markelonis, G. J., et al. (2004). Minocycline inhibits apoptotic death via attenuation of TNF-α expression following iNOS/NO induction by LPS in neuron/glia co-cultures. *J. Neurochem.* 91, 568–578. doi: 10.1111/j.1471-4159.2004.02780.x

Lehnardt, S., Lachance, C., Patrizi, S., Lefebvre, S., Follett, P. L., Jensen, F. E., et al. (2002). The toll-like receptor TLR4 is necessary for lipopolysaccharide-induced oligodendrocyte injury in the CNS. *J. Neurosci.* 22, 2478–2486.

Lisman, J. E. (1997). Bursts as a unit of neuronal information: making unreliable synapses reliable. *Trends Neurosci.* 20, 38–43. doi: 10.1016/S0166-2236(96)10070-9

Maroso, M., Balosso, S., Ravizza, T., Liu, J., Aronica, E., Iyer, A. M., et al. (2010). Toll-like receptor 4 high mobility group box-1 are involved in ictogenesis and can be targeted to reduce seizure. *Nature Med.* 16, 413–420. doi: 10.1038/nm.2127

Nakajima, K., Tohyama, Y., Maeda, S., Kohsaka, S., and Kurihara, T. (2007). Neuronal regulation by which microglia enhance the production of neurotrophic factors for GABAergic, catecholaminergic, and cholinergic neurons. *Neurochem. Int.* 50, 807–820. doi: 10.1016/j.neuint.2007.02.006

Nakamura, Y., Si, Q. S., and Kataoka, K. (1999). Lipopolysaccharide-induced microglia activation in culture: temporal profiles of morphological change and release of cytokines and nitric oxide. *Neurosci. Res.* 35, 95–100. doi: 10.1016/S0168-0102(99)00071-1

Nimmervoll, B., White, R., Yang, J. W., An, S., Henn, C., Sun, J. J., et al. (2012). LPS-induced microglial secretion of TNFα increases activity-dependent neuronal apoptosis in the neonatal cerebral cortex. *Cereb. Cortex* 23, 1742–1755. doi: 10.1093/cercor/bhs156

O'Learly, D. M., Ruff, N. L., and Dyck, R. H. (1994). Development, critical period plasticity, and adult reorganization of mammalian somatosensory systems. *Curr. Opin. Neurobiol.* 4, 535–544. doi: 10.1016/0959-4388(94)90054-X

Palencia, G., Rubio, C., Custodio-Ramirez, V., Paz, C., and Sotelo, J. (2011). Strong anticonvulsant effect of thalidomide on amygdaloid kindling. *Epilepsy Res.* 95, 263–269. doi: 10.1016/j.eplepsyres.2011.04.008

Park, J. S., Svetkauskaite, D., He, Q., Kim, J. Y., Strassheim, D., Ishizaka, A., et al. (2004). Involvement of Toll-like receptors 2 and 4 in cellular activation by high mobility group box 1 protein. *J. Biol. Chem.* 279, 7370–7377. doi: 10.1074/jbc.M306793200

Pascual, O., Achour, S. B., Rostaing, P., Triller, A., and Bessis, A. (2012). Microglia activation triggers astrocyte-mediated modulation of excitatory neurotransmission. *Proc. Natl. Acad. Sci. U.S.A.* 109, E197–E205. doi: 10.1073/pnas.1111098109

Perea, G., Navarrete, M., and Araque, A. (2009). Tripartite synapses: astrocytes process and control synaptic information. *Trends Neurosci.* 32, 421–431. doi: 10.1016/j.tins.2009.05.001

Perry, V. H. (2004). The influence of systemic inflammation on inflammation in the brain: implications for chronic neurodegenerative disease. *Brain Behav. Immun.* 18, 407–441. doi: 10.1016/j.bbi.2004.01.004

Perry, V. H., Nicoll, J. A. R., and Holmes, C. (2010). Microglia in neurodegenerative disease. *Nat. Rev. Neurol.* 6, 193–201. doi: 10.1038/nrneurol.2010.17

Perucca, E., French, J., and Bialer, M. (2007). Development of new antiepileptic drugs: challenges, incentives, and recent advances. *Lancet Neurol.* 6, 793–804. doi: 10.1016/S1474-4422(07)70215-6

Pocock, J. M., and Kettenmann, H. (2007). Neurotransmitter receptors on microglia. *Trends Neurosci.* 30, 527–535. doi: 10.1016/j.tins.2007.07.007

Puia, G., Gullo, F., Dossi, E., Lecchi, M., and Wanke, E. (2012). Novel modulatory effects of neurosteroids and benzodiazepines on excitatory and inhibitory neurons excitability: a multi-electrode array recording study. *Front. Neural Circuits* 6:94. doi: 10.3389/fncir.2012.00094

Sahara, S., Yanagawa, Y., O'Learly, D. M., and Stevens, C. F. (2012). The fraction of cortical GABAergic neurons is constant from near the start of cortical neurogenesis to adulthood. *J. Neurosci.* 32, 4755–4761. doi: 10.1523/JNEUROSCI.6412-11.2012

Sanchez-Vives, N., and McCormick, D. A. (2000). Cellular and network mechanisms of rhythmic recurrent activity in neocortex. *Nat. Neurosci.* 3, 1027–1034. doi: 10.1038/79848

Santello, M., and Volterra, A. (2012). TNFα in synaptic function: switching gears. *Trends Neurosci.* 35, 638–647. doi: 10.1016/j.tins.2012.06.001

Saura, J. (2007). Microglial cells in astroglial culture: a cautionary note. *J. Neuroinflammation* 4, 26. doi: 10.1186/1742-2094-4-26

Sayyah, M., Javad-Pour, M., and Ghazi-Khansari, M. (2003). The bacterial endotoxin lipopolysaccharide enhances seizure susceptibility in mice: involvement of proinflammatory factors: nitric oxide and prostaglandins. *Neuroscience* 122, 1073–1080. doi: 10.1016/j.neuroscience.2003.08.043

Scaffidi, P., Misteli, T., and Bianchi, M. E. (2002). Release of chromatin protein HMGB1 by necrotic cells triggers inflammation. *Nature* 418, 191–195. doi: 10.1038/nature00858

Schafer, D. P., Lehrman, E. K., and Stevens, B. (2013). The "quad-partite" synapse: microglia-synapse interactions in the developing and mature CNS. *Glia* 61, 24–36. doi: 10.1002/glia.22389

Schwartz, M., Shaked, I., Fisher, J., Mizrahi, T., and Schori, H. (2003). Protective autoimmunity against the enemy within: fighting glutamate toxicity. *Trends Neurosci.* 26, 297–302. doi: 10.1016/S0166-2236(03)00126-7

Sheridan, G. K., and Murphy, K. J. (2013). Neuron-glia crosstalk in health and disease: fractalkine and CX_3CR1 take centre stage. *Open Biol.* 3, 130181. doi: 10.1098/rsob.130181

Shieh, C. H., Heinrich, A., Serchov, T., van Calker, D., and Biber, K. (2014). P2X7-dependent, but differentially regulated release of IL-6, CCL2, and TNF-α in cultured mouse microglia. *Glia* 62, 592–607. doi: 10.1002/glia.22628

Stellwagen, D., Beattie, E. C., and Malenka, R. C. (2005). Differential regulation of AMPA receptor and GABA receptor trafficking by tumor necrosis factor-α. *J. Neurosci.* 25, 3219–3328. doi: 10.1523/JNEUROSCI.4486-04.2005

Stellwagen, D., and Malenka, R. C. (2006). Synaptic scaling mediated by glial TNF-α. *Nature* 440, 1054–1059. doi: 10.1038/nature04671

Tancredi, V., D'Arcangelo, G., Grassi, F., Tarroni, P., Palmieri, G., Santoni, A., et al. (1992). Tumor necrosis factor alters synaptic transmission in rat hippocampal slices. *Neurosci. Lett.* 146, 176–178. doi: 10.1016/0304-3940(92)90071-E

Tateno, T., Jimbo, Y., and Robinson, P. C. (2005). Spatio-temporal cholinergic modulation in cultured networks of rat cortical neurons: spontaneous activity. *Neuroscience* 134, 425–437. doi: 10.1016/j.neuroscience.2005.04.049

Tikka, T., Fiebich, B. L., Goldsteins, G., Keinanen, R., and Koistinaho, J. (2001). Minocycline, a tetracycline derivate, is neuroprotective against excitotoxicity by inhibiting activation and proliferation of microglia. *J. Neurosci.* 21, 2580–2588.

Turrigiano, G. G., and Nelson, S. B. (2004). Homeostatic plasticity in the developing nervous system. *Nat. Rev. Neurosci.* 5, 97–107. doi: 10.1038/nrn1327

Valenza, G., Tedesco, L., Lanata, A., De Rossi, D., and Scilingo, E. P. (2013). Novel Spiking Neuron-Astrocyte Networks based on nonlinear transistor-like models of tripartite synapses. *Conf. Proc. IEEE Eng. Med. Biol. Soc.* 2013, 6559–6562. doi: 10.1109/EMBC.2013.6611058

Vezzani, A., Balosso, S., and Ravizza, T. (2008). The role of cytokines in the pathophysiology of epilepsy. *Brain Behav. Immun.* 22, 797–803. doi: 10.1016/j.bbi.2008.03.009

Viviani, B., Boraso, M., Marchetti, N., and Marinovich, M. (2014). Perspectives on neuroinflammation and excitotoxicity: a neurotoxic conspiracy? *Neurotoxicology* 43, 10–20. doi: 10.1016/j.neuro.2014.03.004

Wang, A. L., Yu, A. C. H., Lau, T. G., Lee, C., Wu, L. M., Zhu, X. A., et al. (2005). Minocycline inhibits LPS-induced retinal microglia activation. *Neurochem. Int.* 47, 152–158. doi: 10.1016/j.neuint.2005.04.018

Yrjanheikki, J., Keinanen, R., Pellikka, M., Hokfelt, T., and Koisinaho, J. (1998). Tetracyclines inhibit microglial activation and are neuroprotective in global brain ischemia. *Proc. Natl. Acad. Sci. U.S.A.* 95, 15769–15774. doi: 10.1073/pnas.95.26.15769

5

Interleukin-1 and acute brain injury

Katie N. Murray[1], Adrian R. Parry-Jones[2] and Stuart M. Allan[1]*

[1] Faculty of Life Sciences, University of Manchester, Manchester, UK
[2] Salford Royal NHS Foundation Trust, Salford, UK

Correspondence:
Stuart M. Allan, Faculty of Life Sciences, University of Manchester, AV Hill Building, Manchester M13 9PT, UK
e-mail: stuart.allan@manchester.ac.uk

Inflammation is the key host-defense response to infection and injury, yet also a major contributor to a diverse range of diseases, both peripheral and central in origin. Brain injury as a result of stroke or trauma is a leading cause of death and disability worldwide, yet there are no effective treatments, resulting in enormous social and economic costs. Increasing evidence, both preclinical and clinical, highlights inflammation as an important factor in stroke, both in determining outcome and as a contributor to risk. A number of inflammatory mediators have been proposed as key targets for intervention to reduce the burden of stroke, several reaching clinical trial, but as yet yielding no success. Many factors could explain these failures, including the lack of robust preclinical evidence and poorly designed clinical trials, in addition to the complex nature of the clinical condition. Lack of consideration in preclinical studies of associated co-morbidities prevalent in the clinical stroke population is now seen as an important omission in previous work. These co-morbidities (atherosclerosis, hypertension, diabetes, infection) have a strong inflammatory component, supporting the need for greater understanding of how inflammation contributes to acute brain injury. Interleukin (IL)-1 is the prototypical pro-inflammatory cytokine, first identified many years ago as the endogenous pyrogen. Research over the last 20 years or so reveals that IL-1 is an important mediator of neuronal injury and blocking the actions of IL-1 is beneficial in a number of experimental models of brain damage. Mechanisms underlying the actions of IL-1 in brain injury remain unclear, though increasing evidence indicates the cerebrovasculature as a key target. Recent literature supporting this and other aspects of how IL-1 and systemic inflammation in general contribute to acute brain injury are discussed in this review.

Keywords: interleukin-1, inflammation, acute brain injury, cerebrovasculature

INTRODUCTION

Approximately 15 million people worldwide have a stroke every year, from which one third die and another third are permanently disabled (Corbyn, 2014). Ischemic stroke accounts for 80% of all strokes with the remaining 20% being composed of intracerebral hemorrhage (ICH) and subarachnoid hemorrhage (SAH). Traumatic brain injury (TBI) also falls under the category of acute central nervous system (CNS) injury and its pattern of injury evolves in a similar way to ischemic and hemorrhagic stroke. Currently there is only one drug option available to ischemic stroke patients, the thrombolytic agent recombinant tissue plasminogen activator (tPA), which disperses the clot in the occluded vessel. The primary limitation of tPA is that only 5–13% of the stroke population are eligible for treatment as intravenous (i.v) administration must occur within a 4.5 h time frame of stroke onset for the benefits of the drug to outweigh the risks of hemorrhage (Hacke and Lichy, 2008). Therefore, research over the last two decades has focused on neuroprotective strategies with approximately 1000 compounds being tested preclinically and almost 200 progressing to clinical trials (O'Collins et al., 2006; Minnerup et al., 2012), with no success. Despite these attempts to identify successful stroke treatments, the only pharmacological therapies currently in use are anti-platelet treatments for the general population (Chen et al., 2000) and thrombolysis for the select few (Wardlaw et al., 2012). Similarly, SAH and ICH treatment options are limited to a narrow therapeutic window (Xu et al., 2014; Zhou et al., 2014) thus necessitating an urgent need for new treatment options applicable to a wider spectrum of patients and at extended time points.

In response to these translational failures guidelines were introduced in an attempt to ensure that complete and comprehensive neuroprotection studies were performed before any agent made it to clinical trial i.e., The STAIR criteria (Stroke Therapy Academic Industry Roundtable (STAIR), 1999; Fisher et al., 2009; Albers et al., 2011). Alongside suggestions for improvements to experimental design and conduct, it was also recognized by the STAIR committee that advanced age and prevalent co-morbidities must also be considered and incorporated when modeling ischemic stroke as they increase stroke susceptibility and lead to poorer outcomes (Sieber et al., 2014; Wang et al., 2014). In particular, the contribution of co-morbidities to inflammation prior to and post-stroke is of key importance when determining outcomes after acute CNS injury.

INFLAMMATION AND BRAIN INJURY

Inflammation plays a key detrimental and reparative role in CNS injury and it is widely accepted that inflammatory events prior to and following an insult can have far reaching effects on susceptibility and patient outcome and recovery (VanGilder et al., 2014). Inflammation is an evolutionary-conserved defense strategy of the immune system that can be mounted in response to injury or infection. Acute inflammation is a rapid response to tissue injury and/or pathogens and is traditionally considered a beneficial mechanism to limit damage and evoke tissue repair and resolution of injury (Cuartero et al., 2013). Chronic inflammation conversely is generally associated with dysregulation of the immune system and often manifests itself as systemic inflammatory disease (Elkind, 2010). Ultimately, prolonged or unregulated inflammation, either chronic or acute, is detrimental to health and is particularly damaging if it occurs in close temporal proximity to a CNS insult. Following acute brain injury (e.g., stroke, TBI) a local and systemic inflammatory response is mounted which triggers inflammatory signaling cascades, increases in expression of transcriptional regulators and infiltration and activation of immune cells (Lian et al., 2012; Chu et al., 2014). This inflammatory response evolves over a number of days to amplify the ischemic lesion, but also to initiate tissue repair in the late post-ischemic phase (Iadecola and Anrather, 2011).

THE ROLE OF CYTOKINES IN STROKE

As part of the inflammatory response to brain injury, chemokines and cytokines are secreted from immune cells to trigger a local pro- or anti-inflammatory response on surrounding target cells (Luheshi et al., 2009). Following a CNS insult, multiple cytokines are generated to cause, exacerbate, mediate and/or inhibit cellular injury and repair (Allan et al., 2005). The site of cytokine action is varied and cytokines can be expressed by or act upon glia, neurons, cerebrovascular endothelium and circulating immune cells (Allan and Rothwell, 2001). Under normal basal conditions cytokines are expressed at very low levels which are often difficult to quantify (Hopkins and Rothwell, 1995; Vitkovic et al., 2000). However, following CNS injury they are one of the first mediators relayed to the site of injury (Allan and Rothwell, 2003). The whole range of cytokine families (interleukins (IL), interferons (IFN), tumor necrosis factors (TNF), colony stimulating factors, growth factors and chemokines) have been implicated as contributors to pre-existing risk factors for stroke as well as following reperfusion (Fouda et al., 2013; Zhang et al., 2014). More specifically IL-1, IL-6, IL-10, IL-17, IL-23, TNFα, transforming growth factor β (TGFβ) and IFNγ are seen to increase after stroke (Lakhan et al., 2009), IL-17, IL-23 and IFNγ being associated with exacerbation of stroke in mice (Yilmaz et al., 2006; Shichita et al., 2009), whereas IL-10 and TGFβ are protective (Spera et al., 1998; Zhu et al., 2002). Release of these cytokines generates an inflammatory cascade, resulting in the synthesis of various downstream mediators, including prostaglandin (PG)-E_2, IL-6, nitric oxide (NO), IL-10 and neurotrophins (Pinteaux et al., 2002). IL-1, as the first member of the IL family described, is considered the prototypical inflammatory cytokine. This, together with extensive literature reporting actions of IL-1 in cerebral ischemia, means that this review will focus predominantly on IL-1. Discussion of other inflammatory mediators in stroke can be found in several recent articles—see (Doll et al., 2014) and (Lambertsen et al., 2012).

INTERLEUKIN-1 AND ACUTE BRAIN DAMAGE

IL-1 is a key pro-inflammatory mediator with potent endogenous pyrogenic properties. IL-1 has been implicated in many pathological conditions, both in the periphery (e.g., sepsis, arthritis and autoimmune dysfunction), and centrally (e.g., TBI, SAH, ICH and cerebral ischemia). The two main IL-1 ligands are IL-1α and IL-1β, which show high sequence homology despite being products of different genes (Andrews et al., 1991; **Figure 1**). A third ligand, discovered in 1984, is a naturally occurring competitive antagonist, IL-1 receptor antagonist (IL-1Ra; Dinarello, 1994). This is highly selective and blocks all known actions of IL-1, with no known independent actions (Dinarello, 2011). IL-1 family members are constitutively expressed at low levels in the healthy brain and when released at modest concentrations locally, are not directly neurotoxic *in vitro* or *in vivo* (Lawrence et al., 1998; Rothwell and Luheshi, 2000), but play important roles in normal physiological processes such as development, sleep and synaptic plasticity as well as synaptic pruning and memory formation/consolidation during adulthood (del Rey et al., 2013).

Detrimental effects of IL-1 become evident when CNS injury occurs and there are raised levels of the cytokine. Acute neuronal injuries, such as stroke or TBI, cause a rapid up-regulation of IL-1β, IL-1Ra, IL-1 receptor (IL-1R) I, and IL-1RII expression in rats (Liu et al., 1993; Wang et al., 1997). Expression of IL-1α protein is also seen after cerebral ischemia, as early as 4 h post-reperfusion in microglial cells (Chen et al., 2007; Luheshi et al., 2011). Exogenous administration of recombinant IL-1β, either centrally or systemically, alongside experimental stroke in rodents leads to an exacerbation of ischemic damage (Yamasaki et al., 1995; Stroemer and Rothwell, 1998; McColl et al., 2007). Conversely, disruption of IL-1α and β activity in IL-1α/β knockout (KO) mice resulted in markedly reduced (70%) infarct volumes following experimental stroke (Boutin et al., 2001). Preclinical ICH and SAH studies also report increases in mRNA and protein expression of IL-1 following hemorrhagic injury (Wasserman et al., 2007; Greenhalgh et al., 2012), while clinical studies show that IL-1β promoter polymorphisms are associated with an increased risk of ICH in brain arteriovenous malformation patients (Kim et al., 2009). IL-1Ra has been shown to be safe in small Phase II trials in ischemic stroke (Emsley et al., 2005) and SAH, also resulting in a reduction in inflammatory markers in the circulation and cerebrospinal fluid (Singh et al., 2014). Ongoing clinical studies in larger patient cohorts will confirm the potential of IL-1Ra to move to Phase III efficacy trials.

PRE-EXISTING SYSTEMIC INFLAMMATION AND STROKE INCIDENCE

Harmful effects of IL-1 are not limited to post-stroke inflammation. Accumulating evidence from the clinical and experimental setting suggests that pre-existing inflammation

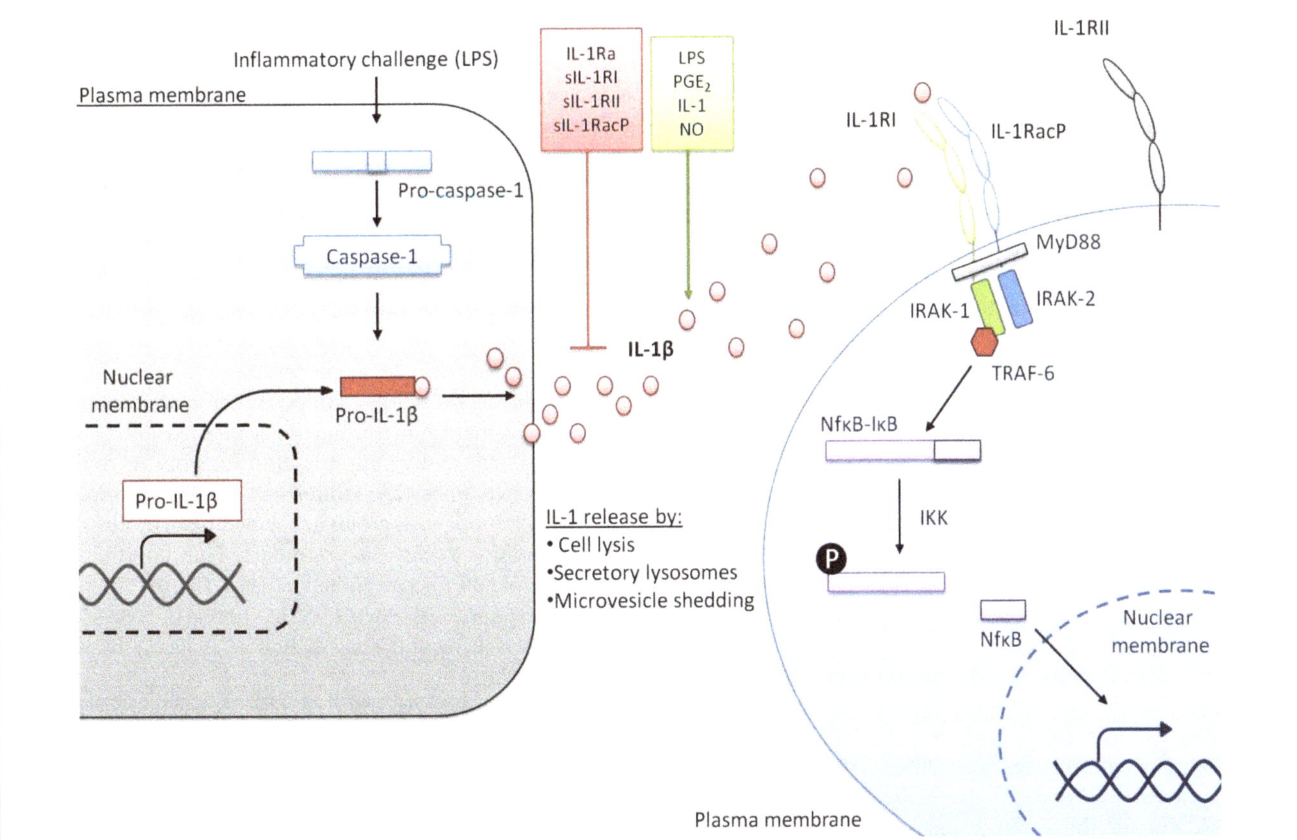

FIGURE 1 | IL-1 signaling pathways. In response to a stimulus such as lipopolysaccharide (LPS) transcription of the gene encoding IL-1β is initiated. IL-1β is made as an inactive precursor protein and caspase-1 cleaves this pro-IL-1β to make the active IL-1β. A variety of factors can promote or inhibit the release of active IL-1β. Once released, IL-1β binds to IL-1RI alongside IL-1 receptor accessory protein (IL-1RAcP) and signal transduction is triggered, including co-localization of myeloid differentiation primary response protein 88 (MyD88), IL-1 receptor associated kinase (IRAK-1) and IRAK-2, recruitment of TNF receptor associated factor 6 (TRAF-6) and activation of nuclear factor kappa B (NFκB) from complex with IκB. Conversely IL-1 receptor type II (IL-1RII) does not induce signal transduction.

and elevated levels of IL-1 can also affect patient susceptibility and severity of CNS injury (McColl et al., 2009; Denes et al., 2010). The overwhelming majority of patients presenting with ischemic or hemorrhagic stroke have one or more risk factors including obesity, hypertension, atherosclerosis, diabetes and infection, which account for 60–80% of stroke risk in the general population (Hankey, 2006; Emsley and Hopkins, 2008). Alongside an increase in susceptibility to stroke, these risk factors also correlate to poorer outcomes both experimentally (Deng et al., 2014; Kim et al., 2014) and clinically (Oppenheimer et al., 1985; Razinia et al., 2007). Evidence indicates that a common element links all of these co-morbidities—namely a raised inflammatory status (Kwan et al., 2013). This pre-existing inflammation can present either chronically or as an acute event such as infection. The importance of these risk factors is highlighted by a study which showed that stroke incidence fell by 29% from 1999 to 2008 and 56 day mortality was reduced from 21% to 12% in 2008 due to better primary management of cardiovascular risk factors with lipid lowering and anti-hypertensive drugs (Lee et al., 2011). It is therefore essential to incorporate these conventional risk factors into preclinical models and to account for their potential actions when treating stroke patients.

Advancing age is the single most important non-modifiable risk factor for stroke with half of all ischemic events occurring in those aged over 75 (Roger et al., 2011). Tight control is usually exerted over the immune system; however, with advanced age this control is lost and there is an increase in serum levels of inflammatory cytokines (Jenny et al., 2002) which increases the vulnerability of the aged brain to stroke. In experimental models of stroke in aged, hypertensive and diabetic animals, an increase in mortality, neurological deficits and infarct volumes are observed (Rewell et al., 2010).

The metabolic syndrome which comprises obesity, dyslipidemia and diabetes is also a risk factor for stroke that has, with societal lifestyle changes, become increasingly prevalent in recent years (Mottillo et al., 2010). Obesity alone is an independent risk factor for stroke and a positive correlation has been observed in multiple ethnic populations and in both sexes, regardless of whether adiposity is measured by body mass index, waist circumference or waist to height proportion (Suk et al., 2003; Yatsuya et al., 2010; Bodenant et al., 2011).

A raised systemic inflammatory profile is a characteristic feature of obesity, evidenced by the raised levels of c-reactive protein (CRP) and IL-6 (Visser et al., 1999; Yudkin et al., 1999). Furthermore, increasing circulating levels of IL-6 and CRP may lead to progressively higher risk of ischemic events (Rost et al., 2001; Miwa et al., 2013). Diabetic patients similarly have higher rates of mortality, more disabling strokes and exhibit impaired recovery following stroke in retrospective and prospective studies when compared to non-diabetic stroke patients (Pulsinelli et al., 1983; Oppenheimer et al., 1985; Woo et al., 1990).

Hypertension is another key modifiable stroke risk factor, with elevated blood pressure (BP) making up 30–40% of all ischemic stroke risk (Lawes et al., 2004). Presence of high BP prior to ischemia also resulted in worse outcome at 10 days and 6 months post-stroke when measured independently of baseline risk factors (Abboud et al., 2006). In experimental models, the harmful effects of obesity, diabetes and hypertension post-stroke have been clearly demonstrated, causing increased ischemic damage, greater disruption of blood brain barrier (BBB) integrity, increased occurrence of hemorrhagic transformation, greater neurological deficits and increased mortality (McColl et al., 2010; Li et al., 2013a,b). This exacerbation in acute injury due to the presence of a pre-existing inflammatory disease has also been seen in a model of ICH in the presence of experimental diabetes. Presence of hyperglycemia increased hematoma expansion and therefore resulted in worse outcome (Liu et al., 2011).

Atherosclerosis is one of the primary contributors to stroke risk due to the rupture and detachment of vascular plaques which can result in thromboembolism (Ohira et al., 2006). Inflammation plays a central role in the initiation and destabilization of atherosclerotic plaques. Unstable plaques have been shown to contain elevated levels of infiltrating leukocytes that express proteolytic enzymes and thrombogenic substances that contribute to the disruption of previously stable plaques (Ross, 1999; Patel et al., 2008; Packard et al., 2009). Experimental studies have utilized anti-inflammatory strategies (e.g., IL-1 neutralization, TNFα antagonism) to show that dampening of the inflammatory response hinders atherosclerotic lesion progression (Braunersreuther et al., 2008; McKellar et al., 2009; Bhaskar et al., 2011).

Infection is another critical risk factor for stroke, with epidemiological studies highlighting an association between bacterial or viral infection and ischemic stroke (Grau et al., 2010). In a study of approximately 19,000 patients from the UK general practice research database, the risk of first time stroke was highest 3 days after diagnosis of infection (Smeeth et al., 2004; Clayton et al., 2008). Further support for a link between infection and stroke is provided by research showing increased deaths attributable to cardiovascular disorders and stroke during respiratory infection epidemics (Eickhoff et al., 1961). Urinary and respiratory tract infections are most commonly associated with increased stroke risk, with *Streptococcus pneumoniae* and influenza both having firm associations (Grau et al., 1995). An increased incidence of hemorrhagic stroke has also been noted following upper respiratory infection due to the increased likelihood of formation and rupture of cerebral aneurisms, leading to SAH (Kunze et al., 2000). Furthermore, in a study examining incidence of infection in ICH patients, those that had infection had significantly larger hemorrhages, poorer National Institutes of Health Stroke Scale scores, raised levels of CRP and were more likely to experience intraventricular hemorrhage extension (Diedler et al., 2009). A causal relationship between stroke and infection is supported by overlap of pathways that are common to both, including inflammation and thrombosis. Platelet activation and aggregation is increased in venous blood samples from patients presenting with stroke and pre-existing infection vs. their non-infectious counterparts thus hinting at a potential common detrimental mechanisms (Zeller et al., 2005). Preclinical data on the relationship between stroke risk and infection are surprisingly sparse with only a small number of studies exploring the effects of infection on stroke outcome. One study showed that human influenza A infected mice had larger infarcts and greater disruption in BBB integrity in comparison to non-infected mice (Muhammad et al., 2011). Additionally, research within our own group has shown that chronic infection with the parasitic *Trichuris muris* model of gut infection prior to ischemic stroke in mice exhibited either a Th1 or Th2 polarized immune response. Mice with a Th1 response showed greater neurological deficits and exacerbation of ischemic brain injury (Dénes et al., 2010).

Common stroke risk factors often co-exist as they can converge on shared pathways (e.g., the inflammatory cascade) and therefore patients who have more than one of these risk factors are at a much greater risk of a severe ischemic event, as pre-existing co-morbidities may act synergistically to exacerbate damage (Howells et al., 2010). Since many of the systemic inflammatory conditions mentioned as risk factors for stroke can be improved by inhibition of IL-1, this suggests a key role for this pro-inflammatory cytokine in altering stroke susceptibility and severity.

IL-1 AND PRE-EXISTING INFLAMMATION

Clinically, elevated IL-1 levels are fundamental to many auto-inflammatory diseases which, as a result, may be improved by IL-1 neutralization (e.g., gout, osteoarthritis and post-myocardial infarction heart failure) (Dinarello, 2011). Growing evidence however, implicates this cytokine in known vascular risk factors for stroke (i.e., atherosclerosis, obesity, diabetes, infection and hypertension), and suggest it is crucial to disease progression in many experimental models of vascular disease (Murray et al., 2013).

IL-1: A VASCULAR RISK FACTOR

In atherosclerosis and obesity, NOD-like receptor protein (NLRP)-3 inflammasome (the inflammasome that controls caspase-1 activity and thus IL-1β processing to its mature form) was a key driving factor in progression of the diseases (Duewell et al., 2010; Vandanmagsar et al., 2011). These results are supported by research in a strain of atherosclerotic-susceptible mice (fed a high-fat diet) crossed with IL-1R1 KO mice. These mice, despite being predisposed to develop atherosclerosis, had a reduced plaque burden and lowered BP due to the ablation of the IL-1R1 and selective loss of IL-1 signaling (Chamberlain et al., 2009). A further study examining the inflammatory state of hypertensive rats following a stroke observed elevated levels of IL-1 which correlated to increased ischemic damage (Liu et al., 1993). In genetic association studies, IL-1 or IL-1Ra gene polymorphisms are associated with increased susceptibility to stroke, atherosclerosis and ICH in humans (Seripa et al., 2003; Um et al., 2003; Worrall et al., 2003; Dziedzic et al., 2005; Rezaii et al., 2009). Further genetic studies assessing the influence of IL-1 genotype status on the risk of cardiovascular disease show that patients with a predisposition to express higher levels of IL-1 were at a significantly higher risk of having coronary artery disease (CAD) due to excess oxidized phospholipids and lipoproteins. This enhanced risk of CAD was not observed in IL-1(-) genotypes (Tsimikas et al., 2014).

IL-1 AND EXAGGERATED BRAIN INJURY

In addition to increasing susceptibility to ischemic stroke, high levels of pre-existing IL-1, exacerbates post-stroke damage. Peripherally-administered lipopolysaccharide (LPS; which produces a robust IL-1 response) has been used to induce systemic inflammation in mice and administration prior to experimental middle cerebral artery occlusion results in a 150% increase in infarct volume when compared to vehicle-treated animals. To further confirm the importance of IL-1 in this model, animals treated with LPS and IL-1Ra had infarct volumes reduced by 60% compared to animals treated with LPS alone (McColl et al., 2007). Pre-existing IL-1 administration also exacerbates acute TBI injury by increasing volume of contusion injury, hippocampal neuronal death and enhancing perivascular neutrophil accumulation (Utagawa et al., 2008). Another example of the damaging effects of acute systemic IL-1 prior to ischemia is seen in models of infection. In mice and rats infected with *Streptococcus pneumoniae*, a robust IL-1 response was induced leading to larger infarct volumes, increased BBB disruption and functional deficits post-stroke. These effects were abrogated by delayed IL-1Ra administration (Dénes et al., 2014). Alongside preclinical evidence, clinical evidence also seems to hint that the presence of a pre-existing, inflammatory infection prior to stroke can impair outcome at later time points, as evidenced by neurological scores (Paganini-Hill et al., 2003; Grau et al., 2010).

The research outlined above indicates that systemic IL-1, whether it pre-existing or post-injury, plays a crucial role in mediating excess acute brain injury, though mechanisms involved remain unclear. As such we propose below a number of mechanisms through which IL-1 may mediate its detrimental actions in acute brain injury.

INFLAMMATION AND THE CEREBROVASCULATURE

During the acute phase of ischemic stroke, inflammation initiates a robust response from many cell types including glial and brain endothelial cells. Considering the vascular nature of stroke and that many of the risk factors that predispose patients to an ischemic insult are characterized by vascular inflammation, it is possible that the brain endothelium is a point of convergence for mechanisms of inflammatory-associated damage. The cerebrovasculature has a number of crucial roles in both physiological and pathological conditions, including regulation of vascular tone (Palomares and Cipolla, 2014). In situations where routes of flow are occluded or cerebral blood flow (CBF) is inadequate as in the case of ischemic and hemorrhagic stroke, intrinsic safeguards, both structural and functional in nature, are in place to maintain and stabilize CBF (Palomares and Cipolla, 2014).

STRUCTURAL ABNORMALITIES ASSOCIATED WITH VASCULAR INFLAMMATION

Under pathological conditions risk factors for stroke have profound effects on cerebrovasculature structure with structural anomalies often being associated with chronic systemic inflammatory diseases (Arsava et al., 2014). In atherosclerosis, plaque formation reduces the internal diameter of vessels and increases the likelihood of thrombus formation and ischemic attack (Bogiatzi et al., 2014). In patients with hypertension, vascular remodeling and hypertrophy is a characteristic feature of the disease and contributes to increased wall thickness, reduced lumen diameter and reduced vascular responsiveness to stimuli (Pabbidi et al., 2013). Furthermore, in a small retrospective study of patients with chronic hyperglycemia, cerebral microvascular remodeling and perfusion deficits were observed in these patients through perfusion computer tomography (Hou et al., 2013). Further studies have also observed vascular asymmetry and a reduction in the number of branches in obese Zucker rats vs. lean Zucker and Wistar rats (Lapi et al., 2013).

FUNCTIONAL ABNORMALITIES ASSOCIATED WITH VASCULAR INFLAMMATION

In addition to changes in the structural architecture of the cerebrovasculature in the presence of systemic inflammation, functional deficits are also apparent. Experimentally, mice fed a high-fat diet for 8 weeks had impaired cerebrovascular function and neurovascular coupling leading to an increase in infarct volume and neurological deficits (Li et al., 2013c). In diabetic rats, CBF responses to sciatic nerve or whisker stimulation were depressed in both type I and type II diabetes (Jackman and Iadecola, 2015) The influence of inflammatory co-morbidities on ischemic penumbra has also been measured in stroke-prone spontaneously hypertensive rats (SHRSP) vs. Wistar Kyoto rats. Results from magnetic resonance imaging (MRI) showed that within 1 h of stroke, SHRSP had significantly more ischemic damage and a smaller penumbra than their normotensive counterparts (McCabe et al., 2009). The expanding perfusion deficit in SHRSP predicts more tissue at risk of infarction, which correlates to poorer clinical outcome. These results have important implications for management of stroke patients with pre-existing hypertension and suggest that ischemic damage could progress at a faster rate in the presence of a disease with an activated inflammatory cascade. It is likely that the vascular risk factors commonly associated with stroke cause cerebral vascular dysfunction (either structural and/or functional), which manifests as inadequate perfusion in brain areas at risk of infarction (the ischemic penumbra). In the clinical setting, perfusion deficits have also been observed in Alzheimer's (Tosun et al., 2009; Austin et al., 2011) and Parkinson's (Takahashi et al., 2010) disease patients and there is a positive correlation between disease progression and larger CBF deficits. Furthermore, cerebral hypoperfusion has been seen in both relapsing-remitting multiple sclerosis (MS) and primary MS (Adhya et al., 2006). Upregulation of vasoactive mediators have also been implicated in postmortem MS brain tissue and hypoperfusion has been observed in MS patients as measured by MRI (D'Haeseleer et al., 2013). Inflammation may therefore contribute to hypoperfusion in both acute and chronic pathologies in preclinical and clinical scenarios.

EFFECTS OF ACUTE IL-1 ON CEREBRAL BLOOD FLOW

The cerebrovascular endothelium is highly responsive to pro-inflammatory stimuli and a primary location of IL-1RI, so it is possible that IL-1 could mediate changes in CBF observed in pathological disease states. Studies in rats have shown that prolonged intracerebroventricular (i.c.v) administration of IL-1 significantly reduced CBF (Maher et al., 2003). During early reperfusion in a rodent model of ischemic stroke a marked reduction in CBF was also observed in animals receiving an intraperitoneal (i.p) injection of IL-1. This same effect was not seen in control stroke animals who did not receive IL-1 (Parry-Jones et al., 2008). Whether effects on CBF reported with i.c.v injection of IL-1 (Maher et al., 2003) are as a result of systemic inflammatory changes is not known, since this was not assessed in the study. However, leakage of substances injected into the cerebral ventricles to the systemic circulation is known so it may be a possibility, especially given that IL-1 was administered over a 2- or 4-week period. A reduction in CBF in the cerebral microcirculation can impinge upon successful reperfusion thus leading to an accelerated collapse of the penumbra and expansion of infarct core. It is therefore possible, that the detrimental role of IL-1 on CBF in the early stages following acute stroke may account for the ability of IL-1 to exacerbate cerebral ischemia (Parry-Jones et al., 2008). In further studies examining this mechanism of IL-1 induced hypoperfusion, acute administration of IL-1 prior to ischemia resulted in a significant perfusion deficit and larger infarct volumes as measured by diffusion-weighted and perfusion-weighted MRI. It was revealed that raised levels of the vasoconstrictor endothelin-1 were present within tissue experiencing hypoperfusion and blockade of the endothelin receptor type A (ETrA) restored CBF and improved infarct volume and functional outcomes. Overall, this indicated acute systemic inflammation interacted with the vasculature to induce changes in CBF which ultimately had a detrimental effect during acute reperfusion (Murray et al., 2014). This hypothesis is further supported by translational studies demonstrating that patients with a history of recent acute infection in the week leading up to their stroke exhibited vascular dysfunction (Pleiner et al., 2004; Bryant et al., 2005). From a peripheral vascular perspective, infection can also transiently impair endothelium-dependent relaxation as observed in children with acute infections (generally upper respiratory tract). Brachial artery flow mediated dilation was measured in a cohort of 600 children suffering from acute infection or recovering from acute infection. Lower brachial artery flow was seen compared to uninfected controls (Charakida et al., 2005). Whilst not examined in the aforementioned human association studies, links between upper respiratory tract infection and high levels of IL-1 have been previously observed. In a study by Dénes et al. the presence of *Streptococcus pneumoniae* infection in mice and rats prior to ischemia significantly exacerbated infarct volume. Delayed administration of IL-1Ra however abolished the infection-induced deficits in functional outcomes and brain injury and vascular activation thus highlighting the detrimental effects of IL-1 on the cerebrovasculature prior to ischemia (Dénes et al., 2014).

CHRONIC IL-1 AND CEREBRAL BLOOD FLOW

Similar mechanisms of inflammation induced vasoconstriction have also been noted in a chronic inflammatory model, the obese Zucker rat in which pressure-induced vasoconstriction was examined. It was observed that these animals exhibited increased myogenic activation and a robust vasoconstrictive response vs. their lean counterparts. This phenomenon was abolished by removal of the endothelium, thus suggesting the endothelium was targeted by systemic inflammation and regulated arterial constriction (Butcher et al., 2013). Furthermore, depletion of macrophages in a hypertensive model improved perfusion however, peripheral arteries did not respond in a similar fashion, suggesting chronic inflammation has brain-specific effects which may not be mirrored in other vascular beds (Pires et al., 2013). Studies have shown that endothelium-dependent relaxation was impaired in type II diabetes in rats and could be restored using ETrA antagonism, thus reinforcing the concept that inflammation-induced vasoconstriction following ischemic stroke may feature in chronic systemic inflammatory conditions (Harris et al., 2008). Changes in the diameter of the cerebral vasculature have also been observed in cases of SAH, stroke, epilepsy and migraine through propagating waves of neuronal depolarization, otherwise known as spreading depolarization (SD; Lauritzen et al., 2011). Inflammatory mediators have also been associated with waves of SD (Urbach et al., 2006), thus reinforcing the hypothesis that inflammation may have a crucial role in determining vessel contractility and tissue perfusion. However, future studies are needed to directly examine the role of chronic inflammation on CBF following stroke and brain injury and to what degree the pro-inflammatory cytokine IL-1 might play in altering vasomotor tone in chronically inflamed cerebrovasculature.

INFLAMMATION AND HYPOPERFUSION: A MECHANICAL ELEMENT?

Following CNS injury, a breach in endothelial integrity has multiple downstream consequences ranging from alterations in endothelial reactivity, vascular tone, pro-coagulant state and inflammatory phenotype (Taka et al., 2002; Clark et al., 2012). The cerebral endothelium is a primary target for neuroinflammatory stimuli due to its capacity to alter vascular tone through chemical and mechanical mechanisms. As discussed above the pro-inflammatory cytokine IL-1 can directly induce expression of vasoactive mediators (e.g., ET-1) which can alter vascular tone through actions on vascular smooth muscle (Moncada and Higgs, 2006; Anfossi et al., 2010). However, the cerebrovasculature can also obstruct CBF following CNS injury by mechanical means.

The role of leukocyte-platelet interactions on CBF

Physical blockade within the cerebrovasculature can be mediated by the interaction between neutrophils and brain endothelial cells. Inflammation can induce an upregulation of adhesion molecules (P-selectin, intercellular adhesion molecule-1 (ICAM-1), vascular cell adhesion molecule-1) and chemokines (IL-8, monocyte chemoattractant protein-1, macrophage inflammatory protein-1) in endothelial cells. Within hours of ischemic injury, circulating neutrophils can either transmigrate between endothelial cells from the blood to the injured tissue or remain adherent to the luminal surface of blood vessels as seen in murine and human post-stroke tissue samples (Enzmann et al., 2013). Neutrophils can release pro-inflammatory mediators which elicit secondary injury to the salvageable ischemic penumbra (Jin et al., 2010; **Figure 2**). Physically, the presence of neutrophils in the microvasculature of the brain under conditions of ischemia and altered perfusion can result in an exaggerated neutrophil accumulation and obstruction in CBF, referred to as the "no re-flow" phenomenon (del Zoppo et al., 1991). In a similar fashion to neutrophils, circulating platelets can also exacerbate ischemic stroke mechanically by impeding CBF. The "no re-flow phenomenon" suggests that the post-stroke complication of hypoperfusion can be attributed to platelet and neutrophil accumulation in microvessels alongside fibrin deposition and obstructive leukocytes (del Zoppo et al., 1991). This accumulation can be reversed in mice receiving anti-glycoprotein (GP) Ib treatment (i.e., to prevent the interaction between platelets and the brain endothelium) thus showing an improvement in post-stroke ischemic CBF (Pham et al., 2011). Furthermore, in transient models of ischemia, anti-leukocyte interventions result in neuroprotection. Using laser-scanning confocal microscopy and laser-Doppler perfusion imaging, neutrophils adhering to the endothelium have been shown to contribute to perfusion deficits following the restoration of CBF (Belayev et al., 2002). Furthermore, treatment with albumin was shown to reverse the adherence and perfusion deficits within the post-capillary microcirculation during the post-ischemic reperfusion period. This mechanical obstruction of CBF by accumulation of platelets and/or neutrophils has also been seen in models of SAH in both dogs and humans (Asano and Sano, 1977; Dóczi, 1985).

In addition to their mechanical effects platelets also have detrimental chemical actions, including the ability to expel their granular contents and to synthesize immune related proteins such as IL-1 (Afshar-Kharghan and Thiagarajan, 2006). Indirectly, platelets can induce an inflammatory response in other cells (e.g., endothelium, microglia) by releasing IL-1 (Hawrylowicz et al., 1991). The important role of activated platelets has been seen in recent research showing that immediately following injury neutrophils recruited to sites of injury can extend a domain to scan for locally activated platelets. Only when productive interactions between platelets and neutrophil projections occur do neutrophils initiate intravascular migration or generate NETs to propel inflammatory responses (Sreeramkumar et al., 2014). This suggests neutrophils and platelets work co-operatively to exacerbate inflammation. *In vivo*, platelets represent a source of IL-1α and it has been proposed that activation of cerebral endothelium via platelet-dependent IL-1 is a crucial step in triggering neutrophil migration to the parenchyma (Thornton et al., 2010). Experimentally, neutralizing platelet GP surface receptors (Le Behot et al., 2014) or use of small molecule inhibitors of GpIIb/IIIa (Lapchak et al., 2002) can improve CBF and functional outcome following ischemic stroke. However, care must be taken when targeting particular GP interactions as some have more potent antithrombotic effects than others (Grüner et al., 2005). Heightened systemic inflammation can also exaggerate platelet adhesion, aggregation and the coagulation cascade (Cao et al., 2009; Granger et al., 2010) which again highlights the pivotal role that inflammatory cascades play in multiple stroke etiologies. Platelet hyperactivity and dysregulation is common to diabetes (Ferroni et al., 2004), hypercholesteremia (Haramaki et al., 2007), hypertension (Gkaliagkousi et al., 2009) and atherosclerosis (Ruggeri, 2003). Thus, platelet and leukocyte interactions are a hallmark of acute and chronic inflammatory diseases and in combination with an ischemic injury may have synergistic detrimental effects.

Another important regulator of CBF are pericytes. Pericytes are contractile cells located on capillaries and have an important role in controlling CBF. In one study exploring the role of pericytes, rat brain slices were exposed to conditions mimicking ischemia, resulting in persistent vasoconstriction and pericyte death (Hall et al., 2014). This pericyte death caused a "rigor mortis" and prolonged vasoconstriction due to adenosine triphosphate (ATP) deprivation that restricts myosin and actin separation and subsequent relaxation. Pericyte dilation and contractility is controlled by various vasoactive mediators and pericytes have the capacity to respond readily to these mediators as they are derived from the smooth muscle cell lineage (Nehls and Drenckhahn, 1993; Pieper et al., 2014). Mechanical obstruction of CBF can also occur due to compression of vessels by progressively edematous neighboring astrocytes (Ito et al., 2011).

Whilst protection of vulnerable new neurons is an important strategy in treating brain injury, stroke is, etiologically, a vascular disorder. It is therefore important to consider the implications of systemic inflammation on the cerebrovasculature and the downstream consequences on CBF.

REPAIR AND RECOVERY POST-STROKE: THE ROLE OF NEUROGENESIS

Aside from modest advancements in neurorehabillitation therapies for stroke survivors there is an absence of effective treatment options beyond the 4.5 h time window that promote any significant recovery. Yet, the brain does command certain endogenous repair processes that are employed following CNS injury to limit cell death and promote neural repair, though this is insufficient to have any major effect in the majority of patients.

A possible driver of functional recovery is post-stroke neurogenesis. Neurogenesis is the generation of new neurons that integrate into pre-existing networks. Contrary to the historical hypothesis that neurons could only form during the developmental periods in early life and were refractory to replication, it is now well established that new neurons are continuously being created in the adult brain. This discovery was aided drastically by the advent of new techniques to track the birth and migration of new neurons (Nowakowski et al., 1989; Paez-Gonzalez et al., 2014). New neurons originate from neural

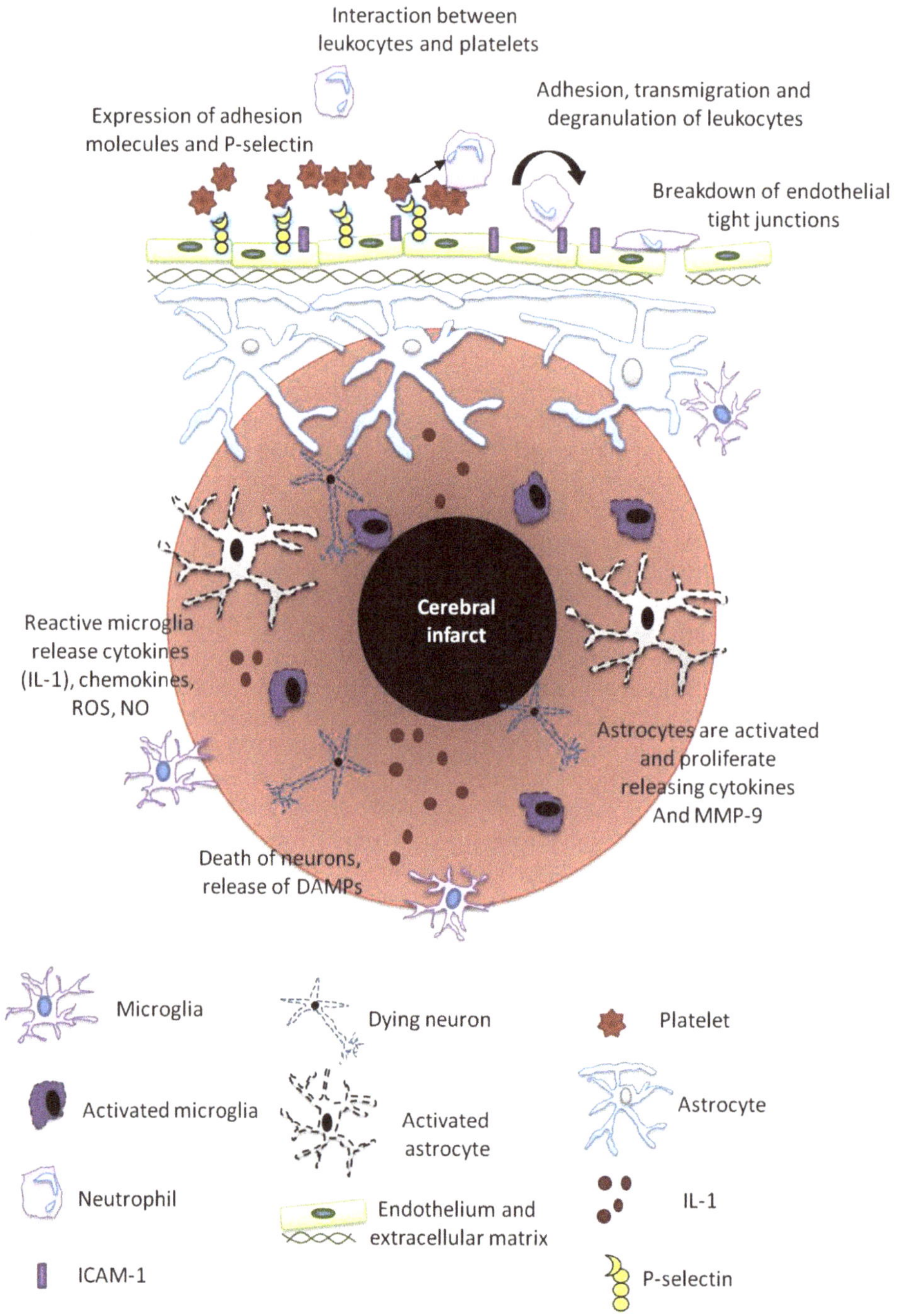

FIGURE 2 | Post-stroke inflammation. Mechanisms of post-stroke inflammation occur via a number of pathways as outlined and include a variety of resident immune cells including microglia, astrocytes, neutrophils, platelets and the cerebral endothelium. These cells release mediators that propagate the inflammatory cascade including reactive oxygen species (ROS), nitric oxide (NO), damage-associated molecular patterns (DAMPs), metalloproteinases (MMPs), ICAM and IL-1.

progenitor cells (NPCs), defined as cells that have the capacity for self-renewal and that can produce multiple distinct cell types (e.g., neurons, astrocytes, oligodendrocytes). Adult neurogenesis is normally restricted to two neurogenic regions: the subventricular zone (SVZ; Reynolds and Weiss, 1992) and subgranular zone (SGZ; Gage et al., 1995) which anatomically house NPCs and functionally control their development. Stroke is a robust trigger of neurogenesis by stimulating NPCs of the SVZ to divide and migrate to the peri-infarct area (Arvidsson et al., 2002; Thored et al., 2006). Treatments that either increase the levels of proliferating NPCs or enhance their survival and migration to the peri-infarct brain lesion would contribute to improved functional recovery and tissue survival after stroke (Nih et al., 2012). However, although ischemic stroke promotes neurogenesis in neurogenic regions and migration of NPCs to sites of injury; most newly generated neurons fail to survive. It is proposed that inflammation associated with ischemic stroke and the pre-existing inflammatory co-morbidities or age may contribute to the high levels of apoptotic death of stroke-generated neuroblasts in preclinical models of ischemia (Seki and Arai, 1995; Kuhn et al., 1996; Kokaia et al., 2006).

INFLAMMATION AND NEUROGENESIS

Mechanisms through which inflammation impairs neurogenesis are poorly understood, due to the range of cells and signaling pathways that can be activated in response to an inflammatory stimulus. Adult neurogenesis is compromised in environments of the brain with mitochondrial dysfunction (Kirby et al., 2009), raised reactive oxygen species (ROS; Zhang et al., 2012), brain irradiation (Monje et al., 2003) and most interestingly, in the presence of activated microglia (Ekdahl et al., 2003; Monje and Palmer, 2003). The connection between reduced neurogenesis and an upregulation in the number and activity of microglia has been observed in response to systemic LPS and results in a 240% increase in the density of detrimental microglial cells in the dentate gyrus (DG), a structure which is essential for learning and memory formation and consolidation. Detrimental actions of microglia on neurogenesis involve production of ROS and NO (Gebicke-Haerter et al., 2001; Moreno-López et al., 2004). Ablation of microglial function using indomethacin (Hoehn et al., 2005) or minocycline (Liu et al., 2007) improves numbers of NPCs after stroke. However, complete inactivation of microglia may not always have positive effects. It has been hypothesized that microglia may be responsive to interactions with CNS-specific T-cells and thus promote NPC proliferation and neuronal survival (Ziv et al., 2006; Schwartz et al., 2009).

Angiogenesis is another important route of tissue repair post-stroke as blocking angiogenesis reduces the localization of immature neurons to peri-infarct tissue (Ohab and Carmichael, 2008). Inflammatory mediators, in particular IL-1 have been implicated in augmenting angiogenic processes. In a study by Pham et al. (2012) IL-1β stimulated oligodendrocytes to produce MMP-9 in the conditioned media. This conditioned media was placed on endothelial cell cultures resulting in a significant increase in endothelial tube formation. This process was mirrored *in vivo* whereby neutralization of IL-1β in a white mater injury model reduced oligodendrocyte MMP-9 expression and thus angiogenesis (Pham et al., 2012). This improvement in angiogenesis post-stroke following IL-1β treatment has also been seen in endothelial progenitor cell (EPC) cultures. Treatment of EPC cultures with the conditioned media from primary rat cortical astrocytes promoted EPC mediated neurovascular remodeling during the post-stroke period (Hayakawa et al., 2012).

ANTI-INFLAMMATORY STRATEGIES TO IMPROVE POST-STROKE NEUROGENESIS

Current drugs e.g., minocycline, that manipulate microglial function often are broad spectrum and unspecific and influence multiple inflammatory pathways essential for the repair phase of stroke recovery. Since neurogenesis may occur for up to a year following stroke, chronic administration of a drug that can inhibit repair may not be ideal. It is therefore important to consider more specific targets of inflammation rather than broad-spectrum drugs to promote neurogenesis after stroke. As indicated earlier IL-1 is implicated in learning and memory and there are numerous studies showing that stress, which involves an elevated inflammatory profile (Banasr et al., 2007) and high levels of IL-1, causes hippocampal dysfunction and a reduction in neurogenesis (Ben Menachem-Zidon et al., 2008; Mathieu et al., 2010). Preclinical data shows that IL-1 exerts anti-neurogeneic properties in chronic stress through up-regulation of NFκB, activator protein (AP)-1 and signal transducer and activator of transcription (STAT)-1 (Pugazhenthi et al., 2013). The actions of IL-1 on neurogenesis have been examined *in vitro* in primary adult hippocampal progenitor cells which possess IL-1RI (Koo and Duman, 2008) and embryonic cortical NPCs (Ajmone-Cat et al., 2010). When the adult hippocampal progenitor cells were treated with IL-1β, there was a reduction in the number of proliferating progenitor cells. Furthermore, this anti-neurogenic effect was found to be mediated by activation of the NFκB signaling pathway, and could be blocked by IL-1Ra (Koo and Duman, 2008). IL-1 also activates the endothelium to produce trophic factors such as vascular endothelial growth factor (VEGF) and insulin-like growth factor (IGF)-1, which are needed for neurogenesis (Anderson et al., 2002; Cao et al., 2004) and is also important in the reparative angiogenic process (Coxon et al., 2002; Voronov et al., 2003; Carmi et al., 2009). However, effects of IL-1 on neurogenesis following acute cerebral ischemia *in vivo* have yet to be elucidated but the potential use of IL-1Ra to improve neurogenesis is an attractive possibility. However, it must be considered that such anti-inflammatory treatments e.g., IL-1Ra, for stroke must be administered within a time frame that does not interfere with the repair process, otherwise there may be detrimental effects (Girard et al., 2014).

POTENTIAL TREATMENT STRATEGIES TARGETING THE IL-1 SYSTEM

Evidence discussed above and in many other articles highlights the IL-1 system as an attractive therapeutic target in the search for treatments for acute CNS injury. Therapeutic interventions include direct targeting of IL-1, antagonism of the IL-1 receptor, use of neutralizing antibodies and inflammasome inhibitors (**Figure 3**). Despite these alternatives, IL-1Ra remains the most widely researched inhibitor of IL-1 actions due to its high specificity and safety. Anakinra, the recombinant form of human IL-1Ra, has a half-life of 4–6 h and is well-tolerated in the patient population, as evidenced by significant research in the rheumatoid arthritis field in which it is a mainstream drug treatment (Mertens and Singh, 2009). Within preclinical stroke studies, the neuroprotective effects of IL-1Ra have been seen in a variety of species e.g., mice, rats and gerbils (Ohtsuki et al., 1996; McColl et al., 2007; Pradillo et al., 2012) and in differing models of ischemia e.g., focal, global, transient and global (Rothwell, 2003). IL-1Ra maintains its neuroprotective effects through a number of routes of administration e.g., i.c.v, i.v and subcutaneously (s.c) (Greenhalgh et al., 2010).

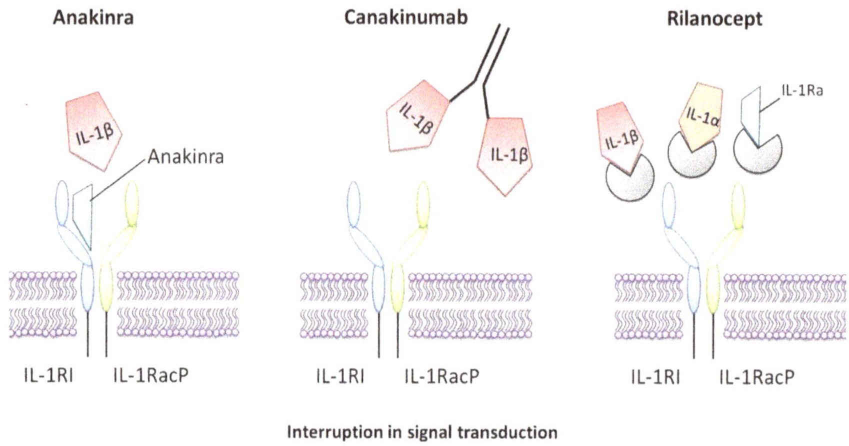

FIGURE 3 | Interleukin-1 inhibitors that are in current clinical use. Anakinra is a recombinant form of human IL-1Ra that directly competes with IL-1 for binding to the IL-1 type I receptor, therefore blocking the biological activity of IL-1. Canakinumab is a human monoclonal antibody that selectively targets IL-1β. Rilonacept is a human dimeric fusion protein that interrupts IL-1 signaling by incorporating components of the IL-1 receptor, thus trapping and sequestering circulating IL-1.

Finally, and perhaps most importantly, IL-1Ra can still inhibit ischemic injury at delayed time points up to 3–4.5 h (Mulcahy et al., 2003) and in co-morbid strains. In a meta-analysis analyzing the effects of IL-1Ra in preclinical models of stroke, IL-1Ra treatment elicited an overall 38% reduction in infarct volume across 17 published studies (Banwell et al., 2009; Parry-Jones et al., 2010). In the clinical arena, results from a randomized, double-blind, placebo-controlled trial of IL-1Ra in acute stroke showed that patients receiving IL-1Ra had lower peripheral white blood cell counts, neutrophil counts, CRP and IL-6 levels. Furthermore, by 3 months, these patients showed some evidence of improved recovery compared to placebo-controlled counterparts, though it is important to realize the study was not powered for such an outcome (Emsley et al., 2005). Further larger scale trials of IL-1Ra in both SAH (ISRCTN25048895) and acute ischemic stroke (ISRCTN74236229) are ongoing. The clinical trial examining the effects of IL-1Ra on inflammatory mediators in SAH has just recruited the final patient and results are expected early in 2015. It is a multi-center, single-blind open label randomized control trial incorporating 140 patients. IL-1Ra was administered twice daily by s.c administration for 21 days in patients presenting within 72 h with aneurismal SAH. Blood samples were taken during this time period to analyze IL-6 and CRP alongside the Glasgow outcome scale. The clinical trial examining the effects of IL-1Ra in ischemic stroke started recruiting in Spring 2014 with participants receiving twice daily, s.c injection of IL-1Ra or placebo. The first injection of IL-1Ra is being given within 6 h of stroke onset with 5 more doses at 12 h intervals for 3 days.

In a clinical trial exploring the role of IL-1β in type II diabetes disease progression, in which patients received IL-1Ra (s.c) once daily for 13 weeks, an improvement in insulin production and glycemic control was observed, along with a reduction in the inflammatory biomarkers, CRP and IL-6 (Larsen et al., 2007). More promising still, in the 39 week follow up study, patients receiving IL-1Ra used 66% less insulin to return to baseline glycemic control levels (Larsen et al., 2009). In a phase II randomized control trial in patients with severe TBI (s.c) administration of IL-1Ra has been shown to be safe, penetrate the brain and to alter the neuroinflammatory response (Helmy et al., 2014).

Clinically, abrogation of IL-1β has also been explored (Yamasaki et al., 1995). Canakinumab is a human monoclonal antibody that selectively targets IL-1β and it has a half-life of 21–28 days (Chakraborty et al., 2012). The use of canakinumab in humans has already been approved for treating arthritis and tested in cryopyrin-associated periodic syndrome (CAPS; Church and McDermott, 2010; Kuemmerle-Deschner et al., 2011; Chakraborty et al., 2013). With this clinical success has come a barrage of research using this anti-IL-1β antibody with much interest in its use in neonatal onset inflammation disease (Sibley et al., 2014), type II diabetes (Howard et al., 2014) and stroke (Ridker et al., 2011). Direct targeting of IL-1 has also been achieved using rilonacept, a human dimeric fusion protein that interferes with IL-1 signaling due to the presence of extracellular components of IL-1RI and IL-1RaP which bind with high affinity to circulating IL-1. This "IL-1 trap" has a half-life of 67 h and has been shown to be safe and effective in CAPS (Goldbach-Mansky et al., 2008; Hoffman et al., 2008). It has been shown that directly targeting IL-1 is a clinically approved strategy for treating auto-immune and autoinflammatory diseases. However further pre-clinical and clinical research is needed if these inhibitors are to be used as therapeutic agents in treating stroke or acute brain injury. Another important consideration when targeting IL-1 is the relative contribution of IL-1α vs. IL-1β. IL-1Ra and rilonacept block the actions of both α and β however canakinumab only targets IL-1β. Historically, IL-1β was considered the primary ligand mediating an exaggerated response to ischemic injury however recent research indicates IL-1α also plays a crucial role in post-stroke pathogenesis and that it may proceed IL-1β expression (Luheshi et al., 2011). In conclusion, it is essential to consider the relative contribution of IL-1α and β to the disease in question, and to identify the time frame in which the anti-inflammatory strategy may be of most benefit.

One of the disadvantages of using IL-1Ra is that BBB penetration is poor due to the large size (kDa) of the macromolar protein. An alternative could be the use of a novel, synthetic peptide called Llantide. This protein is derived from the N-terminal domain of IL-1Ra and therefore mediates its protective effects by binding to IL-1RI and therefore inhibiting NFκB activation and secretion of TNFα from macrophages. The use of this novel peptide in response to an inflammatory challenge e.g., LPS, reduces symptoms of sickness behavior and reduced social depression commonly associated with systemic LPS administration alongside improving plasma levels of IL-10 (Klementiev et al., 2014). Small molecule inhibitors of caspase-1 are protective in experimental models of acute CNS injury (Ross et al., 2007; Suzuki et al., 2009), while neutralization of components of the NLRP1 inflammasome is beneficial in rodent models of ischemic stroke (Fann et al., 2013). Furthermore, ablation of components of the NLRP3 inflammasome are associated with reduced leukocyte infiltration, reduced edema and improvements in neurological function following ICH in mice (Ma et al., 2014). However inhibition of caspase 1 or the inflammasome has yet to be evaluated clinically in stroke.

CONCLUDING REMARKS

A wealth of evidence now exists to show that inflammation is a critical component in cerebral ischemia, by increasing risk and contributing to worse outcome. Conversely, late stage inflammatory processes post-stroke may contribute to brain repair. IL-1 is the first described inflammatory cytokine and has numerous actions that contribute to both injury and repair. Block of IL-1 actions has been demonstrated to be effective in a wide range of clinical conditions, and there is strong experimental evidence to support its role as a key mediator of acute neuronal injury. Ongoing clinical trials in stroke and SAH using IL-1Ra to block the effects of IL-1 will provide further evidence on the potential of IL-1 as a target. Ultimately though this will only be confirmed following successful large Phase III clinical trials of IL-1Ra or alternative inhibitors of IL-1 actions.

ACKNOWLEDGMENTS

This work was supported by the Natalie Kate Moss Trust and Medical Research Council, UK.

REFERENCES

Abboud, H., Labreuche, J., Plouin, F., and Amarenco, P. (2006). High blood pressure in early acute stroke: a sign of a poor outcome? *J. Hypertens.* 24, 381–386. doi: 10.1097/01.hjh.0000200516.33194.e3

Adhya, S., Johnson, G., Herbert, J., Jaggi, H., Babb, J. S., Grossman, R. I., et al. (2006). Pattern of hemodynamic impairment in multiple sclerosis: dynamic susceptibility contrast perfusion MR imaging at 3.0 T. *Neuroimage* 33, 1029–1035. doi: 10.1016/j.neuroimage.2006.08.008

Afshar-Kharghan, V., and Thiagarajan, P. (2006). Leukocyte adhesion and thrombosis. *Curr. Opin. Hematol.* 13, 34–39. doi: 10.1097/01.moh.0000190107.54790.de

Ajmone-Cat, M. A., Cacci, E., Ragazzoni, Y., Minghetti, L., and Biagioni, S. (2010). Pro-gliogenic effect of IL-1alpha in the differentiation of embryonic neural precursor cells in vitro. *J. Neurochem.* 113, 1060–1072. doi: 10.1111/j.1471-4159.2010.06670.x

Albers, G. W., Goldstein, L. B., Hess, D. C., Wechsler, L. R., Furie, K. L., Gorelick, P. B., et al. (2011). Stroke Treatment Academic Industry Roundtable (STAIR) recommendations for maximizing the use of intravenous thrombolytics and expanding treatment options with intra-arterial and neuroprotective therapies. *Stroke* 42, 2645–2650. doi: 10.1161/strokeaha.111.618850

Allan, S. M., and Rothwell, N. J. (2001). Cytokines and acute neurodegeneration. *Nat. Rev. Neurosci.* 2, 734–744. doi: 10.1038/sj.mp.4000223

Allan, S. M., and Rothwell, N. J. (2003). Inflammation in central nervous system injury. *Philos. Trans. R. Soc. Lond. B Biol. Sci.* 358, 1669–1677. doi: 10.1098/rstb.2003.1358

Allan, S. M., Tyrrell, P. J., and Rothwell, N. J. (2005). Interleukin-1 and neuronal injury. *Nat. Rev. Immunol.* 5, 629–640. doi: 10.1038/nri1664

Anderson, M. F., Aberg, M. A. I., Nilsson, M., and Eriksson, P. S. (2002). Insulin-like growth factor-I and neurogenesis in the adult mammalian brain. *Brain Res. Dev. Brain Res.* 134, 115–122. doi: 10.1016/s0165-3806(02)00277-8

Andrews, A. E., Barcham, G. J., Brandon, M. R., and Nash, A. D. (1991). Molecular cloning and characterization of ovine IL-1 alpha and IL-1 beta. *Immunology* 74, 453–460.

Anfossi, G., Russo, I., Doronzo, G., Pomero, A., and Trovati, M. (2010). Adipocytokines in atherothrombosis: focus on platelets and vascular smooth muscle cells. *Mediators Inflamm.* 2010:174341. doi: 10.1155/2010/174341

Arsava, E. M., Vural, A., Akpinar, E., Gocmen, R., Akcalar, S., Oguz, K. K., et al. (2014). The detrimental effect of aging on leptomeningeal collaterals in ischemic stroke. *J. Stroke Cerebrovasc. Dis.* 23, 421–426. doi: 10.1016/j.jstrokecerebrovasdis.2013.03.014

Arvidsson, A., Collin, T., Kirik, D., Kokaia, Z., and Lindvall, O. (2002). Neuronal replacement from endogenous precursors in the adult brain after stroke. *Nat. Med.* 8, 963–970. doi: 10.1038/nm747

Asano, T., and Sano, K. (1977). Pathogenetic role of no-reflow phenomenon in experimental subarachnoid hemorrhage in dogs. *J. Neurosurg.* 46, 454–466. doi: 10.3171/jns.1977.46.4.0454

Austin, B. P., Nair, V. A., Meier, T. B., Xu, G., Rowley, H. A., Carlsson, C. M., et al. (2011). Effects of hypoperfusion in Alzheimer's disease. *J. Alzheimers. Dis.* 26(Suppl. 3), 123–133. doi: 10.3233/JAD-2011-0010

Banasr, M., Valentine, G. W., Li, X.-Y., Gourley, S. L., Taylor, J. R., and Duman, R. S. (2007). Chronic unpredictable stress decreases cell proliferation in the cerebral cortex of the adult rat. *Biol. Psychiatry* 62, 496–504. doi: 10.1016/j.biopsych.2007.02.006

Banwell, V., Sena, E. S., and Macleod, M. R. (2009). Systematic review and stratified meta-analysis of the efficacy of interleukin-1 receptor antagonist in animal models of stroke. *J. Stroke Cerebrovasc. Dis.* 18, 269–276. doi: 10.1016/j.jstrokecerebrovasdis.2008.11.009

Belayev, L., Pinard, E., Nallet, H., Seylaz, J., Liu, Y., Riyamongkol, P., et al. (2002). Albumin therapy of transient focal cerebral ischemia: in vivo analysis of dynamic microvascular responses. *Stroke* 33, 1077–1084. doi: 10.1161/hs0402.105555

Ben Menachem-Zidon, O., Goshen, I., Kreisel, T., Ben Menahem, Y., Reinhartz, E., Ben Hur, T., et al. (2008). Intrahippocampal transplantation of transgenic neural precursor cells overexpressing interleukin-1 receptor antagonist blocks chronic isolation-induced impairment in memory and neurogenesis. *Neuropsychopharmacology* 33, 2251–2262. doi: 10.1038/sj.npp.1301606

Bhaskar, V., Yin, J., Mirza, A. M., Phan, D., Vanegas, S., Issafras, H., et al. (2011). Monoclonal antibodies targeting IL-1 beta reduce biomarkers of atherosclerosis in vitro and inhibit atherosclerotic plaque formation in Apolipoprotein E-deficient mice. *Atherosclerosis* 216, 313–320. doi: 10.1016/j.atherosclerosis.2011.02.026

Bodenant, M., Kuulasmaa, K., Wagner, A., Kee, F., Palmieri, L., Ferrario, M. M., et al. (2011). Measures of abdominal adiposity and the risk of stroke: the MOnica Risk, Genetics, Archiving and Monograph (MORGAM) study. *Stroke* 42, 2872–2877. doi: 10.1161/strokeaha.111.614099

Bogiatzi, C., Hackam, D. G., McLeod, A. I., and Spence, J. D. (2014). Secular trends in ischemic stroke subtypes and stroke risk factors. *Stroke* 45, 3208–3213. doi: 10.1161/strokeaha.114.006536

Boutin, H., LeFeuvre, R. A., Horai, R., Asano, M., Iwakura, Y., and Rothwell, N. J. (2001). Role of IL-1α and IL-1β in ischemic brain damage. *J. Neurosci.* 21, 5528–5534.

Braunersreuther, V., Steffens, S., Arnaud, C., Pelli, G., Burger, F., Proudfoot, A., et al. (2008). A novel RANTES antagonist prevents progression of established atherosclerotic lesions in mice. *Arterioscler. Thromb. Vasc. Biol.* 28, 1090–1096. doi: 10.1161/atvbaha.108.165423

Bryant, A. E., Bayer, C. R., Chen, R. Y. Z., Guth, P. H., Wallace, R. J., and Stevens, D. L. (2005). Vascular dysfunction and ischemic destruction of tissue in Streptococcus pyogenes infection: the role of streptolysin O-induced platelet/neutrophil complexes. *J. Infect. Dis.* 192, 1014–1022. doi: 10.1086/432729

Butcher, J. T., Goodwill, A. G., Stanley, S. C., and Frisbee, J. C. (2013). Differential impact of dilator stimuli on increased myogenic activation of cerebral and skeletal muscle resistance arterioles in obese zucker rats. *Microcirculation* 20, 579–589. doi: 10.1111/micc.12056

Cao, L., Jiao, X., Zuzga, D. S., Liu, Y., Fong, D. M., Young, D., et al. (2004). VEGF links hippocampal activity with neurogenesis, learning and memory. *Nat. Genet.* 36, 827–835. doi: 10.1038/ng1395

Cao, Y.-J., Wang, Y.-M., Zhang, J., Zeng, Y.-J., and Liu, C.-F. (2009). The effects of antiplatelet agents on platelet-leukocyte aggregations in patients with acute cerebral infarction. *J. Thromb. Thrombolysis* 27, 233–238. doi: 10.1007/s11239-007-0190-x

Carmi, Y., Voronov, E., Dotan, S., Lahat, N., Rahat, M. A., Fogel, M., et al. (2009). The role of macrophage-derived IL-1 in induction and maintenance of angiogenesis. *J. Immunol.* 183, 4705–4714. doi: 10.4049/jimmunol.0901511

Chakraborty, A., Tannenbaum, S., Rordorf, C., Lowe, P. J., Floch, D., Gram, H., et al. (2012). Pharmacokinetic and pharmacodynamic properties of canakinumab, a human anti-interleukin-1β monoclonal antibody. *Clin. Pharmacokinet.* 51, e1–e18. doi: 10.2165/11599820-000000000-00000

Chakraborty, A., Van, L. M., Skerjanec, A., Floch, D., Klein, U. R., Krammer, G., et al. (2013). Pharmacokinetic and pharmacodynamic properties of canakinumab in patients with gouty arthritis. *J. Clin. Pharmacol.* 53, 1240–1251. doi: 10.1002/jcph.162

Chamberlain, J., Francis, S., Brookes, Z., Shaw, G., Graham, D., Alp, N. J., et al. (2009). Interleukin-1 regulates multiple atherogenic mechanisms in response to fat feeding. *PLoS One* 4:e5073. doi: 10.1371/journal.pone.0005073

Charakida, M., Donald, A. E., Terese, M., Leary, S., Halcox, J. P., Ness, A., et al. (2005). Endothelial dysfunction in childhood infection. *Circulation* 111, 1660–1665. doi: 10.1161/01.cir.0000160365.18879.1c

Chen, C.-J., Kono, H., Golenbock, D., Reed, G., Akira, S., and Rock, K. L. (2007). Identification of a key pathway required for the sterile inflammatory response triggered by dying cells. *Nat. Med.* 13, 851–856. doi: 10.1038/nm1603

Chen, Z. M., Sandercock, P., Pan, H. C., Counsell, C., Collins, R., Liu, L. S., et al. (2000). Indications for early aspirin use in acute ischemic stroke : a combined analysis of 40 000 randomized patients from the chinese acute stroke trial and the international stroke trial. On behalf of the CAST and IST collaborative groups. *Stroke* 31, 1240–1249. doi: 10.1161/01.str.31.6.1240

Chu, H. X., Kim, H. A., Lee, S., Moore, J. P., Chan, C. T., Vinh, A., et al. (2014). Immune cell infiltration in malignant middle cerebral artery infarction: comparison with transient cerebral ischemia. *J. Cereb. Blood Flow Metab.* 34, 450–459. doi: 10.1038/jcbfm.2013.217

Church, L. D., and McDermott, M. F. (2010). Canakinumab: a human anti-IL-1β monoclonal antibody for the treatment of cryopyrin-associated periodic syndromes. *Expert Rev. Clin. Immunol.* 6, 831–841. doi: 10.1586/eci.10.66

Clark, D., Tuor, U. I., Thompson, R., Institoris, A., Kulynych, A., Zhang, X., et al. (2012). Protection against recurrent stroke with resveratrol: endothelial protection. *PLoS One* 7:e47792. doi: 10.1371/journal.pone.0047792

Clayton, T. C., Thompson, M., and Meade, T. W. (2008). Recent respiratory infection and risk of cardiovascular disease: case-control study through a general practice database. *Eur. Heart J.* 29, 96–103. doi: 10.1093/eurheartj/ehm516

Corbyn, Z. (2014). Statistics: a growing global burden. *Nature* 510, S2–S3. doi: 10.1038/510s2a

Coxon, A., Bolon, B., Estrada, J., Kaufman, S., Scully, S., Rattan, A., et al. (2002). Inhibition of interleukin-1 but not tumor necrosis factor suppresses neovascularization in rat models of corneal angiogenesis and adjuvant arthritis. *Arthritis Rheum.* 46, 2604–2612. doi: 10.1002/art.10546

Cuartero, M. I., Ballesteros, I., Moraga, A., Nombela, F., Vivancos, J., Hamilton, J. A., et al. (2013). N2 neutrophils, novel players in brain inflammation after stroke: modulation by the PPARγ agonist rosiglitazone. *Stroke* 44, 3498–3508. doi: 10.1161/strokeaha.113.002470

del Rey, A., Balschun, D., Wetzel, W., Randolf, A., and Besedovsky, H. O. (2013). A cytokine network involving brain-borne IL-1β, IL-1ra, IL-18, IL-6 and TNFα operates during long-term potentiation and learning. *Brain. Behav. Immun.* 33, 15–23. doi: 10.1016/j.bbi.2013.05.011

del Zoppo, G. J., Schmid-Schönbein, G. W., Mori, E., Copeland, B. R., and Chang, C. M. (1991). Polymorphonuclear leukocytes occlude capillaries following middle cerebral artery occlusion and reperfusion in baboons. *Stroke* 22, 1276–1283. doi: 10.1161/01.str.22.10.1276

D'Haeseleer, M., Beelen, R., Fierens, Y., Cambron, M., Vanbinst, A., Verborgh, C., et al. (2013). Cerebral hypoperfusion in multiple sclerosis is reversible and mediated by endothelin-1. *Proc. Natl. Acad. Sci. U S A* 110, 5654–5658. doi: 10.1073/pnas.1222560110

Dénes, A., Humphreys, N., Lane, T. E., Grencis, R., and Rothwell, N. (2010). Chronic systemic infection exacerbates ischemic brain damage via a CCL5 (regulated on activation, normal T-cell expressed and secreted)-mediated proinflammatory response in mice. *J. Neurosci.* 30, 10086–10095. doi: 10.1523/jneurosci.1227-10.2010

Dénes, Á., Pradillo, J. M., Drake, C., Sharp, A., Warn, P., Murray, K. N., et al. (2014). Streptococcus pneumoniae worsens cerebral ischemia via interleukin 1 and platelet glycoprotein Ibα. *Ann. Neurol.* 75, 670–683. doi: 10.1002/ana.24146

Denes, A., Thornton, P., Rothwell, N. J., and Allan, S. M. (2010). Inflammation and brain injury: acute cerebral ischaemia, peripheral and central inflammation. *Brain. Behav. Immun.* 24, 708–723. doi: 10.1016/j.bbi.2009.09.010

Deng, J., Zhang, J., Feng, C., Xiong, L., and Zuo, Z. (2014). Critical role of matrix metalloprotease-9 in chronic high fat diet-induced cerebral vascular remodelling and increase of ischaemic brain injury in mice†. *Cardiovasc. Res.* 103, 473–484. doi: 10.1093/cvr/cvu154

Diedler, J., Sykora, M., Hahn, P., Rupp, A., Rocco, A., Herweh, C., et al. (2009). C-reactive-protein levels associated with infection predict short- and long-term outcome after supratentorial intracerebral hemorrhage. *Cerebrovasc. Dis.* 27, 272–279. doi: 10.1159/000199465

Dinarello, C. A. (1994). Interleukin-1 antagonists. *J. Interferon Res.* 14, 307. doi: 10.2165/00128413-199308720-00015

Dinarello, C. A. (2011). A clinical perspective of IL-1β as the gatekeeper of inflammation. *Eur. J. Immunol.* 41, 1203–1217. doi: 10.1002/eji.201141550

Dóczi, T. (1985). The pathogenetic and prognostic significance of blood-brain barrier damage at the acute stage of aneurysmal subarachnoid haemorrhage. Clinical and experimental studies. *Acta Neurochir. (Wien)* 77, 110–132. doi: 10.1007/bf01476215

Doll, D. N., Barr, T. L., and Simpkins, J. W. (2014). Cytokines: their role in stroke and potential use as biomarkers and therapeutic targets. *Aging Dis.* 5, 294–306. doi: 10.14336/ad.2014.0500294

Duewell, P., Kono, H., Rayner, K. J., Sirois, C. M., Vladimer, G., Bauernfeind, F. G., et al. (2010). NLRP3 inflammasomes are required for atherogenesis and activated by cholesterol crystals. *Nature* 464, 1357–1361. doi: 10.1038/nature08938

Dziedzic, T., Slowik, A., Pera, J., and Szczudlik, A. (2005). Interleukin 1 beta polymorphism (-511) and risk of stroke due to small vessel disease. *Cerebrovasc. Dis.* 20, 299–303. doi: 10.1159/000087928

Eickhoff, T. C., Sherman, I. L., and Serfling, R. E. (1961). Observations on excess mortality associated with epidemic influenza. *JAMA* 176, 776–782. doi: 10.1001/jama.1961.03040220024005

Ekdahl, C. T., Claasen, J.-H., Bonde, S., Kokaia, Z., and Lindvall, O. (2003). Inflammation is detrimental for neurogenesis in adult brain. *Proc. Natl. Acad. Sci. U S A* 100, 13632–13637. doi: 10.1073/pnas.2234031100

Elkind, M. S. V. (2010). Impact of innate inflammation in population studies. *Ann. N Y Acad. Sci.* 1207, 97–106. doi: 10.1111/j.1749-6632.2010.05736.x

Emsley, H. C., and Hopkins, S. J. (2008). Acute ischaemic stroke and infection: recent and emerging concepts. *Lancet Neurol.* 7, 341–353. doi: 10.1016/s1474-4422(08)70061-9

Emsley, H. C. A., Smith, C. J., Georgiou, R. F., Vail, A., Hopkins, S. J., Rothwell, N. J., et al. (2005). A randomised phase II study of interleukin-1 receptor antagonist in acute stroke patients. *J. Neurol. Neurosurg. Psychiatry* 76, 1366–1372. doi: 10.1136/jnnp.2004.054882

Enzmann, G., Mysiorek, C., Gorina, R., Cheng, Y.-J., Ghavampour, S., Hannocks, M.-J., et al. (2013). The neurovascular unit as a selective barrier to polymorphonuclear granulocyte (PMN) infiltration into the brain after ischemic injury. *Acta Neuropathol.* 125, 395–412. doi: 10.1007/s00401-012-1076-3

Fann, D. Y.-W., Lee, S. Y., Manzanero, S., Tang, S. C., Gelderblom, M., Chunduri, P., et al. (2013). Intravenous immunoglobulin suppresses NLRP1 and NLRP3 inflammasome-mediated neuronal death in ischemic stroke. *Cell Death Dis.* 4:e790. doi: 10.1038/cddis.2013.326

Ferroni, P., Basili, S., Falco, A., and Davì, G. (2004). Platelet activation in type 2 diabetes mellitus. *J. Thromb. Haemost.* 2, 1282–1291. doi: 10.1111/j.1538-7836.2004.00836.x

Fisher, M., Feuerstein, G., Howells, D. W., Hurn, P. D., Kent, T. A., Savitz, S. I., et al. (2009). Update of the stroke therapy academic industry roundtable preclinical recommendations. *Stroke* 40, 2244–2250. doi: 10.1161/strokeaha.108.541128

Fouda, A. Y., Kozak, A., Alhusban, A., Switzer, J. A., and Fagan, S. C. (2013). Anti-inflammatory IL-10 is upregulated in both hemispheres after experimental ischemic stroke: hypertension blunts the response. *Exp. Transl. Stroke Med.* 5:12. doi: 10.1186/2040-7378-5-12

Gage, F. H., Coates, P. W., Palmer, T. D., Kuhn, H. G., Fisher, L. J., Suhonen, J. O., et al. (1995). Survival and differentiation of adult neuronal progenitor cells transplanted to the adult brain. *Proc. Natl. Acad. Sci. U S A* 92, 11879–11883. doi: 10.1073/pnas.92.25.11879

Gebicke-Haerter, P. J., Spleiss, O., Ren, L. Q., Li, H., Dichmann, S., Norgauer, J., et al. (2001). Microglial chemokines and chemokine receptors. *Prog. Brain Res.* 132, 525–532. doi: 10.1016/s0079-6123(01)32100-3

Girard, S., Murray, K. N., Rothwell, N. J., Metz, G. A. S., and Allan, S. M. (2014). Long-term functional recovery and compensation after cerebral ischemia in rats. *Behav. Brain Res.* 270, 18–28. doi: 10.1016/j.bbr.2014.05.008

Gkaliagkousi, E., Corrigall, V., Becker, S., de Winter, P., Shah, A., Zamboulis, C., et al. (2009). Decreased platelet nitric oxide contributes to increased circulating monocyte-platelet aggregates in hypertension. *Eur. Heart J.* 30, 3048–3054. doi: 10.1093/eurheartj/ehp330

Goldbach-Mansky, R., Shroff, S. D., Wilson, M., Snyder, C., Plehn, S., Barham, B., et al. (2008). A pilot study to evaluate the safety and efficacy of the long-acting interleukin-1 inhibitor rilonacept (interleukin-1 Trap) in patients with familial cold autoinflammatory syndrome. *Arthritis Rheum.* 58, 2432–2442. doi: 10.1002/art.23620

Granger, D. N., Rodrigues, S. F., Yildirim, A., and Senchenkova, E. Y. (2010). Microvascular responses to cardiovascular risk factors. *Microcirculation* 17, 192–205. doi: 10.1111/j.1549-8719.2009.00015.x

Grau, A. J., Buggle, F., Heindl, S., Steichen-Wiehn, C., Banerjee, T., Maiwald, M., et al. (1995). Recent infection as a risk factor for cerebrovascular ischemia. *Stroke* 26, 373–379. doi: 10.1161/01.str.26.3.373

Grau, A. J., Urbanek, C., and Palm, F. (2010). Common infections and the risk of stroke. *Nat. Rev. Neurol.* 6, 681–694. doi: 10.1038/nrneurol.2010.163

Greenhalgh, A. D., Brough, D., Robinson, E. M., Girard, S., Rothwell, N. J., and Allan, S. M. (2012). Interleukin-1 receptor antagonist is beneficial after subarachnoid haemorrhage in rat by blocking haem-driven inflammatory pathology. *Dis. Model. Mech.* 5, 823–833. doi: 10.1242/dmm.008557

Greenhalgh, A. D., Galea, J., Dénes, A., Tyrrell, P. J., and Rothwell, N. J. (2010). Rapid brain penetration of interleukin-1 receptor antagonist in rat cerebral ischaemia: pharmacokinetics, distribution, protection. *Br. J. Pharmacol.* 160, 153–159. doi: 10.1111/j.1476-5381.2010.00684.x

Grüner, S., Prostredna, M., Koch, M., Miura, Y., Schulte, V., Jung, S. M., et al. (2005). Relative antithrombotic effect of soluble GPVI dimer compared with anti-GPVI antibodies in mice. *Blood* 105, 1492–1499. doi: 10.1182/blood-2004-06-2391

Hacke, W., and Lichy, C. (2008). Thrombolysis for acute stroke under antiplatelet therapy: safe enough to be beneficial? *Nat. Clin. Pract. Neurol.* 4, 474–475. doi: 10.1038/ncpneuro0867

Hall, C. N., Reynell, C., Gesslein, B., Hamilton, N. B., Mishra, A., Sutherland, B. A., et al. (2014). Capillary pericytes regulate cerebral blood flow in health and disease. *Nature* 508, 55–60. doi: 10.1038/nature13165

Hankey, G. J. (2006). Potential new risk factors for ischemic stroke: what is their potential? *Stroke* 37, 2181–2188. doi: 10.1161/01.str.0000229883.72010.e4

Haramaki, N., Ikeda, H., Takenaka, K., Katoh, A., Sugano, R., Yamagishi, S., et al. (2007). Fluvastatin alters platelet aggregability in patients with hypercholesterolemia: possible improvement of intraplatelet redox imbalance via HMG-CoA reductase. *Arterioscler. Thromb. Vasc. Biol.* 27, 1471–1477. doi: 10.1161/atvbaha.106.128793

Harris, A. K., Elgebaly, M. M., Li, W., Sachidanandam, K., and Ergul, A. (2008). Effect of chronic endothelin receptor antagonism on cerebrovascular function in type 2 diabetes. *Am. J. Physiol. Regul. Integr. Comp. Physiol.* 294, R1213–R1219. doi: 10.1152/ajpregu.00885.2007

Hawrylowicz, C. M., Howells, G. L., and Feldmann, M. (1991). Platelet-derived interleukin 1 induces human endothelial adhesion molecule expression and cytokine production. *J. Exp. Med.* 174, 785–790. doi: 10.1084/jem.174.4.785

Hayakawa, K., Pham, L.-D. D., Katusic, Z. S., Arai, K., and Lo, E. H. (2012). Astrocytic high-mobility group box 1 promotes endothelial progenitor cell-mediated neurovascular remodeling during stroke recovery. *Proc. Natl. Acad. Sci. U S A* 109, 7505–7510. doi: 10.1073/pnas.1121146109

Helmy, A., Guilfoyle, M. R., Carpenter, K. L. H., Pickard, J. D., Menon, D. K., and Hutchinson, P. J. (2014). Recombinant human interleukin-1 receptor antagonist in severe traumatic brain injury: a phase II randomized control trial. *J. Cereb. Blood Flow Metab.* 34, 845–851. doi: 10.1038/jcbfm.2014.23

Hoehn, B. D., Palmer, T. D., and Steinberg, G. K. (2005). Neurogenesis in rats after focal cerebral ischemia is enhanced by indomethacin. *Stroke* 36, 2718–2724. doi: 10.1161/01.str.0000190020.30282.cc

Hoffman, H. M., Throne, M. L., Amar, N. J., Sebai, M., Kivitz, A. J., Kavanaugh, A., et al. (2008). Efficacy and safety of rilonacept (interleukin-1 Trap) in patients with cryopyrin-associated periodic syndromes: results from two sequential placebo-controlled studies. *Arthritis Rheum.* 58, 2443–2452. doi: 10.1002/art.23687

Hopkins, S. J., and Rothwell, N. J. (1995). Cytokines and the nervous system. I: expression and recognition. *Trends Neurosci.* 18, 83–88. doi: 10.1016/0166-2236(95)93881-w

Hou, Q., Zuo, Z., Michel, P., Zhang, Y., Eskandari, A., Man, F., et al. (2013). Influence of chronic hyperglycemia on cerebral microvascular remodeling: an in vivo study using perfusion computed tomography in acute ischemic stroke patients. *Stroke* 44, 3557–3560. doi: 10.1161/strokeaha.113.003150

Howard, C., Noe, A., Skerjanec, A., Holzhauer, B., Wernsing, M., Ligueros-Saylan, M., et al. (2014). Safety and tolerability of canakinumab, an IL-1β inhibitor, in type 2 diabetes mellitus patients: a pooled analysis of three randomised double-blind studies. *Cardiovasc. Diabetol.* 13:94. doi: 10.1186/1475-2840-13-94

Howells, D. W., Porritt, M. J., Rewell, S. S. J., O'Collins, V., Sena, E. S., van der Worp, H. B., et al. (2010). Different strokes for different folks: the rich diversity of animal models of focal cerebral ischemia. *J. Cereb. Blood Flow Metab.* 30, 1412–1431. doi: 10.1038/jcbfm.2010.66

Iadecola, C., and Anrather, J. (2011). The immunology of stroke: from mechanisms to translation. *Nat. Med.* 17, 796–808. doi: 10.1038/nm.2399

Ito, U., Hakamata, Y., Kawakami, E., and Oyanagi, K. (2011). Temporary [corrected] cerebral ischemia results in swollen astrocytic end-feet that compress microvessels and lead to delayed [corrected] focal cortical infarction. *J. Cereb. Blood Flow Metab.* 31, 328–338. doi: 10.1038/jcbfm.2010.97

Jackman, K., and Iadecola, C. (2015). Neurovascular regulation in the ischemic brain. *Antioxid. Redox Signal.* 22, 149–160. doi: 10.1089/ars.2013.5669

Jenny, N. S., Tracy, R. P., Ogg, M. S., Luong, L. A., Kuller, L. H., Arnold, A. M., et al. (2002). In the elderly, interleukin-6 plasma levels and the -174G>C polymorphism are associated with the development of cardiovascular disease. *Arterioscler. Thromb. Vasc. Biol.* 22, 2066–2071. doi: 10.1161/01.atv.0000040224.49362.60

Jin, R., Yang, G., and Li, G. (2010). Inflammatory mechanisms in ischemic stroke: role of inflammatory cells. *J. Leukoc. Biol.* 87, 779–789. doi: 10.1189/jlb.1109766

Kim, H., Hysi, P. G., Pawlikowska, L., Poon, A., Burchard, E. G., Zaroff, J. G., et al. (2009). Common variants in interleukin-1-Beta gene are associated with intracranial hemorrhage and susceptibility to brain arteriovenous malformation. *Cerebrovasc. Dis.* 27, 176–182. doi: 10.1159/000185609

Kim, E., Tolhurst, A. T., and Cho, S. (2014). Deregulation of inflammatory response in the diabetic condition is associated with increased ischemic brain injury. *J. Neuroinflammation* 11:83. doi: 10.1186/1742-2094-11-83

Kirby, D. M., Rennie, K. J., Smulders-Srinivasan, T. K., Acin-Perez, R., Whittington, M., Enriquez, J.-A., et al. (2009). Transmitochondrial embryonic stem cells containing pathogenic mtDNA mutations are compromised in neuronal differentiation. *Cell Prolif.* 42, 413–424. doi: 10.1111/j.1365-2184.2009.00612.x

Klementiev, B., Li, S., Korshunova, I., Dmytriyeva, O., Pankratova, S., Walmod, P. S., et al. (2014). Anti-inflammatory properties of a novel peptide interleukin 1 receptor antagonist. *J. Neuroinflammation* 11:27. doi: 10.1186/1742-2094-11-27

Kokaia, Z., Thored, P., Arvidsson, A., and Lindvall, O. (2006). Regulation of stroke-induced neurogenesis in adult brain-recent scientific progress. *Cereb. Cortex* 16, i16–i17. doi: 10.1093/cercor/bhj174

Koo, J. W., and Duman, R. S. (2008). IL-1beta is an essential mediator of the antineurogenic and anhedonic effects of stress. *Proc. Natl. Acad. Sci. U S A* 105, 751–756. doi: 10.1073/pnas.0708092105

Kuemmerle-Deschner, J. B., Ramos, E., Blank, N., Roesler, J., Felix, S. D., Jung, T., et al. (2011). Canakinumab (ACZ885, a fully human IgG1 anti-IL-1β mAb) induces sustained remission in pediatric patients with cryopyrin-associated periodic syndrome (CAPS). *Arthritis Res. Ther.* 13:R34. doi: 10.1186/ar3266

Kuhn, H. G., Dickinson-Anson, H., and Gage, F. H. (1996). Neurogenesis in the dentate gyrus of the adult rat: age-related decrease of neuronal progenitor proliferation. *J. Neurosci.* 16, 2027–2033.

Kunze, A. K., Annecke, A., Wigger, F., Lichy, C., Buggle, F., Schnippering, H., et al. (2000). Recent infection as a risk factor for intracerebral and subarachnoid hemorrhages. *Cerebrovasc. Dis.* 10, 352–358. doi: 10.1159/000016090

Kwan, J., Horsfield, G., Bryant, T., Gawne-Cain, M., Durward, G., Byrne, C. D., et al. (2013). IL-6 is a predictive biomarker for stroke associated infection and future mortality in the elderly after an ischemic stroke. *Exp. Gerontol.* 48, 960–965. doi: 10.1016/j.exger.2013.07.003

Lakhan, S. E., Kirchgessner, A., and Hofer, M. (2009). Inflammatory mechanisms in ischemic stroke: therapeutic approaches. *J. Transl. Med.* 7:97. doi: 10.1186/1479-5876-7-97

Lambertsen, K. L., Biber, K., and Finsen, B. (2012). Inflammatory cytokines in experimental and human stroke. *J. Cereb. Blood Flow Metab.* 32, 1677–1698. doi: 10.1038/jcbfm.2012.88

Lapchak, P. A., Araujo, D. M., Song, D., and Zivin, J. A. (2002). The nonpeptide glycoprotein IIb/IIIa platelet receptor antagonist SM-20302 reduces tissue plasminogen activator-induced intracerebral hemorrhage after thromboembolic stroke. *Stroke* 33, 147–152. doi: 10.1161/hs0102.100530

Lapi, D., Mastantuono, T., Sapio, D., Paterni, M., and Colantuoni, A. (2013). Pial microvascular responses induced by transient bilateral common carotid artery occlusion in Zucker rats. *Clin. Hemorheol. Microcirc.* 54, 415–429. doi: 10.3233/CH-131763

Larsen, C. M., Faulenbach, M., Vaag, A., Ehses, J. A., Donath, M. Y., and Mandrup-Poulsen, T. (2009). Sustained effects of interleukin-1 receptor antagonist treatment in type 2 diabetes. *Diabetes Care* 32, 1663–1668. doi: 10.2337/dc09-0533

Larsen, C. M., Faulenbach, M., Vaag, A., Vølund, A., Ehses, J. A., Seifert, B., et al. (2007). Interleukin-1-receptor antagonist in type 2 diabetes mellitus. *N. Engl. J. Med.* 356, 1517–1526. doi: 10.1056/NEJMoa065213

Lauritzen, M., Dreier, J. P., Fabricius, M., Hartings, J. A., Graf, R., and Strong, A. J. (2011). Clinical relevance of cortical spreading depression in neurological disorders: migraine, malignant stroke, subarachnoid and intracranial hemorrhage and traumatic brain injury. *J. Cereb. Blood Flow Metab.* 31, 17–35. doi: 10.1038/jcbfm.2010.191

Lawes, C. M. M., Bennett, D. A., Feigin, V. L., and Rodgers, A. (2004). Blood pressure and stroke: an overview of published reviews. *Stroke* 35, 776–785. doi: 10.1161/01.str.0000126208.14181.dd

Lawrence, C. B., Allan, S. M., and Rothwell, N. J. (1998). Interleukin-1beta and the interleukin-1 receptor antagonist act in the striatum to modify excitotoxic brain damage in the rat. *Eur. J. Neurosci.* 10, 1188–1195. doi: 10.1046/j.1460-9568.1998.00136.x

Le Behot, A., Gauberti, M., Martinez De Lizarrondo, S., Montagne, A., Lemarchand, E., Repesse, Y., et al. (2014). GpIbα-VWF blockade restores vessel patency by dissolving platelet aggregates formed under very high shear rate in mice. *Blood* 123, 3354–3363. doi: 10.1182/blood-2013-12-543074

Lee, S., Shafe, A. C. E., and Cowie, M. R. (2011). UK stroke incidence, mortality and cardiovascular risk management 1999–2008: time-trend analysis from the general practice research database. *BMJ Open* 1:e000269. doi: 10.1136/bmjopen-2011-000269

Li, D., Huang, B., Liu, J., Li, L., and Li, X. (2013a). Decreased brain K(ATP) channel contributes to exacerbating ischemic brain injury and the failure of neuroprotection by sevoflurane post-conditioning in diabetic rats. *PLoS One* 8:e73334. doi: 10.1371/journal.pone.0073334

Li, W., Prakash, R., Chawla, D., Du, W., Didion, S. P., Filosa, J. A., et al. (2013b). Early effects of high-fat diet on neurovascular function and focal ischemic brain injury. *Am. J. Physiol. Regul. Integr. Comp. Physiol.* 304, R1001–R1008. doi: 10.1152/ajpregu.00523.2012

Li, W., Qu, Z., Prakash, R., Chung, C., Ma, H., Hoda, M. N., et al. (2013c). Comparative analysis of the neurovascular injury and functional outcomes in experimental stroke models in diabetic Goto-Kakizaki rats. *Brain Res.* 1541, 106–114. doi: 10.1016/j.brainres.2013.10.021

Lian, H., Shim, D. J., Gaddam, S. S. K., Rodriguez-Rivera, J., Bitner, B. R., Pautler, R. G., et al. (2012). IκBα deficiency in brain leads to elevated basal neuroinflammation and attenuated response following traumatic brain injury: implications for functional recovery. *Mol. Neurodegener.* 7:47. doi: 10.1186/1750-1326-7-47

Liu, Z., Fan, Y., Won, S. J., Neumann, M., Hu, D., Zhou, L., et al. (2007). Chronic treatment with minocycline preserves adult new neurons and reduces functional impairment after focal cerebral ischemia. *Stroke* 38, 146–152. doi: 10.1161/01.str.0000251791.64910.cd

Liu, J., Gao, B.-B., Clermont, A. C., Blair, P., Chilcote, T. J., Sinha, S., et al. (2011). Hyperglycemia-induced cerebral hematoma expansion is mediated by plasma kallikrein. *Nat. Med.* 17, 206–210. doi: 10.1038/nm.2295

Liu, T., McDonnell, P. C., Young, P. R., White, R. F., Siren, A. L., Hallenbeck, J. M., et al. (1993). Interleukin-1 beta mRNA expression in ischemic rat cortex. *Stroke* 24, 1746–1750. doi: 10.1161/01.str.24.11.1746

Luheshi, N. M., Kovács, K. J., Lopez-Castejon, G., Brough, D., and Denes, A. (2011). Interleukin-1α expression precedes IL-1β after ischemic brain injury and is localised to areas of focal neuronal loss and penumbral tissues. *J. Neuroinflammation* 8:186. doi: 10.1186/1742-2094-8-186

Luheshi, N. M., Rothwell, N. J., and Brough, D. (2009). Dual functionality of interleukin-1 family cytokines: implications for anti-interleukin-1 therapy. *Br. J. Pharmacol.* 157, 1318–1329. doi: 10.1111/j.1476-5381.2009.00331.x

Ma, Q., Chen, S., Hu, Q., Feng, H., Zhang, J. H., and Tang, J. (2014). NLRP3 inflammasome contributes to inflammation after intracerebral hemorrhage. *Ann. Neurol.* 75, 209–219. doi: 10.1002/ana.24070

Maher, C. O., Anderson, R. E., Martin, H. S., McClelland, R. L., and Meyer, F. B. (2003). Interleukin-1beta and adverse effects on cerebral blood flow during long-term global hypoperfusion. *J. Neurosurg.* 99, 907–912. doi: 10.3171/jns.2003.99.5.0907

Mathieu, P., Piantanida, A. P., and Pitossi, F. (2010). Chronic expression of transforming growth factor-beta enhances adult neurogenesis. *Neuroimmunomodulation* 17, 200–201. doi: 10.1159/000258723

McCabe, C., Gallagher, L., Gsell, W., Graham, D., Dominiczak, A. F., and Macrae, I. M. (2009). Differences in the evolution of the ischemic penumbra in stroke-prone spontaneously hypertensive and Wistar-Kyoto rats. *Stroke* 40, 3864–3868. doi: 10.1161/strokeaha.109.559021

McColl, B. W., Allan, S. M., and Rothwell, N. J. (2009). Systemic infection, inflammation and acute ischemic stroke. *Neuroscience* 158, 1049–1061. doi: 10.1016/j.neuroscience.2008.08.019

McColl, B. W., Rose, N., Robson, F. H., Rothwell, N. J., and Lawrence, C. B. (2010). Increased brain microvascular MMP-9 and incidence of haemorrhagic transformation in obese mice after experimental stroke. *J. Cereb. Blood Flow Metab.* 30, 267–272. doi: 10.1038/jcbfm.2009.217

McColl, B. W., Rothwell, N. J., and Allan, S. M. (2007). Systemic inflammatory stimulus potentiates the acute phase and CXC chemokine responses to experimental stroke and exacerbates brain damage via interleukin-1- and neutrophil-dependent mechanisms. *J. Neurosci.* 27, 4403–4412. doi: 10.1523/jneurosci.5376-06.2007

McKellar, G. E., McCarey, D. W., Sattar, N., and McInnes, I. B. (2009). Role for TNF in atherosclerosis? Lessons from autoimmune disease. *Nat. Rev. Cardiol.* 6, 410–417. doi: 10.1038/nrcardio.2009.57

Mertens, M., and Singh, J. A. (2009). Anakinra for rheumatoid arthritis: a systematic review.. *J. Rheumatol.* 36, 1118–1125. doi: 10.3899/jrheum.090074

Minnerup, J., Sutherland, B. A., Buchan, A. M., and Kleinschnitz, C. (2012). Neuroprotection for stroke: current status and future perspectives. *Int. J. Mol. Sci.* 13, 11753–11772. doi: 10.3390/ijms130911753

Miwa, K., Tanaka, M., Okazaki, S., Furukado, S., Sakaguchi, M., Mochizuki, H., et al. (2013). Association between interleukin-6 levels and first-ever cerebrovascular events in patients with vascular risk factors. *Arterioscler. Thromb. Vasc. Biol.* 33, 400–405. doi: 10.1161/atvbaha.112.300350

Moncada, S., and Higgs, E. A. (2006). The discovery of nitric oxide and its role in vascular biology. *Br. J. Pharmacol.* 147(Suppl. 1), S193–S201. doi: 10.1038/sj.bjp.0706458

Monje, M. L., and Palmer, T. (2003). Radiation injury and neurogenesis. *Curr. Opin. Neurol.* 16, 129–134. doi: 10.1097/00019052-200304000-00002

Monje, M. L., Toda, H., and Palmer, T. D. (2003). Inflammatory blockade restores adult hippocampal neurogenesis. *Science* 302, 1760–1765. doi: 10.1126/science.1088417

Moreno-López, B., Romero-Grimaldi, C., Noval, J. A., Murillo-Carretero, M., Matarredona, E. R., and Estrada, C. (2004). Nitric oxide is a physiological inhibitor of neurogenesis in the adult mouse subventricular zone and olfactory bulb. *J. Neurosci.* 24, 85–95. doi: 10.1523/jneurosci.1574-03.2004

Mottillo, S., Filion, K. B., Genest, J., Joseph, L., Pilote, L., Poirier, P., et al. (2010). The metabolic syndrome and cardiovascular risk a systematic review and meta-analysis. *J. Am. Coll. Cardiol.* 56, 1113–1132. doi: 10.1016/j.jacc.2010.05.034

Muhammad, S., Haasbach, E., Kotchourko, M., Strigli, A., Krenz, A., Ridder, D. A., et al. (2011). Influenza virus infection aggravates stroke outcome. *Stroke* 42, 783–791. doi: 10.1161/STROKEAHA.110.596783

Mulcahy, N. J., Ross, J., Rothwell, N. J., and Loddick, S. A. (2003). Delayed administration of interleukin-1 receptor antagonist protects against transient cerebral ischaemia in the rat. *Br. J. Pharmacol.* 140, 471–476. doi: 10.1038/sj.bjp.0705462

Murray, K. N., Buggey, H. F., Denes, A., and Allan, S. M. (2013). Systemic immune activation shapes stroke outcome. *Mol. Cell. Neurosci.* 53, 14–25. doi: 10.1016/j.mcn.2012.09.004

Murray, K. N., Girard, S., Holmes, W. M., Parkes, L. M., Williams, S. R., Parry-Jones, A. R., et al. (2014). Systemic inflammation impairs tissue reperfusion through endothelin-dependent mechanisms in cerebral ischemia. *Stroke* 45, 3412–3419. doi: 10.1161/strokeaha.114.006613

Nehls, V., and Drenckhahn, D. (1993). The versatility of microvascular pericytes: from mesenchyme to smooth muscle? *Histochemistry* 99, 1–12. doi: 10.1007/bf00268014

Nih, L. R., Deroide, N., Leré-Déan, C., Lerouet, D., Soustrat, M., Levy, B. I., et al. (2012). Neuroblast survival depends on mature vascular network formation after mouse stroke: role of endothelial and smooth muscle progenitor cell co-administration. *Eur. J. Neurosci.* 35, 1208–1217. doi: 10.1111/j.1460-9568.2012.08041.x

Nowakowski, R. S., Lewin, S. B., and Miller, M. W. (1989). Bromodeoxyuridine immunohistochemical determination of the lengths of the cell cycle and the DNA-synthetic phase for an anatomically defined population. *J. Neurocytol.* 18, 311–318. doi: 10.1007/bf01190834

O'Collins, V. E., Macleod, M. R., Donnan, G. A., Horky, L. L., van der Worp, B. H., and Howells, D. W. (2006). 1,026 experimental treatments in acute stroke. *Ann. Neurol.* 59, 467–477. doi: 10.1002/ana.20741

Ohab, J. J., and Carmichael, S. T. (2008). Poststroke neurogenesis: emerging principles of migration and localization of immature neurons. *Neuroscientist* 14, 369–380. doi: 10.1177/1073858407309545

Ohira, T., Shahar, E., Chambless, L. E., Rosamond, W. D., Mosley, T. H., and Folsom, A. R. (2006). Risk factors for ischemic stroke subtypes: the atherosclerosis risk in communities study. *Stroke* 37, 2493–2498. doi: 10.1161/01.str.0000239694.19359.88

Ohtsuki, T., Ruetzler, C. A., Tasaki, K., and Hallenbeck, J. M. (1996). Interleukin-1 mediates induction of tolerance to global ischemia in gerbil hippocampal CA1 neurons. *J. Cereb. Blood Flow Metab.* 16, 1137–1142. doi: 10.1097/00004647-199611000-00007

Oppenheimer, S. M., Hoffbrand, B. I., Oswald, G. A., and Yudkin, J. S. (1985). Diabetes mellitus and early mortality from stroke. *Br. Med. J. (Clin. Res. Ed)* 291, 1014–1015. doi: 10.1136/bmj.291.6505.1349-a

Pabbidi, M. R., Juncos, J., Juncos, L., Renic, M., Tullos, H. J., Lazar, J., et al. (2013). Identification of a region of rat chromosome 1 that impairs the myogenic response and autoregulation of cerebral blood flow in fawn-hooded hypertensive rats. *Am. J. Physiol. Heart Circ. Physiol.* 304, H311–H317. doi: 10.1152/ajpheart.00622.2012

Packard, R. R. S., Lichtman, A. H., and Libby, P. (2009). Innate and adaptive immunity in atherosclerosis. *Semin. Immunopathol.* 31, 5–22. doi: 10.1007/s00281-009-0153-8

Paez-Gonzalez, P., Asrican, B., Rodriguez, E., and Kuo, C. T. (2014). Identification of distinct ChAT(+) neurons and activity-dependent control of postnatal SVZ neurogenesis. *Nat. Neurosci.* 17, 934–942. doi: 10.1038/nn.3734

Paganini-Hill, A., Lozano, E., Fischberg, G., Perez Barreto, M., Rajamani, K., Ameriso, S. F., et al. (2003). Infection and risk of ischemic stroke: differences among stroke subtypes. *Stroke* 34, 452–457. doi: 10.1161/01.str.0000053451.28410.98

Palomares, S. M., and Cipolla, M. J. (2014). Myogenic tone as a therapeutic target for ischemic stroke. *Curr. Vasc. Pharmacol.* 12, 788–800. doi: 10.2174/15701611113116660155

Parry-Jones, A., Boutin, H., Denes, A., McColl, B., Hopkins, S., Allan, S., et al. (2010). Interleukin-1 receptor antagonist in animal models of stroke: a fair summing up? *J. Stroke Cerebrovasc. Dis.* 19, 512–513. doi: 10.1016/j.jstrokecerebrovasdis.2010.01.005

Parry-Jones, A. R., Liimatainen, T., Kauppinen, R. A., Gröhn, O. H. J., and Rothwell, N. J. (2008). Interleukin-1 exacerbates focal cerebral ischemia and reduces ischemic brain temperature in the rat. *Magn. Reson. Med.* 59, 1239–1249. doi: 10.1002/mrm.21531

Patel, A., Jagadesham, V. P., Porter, K. E., Scott, D. J. A., and Carding, S. R. (2008). Characterisation of fractalkine/CX3CL1 and fractalkine receptor (CX3CR1) expression in abdominal aortic aneurysm disease. *Eur. J. Vasc. Endovasc. Surg.* 36, 20–27. doi: 10.1016/j.ejvs.2008.01.014

Pham, L.-D. D., Hayakawa, K., Seo, J. H., Nguyen, M.-N., Som, A. T., Lee, B. J., et al. (2012). Crosstalk between oligodendrocytes and cerebral endothelium contributes to vascular remodeling after white matter injury. *Glia* 60, 875–881. doi: 10.1002/glia.22320

Pham, M., Helluy, X., Kleinschnitz, C., Kraft, P., Bartsch, A. J., Jakob, P., et al. (2011). Sustained reperfusion after blockade of glycoprotein-receptor-Ib in focal cerebral ischemia: an MRI study at 17.6 Tesla. *PLoS One* 6:e18386. doi: 10.1371/journal.pone.0018386

Pieper, C., Marek, J. J., Unterberg, M., Schwerdtle, T., and Galla, H.-J. (2014). Brain capillary pericytes contribute to the immune defense in response to cytokines or LPS in vitro. *Brain Res.* 1550, 1–8. doi: 10.1016/j.brainres.2014.01.004

Pinteaux, E., Parker, L. C., Rothwell, N. J., and Luheshi, G. N. (2002). Expression of interleukin-1 receptors and their role in interleukin-1 actions in murine microglial cells. *J. Neurochem.* 83, 754–763. doi: 10.1046/j.1471-4159.2002.01184.x

Pires, P. W., Girgla, S. S., McClain, J. L., Kaminski, N. E., van Rooijen, N., and Dorrance, A. M. (2013). Improvement in middle cerebral artery structure and endothelial function in stroke-prone spontaneously hypertensive rats after macrophage depletion. *Microcirculation* 20, 650–661. doi: 10.1111/micc.12064

Pleiner, J., Schaller, G., Mittermayer, F., Zorn, S., Marsik, C., Polterauer, S., et al. (2004). Simvastatin prevents vascular hyporeactivity during inflammation. *Circulation* 110, 3349–3354. doi: 10.1161/01.cir.0000147774.90396.ed

Pradillo, J. M., Denes, A., Greenhalgh, A. D., Boutin, H., Drake, C., McColl, B. W., et al. (2012). Delayed administration of interleukin-1 receptor antagonist reduces ischemic brain damage and inflammation in comorbid rats. *J. Cereb. Blood Flow Metab.* 32, 1810–1819. doi: 10.1038/jcbfm.2012.101

Pugazhenthi, S., Zhang, Y., Bouchard, R., and Mahaffey, G. (2013). Induction of an inflammatory loop by interleukin-1β and tumor necrosis factor-α involves NF-kB and STAT-1 in differentiated human neuroprogenitor cells. *PLoS One* 8:e69585. doi: 10.1371/journal.pone.0069585

Pulsinelli, W. A., Levy, D. E., Sigsbee, B., Scherer, P., and Plum, F. (1983). Increased damage after ischemic stroke in patients with hyperglycemia with or without established diabetes mellitus. *Am. J. Med.* 74, 540–544. doi: 10.1016/0002-9343(83)91035-5

Razinia, T., Saver, J. L., Liebeskind, D. S., Ali, L. K., Buck, B., and Ovbiagele, B. (2007). Body mass index and hospital discharge outcomes after ischemic stroke. *Arch. Neurol.* 64, 388–391. doi: 10.1001/archneur.64.3.388

Rewell, S. S. J., Fernandez, J. A., Cox, S. F., Spratt, N. J., Hogan, L., Aleksoska, E., et al. (2010). Inducing stroke in aged, hypertensive, diabetic rats. *J. Cereb. Blood Flow Metab.* 30, 729–733. doi: 10.1038/jcbfm.2009.273

Reynolds, B. A., and Weiss, S. (1992). Generation of neurons and astrocytes from isolated cells of the adult mammalian central nervous system. *Science* 255, 1707–1710. doi: 10.1126/science.1553558

Rezaii, A. A., Hoseinipanah, S. M., Hajilooi, M., Rafiei, A. R., Shikh, N., and Haidari, M. (2009). Interleukin-1 receptor antagonist gene polymorphism and susceptibility to ischemic stroke. *Immunol. Invest.* 38, 220–230. doi: 10.1080/08820130902745146

Ridker, P. M., Thuren, T., Zalewski, A., and Libby, P. (2011). Interleukin-1β inhibition and the prevention of recurrent cardiovascular events: rationale and design of the Canakinumab Anti-inflammatory Thrombosis Outcomes Study (CANTOS). *Am. Heart J.* 162, 597–605. doi: 10.1016/j.ahj.2011.06.012

Roger, V. L., Go, A. S., Lloyd-Jones, D. M., Adams, R. J., Berry, J. D., Brown, T. M., et al. (2011). Heart disease and stroke statistics–2011 update: a report from the american heart association. *Circulation* 123, e18–e209. doi: 10.1161/CIR.0b013e3182009701

Ross, R. (1999). Atherosclerosis–an inflammatory disease. *N. Engl. J. Med.* 340, 115–126. doi: 10.1056/nejm199906173402418

Ross, J., Brough, D., Gibson, R. M., Loddick, S. A., and Rothwell, N. J. (2007). A selective, non-peptide caspase-1 inhibitor, VRT-018858, markedly reduces brain damage induced by transient ischemia in the rat. *Neuropharmacology* 53, 638–642. doi: 10.1016/j.neuropharm.2007.07.015

Rost, N. S., Wolf, P. A., Kase, C. S., Kelly-Hayes, M., Silbershatz, H., Massaro, J. M., et al. (2001). Plasma concentration of C-reactive protein and risk of ischemic stroke and transient ischemic attack: the Framingham study. *Stroke* 32, 2575–2579. doi: 10.1161/hs1101.098151

Rothwell, N. (2003). Interleukin-1 and neuronal injury: mechanisms, modification and therapeutic potential. *Brain. Behav. Immun.* 17, 152–157. doi: 10.1016/s0889-1591(02)00098-3

Rothwell, N. J., and Luheshi, G. N. (2000). Interleukin 1 in the brain: biology, pathology and therapeutic target. *Trends Neurosci.* 23, 618–625. doi: 10.1016/s0166-2236(00)01661-1

Ruggeri, Z. M. (2003). Von Willebrand factor, platelets and endothelial cell interactions. *J. Thromb. Haemost.* 1, 1335–1342. doi: 10.1046/j.1538-7836.2003.00260.x

Schwartz, M., London, A., and Shechter, R. (2009). Boosting T-cell immunity as a therapeutic approach for neurodegenerative conditions: the role of innate immunity. *Neuroscience* 158, 1133–1142. doi: 10.1016/j.neuroscience.2008.12.013

Seki, T., and Arai, Y. (1995). Age-related production of new granule cells in the adult dentate gyrus. *Neuroreport* 6, 2479–2482. doi: 10.1097/00001756-199512150-00010

Seripa, D., Dobrina, A., Margaglione, M., Matera, M. G., Gravina, C., Vecile, E., et al. (2003). Relevance of interleukin-1 receptor antagonist intron-2 polymorphism in ischemic stroke. *Cerebrovasc. Dis.* 15, 276–281. doi: 10.1159/000069497

Shichita, T., Sugiyama, Y., Ooboshi, H., Sugimori, H., Nakagawa, R., Takada, I., et al. (2009). Pivotal role of cerebral interleukin-17-producing gammadeltaT cells in the delayed phase of ischemic brain injury. *Nat. Med.* 15, 946–950. doi: 10.1038/nm.1999

Sibley, C. H., Chioato, A., Felix, S., Colin, L., Chakraborty, A., Plass, N., et al. (2014). A 24-month open-label study of canakinumab in neonatal-onset multisystem inflammatory disease. *Ann. Rheum. Dis.* doi: 10.1136/annrheumdis-2013-204877. [Epub ahead of print].

Sieber, M. W., Guenther, M., Jaenisch, N., Albrecht-Eckardt, D., Kohl, M., Witte, O. W., et al. (2014). Age-specific transcriptional response to stroke. *Neurobiol. Aging* 35, 1744–1754. doi: 10.1016/j.neurobiolaging.2014.01.012

Singh, N., Hopkins, S. J., Hulme, S., Galea, J. P., Hoadley, M., Vail, A., et al. (2014). The effect of intravenous interleukin-1 receptor antagonist on inflammatory mediators in cerebrospinal fluid after subarachnoid haemorrhage: a phase II randomised controlled trial. *J. Neuroinflammation* 11:1. doi: 10.1186/1742-2094-11-1

Smeeth, L., Thomas, S. L., Hall, A. J., Hubbard, R., Farrington, P., and Vallance, P. (2004). Risk of myocardial infarction and stroke after acute infection or vaccination. *N. Engl. J. Med.* 351, 2611–2618. doi: 10.1056/nejmoa041747

Spera, P. A., Ellison, J. A., Feuerstein, G. Z., and Barone, F. C. (1998). IL-10 reduces rat brain injury following focal stroke. *Neurosci. Lett.* 251, 189–192. doi: 10.1016/s0304-3940(98)00537-0

Sreeramkumar, V., Adrover, J. M., Ballesteros, I., Cuartero, M. I., Rossaint, J., Bilbao, I., et al. (2014). Neutrophils scan for activated platelets to initiate inflammation. *Science* 346, 1234–1238. doi: 10.1126/science.1256478

Stroemer, R. P., and Rothwell, N. J. (1998). Exacerbation of ischemic brain damage by localized striatal injection of interleukin-1beta in the rat. *J. Cereb. Blood Flow Metab.* 18, 833–839. doi: 10.1097/00004647-199808000-00003

Stroke Therapy Academic Industry Roundtable (STAIR). (1999). Recommendations for standards regarding preclinical neuroprotective and restorative drug development. *Stroke* 30, 2752–2758. doi: 10.1161/01.str.30.12.2752

Suk, S.-H., Sacco, R. L., Boden-Albala, B., Cheun, J. F., Pittman, J. G., Elkind, M. S., et al. (2003). Abdominal obesity and risk of ischemic stroke: the northern manhattan stroke study. *Stroke* 34, 1586–1592. doi: 10.1161/01.str.0000075294.98582.2f

Suzuki, H., Sozen, T., Hasegawa, Y., Chen, W., and Zhang, J. H. (2009). Caspase-1 inhibitor prevents neurogenic pulmonary edema after subarachnoid hemorrhage in mice. *Stroke* 40, 3872–3875. doi: 10.1161/strokeaha.109.566109

Taka, T., Ohta, Y., Seki, J., Giddings, J. C., and Yamamoto, J. (2002). Impaired flow-mediated vasodilation in vivo and reduced shear-induced platelet reactivity in vitro in response to nitric oxide in prothrombotic, stroke-prone spontaneously hypertensive rats. *Pathophysiol. Haemost. Thromb.* 32, 184–189. doi: 10.1159/000070425

Takahashi, R., Ishii, K., Shimada, K., Ohkawa, S., and Nishimura, Y. (2010). Hypoperfusion of the motor cortex associated with parkinsonism in dementia with Lewy bodies. *J. Neurol. Sci.* 288, 88–91. doi: 10.1016/j.jns.2009.09.033

Thored, P., Arvidsson, A., Cacci, E., Ahlenius, H., Kallur, T., Darsalia, V., et al. (2006). Persistent production of neurons from adult brain stem cells during recovery after stroke. *Stem Cells* 24, 739–747. doi: 10.1634/stemcells.2005-0281

Thornton, P., McColl, B. W., Greenhalgh, A., Denes, A., Allan, S. M., and Rothwell, N. J. (2010). Platelet interleukin-1α drives cerebrovascular inflammation. *Blood* 115, 3632–3639. doi: 10.1182/blood-2009-11-252643

Tosun, D., Schuff, N., and Weiner, M. (2009). An integrated multimodality MR brain imaging study: gray matter tissue loss mediates the association between cerebral hypoperfusion and Alzheimer's disease. *Conf. Proc. IEEE Eng. Med. Biol. Soc.* 2009, 6981–6984. doi: 10.1109/iembs.2009.5333857

Tsimikas, S., Duff, G. W., Berger, P. B., Rogus, J., Huttner, K., Clopton, P., et al. (2014). Pro-inflammatory interleukin-1 genotypes potentiate the risk of coronary artery disease and cardiovascular events mediated by oxidized phospholipids and lipoprotein(a). *J. Am. Coll. Cardiol.* 63, 1724–1734. doi: 10.1016/j.jacc.2013.12.030

Um, J.-Y., Moon, K.-S., Lee, K.-M., and Kim, H.-M. (2003). Interleukin-1 gene cluster polymorphisms in cerebral infarction. *Cytokine* 23, 41–46. doi: 10.1016/s1043-4666(03)00183-2

Urbach, A., Bruehl, C., and Witte, O. W. (2006). Microarray-based long-term detection of genes differentially expressed after cortical spreading depression. *Eur. J. Neurosci.* 24, 841–856. doi: 10.1111/j.1460-9568.2006.04862.x

Utagawa, A., Truettner, J. S., Dietrich, W. D., and Bramlett, H. M. (2008). Systemic inflammation exacerbates behavioral and histopathological consequences of isolated traumatic brain injury in rats. *Exp. Neurol.* 211, 283–291. doi: 10.1016/j.expneurol.2008.02.001

Vandanmagsar, B., Youm, Y.-H., Ravussin, A., Galgani, J. E., Stadler, K., Mynatt, R. L., et al. (2011). The NLRP3 inflammasome instigates obesity-induced inflammation and insulin resistance. *Nat. Med.* 17, 179–188. doi: 10.1038/nm.2279

VanGilder, R. L., Davidov, D. M., Stinehart, K. R., Huber, J. D., Turner, R. C., Wilson, K. S., et al. (2014). C-reactive protein and long-term ischemic stroke prognosis. *J. Clin. Neurosci.* 21, 547–553. doi: 10.1016/j.jocn.2013.06.015

Visser, M., Bouter, L. M., McQuillan, G. M., Wener, M. H., and Harris, T. B. (1999). Elevated C-reactive protein levels in overweight and obese adults. *JAMA* 282, 2131–2135. doi: 10.1001/jama.282.22.2131

Vitkovic, L., Bockaert, J., and Jacque, C. (2000). "Inflammatory" cytokines: neuromodulators in normal brain? *J. Neurochem.* 74, 457–471. doi: 10.1046/j.1471-4159.2000.740457.x

Voronov, E., Shouval, D. S., Krelin, Y., Cagnano, E., Benharroch, D., Iwakura, Y., et al. (2003). IL-1 is required for tumor invasiveness and angiogenesis. *Proc. Natl. Acad. Sci. U S A* 100, 2645–2650. doi: 10.1073/pnas.0437939100

Wang, X., Barone, F. C., Aiyar, N. V., and Feuerstein, G. Z. (1997). Interleukin-1 receptor and receptor antagonist gene expression after focal stroke in rats. *Stroke* 28, 155–161. doi: 10.1161/01.str.28.1.155

Wang, J.-Y., Wang, C.-Y., Huang, Y.-S., Chen, P.-F., Huang, K.-Y., Chou, P., et al. (2014). Increased risk of ischemic stroke after hyperosmolar hyperglycemic state: a population-based follow-up study. *PLoS One* 9:e94155. doi: 10.1371/journal.pone.0094155

Wardlaw, J. M., Murray, V., Berge, E., del Zoppo, G., Sandercock, P., Lindley, R. L., et al. (2012). Recombinant tissue plasminogen activator for acute ischaemic stroke: an updated systematic review and meta-analysis. *Lancet* 379, 2364–2372. doi: 10.1016/S0140-6736(12)60738-7

Wasserman, J. K., Zhu, X., and Schlichter, L. C. (2007). Evolution of the inflammatory response in the brain following intracerebral hemorrhage and effects of delayed minocycline treatment. *Brain Res.* 1180, 140–154. doi: 10.1016/j.brainres.2007.08.058

Woo, J., Lam, C. W., Kay, R., Wong, A. H., Teoh, R., and Nicholls, M. G. (1990). The influence of hyperglycemia and diabetes mellitus on immediate and 3-month morbidity and mortality after acute stroke. *Arch. Neurol.* 47, 1174–1177. doi: 10.1001/archneur.1990.00530110028011

Worrall, B. B., Azhar, S., Nyquist, P. A., Ackerman, R. H., Hamm, T. L., and DeGraba, T. J. (2003). Interleukin-1 receptor antagonist gene polymorphisms in carotid atherosclerosis. *Stroke* 34, 790–793. doi: 10.1161/01.str.0000057815.79289.ec

Xu, H.-L., Garcia, M., Testai, F., Vetri, F., Barabanova, A., Pelligrino, D. A., et al. (2014). Pharmacologic blockade of vascular adhesion protein-1 lessens neurologic dysfunction in rats subjected to subarachnoid hemorrhage. *Brain Res.* 1586, 83–89. doi: 10.1016/j.brainres.2014.08.036

Yamasaki, Y., Matsuura, N., Shozuhara, H., Onodera, H., Itoyama, Y., and Kogure, K. (1995). Interleukin-1 as a pathogenetic mediator of ischemic brain damage in rats. *Stroke* 26, 676–680. doi: 10.1161/01.str.26.4.676

Yatsuya, H., Folsom, A. R., Yamagishi, K., North, K. E., Brancati, F. L., Stevens, J., et al. (2010). Race- and sex-specific associations of obesity measures with ischemic stroke incidence in the Atherosclerosis Risk in Communities (ARIC) study. *Stroke* 41, 417–425. doi: 10.1161/STROKEAHA.109.566299

Yilmaz, G., Arumugam, T. V., Stokes, K. Y., and Granger, D. N. (2006). Role of T lymphocytes and interferon-gamma in ischemic stroke. *Circulation* 113, 2105–2112. doi: 10.1161/circulationaha.105.593046

Yudkin, J. S., Stehouwer, C. D., Emeis, J. J., and Coppack, S. W. (1999). C-reactive protein in healthy subjects: associations with obesity, insulin resistance and endothelial dysfunction: a potential role for cytokines originating from adipose tissue? *Arterioscler. Thromb. Vasc. Biol.* 19, 972–978. doi: 10.1161/01.atv.19.4.972

Zeller, J. A., Lenz, A., Eschenfelder, C. C., Zunker, P., and Deuschl, G. (2005). Platelet-leukocyte interaction and platelet activation in acute stroke with and without preceding infection. *Arterioscler. Thromb. Vasc. Biol.* 25, 1519–1523. doi: 10.1161/01.atv.0000167524.69092.16

Zhang, P., Li, W., Li, L., Wang, N., Li, X., Gao, M., et al. (2012). Treatment with edaravone attenuates ischemic brain injury and inhibits neurogenesis in the subventricular zone of adult rats after focal cerebral ischemia and reperfusion injury. *Neuroscience* 201, 297–306. doi: 10.1016/j.neuroscience.2011.11.005

Zhang, Z.-L., Wu, W.-C., Liu, J.-Q., Yao, Y.-B., Pan, M.-D., Yang, C.-B., et al. (2014). Screening of differentially expressed genes related to ischemic stroke and functional analysis with DNA microarray. *Eur. Rev. Med. Pharmacol. Sci.* 18, 1181–1188.

Zhou, W., Marinescu, M., and Veltkamp, R. (2014). Only very early oxygen therapy attenuates posthemorrhagic edema formation and blood-brain barrier disruption in murine intracerebral hemorrhage. *Neurocrit. Care* doi: 10.1007/s12028-014-0013-9. [Epub ahead of print].

Zhu, Y., Yang, G.-Y., Ahlemeyer, B., Pang, L., Che, X.-M., Culmsee, C., et al. (2002). Transforming growth factor-beta 1 increases bad phosphorylation and protects neurons against damage. *J. Neurosci.* 22, 3898–3909.

Ziv, Y., Ron, N., Butovsky, O., Landa, G., Sudai, E., Greenberg, N., et al. (2006). Immune cells contribute to the maintenance of neurogenesis and spatial learning abilities in adulthood. *Nat. Neurosci.* 9, 268–275. doi: 10.1038/nn1629

6

The role of microglia and myeloid immune cells in acute cerebral ischemia

Corinne Benakis, Lidia Garcia-Bonilla, Costantino Iadecola and Josef Anrather *

Feil Family Brain and Mind Research Institute, Weill Cornell Medical College, New York, NY, USA

****Correspondence:***
Josef Anrather, Feil Family Brain and Mind Research Institute, Weill Cornell Medical College, 407 East 61st Street, RR-409, New York, NY 10065, USA
e-mail: joa2006@med.cornell.edu

The immune response to acute cerebral ischemia is a major contributor to stroke pathobiology. The inflammatory response is characterized by the participation of brain resident cells and peripheral leukocytes. Microglia in the brain and monocytes/neutrophils in the periphery have a prominent role in initiating, sustaining and resolving post-ischemic inflammation. In this review we aim to summarize recent literature concerning the origins, fate and role of microglia, monocytes and neutrophils in models of cerebral ischemia and to discuss their relevance for human stroke.

Keywords: cerebral ischemia, monocytes, microglia, neutrophils, myeloid cells, tissue macrophages

INTRODUCTION

Cerebral ischemia triggers a robust activation of brain resident and peripheral immune cells, which play an active role in the acute and chronic phases of injury, as well as in subsequent reorganization and repair processes (Iadecola and Anrather, 2011; Macrez et al., 2011; Shichita et al., 2012). Numerous experimental studies have depicted the pivotal response of resident microglia, infiltrating monocyte-derived macrophages and neutrophils to either the development of the brain injury or its resolution leading to conflicting interpretation of their protective or deleterious contribution in stroke (Emerich et al., 2002; Chiba and Umegaki, 2013), and ultimately to treatment failure (O'Collins et al., 2006; Smith et al., 2013). Furthermore, discrepancies exist towards the provenance of brain macrophages, that is to say whether they are blood-borne monocytes or resident microglia that further differentiate into macrophages (London et al., 2013). A better understanding of the origin and function of myeloid immune cells populating the ischemic brain may provide the opportunity to manipulate specific subsets for therapeutic benefit. The aims of this review are (a) to summarize the origin and development of leukocytes and resident microglia, (b) to delineate their contribution to ischemic injury based on recent literature, and (c) to assess their therapeutic relevance to human stroke.

ORIGIN AND DEVELOPMENT OF NEUTROPHILS, MONOCYTES AND MICROGLIA

Cerebral ischemia induces a time-dependent recruitment and activation of leukocytes including neutrophils, monocytes and lymphocytes (Iadecola and Anrather, 2011). At the site of injury, macrophage populations consist mainly of activated parenchymal microglia and infiltrating peripheral monocytes that have distinct ontogenesis (London et al., 2013; Prinz and Priller, 2014). Once in the injured tissue, both cell types differentiate into macrophages and may be indistinguishable by classical histological methods since they share similar antigens and morphologies (Prinz and Mildner, 2011). In the next sections, we will summarize recent findings on the origin, fate and function of myeloid immune cells and microglia particularly in the context of acute cerebral ischemia.

ORIGIN AND FATE OF NEUTROPHILS

Neutrophils are innate immune cells and are the first line of defense against microbial infectious agents. They are involved in the phagocytosis, killing and degrading of microorganisms, partly through the generation of reactive oxygen and nitrogen species (ROS/RNS). Neutrophils are generated in the bone marrow (BM) and share with monocytes the common progenitor granulocyte macrophage precursor (GMP; **Figure 1**). Only mature neutrophils are normally released from the BM into circulation, where they exist as circulating and marginated neutrophil pools, primarily in the lung, which can be acutely mobilized for example by adrenergic agonists (Bierman et al., 1951, 1952). After terminal differentiation, under homeostatic conditions, neutrophils remain in the BM for additional 4–6 days before being released into circulation, constituting a BM neutrophil reserve (Craddock et al., 1960). Egress is controlled by the antagonistic activities of C-X-C chemokine receptor type 2 (CXCR2) and CXCR4 receptors. Activation of CXCR2, which binds C-X-C ligand 1 (CXCL1) and CXCL2 chemokines, stimulates BM egress, whereas stromal cell derived CXCL12 (SDF-1) acting on CXCR4 favors retention (Strydom and Rankin, 2013). During neutrophil maturation CXCR2 expression increases, while CXCR4 is downregulated,

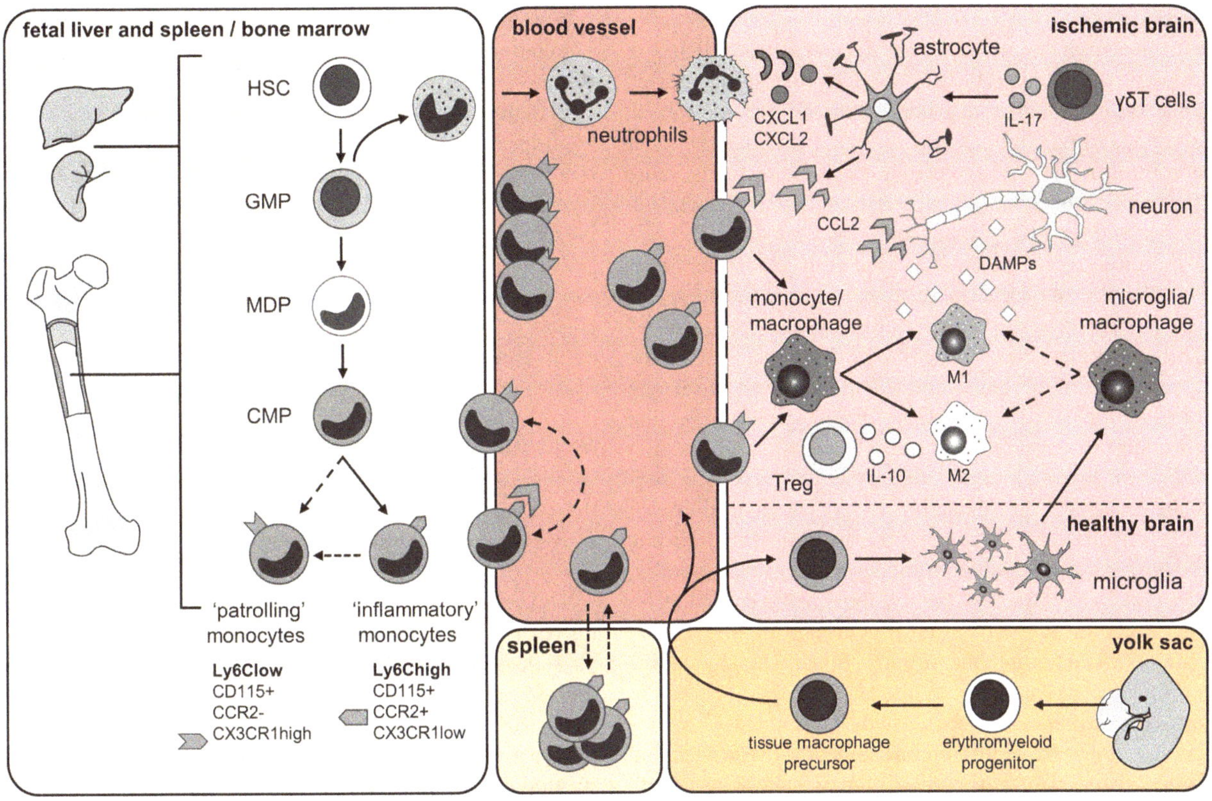

FIGURE 1 | Origin and trafficking of resident microglia and immune cells of myeloid origin. Fetal liver and spleen/bone marrow panel: Monocytes are generated from hematopoietic stem cells (HSCs) in the fetal liver and during adult life in the bone marrow (BM). The granulocyte macrophage precursors (GMP) give rise to immature neutrophils and the macrophage dendritic cell precursors (MDPs). Monocytes develop from hematopoietic stem cells (HSC) after myeloid lineage commitment through a series of increasingly restricted progenitors (GMP, granulocyte/monocyte progenitor; MDP, monocyte/dendritic cell progenitors). The common monocyte progenitor (CMP) is the direct precursors of mature Ly6C^{high} and Ly6C^{low} monocytes. Ly6C^{high} inflammatory monocytes might give rise to circulating Ly6C^{low} monocytes directly, or via a Ly6C^{high} monocyte intermediate. Yolk sac panel: Resident brain microglia have been shown recently to have a different origin than circulating monocytes. During embryonic life, erythroblasts (not shown) and macrophage progenitors are generated in the yolk sac from the common erythro-myeloid progenitor. When the blood circulation is established, macrophage precursors exit the yolk sac and migrate into the developing brain. Embryonic microglia proliferate and are able to renew themselves during gestation and post-natal development as well as in adulthood. Blood vessel and Ischemic brain panels: Few hours after cerebral ischemia onset, mature neutrophils enter the bloodstream upon activation of the CXCR2 receptor and infiltrate the brain in response to chemokines CKLF1 as well as CXCL1 and CXCL2 released by astrocytes. Astrocytic production of these chemokines is dependent upon IL-17 released from brain infiltrating γδT cells. Neutrophils firmly adhere to the endothelium and might either invade the ischemic region or cluster into the perivascular space. During injury, CCL2 is produced by astrocytes, macrophages/microglia and neurons. CCL2 binds its receptor CCR2 expressed by Ly6C^{high} inflammatory monocytes, which promotes their egress from the BM into the blood, and then their recruitment from the blood into the injured tissue. Here, these cells give rise to monocyte-derived DC (not shown) and monocyte-derived macrophage populations, which can further polarize into M1 and M2 macrophages. As the ischemic infarct develops, M1 and M2 macrophages contribute to the exacerbation of the damage or wound healing, respectively. Ly6C^{low} monocytes patrol the blood vessel lumen by associating with the vascular endothelium. Ly6C^{low} monocytes expressing the CX3CR1 receptor are also recruited to sites of inflammation and possibly contribute to wound healing by differentiating into alternatively activated M2 macrophages. Cerebral ischemia/reperfusion leads to the release of damage-associated molecular pattern (DAMP) molecules from dying neurons. These molecules trigger the activation of resident microglia and astrocytes. Activated microglia promote tissue repair by producing trophic factors and by scavenging necrotic cells. Regulatory T lymphocytes (Treg) secreting IL-10 have shown a protective role in cerebral ischemia and might promote macrophage M2 polarization. Spleen panel: An interesting twist to the origin of recruited monocytes during injury has been added by the recent identification of a major monocyte reservoir in the spleen of mice. Following ischemic myocardial injury, splenic monocytes are mobilized to the site of inflammation and participate in tissue injury (Swirski et al., 2009). Dashed arrows represent findings that are not clearly defined yet and need further investigations in context of cerebral ischemia.

which eventually leads to neutrophils egress from the BM. Once in the circulation, neutrophils are thought to be one of the most short-lived cells in the body with circulating half-life of roughly 8 h in humans and 13 h in mice (von Vietinghoff and Ley, 2008; Bugl et al., 2012). As the neutrophil age, CXCR4 receptors become upregulated favoring homing to spleen, liver and BM, wherein neutrophils die by apoptosis and are cleared by resident macrophages. In inflammation, extravasated neutrophils show increased life span of several days and might die as a result of their own cytotoxic molecules by necrosis and by releasing cytotoxic neutrophil extracellular traps (NETs; Yipp et al., 2012).

MONOCYTES, THE BLOOD-BORNE PRECURSORS OF INDUCED TISSUE MACROPHAGES

Similar to neutrophils, monocytes are generated from definitive hematopoietic stem cells (HSC) in the liver and spleen during embryonic development and primarily in the BM after birth (Auffray et al., 2009; Ginhoux and Jung, 2014; **Figure 1**). After lineage commitment they proceed through increasingly more restricted progenitor stages to give rise to mature monocytes that are released into circulation after engagement of the C-C chemokine receptor type 2 (CCR2; Tsou et al., 2007; Hettinger et al., 2013). In the circulation, they can be distinguished from other leukocytes by their myeloid nature, as indicated by (a) high-level expression of CD11b/Mac-1 (a member of the α-integrin family of proteins) and CD115 (colony simulating factor 1 receptor, CSF1R), (b) their phagocytic capacity and (c) their ability to develop into macrophages upon stimulation with CSF-1 *in vitro* (Chitu and Stanley, 2006). There is substantial heterogeneity in circulating monocytes and they can be further divided into functionally distinct subsets according to their surface expression of lymphocyte antigen 6 complex, locus C1 (Ly6C; Swirski et al., 2007; Geissmann et al., 2008), the CCR2 receptor (Geissmann et al., 2003; Prinz and Priller, 2010) and CX3CR1—the high-affinity functional chemokine receptor for fractalkine (Imai et al., 1997). $CD115^+/Ly6C^{high}$ monocytes that express CCR2 are termed "inflammatory" monocytes because they are highly mobile and selectively recruited to inflamed tissues (Auffray et al., 2007; Swirski et al., 2010; Terry et al., 2012). In contrast, $CD115^+/Ly6C^{low}$ monocytes that express CX3CR1 and are negative for CCR2 were initially termed "resident" monocytes because of their longer half-life in circulation and their accumulation in tissues under homeostatic conditions (Geissmann et al., 2003). This subset has been later termed "patrolling" monocytes because of their crawling behavior along the vascular endothelium, and has been shown to orchestrate the disposal of dying or infected endothelial cells (Auffray et al., 2007; Carlin et al., 2013). Their accumulation in the tissue is facilitated by the expression of CX3CR1 that mediates their adhesion and migration (Geissmann et al., 2003). Several reports have proposed that "patrolling" monocytes originate from $CD115^+/Ly6C^{high}$ monocytes in the circulation (Sunderkötter et al., 2004; Lin et al., 2009). However, recent data suggest that $Ly6C^{low}$ monocytes are generated from a myeloid progenitor by the activity of the transcription factor NR4A1 (Nur77) in the BM (Hanna et al., 2011). Additionally, depletion of $CD115^+/Ly6C^{high}$ monocytes in the blood does not affect the numbers of circulating $CD115^+/Ly6C^{low}$ monocytes making it unlikely that $CD115^+/Ly6C^{high}$ cells are the only precursors of "patrolling" monocytes (Geissmann et al., 2008; **Figure 1**).

Under physiological conditions, most $CD115^+/Ly6C^{low}$ crawling monocytes are found within the blood vessels and extravasation rarely occurs. However, in response to tissue damage or infection, these cells extravasate faster than $CD115^+/Ly6C^{high}$ monocytes and are the main TNF producers in the early phase of the inflammatory response (Auffray et al., 2007). In contrast, in a model of myocardial infarction $Ly6C^{high}$ monocytes are the first population to be present in the injured myocardium and display proteolytic and inflammatory functions consistent with a role in tissue damage. $Ly6C^{low}$ monocytes are the predominant population during the resolution phase of the inflammatory response and express repair-promoting proteins such as vascular endothelial growth factor (VEGF; Nahrendorf et al., 2007). The accumulation of $Ly6C^{high}$ and $Ly6C^{low}$ monocytes in inflamed tissues occurs in two phases, although the sequence of infiltration by specific monocyte subsets differs between models, e.g., bacterial infection vs. sterile inflammation (Auffray et al., 2007; Nahrendorf et al., 2007). Thus, $Ly6C^{high}$ and $Ly6C^{low}$ monocytes can have pro- or anti-inflammatory functions depending on the nature of the inflammatory stimulus, the tissue microenvironment and their molecular profile (transcription factors, gene expression, etc.).

MICROGLIA, THE RESIDENT BRAIN MACROPHAGES

In contrast to monocytes, microglia originate exclusively from the yolk sac and colonize the central nervous system (CNS) early during embryonic development before E9 (Ginhoux et al., 2010, 2013; Schulz et al., 2012; Frame et al., 2013). There, yolk sac-derived macrophages proliferate and give rise to mature microglia (**Figure 1**). It seems that microglia are long-lived under physiological conditions and are not normally replaced by BM-derived cells (Alliot et al., 1999; Ajami et al., 2007; Kierdorf et al., 2013a). Recent evidence indicates that microglia homeostasis in adult mice is highly dependent on continuous pro-survival signals provided by the CSF-1 receptor CD115 (Elmore et al., 2014). Blockage of the receptor by selective inhibitors for as little as 7 days resulted in nearly complete depletion of brain microglia. Fast recovery of the microglia population was observed after withdraw of the blocker due to proliferation of brain resident progenitors. These progenitors expressed the neuroectodermal marker Nestin, the hematopoietic marker CD45, the stem cell marker CD34 and stained positive for isolectin B4 (IB4) while being negative for myeloid markers such as ionized calcium binding adapter molecule (Iba1; Elmore et al., 2014). While this is the first study to identify brain-resident microglial progenitors, microglia expansion has been previously described in several disease models. In a model of amyotrophic lateral sclerosis, Solomon et al. characterized the temporal and spatial infiltration of green fluorescent protein (GFP)-BM cells transplanted into lethally irradiated mice. The increased number of spinal cord macrophages following disease onset was attributed to the expansion of resident microglia rather than infiltrated BM-derived precursors (Solomon et al., 2006). Similarly, in experimental autoimmune encephalitis (EAE), Ajami et al. found that blood-borne monocytes transiently infiltrate the spinal cord but do not contribute to the long-term pool of resident microglia (Ajami et al., 2011). Techniques such as parabiosis (Ajami et al., 2007; Ransohoff, 2011), whole body irradiation, head-shielded BM chimeras (Mildner et al., 2011), transgenic mice (Saederup et al., 2010) and fate mapping analysis (Ginhoux et al., 2010) have been instrumental to better discriminate between infiltrating myeloid immune cells and resident microglia. Furthermore, recent data indicate that microglia express a distinctive genetic signature that makes them distinguishable from neurons, astrocytes, oligodendrocytes, and peripheral immune cells including other tissue macrophages. Using transcriptomic and proteomic analysis Butovsky et al. identified several genes that were specifically expressed in CD11b$^+$/CD45^{low} microglia when compared to blood monocytes (Butovsky et al., 2014). Among them, the purinergic receptor P2ry12, the proto-oncogene tyrosine kinase Mertk, and the Fc receptor-like S scavenger receptor Fcrls were exclusively expressed in microglia in brain and spinal cord, and not in peripheral tissue macrophages, e.g., Kupfer cells, alveolar macrophages, etc. P2ry12, Mertk and Fcrls are surface expressed proteins enabling easy antibody-mediated detection in flow cytometric and histological assays. Given that this genetic signature is similar between mice and human microglia, a better differentiation of infiltrating myeloid cells and microglia in human stroke should also be possible. In a model of EAE, expression of these genes was restricted to microglia and was not found in infiltrated monocytes (Butovsky et al., 2014). However, because the analysis was conducted at disease onset, it is not clear whether the signature is retained as the pathology progresses. It remains to be determined whether expression of these marker genes is preserved during all stages of microglial activation, as observed in cerebral ischemia, or whether a similar molecular signature can be acquired by infiltrating monocytes that develop into tissue macrophages. For example, monocytes entering the brain parenchyma could be exposed to a brain-specific environment favoring expression of a microglia-like phenotype. Therefore, a better knowledge of unique genetic signatures and reliable cellular markers would greatly facilitate studies of the origin, function and fate of inflammatory cells in ischemic brain injury.

POLARIZATION OF MONOCYTES- AND MICROGLIA-DERIVED MACROPHAGES

Once in the damaged tissue, CD115$^+$ peripheral-blood monocytes have the ability to differentiate into macrophages and further polarize into several subtypes with specific functions including production of inflammatory molecules and phagocytic activity. Macrophage polarization depends on the type of injury, the nature of the pathogen, the organs involved and interactions with other immune cells. The distinct phenotypes and physiological activities associated with tissue macrophages were mostly described *in vitro* and in non-neuronal tissue, and have only recently been examined in the context of cerebral ischemia. "Classically activated macrophages" or "M1 macrophages" have anti-microbial activity and secrete pro-inflammatory cytokines and reactive oxygen species upon stimulation with interferon-γ (IFNγ) and lipopolysaccharide (LPS; Mills et al., 2000; Gordon and Taylor, 2005; Mosser and Edwards, 2008). On the other hand, "alternative" or M2 macrophages, induced by interleukin-4 (IL-4), IL-10 or transforming growth factor-β (TGF-β), promote anti-inflammatory and reparative processes (Mantovani et al., 2004; Hao et al., 2012; Yang et al., 2014). Several differentially regulated genes have been associated with each polarization state and are used to distinguish between these two populations in mice, including the IgG Fc receptors CD16/32 and inducible nitric oxide synthase (iNOS) for the M1 phenotype, and mannose receptor (CD206), arginase 1 (Arg1), chitinase-like 3 (Chil3 or Ym1), and IL-10 for the M2 phenotype (**Table 1;** Hu et al., 2012; Liu et al., 2013; Murray et al., 2014; Tang et al., 2014).

It must be noted that M1 and M2 are the extreme phenotypes of the broad and heterogeneous activation states of macrophages, and caution is needed in interpreting their multivalent function under pathological conditions (Murray et al., 2014). Recently, the M1/M2 terminology was also applied to activated microglia (Michelucci et al., 2009; David and Kroner, 2011). Exposure of cultured primary microglia to LPS or IFNγ induces a M1-like phenotype with reduced phagocytic activity and expression of iNOS, TNF, IL-1β and IL-6 among others, while IL-4 drives microglia towards a M2-like phenotype with increased Arg1, Ym1 and resistin like α (RELMα, FIZZ1) expression (Michelucci et al., 2009). Others have compared capacity of microglia and blood- or BM-derived macrophages to assume M1 or M2 phenotypes using *in vitro* polarization protocols (Durafourt et al., 2012; Girard et al., 2013). These authors assessed morphology, surface markers, cytokine profile and phagocytic capacity of both polarized blood-borne macrophages and microglia (Durafourt et al., 2012) or compared expression levels of M1/M2 marker genes (Girard et al., 2013). Girard et al. found that both mouse BM-derived macrophages and BV2 microglial cell line displayed a M1 or M2 phenotypes after LPS or IL-4 stimulation, respectively. In contrast, Durafourt et al. found that human microglia was able to respond to both M1 and M2-inducing stimuli, but their M2 gene expression signature was restricted to CD209 and the expression of CD23, CD163, and CD206 was not increased, as observed in M2 polarized macrophages (Durafourt et al., 2012). Although the functional implications remain to be established, these observations highlight important differences between human and mouse microglia. Interestingly, adult human microglia showed higher phagocytic activity and IL-10 expression than macrophages under M1 and M2 conditions, indicating that even in a pro-inflammatory environment microglia can retain anti-inflammatory function, which might be essential for their neuroprotective activity (Durafourt et al., 2012).

CONTRIBUTION OF IMMUNE CELLS OF MYELOID ORIGIN AND MICROGLIA TO CEREBRAL ISCHEMIC INJURY

Acute cerebral ischemia leads to rapid neuronal cell death and activation of resident microglia as well as the infiltration of blood-borne immune cells (Gelderblom et al., 2009; Dénes et al., 2010; **Figure 2**). Activated microglia become phagocytic aiming to clear the damage and promote repair (Faustino et al., 2011). If blood flow is not rapidly restored and ischemic damage develops, injured neurons release damage-associated molecular pattern proteins leading to the secretion of pro-inflammatory mediators and formation of ROS from parenchymal cells (del Zoppo et al., 2000; Shichita et al., 2012; Jackman and Iadecola, 2014). Cytokines and ROS, produced both in the vascular and parenchymal compartments, induce the disruption of the blood brain barrier (BBB) facilitating the infiltration of circulating monocytes, neutrophils and lymphocytes, thereby promoting post-ischemic inflammation (Iadecola and Anrather, 2011; Kleinschnitz et al., 2013; García-Bonilla et al., 2014b). However, neutrophils, as well as monocytes, some T- and B-cells and microglia may also exhibit anti-inflammatory properties that are important for limiting neuronal injury, resolving the inflammation and promoting tissue

Table 1 | Different activation states of neutrophils, circulating monocytes and tissue macrophages in mice.

	Neutrophils	Circulating monocytes		Monocyte-derived macrophages		Resident microglia	
Subsets	N1/N2	"Inflammatory" monocytes	"Patrolling" monocytes	M1	M2 (M2a,b,c)	Surveying microglia	Microglia-derived macrophages
Marker genes	iNOS			iNOS	Arg1, CD206, Chil3 (Ym1)	DAP12	
Receptor expression	$CD45^{high}$ $CD11b^{+}$ $Ly6G^{+}$	$CD45^{high}$ $Ly6C^{high}$ $CD115^{+}$ $CCR2^{+}$ $CX3CR1^{int}$ Ly6G-	$CD45^{high}$ $Ly6C^{low}$ $CD115^{+}$ $CCR2^{-}$ $CX3CR1^{+}$ Ly6G-	$CD45^{high}$ $CD115^{+}$ $CD11b^{+}$ $F4/80^{+}$ CD68 (ED-1) $CCR2^{+}$	$CD45^{high}$ $CD115^{+}$ $CD11b^{+}$ $F4/80^{+}$ CD68 (ED-1) $CX3CR1^{+}$	$CD45^{int}$ $CD11b^{+}$ CX3CR1 $Ibal^{+}$ IB4	$CD45^{high}$ $CD11b^{+}$ $CD115^{+}$ $F4/80^{+}$ CD68 (ED-1) $CX3CR1^{+}$ $Iba1^{+}$ IB4
Activated by [cells]	Platelets, Endothelial cells	Neutrophils, Dying neurons		Th1, NK	Th2	Neurons	Dying neurons
Activated by [molecules]	IL-1α	CCL2		LPS, IFNγ, TNF	IL-4 and IL-13 (M2a), IL-10, Glucocorticoid, TGFβ (M2c), CCL2 (MCP1)		DAMPs, CX3CL1
Function	Neurotoxic (N1), Neuroprotection (N2)	Recruited at sites of inflammation, Precursors of peripheral mononuclear phagocytes	Endothelium integrity	Cytotoxic effect	Phagocytic capacity, Promote neurite outgrowth	Synaptic pruning and remodeling during development, Homeostatic functions	Phagocytosis, Neurotoxicity
Cell products	ROS, NO, RNS, MMP-9, NE	TNF, ROS, NO, IL-1β, Little IL-10	IL-10, VEGF	IL-12, IL-23, TNF, IL-1β, IL-6, ROS	TGFβ, Arg1 and scavenger receptors (M2a), IL-10 (M2c).	TGFβ	IL-1β, TNF, IL-6, Chemokines, IFNγ

The dichotomy in the function of each cell type shown here is an oversimplified view of their activation state. They rather undergo multiple activation phenotypes at a given time making the interpretation of their neuroprotective or/and deleterious effect in cerebral ischemia complex. Whether N1/N2 and M1/M2 phenotypes may apply to neutrophils and microglia, respectively, would need further investigation.

Abbreviations: Arginase 1 (Arg1), Chemokine (C-C motif) ligand 2 (CCL2), C-C chemokine receptor type 2 (CCR2), Chitinase-like 3 (Chil3 or Ym1), CX3C chemokine receptor 1 (CX3CR1), Damage-associated molecular pattern molecules (DAMPs), DNAX activation protein of 12 kDa (DAP12), inducible nitric oxide synthase (iNOS), Interferon gamma (IFNγ), Interleukin-1,4,6,10,12,23 (IL-1, IL-4, IL-6, IL-10, IL-12, IL-23), Ionized calcium binding adaptor molecule 1 (Iba1), Isolectin B4 (IB4), Lipopolysaccharide (LPS), Lymphocyte antigen 6G (Ly6G), Matrix metallopeptidase 9 (MMP-9), monocyte chemotactic protein 1 (MCP1), Natural Killer (NK), Neutrophil elastase (NE), Nitric oxide (NO), Reactive nitrogen species (RNS), Reactive oxygen species (ROS), Transforming growth factor beta (TGF-β), Tumor necrosis factor (TNF), Type 1 T helper (Th1), Type 2 T helper (Th2), Vascular Endothelial Growth Factor (VEGF).

repair (Liesz et al., 2009; Yilmaz and Granger, 2010; Bodhankar et al., 2014). Characterizing the dynamics of leukocyte infiltration after cerebral ischemia is important to understand their functional role and therapeutic potential. Notably, the magnitude and temporal profile of peripheral immune cell infiltration depends upon models of focal cerebral ischemia. For example, permanent ischemia leads to immune cell infiltration as early as 3 h and a more pronounced accumulation of neutrophils compared to transient ischemia (Zhou et al., 2013; Chu et al., 2014b), wherein blood-borne immune cells do not appear in large numbers until 48 h after reperfusion (Stevens et al., 2002; Gelderblom et al., 2009; García-Bonilla et al., 2014b). These differences in the timing of cellular infiltration relative to the development of tissue injury hint at different roles of blood-borne immune cells in these two stroke models. These considerations need to be taken into account when extrapolating findings obtained in animal models to human stroke for therapeutic purposes.

NEUTROPHILS IN BRAIN ISCHEMIA

Neutrophils respond to sterile inflammation, such that induced by brain ischemia, by interacting with endothelial adhesion molecules, mainly selectin family members and intracellular adhesion molecule-1 (ICAM-1), to slow their intravascular movement and induce polarization, which results in firm adhesion to the pro-inflammatory endothelium (Panés et al., 1995, 1999). Rolling and adhesion of leukocytes can be observed *in vivo* as early as 1 h after transient middle cerebral artery (MCA) occlusion and is characterized by neutrophil attachment to the endothelium and increased platelet-neutrophil interactions which is P-selectin and integrin αIIbβ3 dependent (Ishikawa et al., 2004). Due to the proximity of platelets and neutrophils, IL-1α released from activated platelets, might be an early activator of neutrophils (Thornton et al., 2010).

After initial adherence, neutrophils will follow a chemokine and activator gradient produced by the injured tissue. Neutrophils

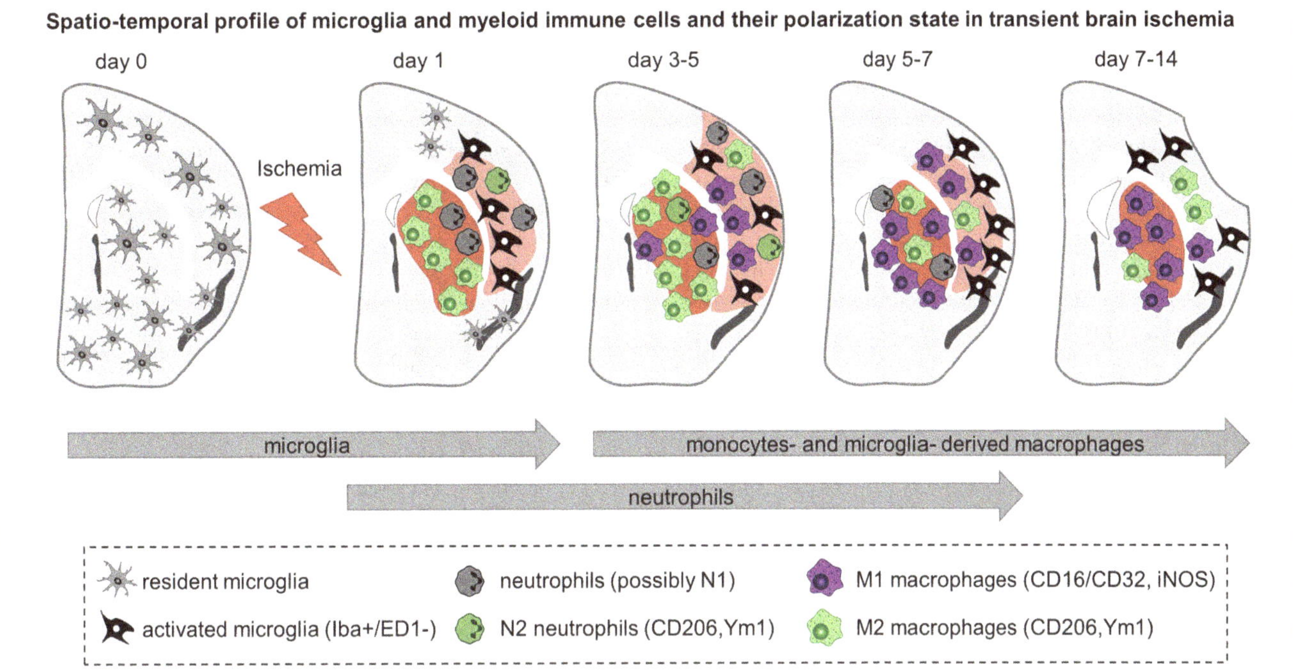

FIGURE 2 | Spatiotemporal profile of myeloid immune cell activation in acute cerebral ischemia. Schematic representation of rodent brain coronal sections through the anterior commissure (bregma = 0) after transient MCA occlusion in C57BL/6 mice. The core of the infarct is represented in red and the peri-infarct area is shown in light red. The evolution of the infarct is based on observations of ours and others and depicted as follow: infarct size becomes detectable 1 day after transient MCA occlusion, is maximal at 3–5 days after ischemia onset and decreases afterwards together with shrinkage of the injured hemisphere and enlargement of the ventricles. Before injury, resident microglia display ramified thin processes and are highly motile. They scan their microenvironment to detect any disturbances. Cerebral ischemia triggers microglia to become activated and to display distinct shapes and expression patterns upon the course of reperfusion. Based on findings depicted here, microglia become activated at the onset of cerebral ischemia—as early as 1 day after injury—and further develop into macrophages. In the core of the infarct, microglia are round-shaped, expressed ED-1 and display a M2 phenotype aimed at phagocytize the cellular debris and clear the damaged tissue. In the peri-infarct region microglia have ramified processes but are negative for the phagocytic marker ED-1. They are present early after injury, peak between 5–7 days and decrease thereafter. Neutrophils are the first myeloid immune cells to invade the brain and might display a N1 or N2 phenotypes. They can be detected in the ischemic region from 1 to 5–7 days after injury. Monocytes infiltrate the ischemic parenchyma after microglia activation and transform into macrophages. Between 3–5 days M2 macrophages are more abundant in the striatum—the core of the infarct—and decline by 2 weeks. In contrast, pro-inflammatory M1 cells are first observed in the peri-infarct of the lesion and increase in number in the core over time and outnumber the M2 macrophages later on. From 3–5 days onwards it is not clear yet whether the so called M1 and M2 macrophages found in the ischemic region are derived preferentially from microglia or infiltrated monocytes and if they have similar functions. Preliminary data suggest that microglia-derived macrophages can proliferate and have greater phagocytic properties than monocytes-derived macrophages.

are the first blood-borne cells found in the ischemic area, reach peak numbers at days 2–4 after transient ischemia and decline thereafter (Gelderblom et al., 2009; García-Bonilla et al., 2014b). The CXCR2 ligands CXCL1 (KC) and CXCL2 (MIP-2α) are the main chemokines responsible for neutrophil extravasation. In the ischemic brain CXCL1 is produced by activated astrocytes in an IL-17 dependent manner (**Figure 1**; Gelderblom et al., 2012). Chemokine-like factor 1 (CKLF1), a recently discovered chemokine, participates in neutrophil recruitment after transient focal ischemia in rats and anti-CKLF1 antibodies diminished neuronal cell death in this model (Kong et al., 2014). The sequence of molecular events regulating neutrophil extravasation remains incompletely understood. CD47, a immunoglobulin superfamily transmembrane glycoprotein expressed on the cell surface of neutrophils, is essential for neutrophil transmigration *in vivo* and *in vitro* (Liu et al., 2001; Su et al., 2008). Accordingly, CD47 deficient mice exhibit reduced brain injury and neutrophil infiltration after transient focal ischemia (Jin et al., 2009).

Endothelial transmigration seems to be essential for the cytotoxic activation of neutrophils (Allen et al., 2012), which is accomplished by induction of ROS production by NADPH oxidase and myeloperoxidase, iNOS dependent nitric oxide generation and concomitant release of RNS, particularly peroxynitrite (Yilmaz and Granger, 2010). Work from our group has shown that iNOS expression in endothelial cells and neutrophils contributes to ischemic brain injury after transient MCA occlusion, but was dispensable for neutrophil recruitment (Iadecola et al., 1997; García-Bonilla et al., 2014a). On the other hand, adoptive transfer of iNOS$^{+/+}$ neutrophils into an iNOS$^{-/-}$ host 24 h after MCA occlusion was sufficient to revert the protection exerted by iNOS deletion (García-Bonilla et al., 2014a). Other potentially neurotoxic molecules released by neutrophils are extracellular proteases. Among them, matrix metalloproteinase 9 (MMP-9), a protease released during neutrophil degranulation, has been shown to contribute to ischemic injury (Romanic et al., 1998). Neutrophil elastase (NE), has also been implicated in brain injury after transient but not permanent focal ischemia (Shimakura et al., 2000; Stowe et al., 2009). There is still debate to what extent neutrophils contribute to post-ischemic inflammation and neuronal cell death. While neutrophil depletion by delivery of anti-neutrophil antibodies was neuroprotective in focal ischemia models (Matsuo et al., 1994), several approaches to limit neutrophil infiltration by cytotoxic drugs or adhesion molecule and chemokine receptor blockade have been unsuccessful (Soriano et al., 1999; Beray-Berthat et al., 2003b; Brait et al., 2011), or have suggested that the contribution of neutrophils to ischemic injury might be brain region specific (Beray-Berthat et al., 2003a). It has also been suggested that neutrophils do not penetrate the ischemic brain tissue but accumulate in the perivascular space after extravasation (Enzmann et al., 2013). However, this finding does not exclude their participation in ischemic injury since neutrophils would be still able release soluble cytotoxic molecules such as ROS, RNS, and proteases, which could induce vascular damage aggravating the ischemia or diffuse into the brain parenchyma causing tissue injury. Indeed, our iNOS BM chimera and adoptive transfer experiments (García-Bonilla et al., 2014b), collectively, support a deleterious role of neutrophils in ischemic brain injury.

FUNCTIONAL POLARIZATION OF NEUTROPHILS IN CEREBRAL ISCHEMIA

In addition to their deleterious effect, neutrophils may also exert neuroprotective functions as recently suggested (Cuartero et al., 2013). In this study it was shown that in a mouse model of permanent focal ischemia the neuroprotective effect of the PPARγ agonist rosiglitazone was abolished in neutrophil depleted animals. Rosiglitazone treatment induced an increase of total number of neutrophils 24 h after ischemia and a shift in the ratio of pro-inflammatory N1 neutrophils to N2 neutrophils shown by increased expression of the M2-marker protein Ym1 (*Chil3*). N2 neutrophils were recently defined as a population of polarized cells with anti-inflammatory phenotype, in accordance to the M1/M2 classification of macrophages, and have been found in tumors where they facilitate tumor growth by inhibiting anti-tumor T cell responses (Fridlender et al., 2009; Mantovani, 2009). Their role in brain ischemia, including the mechanism of neuroprotection, remains to be firmly established, but, analogous to the double-edged role of monocytes/macrophages, neutrophils could also have beneficial effects, perhaps in the repair phase of the injury. For example, neutrophils that undergo apoptosis are ingested by microglia and macrophages, which induce these phagocytic cells to become anti-inflammatory or promote tissue repair (Serhan and Savill, 2005). Therefore, manipulating the polarization state of neutrophils could also have therapeutic relevance.

MONOCYTES AND MICROGLIA IN CEREBRAL ISCHEMIA

Under normal conditions, resident microglia are ramified, have long processes and can be morphologically discerned from macrophages (Nimmerjahn et al., 2005; Boche et al., 2013). Resident microglia can be distinguished from BM-derived monocytes according to their level of CD45 expression: microglia are $CD11b^{+}$ and express intermediate level of CD45 ($CD11b^{+}/CD45^{int}$), whereas monocytes are also positive for CD11b but express high level of CD45 ($CD11b^{+}/CD45^{high}$) (Ford et al., 1995). Monocytes can be further classified as $Ly6C^{high}$ pro-inflammatory monocytes or $Ly6C^{low}$ anti-inflammatory monocytes (David and Kroner, 2011). Upon injury, microglia adopt ameboid morphology and become phagocytic. Activated microglia are commonly identified by the cellular markers: IB4, Iba1, F4/80 or ED-1 (CD68). After cerebral ischemia, microglia display different markers and morphology depending on their localization in the ischemic territory and the course of reperfusion. In the ischemic core microglia have an ameboid shape, are Iba1 positive and ED1 positive and have increased CD11b expression, whereas in the peri-infarct area these cells have shorter processes than in the resting state, are $Iba1^{+}$, but are negative for ED1 (Ito et al., 2001; Morrison and Filosa, 2013). Once microglia differentiate into macrophages they share several antigens and morphological features with hematogenous macrophages (Patel et al., 2013), confounding the interpretation of their origin and ultimately their function in acute cerebral ischemia (Hanisch and Kettenmann, 2007; Hellwig et al., 2013).

Several recent studies have attempted to distinguish microglia from blood-derived macrophages and to define their role in ischemic injury and repair, potentially opening novel therapeutic avenues for the treatment of stroke. To this end, several strategies have been used (Prinz and Priller, 2014). A widely used approach has been to perform BM transplants with fluorescent BM (Tanaka et al., 2003). One drawback to this approach is that whole body irradiation may affect the integrity of the BBB and induce brain cytokine production, creating a permissive environment for brain engraftment of BM-derived immune cells normally not found in the CNS (Mildner et al., 2007). Although head shielding during irradiation or parabiosis may avoid such disturbances, the resulting degree of chimerism (40–50%) is not as high as with whole body irradiation (>90%) (Ginhoux et al., 2013; Prinz and Priller, 2014). The reduced chimerism obtained with these models may not be problematic for cell tracking and fate determination experiments, but it will confound the interpretation of mechanistic studies on the relative contribution of resident and blood-borne immune cells to tissue damage and repair. Recently, it has been shown that chemical BM ablation with busulfan leads to a better rate of blood chimerism with reduced inflammation and myeloid immune cell recruitment in the mouse CNS compared to irradiation (Kierdorf et al., 2013b). However, in our own experience, doses of busulfan that produce a chimerism comparable to irradiation lead to a myeloid immune cell recruitment in brain greater than that seen with irradiation (Sugiyama et al., 2014). Therefore, chemical BM ablation-based approaches require further scrutiny.

Another approach to track blood-borne myeloid cell infiltration into the ischemic area, has been to use ultrasmall superparamagnetic iron oxide particles (USPIO), which labels peripheral phagocytic cells after intravenous injection. USPIO were delivered in one case 5.5 h after permanent MCA occlusion (Rausch et al., 2001) and in an other study 24 h before inducing photothrombotic strokes (Kleinschnitz et al., 2003). Brains were analyzed at different time points after ischemia by magnetic resonance imaging (MRI) and histology. While the temporal profile was slightly different between the two studies, iron particles were detected late in the post-ischemic period, after most of the damage had occurred (Rausch et al., 2001; Kleinschnitz et al., 2003). In a model of neonatal ischemia, microglia—identified as $CD11b^{+}/CD45^{low/int}$ by flow cytometry—were the predominant cell population in the infarct area compared to $CD11b^{+}/CD45^{high}$ monocytes (Denker et al., 2007). A similar pattern was described using GFP-BM chimeric mice. Thus, Schilling et al. found that microglia were the first cells to be activated in the infarcted area, exhibited a more pronounced phagocytic activity and out-numbered GFP-BM monocytes (Schilling et al., 2003, 2005). Collectively, these observations suggest that microglia are likely to be the first cells activated after brain injury, aiming at clearing the cell debris by phagocytosis and contributing to the resolution of inflammation (Neumann et al., 2009). On the other hand, phagocytosis could also contribute to neuronal cell loss after ischemia. For example, it has been suggested that microglia could engulf viable neurons in the ischemic penumbra (Neher et al., 2013). Salvageable neurons would send "eat me" signals to nearby microglia and induce their phagocytosis that further increases brain damage (Neher et al., 2012). In support of this hypothesis, deficiency of the phagocytosis-related receptors Mertk and milk fat globule-EGF factor 8 protein (Mfge8) on microglia promotes functional recovery and reduces brain atrophy in focal infarcts (Neher et al., 2013). On the other hand, deletion of triggering receptor expressed on myeloid cells 2 (TREM2), a receptor expressed on phagocytic microglia and macrophages, did not affect infarct size in a focal ischemia model in mice (Sieber et al., 2013), although TREM2 is essential for their phagocytosis capacity (Takahashi et al., 2007). The molecular mechanisms regulating these microglial behaviors need to be established and may provide new insights into endogenous brain processes regulating injury and repair.

$CCR2^{+}$ MONOCYTES IN CEREBRAL ISCHEMIA

Recruitment of circulating monocytes to the ischemic brain is orchestrated by inflammatory cytokines, de novo-expressed adhesion molecules and chemokines. The monocyte chemoattractant protein (MCP-1, CCL2) and its receptor CCR2 are known to be involved in the inflammatory response of the injured brain after cerebral ischemia (Che et al., 2001; Chu et al., 2014a). After permanent and transient focal ischemia, Gliem et al. found an increase in $Ly6C^{high}$ monocytes at 3 days, whereas the number of $Ly6C^{low}$ monocytes was greatest at 6 days, paralleled by sequential peaks of CCR2 and CX3CR1 mRNA as well as gene expression of the pro- and anti-inflammatory cytokines IL-1β and TGF-β, respectively (Gliem et al., 2012). Furthermore, they demonstrated that selective deletion of CCR2 in BM-derived cells induced a delayed clinical deterioration and hemorrhagic conversion of ischemic infarcts, suggesting a beneficial role of $CCR2^{+}$ monocytes in maintaining the structure of the neurovascular unit (Gliem et al., 2012). Because $CCR2^{+}/Ly6C^{high}$ monocytes can transform into anti-inflammatory $Ly6C^{low}F4/80^{high}$ macrophages, it was suggested that lack of infiltrating $CCR2^{+}$ monocytes results in reduction of anti-inflammatory macrophages at later time points compromising repair mechanisms. However, several other studies demonstrated reduced phagocytic macrophage accumulation in the brain of CCL2 or CCR2 knock-out mice together with smaller infarcts after cerebral artery occlusion (Hughes et al., 2002; Dimitrijevic et al., 2007; Schilling et al., 2009), suggesting a deleterious role of CCR2 monocytes. These discrepancies may reflect the multifunctional roles of $CCR2^{+}$ monocytes, which, while contributing to early brain injury may also enable delayed repair processes.

$CX3CR1^{+}$ MONOCYTES AND MICROGLIA IN CEREBRAL ISCHEMIA

The chemokine CX3CL1 is found on neurons while its receptor CX3CR1 is expressed on microglia and $Ly6C^{low}$ monocytes (Geissmann et al., 2003; Sunnemark et al., 2005; Limatola and Ransohoff, 2014). $CX3CR1^{-/-}$ or $CX3CL1^{-/-}$ mice show reduced brain damage in transient focal ischemia models compared to wild type mice (Soriano et al., 2002; Dénes et al., 2008; Fumagalli et al., 2013), although the effect might not be sustained in time (Gliem et al., 2012). Neuroprotection found in $CX3CR1^{-/-}$ mice following focal cerebral ischemia was correlated with an increase of the M2 macrophage marker genes CD206 and Ym1 and a decrease of M1-iNOS gene expression compared to wild type mice (Fumagalli et al., 2013; Tang et al., 2014). These findings indicate that CX3CR1 deficient mice induce a different pattern of M1/M2 marker expression in the ischemic region. The authors suggest that the lack of CX3CR1 in microglia and infiltrated monocytes favors an anti-inflammatory milieu that protects the brain from infarct development. However, intracerebroventricular delivery of CX3CL1 at the time of MCA occlusion decreased infarct volumes (Cipriani et al., 2011), suggesting that CX3CL1 acts on microglia to reduce their activation state and inhibit the release of inflammatory cytokines (Zujovic et al., 2000; Cardona et al., 2006; Biber et al., 2007). Michaud et al. has recently shown that selective ablation of $Ly6C^{low}/CX3CR1^{+}$ monocytes, thought to preferentially develop into M2 macrophages, does not influence stroke outcome in a hypoxic-ischemic injury model (Michaud et al., 2014). Using $NR4A1^{-/-}$ BM chimeras that lack circulating $Ly6C^{low}/CX3CR1^{+}$ monocytes (Carlin et al., 2013), it was found that structural and functional outcome were not affected. However, brain infiltrating monocytes have not been assessed in this study, and it remains an open question whether $Ly6C^{high}/CCR2^{+}$ monocytes in the brain parenchyma could give rise to $Ly6C^{low}/CX3CR1^{+}$ monocytes/macrophages, even in the absence of the NR4A1 transcription factor.

Using parabiosis of $CX3CR1^{GFP/+}$ mice and wild type partners, Li et al. found that microglia increased gradually during the first week after photothrombotic stroke (Li et al.,

2013). Hypertrophic ameboid microglia were more abundant in the periphery compared to the core of the lesion and many GFP-positive microglia were labeled with the mitotic marker bromodeoxyuridine (Li et al., 2013). In the wild type parabiotic partner, CX3CR1$^{GFP/+}$ infiltrating cells started to populate the brain 5 days after ischemia onset, were less numerous than activated microglia and did not proliferate, suggesting that microglia and monocyte-derived CX3CR1 macrophages are two distinct populations with presumably different roles in cerebral ischemia.

M1 AND M2 PHENOTYPES IN CEREBRAL ISCHEMIA

Recent studies have begun to investigate microglia and macrophage polarization *in vivo*. In a model of permanent focal ischemia, different cell markers were used to characterize the prevalence of phagocytic cells and M2-like phenotype at different time after ischemia (Perego et al., 2011). Soon after injury, ED-1 positive phagocytic cells were present at the border—possibly limiting the expansion of the infarct—whereas Ym1- and CD206-expressing cells were found in the ischemic core. At 7 days, more phagocytic cells invaded the ischemic core where they engulfed neurons. In transient focal ischemia, M2-type gene expression (CD206, Arg1, CCL22, Ym1/2, IL-10, and TGF-β) was first apparent from 1 to 3 days after ischemia, peaked at 3–5 days, was reduced at 7 days and returned to pre-injury levels by day 14. M1-type genes (iNOS, CD11b, CD16, CD32, and CD86) were gradually increased from day 3 and remained elevated for 14 days after ischemia (Hu et al., 2012). The M1/M2 phenotype was also assessed in *in vitro* models of ischemic injury using microglia and neuronal co-culture. M1-polarized microglia/macrophages exacerbate neuronal death compared with M2 cells (Hu et al., 2012; Girard et al., 2013). Hu et al. suggested that early expression of M2 genes may contribute to neuroprotection by enhancing the phagocytosis of dead cells, removal of tissue debris and promote recovery. At later stages, cells displaying a M1 phenotype may induce pro-inflammatory mediators and exacerbate neuronal death. Therefore, limiting such M2 to M1 shift and promoting M2 polarization could be a potential therapeutic strategy (Hu et al., 2012). *In vitro* experiments have to be interpreted with caution because microglia are commonly derived from neonatal tissue and develop in a culture environment that cannot recapitulate the maturation process that occurs *in vivo* (Hellwig et al., 2013). Importantly, the gene expression signature characteristic for adult brain microglia is lost in primary neonatal microglia cultures as well as in microglial cell lines including BV2 and N9 cells (Butovsky et al., 2014). Thus, *in vivo* translation of findings obtained with *in vitro* polarization models might not be easily achieved. Desestret et al. administered differentiated BM-derived M2 macrophages 4 days after cerebral ischemia by intravenous injection. M2 macrophages failed to induce protection or improve behavioral outcome (Desestret et al., 2013). On the other hand, Girard et al. have proposed that M1 and M2 BM-derived macrophages promote cell death *in vitro*, whereas M2 microglia is neuroprotective. However, microglia does not display a classic M1 and M2 phenotypes after MCA occlusion (Girard et al., 2013). The ability of microglia to differentiate into multiple macrophage-related phenotypes depending on their microenvironment highlights the complexity of their response to cerebral ischemia (Taylor and Sansing, 2013).

A ROLE FOR SPLENIC MONOCYTES IN BRAIN ISCHEMIA?

The discovery of a splenic monocyte reservoir in adult mice, that is mobilized following ischemic myocardial injury (Swirski et al., 2009), has sparked renewed interest in the role of the spleen in brain ischemia. Previous studies have shown that splenocytes respond to cerebral ischemia by producing large amounts of inflammatory mediators early after injury (Offner et al., 2006b), followed later by an increase of blood monocytes and splenic regulatory T cells, that are thought to dampen the inflammatory response (Offner et al., 2006a). In accordance with these findings, chronic splenectomy (Ajmo et al., 2008) or acute spleen irradiation (Ostrowski et al., 2012) have been performed in rats to inhibit systemic inflammatory responses after stroke. Although the studies differed in the ischemic model, i.e., permanent vs. transient ischemia, both studies observed neuroprotection together with a decrease of immune cell counts in the ischemic region. In addition, post-stroke treatment with the antibacterial agent moxifloxacin (MFX) reduced peripheral infection and infarct size in animal models of stroke (Meisel et al., 2004; Bao et al., 2010). In MFX-treated mice the percentage of the splenic pro-inflammatory Ly6C^{high} monocytes was reduced compared to vehicle animals 7 days after stroke, together with reduced expression of CCR2 in the spleen and the brain (Bao et al., 2010). These studies suggest that interventions aiming at reducing systemic inflammation, specifically by targeting splenocytes, could lead to a reduction of brain immune cell infiltration and neuroprotection. However, these reports did not assess whether leukocytes, specifically monocytes, found in the brain originate from the spleen and contribute directly to stroke outcome. For instance, Ajmo et al. did not find alteration of immune cell counts in peripheral blood following MCA occlusion in sham or splenectomized animals, while spleen irradiation after MCA occlusion resulted in a drop of circulating lymphocytes, but failed to lower blood monocytes and neutrophils (Ajmo et al., 2008; Ostrowski et al., 2012). Thus it is not clear whether peripheral immune cells are mobilized from the spleen into the brain and contribute directly to stroke outcome. Recently, Kim et al. analyzed the temporal profile of brain infiltrating Ly6C^{high} and Ly6C^{low} monocytes after focal ischemic injury in acutely splenectomized mice (Kim et al., 2014). In sham mice, they found that brain ischemia induced a reduction of both monocytes subsets in the spleen that temporally correlated with their increase in the ischemic brain. In splenectomized mice, brain Ly6C^{high} and Ly6C^{low} monocytes were reduced at 1 and 3 days after stroke compared to sham surgery. However no difference in infarct size was observed between groups (Kim et al., 2014). While this study did not directly track splenic monocytes and the findings remain correlative, it suggests that the spleen might contribute both Ly6C^{high} and Ly6C^{low} monocytes after brain ischemia. The failure to observe neuroprotection in this model might be related to simultaneous reduction of both monocyte subsets, thus balancing the loss of deleterious Ly6C^{high} monocytes with the loss of beneficial Ly6C^{low} monocytes, which might be involved in resolution of the inflammation and tissue repair (Shechter et al., 2013).

MYELOID IMMUNE CELLS IN HUMAN STROKE

TEMPORAL PROFILE OF MYELOID IMMUNE CELL ACTIVATION AND INFILTRATION

Histological analysis of autopsy material from patients allowed to draw a temporal profile of cellular events from 1 day after stroke onset to several years (Chuaqui and Tapia, 1993; Mena et al., 2004). Astrogliosis was observed within the first day of cerebral infarct development together with neutrophils, which were observed in 81% of cases between 3–37 days after stroke onset (Mena et al., 2004). This active inflammatory phase was accompanied by tissue necrosis and infiltration of inflammatory cells such as mononuclear cells and macrophages, which were not observed during the first 2 days after stroke onset. Interestingly, inflammatory mononuclear cells and macrophages persisted up to 53 years and were found in the majority of late stage specimens while neutrophils were absent (Mena et al., 2004). Although the temporal sequence and type of cells in the infarct are similar in rodents and humans (Gelderblom et al., 2009), the chronology of events seems to be more delayed and more spread out in time in humans.

Advanced imaging techniques to visualize post-ischemic inflammation and leukocyte infiltration are increasingly being employed in the clinical setting. Visualization of infiltrated macrophages in stroke patients was performed by USPIO-MRI (Saleh et al., 2004, 2007; Cho et al., 2007). In all patients tested, an increase signal of USPIO was observed by MRI in the brain parenchyma (Saleh et al., 2004). Only a minority of patients that received USPIO between 24 h and 96 h after symptom onset showed a positive signal in the brain (Cho et al., 2007; Saleh et al., 2007). However, iron-positive cells detected in the brain cannot represent only monocytes since activated microglia can engulf iron particles as well (Oude Engberink et al., 2008; Desestret et al., 2009). Injection of iron oxide monocytes labeled *ex vivo* allowed to follow their brain infiltration in experimental models of stroke (see previous section) (Stroh et al., 2006; Oude Engberink et al., 2008). Similarly, the use of *ex vivo* monocyte labeling in humans may increase our understanding of the temporal pattern of blood-borne cell infiltration after stroke. Positron emission tomography (PET) has been used to label inflammatory cells in stroke patients using the radioligands $^{11}C(R)$-PK11195 for the translocator protein 18kDa (TSPO), commonly used as a microglial marker (Stephenson et al., 1995; Cagnin et al., 2007). Analysis in patients showed an increase of the marker between 3 and 150 days after stroke (Gerhard et al., 2005). Positive labeling was observed early after ischemia, initially at the periphery of the lesion, then in the infarct core and eventually in peri-infarct regions (Gerhard et al., 2005; Thiel and Heiss, 2011). Altogether, the time of magnetic particles or radiolabelled agents infusion might be critical to discriminate resident microglia from immune cells of myeloid origin (Deddens et al., 2012). However, a limitation is that these techniques of brain macrophage visualization do not permit to differentiate between their different subtypes and activation states (Weissleder et al., 2014).

MONOCYTE SUBSETS IN PATIENTS WITH CEREBRAL ISCHEMIA

In human three distinct blood monocytes can be distinguished relative to the expression of the receptor CD14 (LPS co-receptor) and CD16 (Fcγ receptor III). The majority of human "classical" monocytes express high level of CD14 and are negative for CD16 ($CD14^{++}/CD16^{-}$), whereas the minor subtypes express CD16 and can be either $CD14^{high}$ ($CD14^{++}/CD16^{+}$) or $CD14^{low}$ ($CD14^{dim}/CD16^{+}$), also known as intermediate and non-classical monocytes, respectively (Ziegler-Heitbrock, 1996; Ziegler-Heitbrock et al., 2010). The classical monocytes $CD14^{+}/CD16^{-}$ share some features with the murine $Ly6C^{high}$ monocytes such as the high expression of the chemokine receptor CCR2 (Weber et al., 2000), whereas $CD16^{+}$ cells express CX3CR1 similar to mouse $Ly6C^{low}$ monocytes (Merino et al., 2011). However, the pro- or anti-inflammatory functions of these different monocyte subsets depend on the inflammatory context and, as in the mouse, a strict association of phenotype and function can not be established (Gordon and Taylor, 2005; Ziegler-Heitbrock, 2007; Merino et al., 2011). For example, blood monocyte subsets from healthy donors showed different pattern of response when stimulated with LPS (Frankenberger et al., 1996; Skrzeczyńska-Moncznik et al., 2008). $CD14^{dim}/CD16^{+}$ monocytes were found to produce more TNF compared to $CD14^{high}/CD16^{+}$ and $CD14^{high}/CD16^{-}$ monocytes, whereas $CD14^{high}/CD16^{+}$ were the main source for IL-10, (Belge et al., 2002; Skrzeczyńska-Moncznik et al., 2008).

Similar to the mouse (Offner et al., 2006b), stroke has a significant impact on the peripheral immune system in humans (Kamel and Iadecola, 2012). Although there is significant immunosuppression in acute stroke (Meisel et al., 2005; Chamorro et al., 2006), a significant increase of circulating monocytes has also been reported (Losy and Zaremba, 2001). The different subtypes of blood monocytes were investigated in patients following stroke and were correlated with outcome severity (Urra et al., 2009). The $CD14^{high}/CD16^{+}$ subset was increased 48 h after admission, while a parallel decrease in the $CD14^{dim}/CD16^{+}$ subtype was observed. An increase in classical $CD14^{high}/CD16^{-}$ monocytes was associated with poor outcome, whereas increased $CD16^{+}$ monocytes were linked to a better prognosis (Urra et al., 2009). CD14 expressing cells were observed in brain tissue from patients with focal infarction as early as 1 day and persisted for months after ischemia (Beschorner et al., 2002), suggesting a long-term involvement in inflammatory processes at the site of injury.

There is still a large knowledge gap about human microglia and immune cells of myeloid origin regarding their activation state, spatiotemporal distribution in the brain and, ultimately, about their role in acute cerebral ischemia. Advanced brain imaging modalities in humans and new cerebral ischemic models more representative of human stroke would help enhance our understanding of the inflammatory processes occurring in acute cerebral ischemia and to test therapeutic strategies directed at manipulating their beneficial or deleterious effects.

TARGETING INFLAMMATION AS THERAPEUTIC STRATEGIES

The only successful treatment for ischemic stroke is thrombolysis with tissue plasminogen activator (tPA), which, due to the narrow therapeutic window (<4.5 h) (Hacke et al., 2008) and safety concerns, is administered to less than 5% of patients (Fonarow et al., 2011). Different strategies aimed at preventing the inflammatory response after cerebral ischemia have been successful in rodent models. Ischemic damage was shown to be attenuated, among others, by inhibition of microglial activation using the immunomodulatory antibiotic minocycline, systemic T lymphocytes depletion using sphingosine 1-phosphate receptor agonist (FTY720), diminishing free radical generating and pro-inflammatory enzymes, such as iNOS or cyclooxygenase-2, inhibition of cytokines secretion, or targeting adhesion molecules (for reviews, Dirnagl et al., 1999; Iadecola and Alexander, 2001; Wang, 2005; Jordán et al., 2008).

Unfortunately attempts to translate anti-inflammatory therapeutic interventions into the clinics have been more disappointing than promising (O'Collins et al., 2006; Moskowitz et al., 2010). The selective IL-1 receptor antagonist, IL1-ra, which limits the pro-inflammatory action of IL-1, has been tested in randomized patients with acute stroke (Emsley et al., 2005). Despite a conclusive phase II study no recent publications have reported the recombinant human IL1-ra as a therapeutic agent for acute stroke. Strategies to inhibit neutrophil infiltration have been tested in clinical trials. Treatment with the murine mono-clonal anti-ICAM-1 in the Enlimomab trial (Enlimomab Acute Stroke Trial Investigators, 2001) or UK-279,276 (neutrophil inhibitory factor) have failed to improve recovery in acute ischemic stroke patients (Krams et al., 2003). Likewise, NXY-059, a nitrone-based free radical trapping agent, has not demonstrated any benefits in stroke clinical trials (Shuaib et al., 2007). The granulocyte colony-stimulating factor (G-CSF), that stimulates proliferation, survival, and maturation of BM-derived cells, has shown neuroprotective effect in models of transient focal ischemia by inducing mobilization of haemopoietic stem cells, by having anti-apoptotic and anti-inflammatory properties, as well as by promoting neuronal differentiation and angiogenesis (Komine-Kobayashi et al., 2006; England et al., 2009). However, recent results from a large phase IIb trial (AXIS-2) was not able to detect clinical efficacy in acute ischemic stroke patients (Ringelstein et al., 2013).

Reasons for failure have been discussed extensively in the literature and might include ambivalent roles of post-stroke inflammation as well as functional differences between rodent and human immune systems, patient inclusion criteria, timing of intervention, evaluation of efficacy, pharmacokinetic issues and side effects such as promoting infections and fever (for review, Dirnagl, 2006; Endres et al., 2008). Before translating experimental findings into therapies that target the immune system in stroke patients, there is a need to better understand the spatiotemporal profile and functional states of immune cells involved in ischemic brain injury in humans. A better insight in these aspects is crucial for planning future clinical trials targeting post-ischemic inflammation.

CONCLUDING REMARKS

The surprising plasticity of myeloid immune cells and microglia in their response to tissue injury highlights the need for further research to define spatiotemporal profiles of their distinct subsets in ischemic brain injury. Given the neuroprotective potential of some of these subsets, it has become clear that inhibiting inflammation in general or indiscriminately blocking leukocyte access to the brain might not be a viable therapeutic approach. The failure of clinical trials that targeted post-ischemic leukocyte recruitment might be in part explained by the indiscriminate nature of these approaches and a lack of a nuanced understanding of the impact of inflammation on damage and repair processes in the post-ischemic brain. Our understanding of the behavior of myeloid immune cells and microglia in ischemic stroke is still limited. Key questions to be addressed in future research include the transcriptomic and proteomic characterization of myeloid immune cell subsets at different stages of brain ischemia, the mechanism of monocytes, neutrophils and microglia polarization in the ischemic environment, and the neural and humoral signals generated by the ischemic brain to modulate peripheral immune cell activation and mobilization. Answering some of these questions would provide the knowledge base needed to design more specific immunotherapies for the treatment of ischemic stroke.

ACKNOWLEDGMENTS

This work was supported by National Institutes of Health (NIH) Grants NS34179 (Costantino Iadecola) and NS081179 (Josef Anrather). Corinne Benakis was supported by grant P3SMP3 148367 from the Swiss National Science Foundation and the Swiss Foundation for Grants in Biology and Medicine (SFGBM).

REFERENCES

Ajami, B., Bennett, J. L., Krieger, C., McNagny, K. M., and Rossi, F. M. V. (2011). Infiltrating monocytes trigger EAE progression, but do not contribute to the resident microglia pool. *Nat. Neurosci.* 14, 1142–1149. doi: 10.1038/nn.2887

Ajami, B., Bennett, J. L., Krieger, C., Tetzlaff, W., and Rossi, F. M. V. (2007). Local self-renewal can sustain CNS microglia maintenance and function throughout adult life. *Nat. Neurosci.* 10, 1538–1543. doi: 10.1038/nn2014

Ajmo, C. T., Vernon, D. O. L., Collier, L., Hall, A. A., Garbuzova-Davis, S., Willing, A., et al. (2008). The spleen contributes to stroke-induced neurodegeneration. *J. Neurosci. Res.* 86, 2227–2234. doi: 10.1002/jnr.21661

Allen, C., Thornton, P., Denes, A., McColl, B. W., Pierozynski, A., Monestier, M., et al. (2012). Neutrophil cerebrovascular transmigration triggers rapid neurotoxicity through release of proteases associated with decondensed DNA. *J. Immunol.* 189, 381–392. doi: 10.4049/jimmunol.1200409

Alliot, F., Godin, I., and Pessac, B. (1999). Microglia derive from progenitors, originating from the yolk sac and which proliferate in the brain. *Brain Res. Dev. Brain Res.* 117, 145–152. doi: 10.1016/s0165-3806(99)00113-3

Auffray, C., Fogg, D., Garfa, M., Elain, G., Join-Lambert, O., Kayal, S., et al. (2007). Monitoring of blood vessels and tissues by a population of monocytes with patrolling behavior. *Science* 317, 666–670. doi: 10.1126/science.1142883

Auffray, C., Sieweke, M. H., and Geissmann, F. (2009). Blood monocytes: development, heterogeneity and relationship with dendritic cells. *Annu. Rev. Immunol.* 27, 669–692. doi: 10.1146/annurev.immunol.021908.132557

Bao, Y., Kim, E., Bhosle, S., Mehta, H., and Cho, S. (2010). A role for spleen monocytes in post-ischemic brain inflammation and injury. *J. Neuroinflammation.* 7:92. doi: 10.1186/1742-2094-7-92

Belge, K. U., Dayyani, F., Horelt, A., Siedlar, M., Frankenberger, M., Frankenberger, B., et al. (2002). The proinflammatory CD14+ CD16+ DR++ monocytes are a major source of TNF. *J. Immunol.* 168, 3536–3542. doi: 10.4049/jimmunol.168.7.3536

Beray-Berthat, V., Croci, N., Plotkine, M., and Margaill, I. (2003a). Polymorphonuclear neutrophils contribute to infarction and oxidative stress in the cortex but not in the striatum after ischemia-reperfusion in rats. *Brain Res.* 987, 32–38. doi: 10.1016/s0006-8993(03)03224-4

Beray-Berthat, V., Palmier, B., Plotkine, M., and Margaill, I. (2003b). Neutrophils do not contribute to infarction, oxidative stress and NO synthase activity in severe brain ischemia. *Exp. Neurol.* 182, 446–454. doi: 10.1016/s0014-4886(03)00106-7

Beschorner, R., Schluesener, H. J., Gözalan, F., Meyermann, R., and Schwab, J. M. (2002). Infiltrating CD14+ monocytes and expression of CD14 by activated parenchymal microglia/macrophages contribute to the pool of CD14+ cells in ischemic brain lesions. *J. Neuroimmunol.* 126, 107–115. doi: 10.1016/s0165-5728(02)00046-2

Biber, K., Neumann, H., Inoue, K., and Boddeke, H. W. G. M. (2007). Neuronal 'On' and 'Off' signals control microglia. *Trends Neurosci.* 30, 596–602. doi: 10.1016/j.tins.2007.08.007

Bierman, H. R., Kelly, K. H., Cordes, F. L., Byron, R. L. Jr., Polhemus, J. A., and Rappoport, S. (1952). The release of leukocytes and platelets from the pulmonary circulation by epinephrine. *Blood* 7, 683–692.

Bierman, H. R., Kelly, K. H., King, F. W., and Petrakis, N. L. (1951). The pulmonary circulation as a source of leucocytes and platelets in man. *Science* 114, 276–277. doi: 10.1126/science.114.2959.276

Boche, D., Perry, V. H., and Nicoll, J. A. R. (2013). Review: activation patterns of microglia and their identification in the human brain. *Neuropathol. Appl. Neurobiol.* 39, 3–18. doi: 10.1111/nan.12011

Bodhankar, S., Chen, Y., Vandenbark, A. A., Murphy, S. J., and Offner, H. (2014). Treatment of experimental stroke with IL-10-producing B-cells reduces infarct size and peripheral and CNS inflammation in wild-type B-cell-sufficient mice. *Metab. Brain Dis.* 29, 59–73. doi: 10.1007/s11011-013-9474-3

Brait, V. H., Rivera, J., Broughton, B. R. S., Lee, S., Drummond, G. R., and Sobey, C. G. (2011). Chemokine-related gene expression in the brain following ischemic stroke: no role for CXCR2 in outcome. *Brain Res.* 1372, 169–179. doi: 10.1016/j.brainres.2010.11.087

Bugl, S., Wirths, S., Müller, M. R., Radsak, M. P., and Kopp, H.-G. (2012). Current insights into neutrophil homeostasis. *Ann. N Y Acad. Sci.* 1266, 171–178. doi: 10.1111/j.1749-6632.2012.06607.x

Butovsky, O., Jedrychowski, M. P., Moore, C. S., Cialic, R., Lanser, A. J., Gabriely, G., et al. (2014). Identification of a unique TGF-β-dependent molecular and functional signature in microglia. *Nat. Neurosci.* 17, 131–143. doi: 10.1038/nn.3599

Cagnin, A., Kassiou, M., Meikle, S. R., and Banati, R. B. (2007). Positron emission tomography imaging of neuroinflammation. *Neurotherapeutics* 4, 443–452. doi: 10.1016/j.nurt.2007.04.006

Cardona, A. E., Pioro, E. P., Sasse, M. E., Kostenko, V., Cardona, S. M., Dijkstra, I. M., et al. (2006). Control of microglial neurotoxicity by the fractalkine receptor. *Nat. Neurosci.* 9, 917–924. doi: 10.1038/nn1715

Carlin, L. M., Stamatiades, E. G., Auffray, C., Hanna, R. N., Glover, L., Vizcay-Barrena, G., et al. (2013). Nr4a1-dependent Ly6C(low) monocytes monitor endothelial cells and orchestrate their disposal. *Cell* 153, 362–375. doi: 10.1016/j.cell.2013.03.010

Chamorro, A., Amaro, S., Vargas, M., Obach, V., Cervera, A., Torres, F., et al. (2006). Interleukin 10, monocytes and increased risk of early infection in ischaemic stroke. *J. Neurol. Neurosurg. Psychiatry* 77, 1279–1281. doi: 10.1136/jnnp.2006.100800

Che, X., Ye, W., Panga, L., Wu, D. C., and Yang, G. Y. (2001). Monocyte chemoattractant protein-1 expressed in neurons and astrocytes during focal ischemia in mice. *Brain Res.* 902, 171–177. doi: 10.1016/s0006-8993(01)02328-9

Chiba, T., and Umegaki, K. (2013). Pivotal roles of monocytes/macrophages in stroke. *Mediators Inflamm.* 2013, 1–10. doi: 10.1155/2013/759103

Chitu, V., and Stanley, E. R. (2006). Colony-stimulating factor-1 in immunity and inflammation. *Curr. Opin. Immunol.* 18, 39–48. doi: 10.1016/j.coi.2005.11.006

Cho, T.-H., Nighoghossian, N., Wiart, M., Desestret, V., Cakmak, S., Berthezene, Y., et al. (2007). USPIO-enhanced MRI of neuroinflammation at the sub-acute stage of ischemic stroke: preliminary data. *Cerebrovasc. Dis.* 24, 544–546. doi: 10.1159/000111222

Chu, H. X., Arumugam, T. V., Gelderblom, M., Magnus, T., Drummond, G. R., and Sobey, C. G. (2014a). Role of CCR2 in inflammatory conditions of the central nervous system. *J. Cereb. Blood Flow Metab.* 34, 1425–1429. doi: 10.1038/jcbfm.2014.120

Chu, H. X., Kim, H. A., Lee, S., Moore, J. P., Chan, C. T., Vinh, A., et al. (2014b). Immune cell infiltration in malignant middle cerebral artery infarction: comparison with transient cerebral ischemia. *J. Cereb. Blood Flow Metab.* 34, 450–459. doi: 10.1038/jcbfm.2013.217

Chuaqui, R., and Tapia, J. (1993). Histologic assessment of the age of recent brain infarcts in man. *J. Neuropathol. Exp. Neurol.* 52, 481–489. doi: 10.1097/00005072-199309000-00006

Cipriani, R., Villa, P., Chece, G., Lauro, C., Paladini, A., Micotti, E., et al. (2011). CX3CL1 is neuroprotective in permanent focal cerebral ischemia in rodents. *J. Neurosci.* 31, 16327–16335. doi: 10.1523/JNEUROSCI.3611-11.2011

Craddock, C. G., Perry, S., Ventzke, L. E., and Lawrence, J. S. (1960). Evaluation of marrow granulocytic reserves in normal and disease states. *Blood* 15, 840–855.

Cuartero, M. I., Ballesteros, I., Moraga, A., Nombela, F., Vivancos, J., Hamilton, J. A., et al. (2013). N2 neutrophils, novel players in brain inflammation after stroke: modulation by the PPARγ agonist rosiglitazone. *Stroke* 44, 3498–3508. doi: 10.1161/STROKEAHA.113.002470

David, S., and Kroner, A. (2011). Repertoire of microglial and macrophage responses after spinal cord injury. *Nat. Rev. Neurosci.* 12, 388–399. doi: 10.1038/nrn3053

Deddens, L. H., Van Tilborg, G. A. F., Mulder, W. J. M., de Vries, H. E., and Dijkhuizen, R. M. (2012). Imaging neuroinflammation after stroke: current status of cellular and molecular MRI strategies. *Cerebrovasc. Dis.* 33, 392–402. doi: 10.1159/000336116

del Zoppo, G., Ginis, I., Hallenbeck, J. M., and Iadecola, C. (2000). Inflammation and stroke: putative role for cytokines, adhesion molecules and iNOS in brain response to ischemia. *Brain Pathol.* 10, 95–112. doi: 10.1111/j.1750-3639.2000.tb00247.x

Dénes, A., Ferenczi, S., Halász, J., Környei, Z., and Kovács, K. J. (2008). Role of CX3CR1 (fractalkine receptor) in brain damage and inflammation induced by focal cerebral ischemia in mouse. *J. Cereb. Blood Flow Metab.* 28, 1707–1721. doi: 10.1038/jcbfm.2008.64

Dénes, A., Thornton, P., Rothwell, N. J., and Allan, S. M. (2010). Inflammation and brain injury: acute cerebral ischaemia, peripheral and central inflammation. *Brain Behav. Immun.* 24, 708–723. doi: 10.1016/j.bbi.2009.09.010

Denker, S. P., Ji, S., Dingman, A., Lee, S. Y., Derugin, N., Wendland, M. F., et al. (2007). Macrophages are comprised of resident brain microglia not infiltrating peripheral monocytes acutely after neonatal stroke. *J. Neurochem.* 100, 893–904. doi: 10.1111/j.1471-4159.2006.04162.x

Desestret, V., Brisset, J.-C., Moucharrafie, S., Devillard, E., Nataf, S., Honnorat, J., et al. (2009). Early-stage investigations of ultrasmall superparamagnetic iron oxide-induced signal change after permanent middle cerebral artery occlusion in mice. *Stroke* 40, 1834–1841. doi: 10.1161/STROKEAHA.108.531269

Desestret, V., Riou, A., Chauveau, F., Cho, T.-H., Devillard, E., Marinescu, M., et al. (2013). In vitro and in vivo models of cerebral ischemia show discrepancy in therapeutic effects of M2 macrophages. *PLoS One* 8:e67063. doi: 10.1371/journal.pone.0067063

Dimitrijevic, O. B., Stamatovic, S. M., Keep, R. F., and Andjelkovic, A. V. (2007). Absence of the chemokine receptor CCR2 protects against cerebral ischemia/reperfusion injury in mice. *Stroke* 38, 1345–1353. doi: 10.1161/01.str.0000259709.16654.8f

Dirnagl, U. (2006). Bench to bedside: the quest for quality in experimental stroke research. *J. Cereb. Blood Flow Metab.* 26, 1465–1478. doi: 10.1038/sj.jcbfm.9600298

Dirnagl, U., Iadecola, C., and Moskowitz, M. A. (1999). Pathobiology of ischaemic stroke: an integrated view. *Trends Neurosci.* 22, 391–397. doi: 10.1016/s0166-2236(99)01401-0

Durafourt, B. A., Moore, C. S., Zammit, D. A., Johnson, T. A., Zaguia, F., Guiot, M.-C., et al. (2012). Comparison of polarization properties of human adult microglia and blood-derived macrophages. *Glia* 60, 717–727. doi: 10.1002/glia.22298.p02.102

Elmore, M. R. P., Najafi, A. R., Koike, M. A., Dagher, N. N., Spangenberg, E. E., Rice, R. A., et al. (2014). Colony-stimulating factor 1 receptor signaling is necessary for microglia viability, unmasking a microglia progenitor cell in the adult brain. *Neuron* 82, 380–397. doi: 10.1016/j.neuron.2014.02.040

Emerich, D. F., Dean, R. L., and Bartus, R. T. (2002). The role of leukocytes following cerebral ischemia: pathogenic variable or bystander reaction to emerging infarct? *Exp. Neurol.* 173, 168–181. doi: 10.1006/exnr.2001.7835

Emsley, H. C. A., Smith, C. J., Georgiou, R. F., Vail, A., Hopkins, S. J., Rothwell, N. J., et al. (2005). A randomised phase II study of interleukin-1 receptor antagonist in acute stroke patients. *J. Neurol. Neurosurg. Psychiatry.* 76, 1366–1372. doi: 10.1136/jnnp.2004.054882

Endres, M., Engelhardt, B., Koistinaho, J., Lindvall, O., Meairs, S., Mohr, J. P., et al. (2008). Improving outcome after stroke: overcoming the translational roadblock. *Cerebrovasc. Dis.* 25, 268–278. doi: 10.1159/000118039

England, T. J., Gibson, C. L., and Bath, P. M. W. (2009). Granulocyte-colony stimulating factor in experimental stroke and its effects on infarct size and functional outcome: a systematic review. *Brain Res. Rev.* 62, 71–82. doi: 10.1016/j.brainresrev.2009.09.002

Enlimomab Acute Stroke Trial Investigators. (2001). Use of anti-ICAM-1 therapy in ischemic stroke results of the Enlimomab Acute Stroke Trial. *Neurology* 57, 1428–1434. doi: 10.1212/wnl.57.8.1428

Enzmann, G., Mysiorek, C., Gorina, R., Cheng, Y.-J., Ghavampour, S., Hannocks, M.-J., et al. (2013). The neurovascular unit as a selective barrier to polymorphonuclear granulocyte (PMN) infiltration into the brain after ischemic injury. *Acta Neuropathol.* 125, 395–412. doi: 10.1007/s00401-012-1076-3

Faustino, J. V., Wang, X., Johnson, C. E., Klibanov, A., Derugin, N., Wendland, M. F., et al. (2011). Microglial cells contribute to endogenous brain defenses after acute neonatal focal stroke. *J. Neurosci.* 31, 12992–13001. doi: 10.1523/JNEUROSCI.2102-11.2011

Fonarow, G. C., Smith, E. E., Saver, J. L., Reeves, M. J., Bhatt, D. L., Grau-Sepulveda, M. V., et al. (2011). Timeliness of tissue-type plasminogen activator therapy in acute ischemic stroke: patient characteristics, hospital factors and outcomes associated with door-to-needle times within 60 minutes. *Circulation* 123, 750–758. doi: 10.1161/CIRCULATIONAHA.110.974675

Ford, A. L., Goodsall, A. L., Hickey, W. F., and Sedgwick, J. D. (1995). Normal adult ramified microglia separated from other central nervous system macrophages by flow cytometric sorting. Phenotypic differences defined and direct ex vivo antigen presentation to myelin basic protein-reactive CD4+ T cells compared. *J. Immunol.* 154, 4309–4321.

Frame, J. M., McGrath, K. E., and Palis, J. (2013). Erythro-myeloid progenitors: "definitive" hematopoiesis in the conceptus prior to the emergence of hematopoietic stem cells. *Blood Cells Mol. Dis.* 51, 220–225. doi: 10.1016/j.bcmd.2013.09.006

Frankenberger, M., Sternsdorf, T., Pechumer, H., Pforte, A., and Ziegler-Heitbrock, H. W. (1996). Differential cytokine expression in human blood monocyte subpopulations: a polymerase chain reaction analysis. *Blood* 87, 373–377.

Fridlender, Z. G., Sun, J., Kim, S., Kapoor, V., Cheng, G., Ling, L., et al. (2009). Polarization of tumor-associated neutrophil phenotype by TGF-beta: "N1" versus "N2" TAN. *Cancer Cell* 16, 183–194. doi: 10.1016/j.ccr.2009.06.017

Fumagalli, S., Perego, C., Ortolano, F., and de Simoni, M.-G. (2013). CX3CR1 deficiency induces an early protective inflammatory environment in ischemic mice. *Glia* 61, 827–842. doi: 10.1002/glia.22474

García-Bonilla, L., Benakis, C., Moore, J., Iadecola, C., and Anrather, J. (2014a). Immune mechanisms in cerebral ischemic tolerance. *Front. Neurosci.* 8:44. doi: 10.3389/fnins.2014.00044

García-Bonilla, L., Moore, J. M., Racchumi, G., Zhou, P., Butler, J. M., Iadecola, C., et al. (2014b). Inducible nitric oxide synthase in neutrophils and endothelium contributes to ischemic brain injury in mice. *J. Immunol.* 193, 2531–2537. doi: 10.4049/jimmunol.1400918

Geissmann, F., Auffray, C., Palframan, R., Wirrig, C., Ciocca, A., Campisi, L., et al. (2008). Blood monocytes: distinct subsets, how they relate to dendritic cells and their possible roles in the regulation of T-cell responses. *Immunol. Cell Biol.* 86, 398–408. doi: 10.1038/icb.2008.19

Geissmann, F., Jung, S., and Littman, D. R. (2003). Blood monocytes consist of two principal subsets with distinct migratory properties. *Immunity* 19, 71–82. doi: 10.1016/s1074-7613(03)00174-2

Gelderblom, M., Leypoldt, F., Steinbach, K., Behrens, D., Choe, C.-U., Siler, D. A., et al. (2009). Temporal and spatial dynamics of cerebral immune cell accumulation in stroke. *Stroke* 40, 1849–1857. doi: 10.1161/STROKEAHA.108.534503

Gelderblom, M., Weymar, A., Bernreuther, C., Velden, J., Arunachalam, P., Steinbach, K., et al. (2012). Neutralization of the IL-17 axis diminishes neutrophil invasion and protects from ischemic stroke. *Blood* 120, 3793–3802. doi: 10.1182/blood-2012-02-412726

Gerhard, A., Schwarz, J., Myers, R., Wise, R., and Banati, R. B. (2005). Evolution of microglial activation in patients after ischemic stroke: a [11C](R)-PK11195 PET study. *Neuroimage* 24, 591–595. doi: 10.1016/j.neuroimage.2004.09.034

Ginhoux, F., Greter, M., Leboeuf, M., Nandi, S., See, P., Gokhan, S., et al. (2010). Fate mapping analysis reveals that adult microglia derive from primitive macrophages. *Science* 330, 841–845. doi: 10.1126/science.1194637

Ginhoux, F., and Jung, S. (2014). Monocytes and macrophages: developmental pathways and tissue homeostasis. *Nat. Rev. Immunol.* 14, 392–404. doi: 10.1038/nri3671

Ginhoux, F., Lim, S., Hoeffel, G., Low, D., and Huber, T. (2013). Origin and differentiation of microglia. *Front. Cell. Neurosci.* 7:45. doi: 10.3389/fncel.2013.00045

Girard, S., Brough, D., Lopez-Castejon, G., Giles, J., Rothwell, N. J., and Allan, S. M. (2013). Microglia and macrophages differentially modulate cell death after brain injury caused by oxygen-glucose deprivation in organotypic brain slices. *Glia* 61, 813–824. doi: 10.1002/glia.22478

Gliem, M., Mausberg, A. K., Lee, J.-I., Simiantonakis, I., Van Rooijen, N., Hartung, H.-P., et al. (2012). Macrophages prevent hemorrhagic infarct transformation in murine stroke models. *Ann. Neurol.* 71, 743–752. doi: 10.1002/ana.23529

Gordon, S., and Taylor, P. R. (2005). Monocyte and macrophage heterogeneity. *Nat. Rev. Immunol.* 5, 953–964. doi: 10.1038/nri1733

Hacke, W., Kaste, M., Bluhmki, E., Brozman, M., Dávalos, A., Guidetti, D., et al. (2008). Thrombolysis with alteplase 3 to 4.5 hours after acute ischemic stroke. *N. Engl. J. Med.* 359, 1317–1329. doi: 10.1056/NEJMoa0804656

Hanisch, U.-K., and Kettenmann, H. (2007). Microglia: active sensor and versatile effector cells in the normal and pathologic brain. *Nat. Neurosci.* 10, 1387–1394. doi: 10.1038/nn1997

Hanna, R. N., Carlin, L. M., Hubbeling, H. G., Nackiewicz, D., Green, A. M., Punt, J. A., et al. (2011). The transcription factor NR4A1 (Nur77) controls bone marrow differentiation and the survival of Ly6C- monocytes. *Nat. Immunol.* 12, 778–785. doi: 10.1038/ni.2063

Hao, N.-B., Lü, M.-H., Fan, Y.-H., Cao, Y.-L., Zhang, Z.-R., and Yang, S.-M. (2012). Macrophages in tumor microenvironments and the progression of tumors. *Clin. Dev. Immunol.* 2012, 1–11. doi: 10.1155/2012/948098

Hellwig, S., Heinrich, A., and Biber, K. (2013). The brain's best friend: microglial neurotoxicity revisited. *Front. Cell. Neurosci.* 7:71. doi: 10.3389/fncel.2013.00071

Hettinger, J., Richards, D. M., Hansson, J., Barra, M. M., Joschko, A.-C., Krijgsveld, J., et al. (2013). Origin of monocytes and macrophages in a committed progenitor. *Nat. Immunol.* 14, 821–830. doi: 10.1038/ni.2638

Hu, X., Li, P., Guo, Y., Wang, H., Leak, R. K., Chen, S., et al. (2012). Microglia/macrophage polarization dynamics reveal novel mechanism of injury expansion after focal cerebral ischemia. *Stroke* 43, 3063–3070. doi: 10.1161/STROKEAHA.112.659656

Hughes, P. M., Allegrini, P. R., Rudin, M., Perry, V. H., Mir, A. K., and Wiessner, C. (2002). Monocyte chemoattractant protein-1 deficiency is protective in a murine stroke model. *J. Cereb. Blood Flow Metab.* 22, 308–317. doi: 10.1097/00004647-200203000-00008

Iadecola, C., and Alexander, M. (2001). Cerebral ischemia and inflammation. *Curr. Opin. Neurol.* 14, 89–94. doi: 10.1097/00019052-200102000-00014

Iadecola, C., and Anrather, J. (2011). The immunology of stroke: from mechanisms to translation. *Nat. Med.* 17, 796–808. doi: 10.1038/nm.2399

Iadecola, C., Zhang, F., Casey, R., Nagayama, M., and Ross, M. E. (1997). Delayed reduction of ischemic brain injury and neurological deficits in mice lacking the inducible nitric oxide synthase gene. *J. Neurosci.* 17, 9157–9164.

Imai, T., Hieshima, K., Haskell, C., Baba, M., Nagira, M., Nishimura, M., et al. (1997). Identification and molecular characterization of fractalkine receptor CX3CR1, which mediates both leukocyte migration and adhesion. *Cell* 91, 521–530. doi: 10.1016/s0092-8674(00)80438-9

Ishikawa, M., Cooper, D., Arumugam, T. V., Zhang, J. H., Nanda, A., and Granger, D. N. (2004). Platelet-leukocyte-endothelial cell interactions after middle cerebral artery occlusion and reperfusion. *J. Cereb. Blood Flow Metab.* 24, 907–915. doi: 10.1097/01.wcb.0000132690.96836.7f

Ito, D., Tanaka, K., Suzuki, S., Dembo, T., and Fukuuchi, Y. (2001). Enhanced expression of Iba1, ionized calcium-binding adapter molecule 1, after transient focal cerebral ischemia in rat brain. *Stroke* 32, 1208–1215. doi: 10.1161/01.str.32.5.1208

Jackman, K., and Iadecola, C. (2014). Neurovascular regulation in the ischemic brain. *Antioxid. Redox Signal.* doi: 10.1089/ars.2013.5669. [Epub ahead of print].

Jin, G., Tsuji, K., Xing, C., Yang, Y.-G., Wang, X., and Lo, E. H. (2009). CD47 gene knockout protects against transient focal cerebral ischemia in mice. *Exp. Neurol.* 217, 165–170. doi: 10.1016/j.expneurol.2009.02.004

Jordán, J., Segura, T., Brea, D., Galindo, M. F., and Castillo, J. (2008). Inflammation as therapeutic objective in stroke. *Curr. Pharm. Des.* 14, 3549–3564. doi: 10.2174/138161208786848766

Kamel, H., and Iadecola, C. (2012). Brain-immune interactions and ischemic stroke: clinical implications. *Arch. Neurol.* 69, 576–581. doi: 10.1001/archneurol.2011.3590

Kierdorf, K., Erny, D., Goldmann, T., Sander, V., Schulz, C., Perdiguero, E. G., et al. (2013a). Microglia emerge from erythromyeloid precursors via Pu.1- and Irf8-dependent pathways. *Nat. Neurosci.* 16, 273–280. doi: 10.1038/nn.3318

Kierdorf, K., Katzmarski, N., Haas, C. A., and Prinz, M. (2013b). Bone marrow cell recruitment to the brain in the absence of irradiation or parabiosis bias. *PLoS One* 8:e58544. doi: 10.1371/journal.pone.0058544

Kim, E., Yang, J., Beltran, C. D., and Cho, S. (2014). Role of spleen-derived monocytes/macrophages in acute ischemic brain injury. *J. Cereb. Blood Flow Metab.* 34, 1411–1419. doi: 10.1038/jcbfm.2014.101

Kleinschnitz, C., Bendszus, M., Frank, M., Solymosi, L., Toyka, K. V., and Stoll, G. (2003). In vivo monitoring of macrophage infiltration in experimental ischemic brain lesions by magnetic resonance imaging. *J. Cereb. Blood Flow Metab.* 23, 1356–1361. doi: 10.1097/01.wcb.0000090505.76664.db

Kleinschnitz, C., Kraft, P., Dreykluft, A., Hagedorn, I., Göbel, K., Schuhmann, M. K., et al. (2013). Regulatory T cells are strong promoters of acute ischemic stroke in mice by inducing dysfunction of the cerebral microvasculature. *Blood* 121, 679–691. doi: 10.1182/blood-2012-04-426734

Komine-Kobayashi, M., Zhang, N., Liu, M., Tanaka, R., Hara, H., Osaka, A., et al. (2006). Neuroprotective effect of recombinant human granulocyte colony-stimulating factor in transient focal ischemia of mice. *J. Cereb. Blood Flow Metab.* 26, 402–413. doi: 10.1038/sj.jcbfm.9600195

Kong, L. L., Wang, Z. Y., Han, N., Zhuang, X. M., Wang, Z. Z., Li, H., et al. (2014). Neutralization of chemokine-like factor 1, a novel C-C chemokine, protects against focal cerebral ischemia by inhibiting neutrophil infiltration via MAPK pathways in rats. *J. Neuroinflammation* 11:112. doi: 10.1186/1742-2094-11-112

Krams, M., Lees, K. R., Hacke, W., Grieve, A. P., Orgogozo, J.-M., Ford, G. A., et al. (2003). Acute Stroke Therapy by Inhibition of Neutrophils (ASTIN): an adaptive dose-response study of UK-279,276 in acute ischemic stroke. *Stroke* 34, 2543–2548. doi: 10.1161/01.str.0000092527.33910.89

Li, T., Pang, S., Yu, Y., Wu, X., Guo, J., and Zhang, S. (2013). Proliferation of parenchymal microglia is the main source of microgliosis after ischaemic stroke. *Brain* 136, 3578–3588. doi: 10.1093/brain/awt287

Liesz, A., Suri-Payer, E., Veltkamp, C., Doerr, H., Sommer, C., Rivest, S., et al. (2009). Regulatory T cells are key cerebroprotective immunomodulators in acute experimental stroke. *Nat. Med.* 15, 192–199. doi: 10.1038/nm.1927

Limatola, C., and Ransohoff, R. M. (2014). Modulating neurotoxicity through CX3CL1/CX3CR1 signaling. *Front. Cell. Neurosci.* 8:229. doi: 10.3389/fncel.2014.00229

Lin, S. L., Castaño, A. P., Nowlin, B. T., Lupher, M. L., and Duffield, J. S. (2009). Bone marrow Ly6Chigh monocytes are selectively recruited to injured kidney and differentiate into functionally distinct populations. *J. Immunol.* 183, 6733–6743. doi: 10.4049/jimmunol.0901473

Liu, C., Li, Y., Yu, J., Feng, L., Hou, S., Liu, Y., et al. (2013). Targeting the shift from M1 to M2 macrophages in experimental autoimmune encephalomyelitis mice treated with fasudil. *PLoS One* 8:e54841. doi: 10.1371/journal.pone.0054841

Liu, Y., Merlin, D., Burst, S. L., Pochet, M., Madara, J. L., and Parkos, C. A. (2001). The role of CD47 in neutrophil transmigration. Increased rate of migration correlates with increased cell surface expression of CD47. *J. Biol. Chem.* 276, 40156–40166. doi: 10.1074/jbc.m104138200

London, A., Cohen, M., and Schwartz, M. (2013). Microglia and monocyte-derived macrophages: functionally distinct populations that act in concert in CNS plasticity and repair. *Front. Cell. Neurosci.* 7:34. doi: 10.3389/fncel.2013.00034

Losy, J., and Zaremba, J. (2001). Monocyte chemoattractant protein-1 is increased in the cerebrospinal fluid of patients with ischemic stroke. *Stroke* 32, 2695–2696. doi: 10.1161/hs1101.097380

Macrez, R., Ali, C., Toutirais, O., Le Mauff, B., Defer, G., Dirnagl, U., et al. (2011). Stroke and the immune system: from pathophysiology to new therapeutic strategies. *Lancet Neurol.* 10, 471–480. doi: 10.1016/s1474-4422(11)70066-7

Mantovani, A. (2009). The yin-yang of tumor-associated neutrophils. *Cancer Cell* 16, 173–174. doi: 10.1016/j.ccr.2009.08.014

Mantovani, A., Sica, A., Sozzani, S., Allavena, P., Vecchi, A., and Locati, M. (2004). The chemokine system in diverse forms of macrophage activation and polarization. *Trends Immunol.* 25, 677–686. doi: 10.1016/j.it.2004.09.015

Matsuo, Y., Onodera, H., Shiga, Y., Nakamura, M., Ninomiya, M., Kihara, T., et al. (1994). Correlation between myeloperoxidase-quantified neutrophil accumulation and ischemic brain injury in the rat. Effects of neutrophil depletion. *Stroke* 25, 1469–1475. doi: 10.1161/01.str.25.7.1469

Meisel, C., Prass, K., Braun, J., Victorov, I., Wolf, T., Megow, D., et al. (2004). Preventive antibacterial treatment improves the general medical and neurological outcome in a mouse model of stroke. *Stroke* 35, 2–6. doi: 10.1161/01.str.0000109041.89959.4c

Meisel, C., Schwab, J. M., Prass, K., Meisel, A., and Dirnagl, U. (2005). Central nervous system injury-induced immune deficiency syndrome. *Nat. Rev. Neurosci.* 6, 775–786. doi: 10.1038/nrn1765

Mena, H., Cadavid, D., and Rushing, E. J. (2004). Human cerebral infarct: a proposed histopathologic classification based on 137 cases. *Acta Neuropathol.* 108, 524–530. doi: 10.1007/s00401-004-0918-z

Merino, A., Buendia, P., Martin-Malo, A., Aljama, P., Ramirez, R., and Carracedo, J. (2011). Senescent CD14+CD16+ monocytes exhibit proinflammatory and proatherosclerotic activity. *J. Immunol.* 186, 1809–1815. doi: 10.4049/jimmunol.1001866

Michaud, J.-P., Pimentel-Coelho, P. M., Tremblay, Y., and Rivest, S. (2014). The impact of Ly6Clow monocytes after cerebral hypoxia-ischemia in adult mice. *J. Cereb. Blood Flow Metab.* 34, e1–e9. doi: 10.1038/jcbfm.2014.80

Michelucci, A., Heurtaux, T., Grandbarbe, L., Morga, E., and Heuschling, P. (2009). Characterization of the microglial phenotype under specific pro-inflammatory and anti-inflammatory conditions: effects of oligomeric and fibrillar amyloid-beta. *J. Neuroimmunol.* 210, 3–12. doi: 10.1016/j.jneuroim.2009.02.003

Mildner, A., Schlevogt, B., Kierdorf, K., Böttcher, C., Erny, D., Kummer, M. P., et al. (2011). Distinct and non-redundant roles of microglia and myeloid subsets in mouse models of Alzheimer's disease. *J. Neurosci.* 31, 11159–11171. doi: 10.1523/JNEUROSCI.6209-10.2011

Mildner, A., Schmidt, H., Nitsche, M., Merkler, D., Hanisch, U.-K., Mack, M., et al. (2007). Microglia in the adult brain arise from Ly-6ChiCCR2+ monocytes only under defined host conditions. *Nat. Neurosci.* 10, 1544–1553. doi: 10.1038/nn2015

Mills, C. D., Kincaid, K., Alt, J. M., Heilman, M. J., and Hill, A. M. (2000). M-1/M-2 macrophages and the Th1/Th2 paradigm. *J. Immunol.* 164, 6166–6173. doi: 10.4049/jimmunol.164.12.6166

Morrison, H. W., and Filosa, J. A. (2013). A quantitative spatiotemporal analysis of microglia morphology during ischemic stroke and reperfusion. *J. Neuroinflammation* 10:4. doi: 10.1186/1742-2094-10-4

Moskowitz, M. A., Lo, E. H., and Iadecola, C. (2010). The science of stroke: mechanisms in search of treatments. *Neuron* 67, 181–198. doi: 10.1016/j.neuron.2010.07.002

Mosser, D. M., and Edwards, J. P. (2008). Exploring the full spectrum of macrophage activation. *Nat. Rev. Immunol.* 8, 958–969. doi: 10.1038/nri2448

Murray, P. J., Allen, J. E., Biswas, S. K., Fisher, E. A., Gilroy, D. W., Goerdt, S., et al. (2014). Macrophage activation and polarization: nomenclature and experimental guidelines. *Immunity* 41, 14–20. doi: 10.1016/j.immuni.2014.06.008

Nahrendorf, M., Swirski, F. K., Aikawa, E., Stangenberg, L., Wurdinger, T., Figueiredo, J.-L., et al. (2007). The healing myocardium sequentially mobilizes two monocyte subsets with divergent and complementary functions. *J. Exp. Med.* 204, 3037–3047. doi: 10.1084/jem.20070885

Neher, J. J., Emmrich, J. V., Fricker, M., Mander, P. K., Théry, C., and Brown, G. C. (2013). Phagocytosis executes delayed neuronal death after focal brain ischemia. *Proc. Natl. Acad. Sci. U S A* 110, E4098–E4107. doi: 10.1073/pnas.1308679110

Neher, J. J., Neniskyte, U., and Brown, G. C. (2012). Primary phagocytosis of neurons by inflamed microglia: potential roles in neurodegeneration. *Front. Pharmacol.* 3:27. doi: 10.3389/fphar.2012.00027

Neumann, H., Kotter, M. R., and Franklin, R. J. M. (2009). Debris clearance by microglia: an essential link between degeneration and regeneration. *Brain* 132, 288–295. doi: 10.1093/brain/awn109

Nimmerjahn, A., Kirchhoff, F., and Helmchen, F. (2005). Resting microglial cells are highly dynamic surveillants of brain parenchyma in vivo. *Science* 308, 1314–1318. doi: 10.1126/science.1110647

O'Collins, V. E., Macleod, M. R., Donnan, G. A., Horky, L. L., van der Worp, B. H., and Howells, D. W. (2006). 1,026 experimental treatments in acute stroke. *Ann. Neurol.* 59, 467–477. doi: 10.1002/ana.20741

Offner, H., Subramanian, S., Parker, S. M., Afentoulis, M. E., Vandenbark, A. A., and Hurn, P. D. (2006b). Experimental stroke induces massive, rapid activation of the peripheral immune system. *J. Cereb. Blood Flow Metab.* 26, 654–665. doi: 10.1038/sj.jcbfm.9600217

Offner, H., Subramanian, S., Parker, S. M., Wang, C., Afentoulis, M. E., Lewis, A., et al. (2006a). Splenic atrophy in experimental stroke is accompanied by increased regulatory T cells and circulating macrophages. *J. Immunol.* 176, 6523–6531. doi: 10.4049/jimmunol.176.11.6523

Ostrowski, R. P., Schulte, R. W., Nie, Y., Ling, T., Lee, T., Manaenko, A., et al. (2012). Acute splenic irradiation reduces brain injury in the rat focal ischemic stroke model. *Transl. Stroke Res.* 3, 473–481. doi: 10.1007/s12975-012-0206-5

Oude Engberink, R. D., Blezer, E. L., Hoff, E. I., van der Pol, S. M., van der Toorn, A., Dijkhuizen, R. M., et al. (2008). MRI of monocyte infiltration in an animal model of neuroinflammation using SPIO-labeled monocytes or free USPIO. *J. Cereb. Blood Flow Metab.* 28, 841–851. doi: 10.1038/sj.jcbfm.9600580

Panés, J., Perry, M. A., Anderson, D. C., Manning, A., Leone, B., Cepinskas, G., et al. (1995). Regional differences in constitutive and induced ICAM-1 expression in vivo. *Am. J. Physiol.* 269, H1955–H1964.

Panés, J., Perry, M., and Granger, D. N. (1999). Leukocyte-endothelial cell adhesion: avenues for therapeutic intervention. *Br. J. Pharmacol.* 126, 537–550. doi: 10.1038/sj.bjp.0702328

Patel, A. R., Ritzel, R., McCullough, L. D., and Liu, F. (2013). Microglia and ischemic stroke: a double-edged sword. *Int. J. Physiol. Pathophysiol. Pharmacol.* 5, 73–90.

Perego, C., Fumagalli, S., and de Simoni, M.-G. (2011). Temporal pattern of expression and colocalization of microglia/macrophage phenotype markers following brain ischemic injury in mice. *J. Neuroinflammation* 8:174. doi: 10.1186/1742-2094-8-174

Prinz, M., and Mildner, A. (2011). Microglia in the CNS: immigrants from another world. *Glia* 59, 177–187. doi: 10.1002/glia.21104

Prinz, M., and Priller, J. (2010). Tickets to the brain: role of CCR2 and CX3CR1 in myeloid cell entry in the CNS. *J. Neuroimmunol.* 224, 80–84. doi: 10.1016/j.jneuroim.2010.05.015

Prinz, M., and Priller, J. (2014). Microglia and brain macrophages in the molecular age: from origin to neuropsychiatric disease. *Nat. Rev. Neurosci.* 15, 300–312. doi: 10.1038/nrn3722

Ransohoff, R. M. (2011). Microglia and monocytes: 'tis plain the twain meet in the brain. *Nat. Neurosci.* 14, 1098–1100. doi: 10.1038/nn.2917

Rausch, M., Sauter, A., Fröhlich, J., Neubacher, U., Radü, E. W., and Rudin, M. (2001). Dynamic patterns of USPIO enhancement can be observed in macrophages after ischemic brain damage. *Magn. Reson. Med.* 46, 1018–1022. doi: 10.1002/mrm.1290.abs

Ringelstein, E. B., Thijs, V., Norrving, B., Chamorro, A., Aichner, F., Grond, M., et al. (2013). Granulocyte colony-stimulating factor in patients with acute ischemic stroke: results of the AX200 for Ischemic Stroke trial. *Stroke* 44, 2681–2687. doi: 10.1161/STROKEAHA.113.001531

Romanic, A. M., White, R. F., Arleth, A. J., Ohlstein, E. H., and Barone, F. C. (1998). Matrix metalloproteinase expression increases after cerebral focal ischemia in rats inhibition of matrix metalloproteinase-9 reduces infarct size. *Stroke* 29, 1020–1030. doi: 10.1161/01.str.29.5.1020

Saederup, N., Cardona, A. E., Croft, K., Mizutani, M., Cotleur, A. C., Tsou, C.-L., et al. (2010). Selective chemokine receptor usage by central nervous system myeloid cells in CCR2-red fluorescent protein knock-in mice. *PLoS One* 5:e13693. doi: 10.1371/journal.pone.0013693

Saleh, A., Schroeter, M., Jonkmanns, C., Hartung, H.-P., Mödder, U., and Jander, S. (2004). In vivo MRI of brain inflammation in human ischaemic stroke. *Brain* 127, 1670–1677. doi: 10.1093/brain/awh191

Saleh, A., Schroeter, M., Ringelstein, A., Hartung, H.-P., Siebler, M., Mödder, U., et al. (2007). Iron oxide particle-enhanced MRI suggests variability of brain inflammation at early stages after ischemic stroke. *Stroke* 38, 2733–2737. doi: 10.1161/strokeaha.107.481788

Schilling, M., Besselmann, M., Leonhard, C., Mueller, M., Ringelstein, E. B., and Kiefer, R. (2003). Microglial activation precedes and predominates over macrophage infiltration in transient focal cerebral ischemia: a study in green fluorescent protein transgenic bone marrow chimeric mice. *Exp. Neurol.* 183, 25–33. doi: 10.1016/s0014-4886(03)00082-7

Schilling, M., Besselmann, M., Müller, M., Strecker, J. K., Ringelstein, E. B., and Kiefer, R. (2005). Predominant phagocytic activity of resident microglia over hematogenous macrophages following transient focal cerebral ischemia: an investigation using green fluorescent protein transgenic bone marrow chimeric mice. *Exp. Neurol.* 196, 290–297. doi: 10.1016/j.expneurol.2005.08.004

Schilling, M., Strecker, J.-K., Ringelstein, E. B., Schäbitz, W.-R., and Kiefer, R. (2009). The role of CC chemokine receptor 2 on microglia activation and blood-borne cell recruitment after transient focal cerebral ischemia in mice. *Brain Res.* 1289, 79–84. doi: 10.1016/j.brainres.2009.06.054

Schulz, C., Gomez Perdiguero, E., Chorro, L., Szabo-Rogers, H., Cagnard, N., Kierdorf, K., et al. (2012). A lineage of myeloid cells independent of Myb and hematopoietic stem cells. *Science* 336, 86–90. doi: 10.1126/science.1219179

Serhan, C. N., and Savill, J. (2005). Resolution of inflammation: the beginning programs the end. *Nat. Immunol.* 6, 1191–1197. doi: 10.1038/ni1276

Shechter, R., Miller, O., Yovel, G., Rosenzweig, N., London, A., Ruckh, J., et al. (2013). Recruitment of beneficial M2 macrophages to injured spinal cord is orchestrated by remote brain choroid plexus. *Immunity* 38, 555–569. doi: 10.1016/j.immuni.2013.02.012

Shichita, T., Sakaguchi, R., Suzuki, M., and Yoshimura, A. (2012). Post-ischemic inflammation in the brain. *Front. Immunol.* 3:132. doi: 10.3389/fimmu.2012.00132

Shimakura, A., Kamanaka, Y., Ikeda, Y., Kondo, K., Suzuki, Y., and Umemura, K. (2000). Neutrophil elastase inhibition reduces cerebral ischemic damage in the middle cerebral artery occlusion. *Brain Res.* 858, 55–60. doi: 10.1016/s0006-8993(99)02431-2

Shuaib, A., Lees, K. R., Lyden, P., Grotta, J., Dávalos, A., Davis, S. M., et al. (2007). NXY-059 for the treatment of acute ischemic stroke. *N. Engl. J. Med.* 357, 562–571. doi: 10.1056/NEJMoa070240

Sieber, M. W., Jaenisch, N., Brehm, M., Guenther, M., Linnartz-Gerlach, B., Neumann, H., et al. (2013). Attenuated inflammatory response in triggering receptor expressed on myeloid cells 2 (TREM2) knock-out mice following stroke. *PLoS One* 8:e52982. doi: 10.1371/journal.pone.0052982

Skrzeczyńska-Moncznik, J., Bzowska, M., Loseke, S., Grage-Griebenow, E., Zembala, M., and Pryjma, J. (2008). Peripheral blood CD14highCD16+ monocytes are main producers of IL-10. *Scand. J. Immunol.* 67, 152–159. doi: 10.1111/j.1365-3083.2007.02051.x

Smith, C. J., Lawrence, C. B., Rodriguez-Grande, B., Kovács, K. J., Pradillo, J. M., and Dénes, A. (2013). The immune system in stroke: clinical challenges and their translation to experimental research. *J. Neuroimmune Pharmacol.* 8, 867–887. doi: 10.1007/s11481-013-9469-1

Solomon, J. N., Lewis, C.-A. B., Ajami, B., Corbel, S. Y., Rossi, F. M. V., and Krieger, C. (2006). Origin and distribution of bone marrow-derived cells in the central nervous system in a mouse model of amyotrophic lateral sclerosis. *Glia* 53, 744–753. doi: 10.1002/glia.20331

Soriano, S. G., Amaravadi, L. S., Wang, Y. F., Zhou, H., Yu, G. X., Tonra, J. R., et al. (2002). Mice deficient in fractalkine are less susceptible to cerebral ischemia-reperfusion injury. *J. Neuroimmunol.* 125, 59–65. doi: 10.1016/s0165-5728(02)00033-4

Soriano, S. G., Wang, Y. F., Wagner, D. D., and Frenette, P. S. (1999). P- and E-selectin-deficient mice are susceptible to cerebral ischemia-reperfusion injury. *Brain Res.* 835, 360–364. doi: 10.1016/s0006-8993(99)01637-6

Stephenson, D. T., Schober, D. A., Smalstig, E. B., Mincy, R. E., Gehlert, D. R., and Clemens, J. A. (1995). Peripheral benzodiazepine receptors are colocalized with activated microglia following transient global forebrain ischemia in the rat. *J. Neurosci.* 15, 5263–5274.

Stevens, S. L., Bao, J., Hollis, J., Lessov, N. S., Clark, W. M., and Stenzel-Poore, M. P. (2002). The use of flow cytometry to evaluate temporal changes in inflammatory cells following focal cerebral ischemia in mice. *Brain Res.* 932, 110–119. doi: 10.1016/s0006-8993(02)02292-8

Stowe, A. M., Adair-Kirk, T. L., Gonzales, E. R., Perez, R. S., Shah, A. R., Park, T. S., et al. (2009). Neutrophil elastase and neurovascular injury following focal stroke and reperfusion. *Neurobiol. Dis.* 35, 82–90. doi: 10.1016/j.nbd.2009.04.006

Stroh, A., Zimmer, C., Werner, N., Gertz, K., Weir, K., Kronenberg, G., et al. (2006). Tracking of systemically administered mononuclear cells in the ischemic brain by high-field magnetic resonance imaging. *Neuroimage* 33, 886–897. doi: 10.1016/j.neuroimage.2006.07.009

Strydom, N., and Rankin, S. M. (2013). Regulation of circulating neutrophil numbers under homeostasis and in disease. *J. Innate Immun.* 5, 304–314. doi: 10.1159/000350282

Su, X., Johansen, M., Looney, M. R., Brown, E. J., and Matthay, M. A. (2008). CD47 deficiency protects mice from lipopolysaccharide-induced acute lung injury and Escherichia coli pneumonia. *J. Immunol.* 180, 6947–6953. doi: 10.4049/jimmunol.180.10.6947

Sugiyama, Y., Faraco, G., Iadecola, C., and Anrather, J. (2014). "Regional and phenotypic differences in hematogenous cells repopulating the brain after irradiation or chemotherapy-based myeloablative approaches for bone marrow transplantation," in *Society for Neuroscience Annual Meeting* (Washington, DC), Abstract.

Sunderkötter, C., Nikolic, T., Dillon, M. J., van Rooijen, N., Stehling, M., Drevets, D. A., et al. (2004). Subpopulations of mouse blood monocytes differ in maturation stage and inflammatory response. *J. Immunol.* 172, 4410–4417. doi: 10.4049/jimmunol.172.7.4410

Sunnemark, D., Eltayeb, S., Nilsson, M., Wallström, E., Lassmann, H., Olsson, T., et al. (2005). CX3CL1 (fractalkine) and CX3CR1 expression in myelin oligodendrocyte glycoprotein-induced experimental autoimmune encephalomyelitis: kinetics and cellular origin. *J. Neuroinflammation* 2:17. doi: 10.1186/1742-2094-2-17

Swirski, F. K., Libby, P., Aikawa, E., Alcaide, P., Luscinskas, F. W., Weissleder, R., et al. (2007). Ly-6Chi monocytes dominate hypercholesterolemia-associated monocytosis and give rise to macrophages in atheromata. *J. Clin. Invest.* 117, 195–205. doi: 10.1172/jci29950

Swirski, F. K., Nahrendorf, M., Etzrodt, M., Wildgruber, M., Cortez-Retamozo, V., Panizzi, P., et al. (2009). Identification of splenic reservoir monocytes and their deployment to inflammatory sites. *Science* 325, 612–616. doi: 10.1126/science.1175202

Swirski, F. K., Wildgruber, M., Ueno, T., Figueiredo, J.-L., Panizzi, P., Iwamoto, Y., et al. (2010). Myeloperoxidase-rich Ly-6C+ myeloid cells infiltrate allografts and contribute to an imaging signature of organ rejection in mice. *J. Clin. Invest.* 120, 2627–2634. doi: 10.1172/JCI42304

Takahashi, K., Prinz, M., Stagi, M., Chechneva, O., and Neumann, H. (2007). TREM2-transduced myeloid precursors mediate nervous tissue debris clearance and facilitate recovery in an animal model of multiple sclerosis. *PLoS Med.* 4:e124. doi: 10.1371/journal.pmed.0040124

Tanaka, R., Komine-Kobayashi, M., Mochizuki, H., Yamada, M., Furuya, T., Migita, M., et al. (2003). Migration of enhanced green fluorescent protein expressing bone marrow-derived microglia/macrophage into the mouse brain following permanent focal ischemia. *Neuroscience* 117, 531–539. doi: 10.1016/s0306-4522(02)00954-5

Tang, Z., Gan, Y., Liu, Q., Yin, J.-X., Liu, Q., Shi, J., et al. (2014). CX3CR1 deficiency suppresses activation and neurotoxicity of microglia/macrophage in experimental ischemic stroke. *J. Neuroinflammation* 11:26. doi: 10.1186/1742-2094-11-26

Taylor, R. A., and Sansing, L. H. (2013). Microglial responses after ischemic stroke and intracerebral hemorrhage. *Clin. Dev. Immunol.* 2013:746068. doi: 10.1155/2013/746068

Terry, R. L., Getts, D. R., Deffrasnes, C., van Vreden, C., Campbell, I. L., and King, N. J. C. (2012). Inflammatory monocytes and the pathogenesis of viral encephalitis. *J. Neuroinflammation* 9:270. doi: 10.1186/1742-2094-9-270

Thiel, A., and Heiss, W.-D. (2011). Imaging of microglia activation in stroke. *Stroke* 42, 507–512. doi: 10.1161/STROKEAHA.110.598821

Thornton, P., McColl, B. W., Greenhalgh, A., Dénes, A., Allan, S. M., and Rothwell, N. J. (2010). Platelet interleukin-1alpha drives cerebrovascular inflammation. *Blood* 115, 3632–3639. doi: 10.1182/blood-2009-11-252643

Tsou, C.-L., Peters, W., Si, Y., Slaymaker, S., Aslanian, A. M., Weisberg, S. P., et al. (2007). Critical roles for CCR2 and MCP-3 in monocyte mobilization from bone marrow and recruitment to inflammatory sites. *J. Clin. Invest.* 117, 902–909. doi: 10.1172/jci29919

Urra, X., Villamor, N., Amaro, S., Gómez-Choco, M., Obach, V., Oleaga, L., et al. (2009). Monocyte subtypes predict clinical course and prognosis in human stroke. *J. Cereb. Blood Flow Metab.* 29, 994–1002. doi: 10.1038/jcbfm.2009.25

von Vietinghoff, S., and Ley, K. (2008). Homeostatic regulation of blood neutrophil counts. *J. Immunol.* 181, 5183–5188. doi: 10.4049/jimmunol.181.8.5183

Wang, X. (2005). Investigational anti-inflammatory agents for the treatment of ischaemic brain injury. *Expert Opin. Investig. Drugs* 14, 393–409. doi: 10.1517/13543784.14.4.393

Weber, C., Belge, K. U., von Hundelshausen, P., Draude, G., Steppich, B., Mack, M., et al. (2000). Differential chemokine receptor expression and function in human monocyte subpopulations. *J. Leukoc. Biol.* 67, 699–704.

Weissleder, R., Nahrendorf, M., and Pittet, M. J. (2014). Imaging macrophages with nanoparticles. *Nat. Mater.* 13, 125–138. doi: 10.1038/nmat3780

Yang, J., Zhang, L., Yu, C., Yang, X.-F., and Wang, H. (2014). Monocyte and macrophage differentiation: circulation inflammatory monocyte as biomarker for inflammatory diseases. *Biomark. Res.* 2:1. doi: 10.1186/2050-7771-2-1

Yilmaz, G., and Granger, D. N. (2010). Leukocyte recruitment and ischemic brain injury. *Neuromolecular. Med.* 12, 193–204. doi: 10.1007/s12017-009-8074-1

Yipp, B. G., Petri, B., Salina, D., Jenne, C. N., Scott, B. N. V., Zbytnuik, L. D., et al. (2012). Infection-induced NETosis is a dynamic process involving neutrophil multitasking in vivo. *Nat. Med.* 18, 1386–1393. doi: 10.1038/nm.2847

Zhou, W., Liesz, A., Bauer, H., Sommer, C., Lahrmann, B., Valous, N., et al. (2013). Postischemic brain infiltration of leukocyte subpopulations differs among murine permanent and transient focal cerebral ischemia models. *Brain Pathol.* 23, 34–44. doi: 10.1111/j.1750-3639.2012.00614.x

Ziegler-Heitbrock, H. W. (1996). Heterogeneity of human blood monocytes: the CD14+CD16+ subpopulation. *Immunol. Today* 17, 424–428. doi: 10.1016/0167-5699(96)10029-3

Ziegler-Heitbrock, L. (2007). The CD14+ CD16+ blood monocytes: their role in infection and inflammation. *J. Leukoc. Biol.* 81, 584–592. doi: 10.1189/jlb.0806510

Ziegler-Heitbrock, L., Ancuta, P., Crowe, S., Dalod, M., Grau, V., Hart, D. N., et al. (2010). Nomenclature of monocytes and dendritic cells in blood. *Blood* 116, e74–e80. doi: 10.1182/blood-2010-02-258558

Zujovic, V., Benavides, J., Vigé, X., Carter, C., and Taupin, V. (2000). Fractalkine modulates TNF-α secretion and neurotoxicity induced by microglial activation. *Glia* 29, 305–315. doi: 10.1002/(sici)1098-1136(20000215)29:4<305::aid-glia2>3.3.co;2-m

7

Versatility of the complement system in neuroinflammation, neurodegeneration and brain homeostasis

Franca Orsini[1], Daiana De Blasio[1,2], Rosalia Zangari[1,3], Elisa R. Zanier[1] and Maria-Grazia De Simoni[1]*

[1] Department of Neuroscience, IRCCS – Istituto di Ricerche Farmacologiche Mario Negri, Milan, Italy
[2] Department of Experimental and Clinical Sciences, University of Chieti, Pescara, Italy
[3] Department of Anesthesia and Critical Care Medicine, Fondazione IRCCS Ca' Granda Ospedale Maggiore Policlinico, University of Milan, Milan, Italy

Correspondence:
Maria-Grazia De Simoni, Department of Neuroscience, IRCCS – Istituto di Ricerche Farmacologiche Mario Negri, Via G. La Masa 19, 20156 Milan, Italy
e-mail: desimoni@marionegri.it

The immune response after brain injury is highly complex and involves both local and systemic events at the cellular and molecular level. It is associated to a dramatic over-activation of enzyme systems, the expression of proinflammatory genes and the activation/recruitment of immune cells. The complement system represents a powerful component of the innate immunity and is highly involved in the inflammatory response. Complement components are synthesized predominantly by the liver and circulate in the bloodstream primed for activation. Moreover, brain cells can produce complement proteins and receptors. After acute brain injury, the rapid and uncontrolled activation of the complement leads to massive release of inflammatory anaphylatoxins, recruitment of cells to the injury site, phagocytosis and induction of blood brain barrier (BBB) damage. Brain endothelial cells are particularly susceptible to complement-mediated effects, since they are exposed to both circulating and locally synthesized complement proteins. Conversely, during neurodegenerative disorders, complement factors play distinct roles depending on the stage and degree of neuropathology. In addition to the deleterious role of the complement, increasing evidence suggest that it may also play a role in normal nervous system development (wiring the brain) and adulthood (either maintaining brain homeostasis or supporting regeneration after brain injury). This article represents a compendium of the current knowledge on the complement role in the brain, prompting a novel view that complement activation can result in either protective or detrimental effects in brain conditions that depend exquisitely on the nature, the timing and the degree of the stimuli that induce its activation. A deeper understanding of the acute, subacute and chronic consequences of complement activation is needed and may lead to new therapeutic strategies, including the ability of targeting selective step in the complement cascade.

Keywords: complement system, therapeutic targets, endothelium, stroke, traumatic brain injury, Alzheimer's disease, brain homeostasis

THE COMPLEMENT SYSTEM: A BACKGROUND

In 1891, Buchner et al. discovered and reported a heat labile factor able to kill bacteria in blood, naming it "alexin" (in Greek, means "to ward off") (Ehrlich and Morgenroth, 1899; Buchner, 1981; Nesargikar et al., 2012). Bordet subsequently demonstrated that immune lysis requires the presence of two factors: a heat-labile lytic factor similar to "alexin" and a heat-stable factor, which he termed "sensitizer" (now known to be the antibody) (Morgan, 1990; Nesargikar et al., 2012). In 1899, Paul Ehrlich refined this theory describing the requirement for a supplementary molecule, named "the complement" (which replaced the historical term "alexin") necessary to induce antibody-induced

Abbreviations: AD, Alzheimer's disease; ALS, amyotrophic lateral sclerosis; AP, alternative pathway; Aβ, Amyloid-β; BBB, blood brain barrier; C1-INH, C1 inhibitor; C3aR, C3a receptor; C5aR, C5a receptor (also known as CD88); CCI, cortical controlled impact; CL-11, collectin-11; CNS, central nervous system; CP, classical pathway; CRP, C-reactive protein; CSF, cerebrospinal fluid; CVF, cobra venom factor; DAMPs, damage-associated molecular patterns; dLGN, dorsal lateral geniculate nucleus; hAPP, human amyloid precursor protein; HUVECs, human umbilical vein endothelial cells; ICAM-1, intercellular adhesion molecule-1; LP, lectin pathway; MAC, membrane attack complex; MASPs, MBL-associated serine proteases; MBL, mannose binding lectin; MCP-1, monocyte chemotactic protein-1; NFL, neurofilament subunit protein; NGF, nerve growth factor; NPCs, neural stem and progenitor cells; PAMPs, pathogen-associated molecular patterns; PARs, protease activated receptors; PD, Parkinson's disease; RANTES, regulated on activation normal T cell expressed and secreted; RGCs, retinal ganglion cells; SAH, aneurysmal subarachnoid haemorrhage; SOD1, superoxide dismutase 1; SVZ, subventricular zone; TBI, traumatic brain injury; tMCAo, transient middle cerebral artery occlusion; TP, terminal pathway; VCAM-1, vascular cell adhesion protein-1; WT, wild type.

bacterial lysis. Over one hundred years later, the role of the complement system is known to extend well-beyond that of a supplementary molecule. This physiological system is now recognized as an extremely potent component of the defense cascade of innate immunity, able not only to scavenge pathogens and antigens but also to respond to endogenous so called danger signals. Numerous experimental and clinical studies have recently demonstrated the involvement of this system in different acute and chronic pathological conditions, highlighting the importance of complement as a crucial factor in the activation and control of the generalized immune response. In addition, beyond elimination of potentially toxic molecules, its contribution to diverse homeostatic processes, such as lipid metabolism, angiogenesis, tissue modeling and maintenance has been recently proposed.

The complement system consists of more than 30 fluid-phase and cell-associated proteins (Wagner and Frank, 2010), each with different functions including, but not limited to, initiator molecules, substrates, regulators, inhibitors and receptors for complement proteins. The activation of the complement system can be triggered by exogenous and/or endogenous danger signals (pathogen-associated molecular patterns—PAMPs and/or damage-associated molecular patterns—DAMPs respectively) through the classical (CP), lectin (LP) or alternative pathway (AP). These pathways are each activated by different types of danger signals but share the same cascade-like activation system consisting of a number of proteolytic reactions, during which an inactivated protein is cleaved into smaller and active peptide fragments (see **Figure 1**). Briefly, the CP is activated through the binding of C1q to antigen-antibody complexes or directly by specific molecules including β-amyloid, C reactive protein (CRP), DNA and/or apoptotic bodies. The LP is activated through different pattern recognition receptors, including, in humans, mannose binding lectin (MBL), ficolin-1, ficolin-2 and ficolin-3 and collectin-11 (CL-11). These lectin molecules bind to high-density arrays of mannose, fucose and N-acetylated sugars exposed by pathogens or by altered host cells. The activation of the AP is driven by the spontaneous hydrolysis of circulating C3 (tick-over process) into C3(H_2O) on cellular surfaces. In addition, another complement activation pathway, named the extrinsic pathway, that is driven by serine protease components of the coagulation system, has been described (Huber-Lang et al., 2006). Increasing evidence suggests an intimate but not yet fully disclosed interaction between the complement and coagulation cascades which is particularly relevant in cerebrovascular disease, in which the balance between coagulation and fibrinolysis may be clinically manipulated for therapeutic purposes. All these pathways, converging on the C5 convertase formation (see **Figure 1**), activate a common cascade (named the terminal pathway, TP) through the cleavage of C5 into C5a and C5b. The former, along with C3a (generated by up-stream cleavage of C3), functions as anaphylatoxins, inducing a potent inflammatory response and stimulating the recruitment of peripheral immune cells. The latter fragment (C5b) binds to the targeted cell, allowing the assembly of C6, C7, C8 and C9 into a pore called membrane attack complex (C5b-9 or MAC), that causes the direct cellular lysis. Another critical consequence of complement activation is that many of these cleavage products, such as C3b and C4b as well as C5b, work as opsonins to trigger an overactivation of the phagocytic response. In addition, complement components are able to orchestrate an immune reaction by communicating with multiple immune cells through different receptors, thereby leading to robust local and systemic inflammatory responses (Ricklin and Lambris, 2007).

The complement system is also endowed with highly sophisticated regulatory mechanisms that serve to finely tune its physiological function (Ricklin and Lambris, 2007). The complement regulatory molecules are classified as fluid-phase or membrane-bound regulators (**Table 1**). One of the most well-studied circulating complement regulators is C1 inhibitor (C1-INH), a serine-protease that acts to inactivate the C1q/C1r/C1s and the MBL/MASP-1/MASP-2 complex. At high concentrations, C1-INH may also inactivate C3b generated by the AP (Wagner and Frank, 2010) as well as molecules associated with the kinin, fibrinolytic and coagulation systems (e.g., factor XII and IX) (Ehrnthaller et al., 2011).

The complement system also comprises a wide array of specific receptors for complement proteins by which the system induces phagocytosis and triggers the inflammatory response via direct communication with immune cells (Ricklin et al., 2010). The most important complement receptors include: (1) C1q receptors (gC1qR, C1qRp and cC1qR) that have been associated with the phagocytic process; (2) the integrin receptors, including complement receptor 3 (CR3, also known as CD11b/CD18) and 4 (CR4, also known as CD11c-CD18) that bind to iC3b fragment (a complement product coming from a further cleavage of C3b) to further promote cellular phagocytosis, cytokine responses, leukocyte trafficking and synapse formation; (3) C3a (C3aR) and C5a (C5aR or CD88) receptors that trigger a sustained proinflammatory signaling. Overall the role of the complement receptors is still to be fully elucidated.

SOURCES AND COMPARTMENTS OF ACTIVATION

SOURCES IN HEALTH AND BRAIN INJURY

Complement proteins account for approximately 4% of total blood proteins. Physiologically, they monitor the blood and the cell surfaces and are constantly primed for activation when potential threats are detected. The liver represents the major source of complement components released into the systemic circulation, and hepatocytes are known to be capable of synthesizing the myriad classes of complement proteins (Morgan and Gasque, 1997; Brennan et al., 2012). Other cell types, such as fibroblasts, monocytes, epithelial and endothelial cells and, most notably, all brain cell populations, are programmed to produce selected complement factors. The adult brain, once considered immunologically privileged, is subjected to considerable immune surveillance and possesses its own immune competence. Current evidence suggests that astrocytes, neurons, microglia and oligodendrocytes are all able to directly synthesize several factors, regulators and receptors for complement proteins (Woodruff et al., 2010; Veerhuis et al., 2011). Neurons, astrocytes and microglia can produce complement initiators such as C1q (Stevens et al., 2007) and C3, receptors such as C3aR and C5aR as well as inhibitors such as C1-INH and CD59, although other complement proteins can be specifically produced by the different brain cells. Under normal conditions,

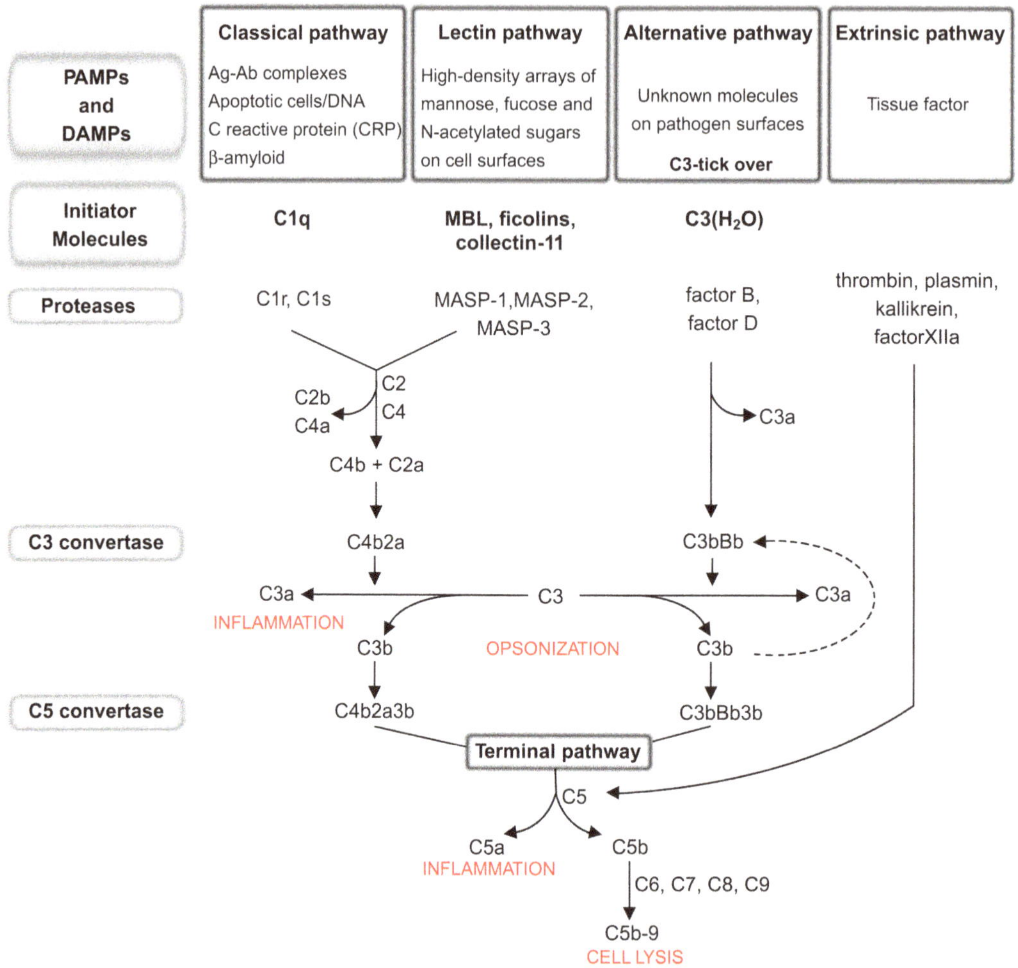

FIGURE 1 | The complement system: an overview. Classical pathway (CP): C1q, the CP initiator, recognizes and binds antigen-antibody complexes or specific molecules, including β-amyloid, C reactive protein (CRP), DNA and apoptotic bodies. After binding, the C1r and C1s proteases subsequently cleave C4 and C2 to generate C4a, C4b, C2a, C2b, permitting the formation of C4b2a (CP C3 convertase). This complex cleaves C3 into C3a, which, in turn, acts as potent anaphylatoxin, and C3b that binds to the complex forming the C4b2a3b protein block (CP C5 convertase). **Lectin pathway (LP):** MBL, ficolin-1, ficolin-2, ficolin-3 and collectin-11, the LP initiators, recognize and bind high-density arrays of mannose, fucose and N-acetylated sugars exposed by pathogens or by self-altered cells. After binding, the MBL-associated serine proteases (MASPs), MASP-1 and -2, associated in complex with the above recognition molecules (MBL/ficolins), cleave C4 and C2, thereby forming C3 convertase and C5 convertase in a similar manner to that of the CP (Ehrnthaller et al., 2011). The role of the third serine protease, called MASP-3, remains unclear (Kjaer et al., 2013). **Alternative pathway (AP):** the activation of the AP is driven by a spontaneous hydrolysis of circulating C3 (called tick-over process) to form C3(H_2O). This molecule then associates factor B and factor D to form C3bBb (AP C3 convertase). Similar to the C3 convertase generated in the CP and LP, this complex splits C3 into C3a and C3b, with the latter creating a new C3 convertase (AP amplification loop, dotted line), and/or binding C3 convertase already present to create the C3bBb3b complex (AP C5 convertase). **Extrinsic pathway:** the recent characterization of this activation pathway suggests that it is driven by activated proteolytic enzymes, including thrombin, plasmin, kallikrein, factor XIIa. Thrombin possesses its own C5 convertase activity and, under undefined conditions, has been shown to have the capacity to directly cleave C5 to generate the correspondent active fragments (Huber-Lang et al., 2006). Recently, it has been shown that the coagulation serine proteases are likewise able to cleave C3 (Markiewski et al., 2007; Amara et al., 2010). **Terminal pathway:** CP, AP, LP and the extrinsic pathway all converge at C5 convertase formation, activating a common cascade through the cleavage of C5 into the anaphylatoxin C5a and the active C5b. Finally, (1) C3b fragment binds the targeted cell allowing the assembly of C6, C7, C8 and C9 in a pore called membrane attack complex (C5b-9 or MAC), that causes the direct lysis of the cell; (2) many fragments, such as C3b and C4b as well as C5b, work as opsonins triggering an overactivation of the phagocytic response; (3) altogether complement components are able to orchestrate an adaptative immune reaction by communicating with multiple immune cells (Ricklin and Lambris, 2007) through different receptors, leading to a robust local and systemic inflammatory response.

complement synthesis in brain cells is low and is believed to be involved in physiological processes during brain development and homeostasis (vide infra). Following cellular injury and damage, complement synthesis in brain cells can markedly increase and contribute to tissue damage (Woodruff et al., 2010). The activation of the complement system has been extensively

Table 1 | Main complement regulators.

Regulator	Abbreviation	Target pathway	Functions
Fluid phase regulators:			
C1-inhibitor	C1-INH	CP and LP	Inhibits C1r, C1s, MASP-1 and MASP-2 proteolytic activities
MBL/ficolin-associated protein 1	MAP-1	LP	Binds MBL and ficolins and inhibits C4 deposition
Factor I	FI	CP, LP and AP	Cleaves C3b and C4b in their inactive fragments
C4 binding protein	C4BP	CP and LP	Accelerates decay of classical and lectin C3 convertase along with FI
Factor H	FH	AP	Accelerates decay of alternative C3 convertase along with FI
Carboxypeptidase N		CP, LP and AP	Inactivates C3a and C5a anaphylatoxin
Membrane-bound regulators:			
CR1		CP, LP and AP	Binds C3b,C4b and C1q to promote phagocytosis of immune-complexes and accelerates decay of convertases
CD46		CP, LP and AP	Binds C3b and C4b accelerating decay of C3 convertase, cofactor for FI
CD55		CP, LP and AP	Accelerates decay of C3 convertases
Complement receptor 1-related protein y	Crry	CP, LP and AP	Cleaves C3b and C4b inhibiting C3 convertases formation, cofactor for FI
CD59		CP, LP and AP	Binds C8 and C9 preventing the assembly of C5b-9 lytic complex

CP, classical pathway; LP, lectin pathway; AP, alternative pathway.

demonstrated in both chronic neurodegenerative and acute neuroinflammatory central nervous system (CNS) conditions, with neurons showing selective vulnerability to complement mediated damage (Singhrao et al., 2000), most likely due to their low basal expression of cell-membrane associated complement regulators (e.g., CD55 and CD46). However, distinctive kinetics of complement activation between chronic neurodegeneration and acute brain injury and neuroinflammatory insults occur. In neurodegenerative disorders, local complement biosynthesis and uncontrolled complement activation in the tissue are crucial for contributing to neuronal loss and local inflammation, with blood brain barrier (BBB) injury appearing during the disease chronic stages (Gasque et al., 2000). Conversely, one common feature of acute brain injuries, such as stroke, subarachnoid hemorrhage and brain trauma, includes early and severe BBB breakdown. Thus, in addition to complement proteins and regulators produced locally in the tissue, brain parenchyma immediately following acute injury is rapidly invaded by a number of inflammatory cells and molecules, including complement proteins circulating in high concentration in blood (Brennan et al., 2012). Although this process is essential for triggering the removal of cellular debris, when over-activated, it may severely affect neuronal and glial integrity in cells spared at the time of the primary injury.

THE BRAIN ENDOTHELIUM: A CRITICAL COMPARTMENT OF ACTION

Brain vascular endothelial cells are major players in this cascade of events. They represent the physical barrier between the periphery and the brain parenchyma and since they are continuously exposed to blood-derived complement effectors, they remain a target of circulating active complement molecules (Bossi et al., 2011). In response to stress signals, endothelial cells may expose DAMPs to become selective targets for complement initiators. Endothelial cells can also produce selected complement components, subsequently increasing the local availability and cell toxicity of these molecules. The complement-mediated endothelial damage promotes BBB leakage with a subsequent influx of active complement fragments and cytokines, as well as immune cells into the injured brain tissue with amplification of local inflammation (**Figure 2**). Endothelial cells may therefore play a central role in triggering/modulating local complement activation and in the partition of complement components from blood to brain.

C1q is known to directly bind endothelial cells (Yin et al., 2007; Bossi et al., 2008) inducing the expression of adhesion molecules, such as E-selectin, intercellular adhesion molecule-1 (ICAM-1) and vascular cell adhesion protein-1 (VCAM-1; Lozada et al., 1995), and the release of chemokines and cytokines, such as IL-8, monocyte chemotactic protein-1 (MCP-1) and IL-6 (van den Berg et al., 1998). It has been reported that C1q and MBL compete for the binding to endothelial surfaces (Oroszlán et al., 2007). MBL deposition on endothelial cells has been demonstrated independently from C1q, both in *in vitro* and *in vivo* settings and is known to occur after oxidative stress on human umbilical vein endothelial cells (HUVECs), accompanied with iC3b deposition. Furthermore, MBL and iC3b deposition are reduced in the presence of functionally inhibitor anti-MBL antibodies (Collard et al., 2000) suggesting that MBL adhesion on endothelial cells mediates complement activation. It has also been proposed that MBL deposition is driven by increased endothelial expression of cytokeratin 1 after hypoxia, since anti-cytokeratin treatment is able to attenuate MBL and iC3b presence on HUVECs under the same conditions (Collard et al., 2001). Although the specific MBL-binding molecules expressed by damaged endothelial cells remain unclear, MBL deposition has been demonstrated *in vivo* in different organs, such as heart (Pavlov et al., 2012), kidney (Møller-Kristensen et al., 2005; Castellano et al., 2010), intestine (McMullen et al., 2006) and brain (Gesuete et al., 2009; Orsini et al., 2012) following ischemia reperfusion injury. MBL deposition also occurs after both human and experimental traumatic brain injury (TBI; Longhi et al.,

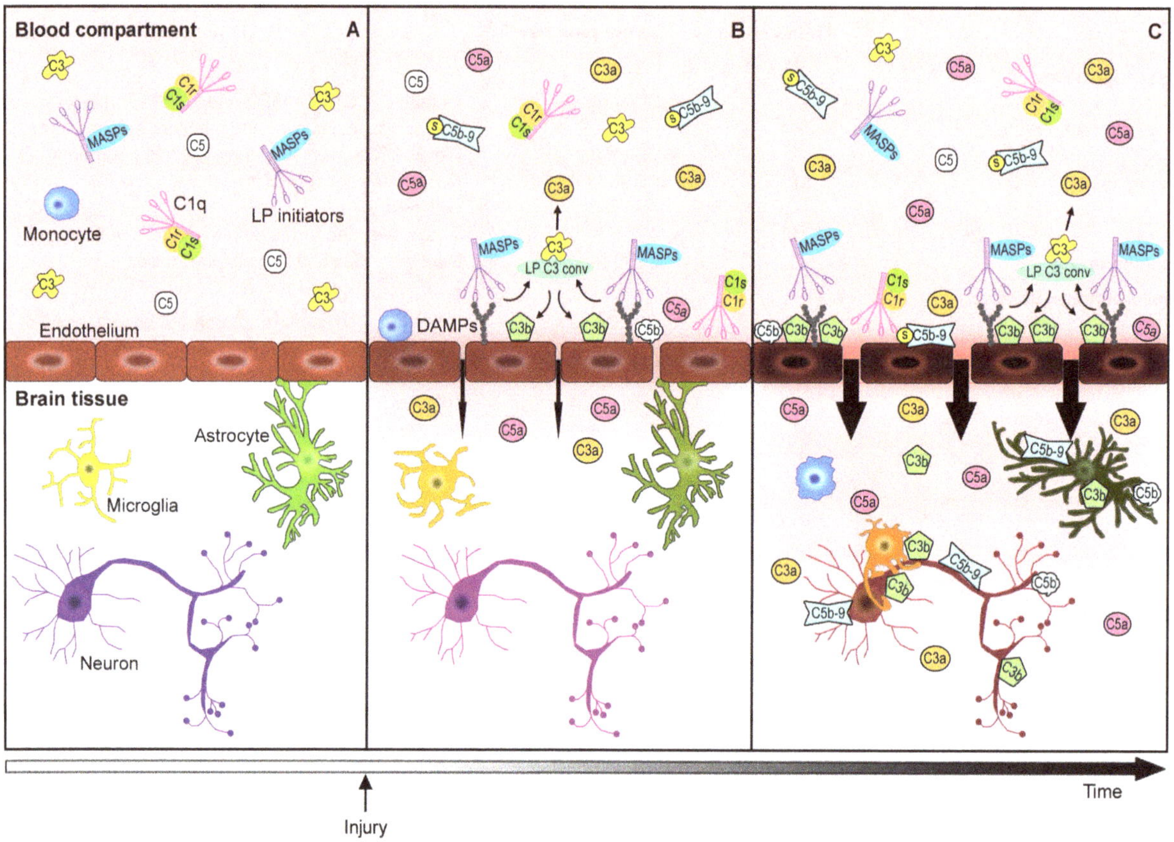

FIGURE 2 | Complement-mediated endothelial damage: working hypothesis. Healthy brain endothelial cells physically isolate the brain parenchyma from the blood compartment. Under physiological conditions, complement proteins, such as C1q, LP initiators, C3 and C5, monitor the blood and the cell surfaces for potential threats **(A)**. The additional complement factors that normally circulate in the bloodstream, have been omitted in this figure for purposes of clarity and simplification. When a cerebrovascular injury occurs **(B)**, endothelial cells may change their glycosylation profile, leading to the exposure of high density arrays of sugar (DAMPs). LP initiators, through their carbohydrate recognition domains, can recognize and bind altered endothelial cells, leading to LP complement activation **(B)**. Complement activated fragments trigger the expression of adhesion molecules and the release of chemokines and cytokines (not shown) on endothelial cells, resulting in the worsening of the BBB leakage **(B→C)**. The injured brain parenchyma is then rapidly invaded by the full immune arsenal, including the complement proteins, cytokines and immune cells (e.g., monocytes) belonging to the blood compartment, leading to amplification of local damage **(C)**. The overactivation of the complement system in brain tissue leads to: (1) a potent inflammatory response and the recruitment of peripheral immune cells mediated by C3a and C5a anaphylatoxins, (2) direct lysis of neurons and other brain cells, including those that are potentially savable, by C5b-9, (3) opsonization with subsequent microglia/macrophage phagocytosis of the target cells by C3b and C5b. This schema proposes a key role for endothelial cells in triggering local LP complement activation and suggests that targeting the peripheral compartment may represent effective strategy for brain protection from injury and different acute CNS diseases.

2014), suggesting that this response represents one of several toxic events after trauma (**Figure 2**). Another protein belonging to the LP, the serine protease MASP-1, is currently under evaluation for its effect on endothelium. It has been demonstrated that MASP-1 induces p38- mitogen-activated protein kinases (MAPK) activation, NFkappaB signaling and Ca^{2+} mobilization in HUVECs, inducing IL-6 and IL-8 production (Jani et al., 2014) as well as E-selectin expression (Dobó et al., 2014). MASP-1, like thrombin, also activates endothelial cells directly by cleaving the protease activated receptors (PARs; Megyeri et al., 2009). Other complement components have been demonstrated to interact with endothelial cells and promote vascular toxicity. For example, anaphylotoxin C3a and C5a may interact with the corresponding receptors on endothelial cells (Van Beek et al., 2000) inducing cytoskeletal modifications (Schraufstatter et al., 2002; Bossi et al., 2011) and increasing mRNA levels of IL-8, IL-1β and RANTES (regulated on activation normal T cell expressed and secreted) (Monsinjon et al., 2003). In addition, C3 knock-out (C3-/-) mice showed reduced immune complex-mediated vascular leakage when compared to wild type (WT) mice (Lister et al., 2007; Bossi et al., 2011), even though a direct toxic effect of C3a on endothelial cells has not been demonstrated (Schraufstatter et al., 2002). The same authors reported that C5a induces endothelial cells shrinkage with subsequent increased vascular permeability. The vascular properties of C5a have also been reported in an endotoxin-induced permeability model, in which C5aR-siRNA was able to limit the vascular leakage (Liu et al., 2010). In addition to the effects on the aforementioned complement components, TP proteins can lead to vascular dysfunction. For example, the circulating soluble C5b-9 (sC5b-9), a cytotoxic inactive complex formed by C5b-9 terminal lytic complex associated with soluble regulators, induced vascular leakage on HUVECs and in an *in vivo* model of mesenteric microvessel permeability (Tedesco et al., 1997; Bossi et al., 2004).

Taken together, these data suggest that protein products derived from complement activation can act on endothelial cells and shift, via different mechanisms, endothelial activation towards a toxic phenotype with associated increased vascular permeability.

THE DISRUPTIVE OVERWHELMING POWER OF COMPLEMENT IN ACUTE NEUROINFLAMMATORY BRAIN CONDITIONS

Stroke and TBI represent two major types of acute neuroinflammatory brain conditions. Stroke remains the third leading cause of death worldwide and the first cause of long-term disability in Europe (Corbyn, 2014), while TBI remains the principal cause of death and disability in active young adults today (Lingsma et al., 2010). Moreover, TBI has been proposed to be an independent risk factor for stroke (Burke et al., 2013). Fewer than 10% of stroke patients are eligible for treatment with tissue-type plasminogen activator, the only current therapy available, to date. Despite the creation of increasingly widespread networks of organized acute stroke units, a high proportion of hospitalized stroke patients survive with permanent neurological impairment and disability. Similarly, no treatment is currently available for TBI and surviving patients often report severe and/or prolonged disabilities. Although stroke and TBI share important molecular and cellular pathogenic mechanisms leading to the progression of damage, due to the different nature of the primary insult, they are also associated with specific cellular vulnerability and activation of distinct pathogenic cascades. We will focus on these two conditions that induce profound alterations of both central and peripheral immune system (Bellavance and Rivest, 2012; Chamorro et al., 2012), review the available data on the disruptive overwhelming power of complement in acute brain injury and summarize both the common and divergent relevant cellular and molecular mediators which represent candidates for the development of novel targeted therapeutic strategies.

STROKE

Evidence of complement system activation

A role for the complement system in ischemia/reperfusion injury was first suggested by Hill and Ward (1971), who demonstrated the presence of C3-cleavage factors with chemotactic activity in damaged rat myocardial tissue. Activation of the complement system after ischemia/reperfusion injury in different organs such as heart, kidney, intestine and brain has been subsequently documented (Arumugam et al., 2009; Cervera et al., 2010; Orsini et al., 2012), suggesting that complement represents a common but key mechanism involved in the exacerbation of tissue damage after ischemia.

In stroke patients, activation of the complement system has been documented in plasma or serum samples as well as in post-mortem brain tissues. Specifically, C3a and C5a plasma levels were shown to increase post-stroke, reaching peak values at days 1 and 14 respectively (Mocco et al., 2006b). Follow-up studies have extended these observations, documenting an increase in C3 and C3a plasma levels in patients with small vessel disease or cardioembolic stroke when compared to controls, and additionally demonstrating a positive correlation between their levels and unfavorable outcome in cardioembolic stroke (Stokowska et al., 2013). Acute (day 1–2) plasma sC5b-9 levels in patients with either ischemic or hemorrhagic stroke have been shown to be significantly increased when compared to non-stroke controls (Széplaki et al., 2009; Zanier et al., 2014) and shown to increase over time during post-stroke recovery (Pedersen et al., 2004). In a cohort of mild stroke patients, Mocco et al. (2006b), observed decreased plasma sC5b-9 levels when compared to non-stroke controls. These data highlight that interpretation of alterations in systemic concentrations of complement factors is not straightforward, since injury severity or timing issues may markedly affect plasma dynamics of complement activation products. Furthermore, caution must be observed when interpreting the clinical data, since both an increase and decrease of circulating complement factors may be regarded as indicator of complement activation reflecting either increased synthesis or increased consumption/deposition.

In addition to the analysis of circulating factors, the presence of differing complement proteins in post-mortem brain tissues of human stroke patients has also been investigated, providing important information regarding the specific cell population associated with the expression or deposition of selective factors. Immunohistochemical analysis of human brain tissue has revealed that expression of factors, such as C1q, C4d, C3c and C9, is detectable in neurons in ischemic brain regions but absent in non-stroke control tissues (Pedersen et al., 2009). C1q immunostaining was associated with microglial cells, while C3c and C9 staining were associated both with microglia and astrocytes in necrotic areas. Existing data concerning C5b-9 complex is more controversial, with some authors finding no deposition of this factor in ischemic brain tissue (Pedersen et al., 2009), while others reporting increased C5b-9 and C3d immunoreactivity in infarcted areas (Lindsberg et al., 1996). Additionally, immunopositivity for the regulators CD59 and CD55 (**Table 1**) which is present in healthy controls, is undetectable in ischemic brains (Pedersen et al., 2009), suggesting that down-regulation of these molecules may contribute to ischemic pathology.

Additional information concerning the role of key complement mediators in brain ischemia comes from experimental animal studies. The earliest studies were performed using cobra venom factor (CVF) that induces non-selective but total complement depletion. Rats treated with CVF 1 day before transient middle cerebral artery occlusion (tMCAo), showed higher reactive hyperaemia and better preservation of somatosensory evoked potentials when compared to vehicle-treated rats (Vasthare et al., 1998). A subsequent study demonstrated reduced cerebral infarct volume and atrophy in adult and neonatal rats following CVF administration (Figueroa et al., 2005). In contrast, other studies testing the efficacy of prophylactic CVF administration failed to show any protective effect in a thromboembolic stroke model in rabbits (Lew et al., 1999) or in an hypoxia/ischemia model in immature rats (Lassiter et al., 2001). The species selection and the differences in stroke models may explain, in part, these discordant observations. However, these data also suggest that full complement depletion may not be an optimal therapeutic strategy and that more targeted manipulation aimed at inhibiting/deleting selective complement components should be evaluated. To this end, studies concerning the inhibition of downstream-cascade complement proteins have been conducted to elucidate their specific contribution in mediating brain damage after ischemia. C3-/- ischemic mice showed better neurological scores, reduced ischemic volume, granulocyte infiltration and oxidative stress when compared to WT mice subjected to cerebral ischemia, confirming the deleterious effects of complement system activation in this condition (Atkinson et al., 2006; Mocco et al., 2006a). Furthermore, the expression of C3aR has been shown to increase after cerebral ischemia (Barnum et al., 2002) and its pharmacological inhibition with a C3aR antagonist conferred protection of anatomical damage associated with reduced endothelial ICAM-1 staining (Ducruet et al., 2008).

The precise role of C5 in brain ischemic injury remains unclear. Recent *in vitro* data has shown that brain ischemia, mimicked by oxygen-glucose deprivation, induces the cleavage of the C5 expressed by neurons leading to apoptotic cell death signaling (Pavlovski et al., 2012). *In vivo* studies have shown disparate results depending on post-stroke evaluation time points. Twenty-four hours after ischemic onset, Mocco et al. found no effect on neurological scores or ischemic volume in C5 knock-out mice (C5-/-) when compared to WT mice (Mocco et al., 2006a). Conversely, Arumugam et al. reported improved functional outcome with reduced brain damage in C5-/- compared with their WT littermates, when assessed 72 h after injury (Arumugam et al., 2007). Brain expression of C5aR increases in mice after cerebral ischemia (Barnum et al., 2002) and although the administration of C5aR antagonist elicited only a slight improvement in neurological deficits and infarct volume in 60 min tMCAo mice (Arumugam et al., 2007), more clear cut protective effects on neurological deficits and infarct volume were observed after 45 min tMCAo (Kim et al., 2008).

The deleterious role of terminal complement pathway activation has been assessed in experimental stroke models using a variety of strategies. The first was to investigate the susceptibility of C6 knock-out mice (C6-/-) to ischemic brain damage. No differences concerning either neurological deficits or ischemic damage were observed in C6-/- compared to WT mice (Elvington et al., 2012). The second strategy was aimed at studying the susceptibility to ischemia in CD59 knock-out mice (CD59-/-), which lack this important endogenous membrane-bound inhibitor of C5b-9 formation (see **Table 1**). Three days after 30 min tMCAo, CD59-/- showed increased infarct volume, greater neurological deficits and increased brain swelling compared to injured WT mice, indicating that CD59 may exert a protective role by inhibiting the C5b-9 assembly on damaged target cells. In contrast, there were no differences on those outcomes between the two strains when the mice were subjected to 60 min tMCAo followed by 2 days of reperfusion, despite the increase in the number of terminal-dUTP-nick end labeled (TUNEL)-positive cells in CD59-/- compared to WT (Harhausen et al., 2010). In addition, the differences observed were restricted to male mice, while no effects were found in female mice (Harhausen et al., 2010). The most recent strategy has been to investigate the role of CD55 regulator (see **Table 1**) after ischemic brain insults. Primary cortical rat neurons were exposed to hypoxia-like conditions, mimicked by NaCN exposure, and incubated with or without the complement inhibitor CD55. The complement inhibitor prevented dendritic spine loss induced by hypoxia and increased cell viability following the hypoxic insult. In addition, CD55 treatment attenuated the increase of C3 and C3aR neuronal expression, as well as the generation of C3a and C5b-9 triggered by hypoxemia (Mack et al., 2006; Wang et al., 2010). Taken together, these different strategies combine to suggest an involvement of the terminal complement pathway activation in inducing cerebral damage after ischemia.

Distinct roles of activation pathways

Further research has been performed on the initiators of the complement cascade to better clarify the specific contribution of the different activation stimuli. It has been demonstrated that C1q, the initiator of the CP, is present on neuronal cell bodies and in cellular debris beginning 6 h after tMCAo (Mack et al., 2006). Furthermore, widespread C1q biosynthesis has been detected in rat microglia, but not in astrocytes or neurons, 24 h after global cerebral ischemia (Schäfer et al., 2000). Nevertheless, we and others have demonstrated that C1q knock-out (C1q-/-) mice were not protected against brain ischemia (De Simoni et al., 2003; Mocco et al., 2006a), suggesting that this component of the complement cascade does not directly induce post-ischemic neuronal damage. Conversely, neonatal C1q-/- mice subjected to hypoxic/ischemic brain injury showed a reduction of infarct volume, neurological deficits, C3 deposition and granulocytes infiltration in infracted areas compared to WT mice (Ten et al., 2005). The apparent discrepancy regarding the C1q role after adult vs. neonatal ischemic injury might be explained by differing age-dependent complement susceptibility. Indeed, it has been demonstrated that a developmentally-related increase in C1q, FB, C3, C4 and C5 expression occurs up to 24 months in mice (Reichwald et al., 2009; Stephan et al., 2013). Although no data are available regarding the expression of C1q, C1q receptors or complement regulators in newborn mice, it is known that C1q is extremely important during neuronal wiring and synapse elimination (vide infra and see Stephan et al., 2012), suggesting a higher susceptibility/sensitivity to C1q-mediated effects in newborn vs. adult neurons.

C1-INH, with its ability to bind and inactivate C1r and C1s, has been suggested to be one of the major regulators of the CP (Ziccardi, 1981). However, subsequent studies (Davis et al., 2010) have demonstrated that this molecule is able to inhibit both the classical and the LPs. Furthermore, it has been shown that C1-INH possesses a greater ability to inactivate MASP-2 than classical proteases, suggesting that the LP might be a more relevant target for C1-INH compared to the CP (Kerr et al., 2008). Additional studies have shown that exogenous administration of C1-INH was protective in a variety of brain ischemia experimental models (Heimann et al., 1999; Akita et al., 2003; De Simoni et al., 2003, 2004; Storini et al., 2005; Gesuete et al., 2009; Heydenreich et al., 2012). We have reported that mice subjected to cerebral ischemia and treated with C1-INH showed reduced ischemic volume, neurological deficits, degenerating cells and leukocytes infiltration in the damaged parenchyma when compared to saline-treated ischemic mice (De Simoni et al., 2004). The protective effects elicited by C1-INH administration were associated with reduced mRNA expression of endothelial adhesion molecules, including P-selectin and ICAM-1, normally induced by ischemic injury (Storini et al., 2005). More recently, Heydenreich et al. reported that C1-INH administration resulted in a significant reduction of BBB leakage compared to saline in ischemic mice (Heydenreich et al., 2012). In order to better understand the molecular targets of C1-INH, we analyzed the effect of C1-INH administration in C1q-/- mice subjected to cerebral ischemia. Although adult C1q-/- mice were not protected from ischemic injury, C1-INH was effective in reducing the ischemic volume in C1q deprived mice, suggesting that C1-INH protective effects are not mediated by the CP. Taken together, this recent evidence supports the hypothesis for a central role of LP in C1-INH mediated protection, since: (1) C1-INH binds MBL with high affinity *in vitro*, (2) C1-INH and MBL co-localize on ischemic endothelium *in vivo*; and (3) C1-INH administration reduces the levels of functional MBL/MASP-2 complexes in the plasma of ischemic mice (Gesuete et al., 2009).

Detailed analysis of the MBL gene in humans reveals that a surprisingly high percentage of individuals (15–30% of the Caucasian population) carry MBL polymorphisms leading to low circulating MBL levels. Notably, in 2 independent studies, MBL deficiency has been associated with favorable outcome in stroke patients (Cervera et al., 2010; Osthoff et al., 2011) providing an additional rationale for the development of further studies to better understand the specific pathogenic role of MBL and of the other LP activators in stroke. In mice subjected to cerebral ischemia, MBL deficiency was associated with reduced neurological deficits, brain lesion and C3 deposition compared to WT mice during the acute post-injury phase (Cervera et al., 2010; Orsini et al., 2012). However, 7 days after the insult, MBL knockout mice (MBL-/-) did not show any evidence of neuronal protection, indicating that MBL may be necessary during tissue repair processes (Ducruet et al., 2011), suggesting that transient MBL inhibition may be a desirable and efficacious therapeutic strategy. Recently, we have demonstrated that pharmacological inhibition of MBL is highly protective in models of cerebral ischemia, possessing a wide window of efficacy both in mice and rats. We have reported that: (1) treatment with Polyman2, a dendrimeric molecule binding MBL with high affinity, induced a reduction of neurological deficits and ischemic volume when administered up to 24 h after induction of injury in mice; and (2) a functional inhibitory neutralizing antibody against MBL induced a long-lasting (up to 1 month) reduction of neurological deficits and ischemic volume when administered 18 h after ischemia in rats (Orsini et al., 2012). In addition, we have demonstrated that MBL was deposited specifically along the luminal side of ischemic vessels, up to 48 h post-injury. We hypothesize that the wide therapeutic window observed may be the result of targeting this long-lasting pathogenic cascade within ischemic endothelium (**Figure 2**). More recently, it has been proposed that MBL contributes to cerebral damage by promoting local microvascular thrombosis after ischemia in mice (de la Rosa et al., 2014). In these studies, MBL-/- mice showed significantly improved recovery of regional blood flow at 6 h and reduced fibrinogen levels in the ischemic tissue 24 h after tMCAo when compared to ischemic WT mice. Moreover, the administration of argatroban, a thrombin inhibitor, significantly reduced neurological deficits and ischemic volume in ischemic WT but not in MBL-/- mice, suggesting that the deleterious effects of MBL in the ischemic brain are partially mediated by thrombin activation. Additionally, MASP-1 and thrombin both share common targets, including PARs, on endothelial cells (Megyeri et al., 2009), suggestive of close interplay between LP and extrinsic pathway. The existing data underscore the need for further elucidation of the specific interaction between complement and coagulation systems and its relevance to injury progression in acute brain injury.

As previously stated, in addition to MBL, other activators of LP like ficolins and CL-11 exist that may be relevant in stroke. Available evidence indicate that among the currently-identified LP initiators, ficolin-3 exhibits the highest blood concentration and activation capacity in humans (Hummelshoj et al., 2008). In ischemic stroke patients, serum levels of ficolin-2 and ficolin-3 have been shown to be significantly decreased compared to non-ischemic controls, indicating that ficolins may be consumed during the acute phases of ischemic pathology. Perhaps more importantly, only ficolin-3 levels inversely correlate with the stroke severity at admission (7–8 h) and with outcome at 3–4 days (Füst et al., 2011), suggesting that ficolin-3 contributes to the pathogenic processes of cerebral ischemia. We have recently demonstrated that the LP pathway is activated after aneurysmal subarachnoid hemorrhage (SAH) in patients, and that plasma concentrations of ficolin-3 reflect both the severity of brain injury evaluated by clinical and structural parameters and the extent of SAH-associated brain complications (Zanier et al., 2014). In this rare stroke subtype characterized by the bleeding of an intracranial aneurysm, brain ischemia is generally believed to be the main determinant of unfavorable outcome in the acute phase, occurring as result of initial intracranial bleeding and/or at delayed stages as a consequence of vasospasm. One explanation for the decrease of ficolin-3 and functional LP activity is the consumption of this protein in the course of SAH-related events. LP initiators can recognize and bind damage-associated molecular patterns exposed by dying or reversibly damaged cells through their carbohydrate recognition domain. After stroke, injured endothelial cells may change their glycosylation profile, thereby becoming the earliest suitable targets for LP initiators. Overall, these data argue for a major role of the LP, rather than the CP, in complement-mediated toxic effects after stroke and support the concept that the LP may be selectively targeted to control injury progression in brain ischemia.

The contribution of the AP following brain ischemia is, to date, poorly understood. The major difficultly in assessing the contribution of the AP to ischemic damage is that its main activating protein C3, belongs not exclusively to the AP but also to CP and LP. However, recent strategies have been developed to obtain selective AP inhibition. Elvington et al. (2012) recently employed both FB knock-out mice (FB-/-) and the administration of CR2-fH, a specific inhibitor of the AP, in WT mice and reported that FB-/- and CR2-fH-treated mice displayed significant improvement in neurological scores, smaller ischemic volume, reduced P-selectin expression, neutrophil infiltration and microthrombi formation compared to WT or vehicle-treated animals. Interestingly, FB-/- and CR2-fH-treated mice showed less pronounced protective effects when compared to mice knockout for both C1q and MBL (C1q/MBL-/-) or WT mice treated with CR2-Crry, which inhibits not only the alternative but the whole activation pathways. In addition, FB-/- and CR2-fH-treated mice, but not C1q/MBL-/- mice, showed increased brain C3d deposition, supporting the hypothesis that the AP is not sufficient *per se* to initiate post-ischemic complement activation (Elvington et al., 2012). Thus overall the AP does not initiate full complement activation but appears to contribute to the propagation of cerebral injury via amplification of the other cascades.

TRAUMATIC BRAIN INJURY

Evidence of complement system activation

The involvement of the complement system in TBI began to be studied in the early 1990s. Although our current knowledge is limited when compared to that of stroke, evidence has accumulated from both clinical and experimental studies allowing for the identification of critical complement-associated factors as mediators of the pathophysiological sequelae of TBI.

A role for complement after TBI in patients has been suggested by studies of cerebrospinal fluid (CSF; Kossmann et al., 1997; Stahel et al., 2001) and cerebral contused tissue (Bellander et al., 2001; Longhi et al., 2014). Following TBI, C3 and FB levels were 20 and 4 times higher in CSF than those found in controls, respectively (Kossmann et al., 1997). Moreover, C5b-9 levels were 1800-fold increased in TBI patients compared to non-injured controls, suggestive of full activation of complement in TBI (Stahel et al., 2001). Additionally, in contused brain tissue, immunoreactivity for complement C3b, C3d and C5b-9 was increased on neuronal cell surfaces (Bellander et al., 2001), while no staining was detected in control tissue. These observations suggest that complement activation occurs in brain cells following TBI, possibly leading to an exacerbation of cerebral damage after the initial (primary) injury. Extensive BBB damage in patients following moderate to severe TBI may suggest that the major source of complement factors may be the vascular compartment, rather than intraparenchymal expression (Kossmann et al., 1997).

Additional evidence for the role of complement in TBI comes from several experimental animal models. The first study on the effect of global complement inhibition in TBI employed soluble CR1 (sCR1), a molecule that inhibits all complement activation pathways by preventing the C3-convertase formation. Rats pre-treated with sCR1 displayed a 41% reduction in neutrophil extravasation following TBI, suggesting that complete complement system inhibition may attenuate vascular permeability (Kaczorowski et al., 1995). Additionally, mice over-expressing soluble Crry (sCryy, see **Table 1**), a C3 convertase inhibitor, showed reduced BBB leakage and neurobehavioral deficits after weight drop brain injury when compared to brain-injured WT mice (Rancan et al., 2003). In this study, exogenous administration of Crry-IgG (Crry fused with IgG1Fc for bioavailability purpose) in brain-injured WT mice resulted in an attenuation of neurological deficits at 4 and 24 h after TBI and a reduction of neuronal loss in the hippocampus at 4 h compared with vehicle-treatment (Rancan et al., 2003). Treatment with Crry-IgG not only prevented C3 convertase activation, but also induced an up-regulation of both complement-regulatory genes (C1-INH, CD55 and CD59, see **Table 1**) and the anti-apoptotic Bcl-2 gene (Leinhase et al., 2006). Although Crry may represent a promising pharmacological treatment in the early phase after TBI, further studies are needed to elucidate its protective mechanism of action (Leinhase et al., 2006). Thus, similarly to what found in stroke models, also in TBI C3 convertase may represent a therapeutical target.

The specific role of C3 in TBI has been assessed in C3-/- mice subjected to cortical controlled impact (CCI) brain injury. Although brain-injured C3-/- mice did not differ from brain-injured WT with respect to pre- or post-injury motor and cognitive performance and brain lesion size after trauma, neutrophil recruitment was shown to decrease in these knock-out mice by approximately 50% (You et al., 2007). Additional effects were observed in C3-/- mice subjected to a traumatic cryoinjury model, which mimics several aspects of the TBI pathology, including BBB opening and brain edema. Using this model, investigators reported decreased lesion volume and vascular damage associated with reduced hemorrhage and neutrophil recruitment sustained by a diminished proinflammatory gene expression (RANTES, Eotaxin, MCP-1 and migration inhibitory factor, MIF) in brain-injured C3-/- mice (Sewell et al., 2004). Although these contrasting data do not permit a clear understanding of the exact role of C3 after TBI, the provocative observations, to date, argue for continued work in this area.

The effect of TP over-activation has been studied in experimental TBI using multiple approaches that have consistently demonstrated a detrimental role for this pathway in TBI. In C5-/- mice or in WT mice treated with C5aR antagonist, a significant reduction of neutrophil extravasation after brain cryoinjury was observed when compared to brain-injured control mice. Since the degree of reduction was incomplete (only reaching 35%), other complement chemoattractant molecules (e.g., C3a) may play a more predominant role in regulating this process in TBI (Sewell et al., 2004). Furthermore, after weight-drop TBI, administration of a C5-binding protein complement inhibitor (OmCI, administered up to 15 min after injury), which blocks the generation of both C5a and C5b-9 (Fluiter et al., 2014), reduced neurological deficits, weight loss, C9 immunostaining and microglia/macrophage activation compared with vehicle treatment (Fluiter et al., 2014). OmCI treatment was also associated with decreased neuronal apoptosis and axonal loss. Since protective effects of OmCI treatment are known to be associated with both C5a and C5b-9 inhibition, in order to better understand the specific contribution of down-stream C5b-9, its synthesis was subsequently prevented via the administration of C6 mRNA antisense oligonucleotide. Similar neuroprotective results were obtained to those observed after OmCI treatment (Fluiter et al., 2014). These data highlight the potential role of C5b-9 (vs C5/C5a) as a major mediator of complement-mediated damage after TBI. However, to date, a selective C5 inhibitory strategy has not been evaluated experimentally using a clinically relevant TBI model. The role of C5b-9 formation has also been investigated using CD59-/- mice (see **Table 1**). Following weight-drop brain injury, CD59 gene expression was observed to be up-regulated in WT mice, suggestive of the activation of a neuronal protective mechanism against lysis. Brain-injured CD59-/- mice showed increased neurobehavioral deficits and neuronal cell death when compared to brain-injured WT mice, suggesting that CD59 plays a direct role in protecting the brain after TBI, possibly by inhibition of C5b-9 formation, as previously described for stroke (Stahel et al., 2009). Overall, these studies underscore a role for full complement activation in the exacerbation of inflammatory processes leading to neurobehavioral and anatomical damage after TBI and brain ischemia.

Distinct roles of activation pathways

Beyond our understanding of the relevance of the end-stage complement components in the pathobiological sequelae of TBI, additional studies have begun to address the significance of the activation of specific complement pathways. C4 is an intermediate complement substrate belonging to both CP and LP activation. Knock-out mice for this complement factor (C4-/-) showed improved motor deficits and less post-injury damage after CCI brain injury when compared to injured WT. Similarly, administration of human C4 reversed the motor recovery in C4-/- mice. These data, demonstrating that C4 impairs the recovery of posttraumatic motor deficits and contributes to brain tissue damage (You et al., 2007), suggest that CP and LP are both involved in the pathogenesis of TBI.

In contused tissue from TBI patients, C1q immunoreactivity was found on microglia/macrophage and astrocyte cell surfaces close to the border zone of brain contusions (Bellander et al., 2001). In mice, C1q gene expression increased both at 1 and 4 days after CCI. However, C1q-/- mice did not show an amelioration of neurobehavioral deficits and a reduction of tissue damage after brain trauma compared to injured WT mice suggesting that inhibition of C1q does not lead to neuroprotective effects in TBI (You et al., 2007). These observations support those observed following cerebral ischemia and suggest that C1q does not represent a major target for treatment of acute brain pathology following CNS injury.

Similarly to what has been reported for stroke, C1-INH (**Table 1**) has been revealed to possess neuroprotective properties in TBI. Mice injected with C1-INH at 10 min or 1 h after CCI brain injury showed a significant and long lasting improvement of motor function over 4 weeks post-injury. Furthermore, mice treated at 10 min showed improved cognitive outcome with a concomitant decrease in lesion volume. These data demonstrate that C1-INH may be protective via the modulation of early mechanisms of secondary damage after TBI (Longhi et al., 2009). Insight concerning the putative mechanisms of action of C1-INH, obtained from experimental stroke studies (vide supra) further supports a focus on the role of LP in TBI. We therefore investigated the MBL presence in both human and experimental TBI. In TBI patients, we demonstrated that MBL immunostaining was present inside and around brain vessels in contused brain tissue removed both early (<6 h) or late (4–5 d) following TBI. Conversely, MBL staining was absent in control patients (Longhi et al., 2014). Similarly, in mice subjected to CCI brain injury, MBL was distributed inside and around brain vessels, visible up to 1 week after CCI, possibly representing a long lasting event after trauma (Longhi et al., 2014). The effect of MBL deletion has been investigated in MBL-/- mice who showed increased degenerating cells in hippocampus 6 h after mild CCI brain injury with an exacerbation of neurobehavioral deficits 1 week post-injury compared to brain-injured WT mice (Yager et al., 2008). Conversely, when studied up to 5 weeks after severe CCI brain injury, MBL-/- mice displayed better neurobehavioral outcome beginning from the second up to the forth week after injury when compared to WT. These behavioral improvements were associated with reduced neuronal cell loss at 5 weeks (Longhi et al., 2014). These findings suggest that MBL absence may lead either to attenuation of mechanisms of secondary brain damage or to the activation of reparative/regenerative processes that occur at more chronic time points after injury (Longhi et al., 2014). Similar to what has been described in models of stroke, increasing evidence highlight the major contribution of the LP, rather than the CP, in mediating secondary damage after TBI and suggest that LP initiators are a viable therapeutic target for future study to limit tissue damage and cell loss following acute CNS injury.

Similar to studies in brain ischemia, few studies have been performed regarding the role of the AP in TBI, to date. FB-/- mice were reported to exhibit a robust decrease of C5a serum levels at 4 h, 24 h and 7 d after weight-drop brain injury, suggesting that AP activation contributes to overall complement activation. In addition, FB-/- mice showed less neuronal death compared to brain-injured WT at 7 days post-injury (Leinhase et al., 2006). Additional studies have investigated the effect of anti-factor B antibody administration which effectively reduces the activation of the AP. Treatment with this compound conferred protection against TBI-induced neuronal cell death, but did not improve neurological deficits when compared to vehicle treatment. This discrepancy was likely due to the lack of sensitivity of the neurological tests employed to detect subtle changes in behavioral performance (Leinhase et al., 2007). In summary, activation of the AP in the setting of TBI appears to have a detrimental effect on pathological and neurobehavioral outcome, although it remains unclear whether this system plays a key role in triggering the full complement activation.

NEURODEGENERATIVE DISORDERS: THE EVIDENCE OF A DELICATE BALANCE BETWEEN COMPLEMENT MEDIATED PROTECTIVE AND TOXIC EFFECTS

Neurodegenerative disorders are defined as hereditary or sporadic conditions caused by progressive loss of neuronal structures and functions, until neuronal cell death. Many neurodegenerative conditions, including Alzheimer's disease (AD), Parkinson's disease (PD) and amyotrophic lateral sclerosis (ALS), occur as a result of this progressive neurodegenerative processes. Despite they arise from different molecular aberrations, they show important similarities in the pathogenic cellular mechanisms (e.g., protein misfolding, defective protein degradation pathways and mitochondrial dysfunction) and in the immune response (complement system and immune cell activation associated with inflammation). Currently there are no drugs able to slow the progression of these disorders.

Among the neurodegenerative disorders, AD is the most common one. Thirty six million people worldwide were estimated to be living with dementia in 2010, a number expected to reach 115 million people by 2050 (Hugo and Ganguli, 2014). We will focus on the complex, versatile role of the complement system in AD outlining emerging evidence that show either beneficial or detrimental effects of this system depending on the disease stage. Additionally we will discuss the limited data available on PD and ALS pathology. A deeper knowledge on the role of the complement system in neurodegenerative disorders may lead to new therapeutic options.

ALZHEIMER'S DISEASE

Evidence of complement system activation

Since the early 1980s, the full range of classical and AP activation, involving all steps of the cascade through TP, has been described to be associated with AD (Meraz-Ríos et al., 2013).

In humans, multiple isoforms of complement factors have been reported to be present in the CSF of AD patients. Differences in patterns of complement factor expression between normal controls and AD patients have also been reported at different stages of the pathology, suggestive of a distinctive temporal pattern of complement protein expression in relation to amyloid-β (Aβ) plaque deposition and Aβ plaque maturation. CSF levels of C1q, C3d and C4d have been found to increase during the early stages of AD during Aβ formation, showing a positive correlation with total plaque number from very mild to severe clinical cases (Finehout et al., 2005; Wang et al., 2011; Daborg et al., 2012). In post mortem studies comparing young, middle aged and old cases, similar results have been obtained (Stoltzner et al., 2000), documenting increased brain immunoreactivity for complement proteins with age (Stoltzner et al., 2000; Veerhuis et al., 2003; Fonseca et al., 2004a; Zanjani et al., 2005). The CP initiator C1q has been found to be up-regulated up to 80-fold in areas of human AD brains showing pathological neurodegeneration (Yasojima et al., 1999), a relevant observation in view of the fact that C1q is known to bind directly Aβ fibrils (fAβ) and neurofibrillary tangles (Rogers et al., 1992; Jiang et al., 1994; Shen et al., 2001; Webster et al., 2001; Veerhuis et al., 2003), underscoring the need for a deeper understanding of the C1q specific role in AD pathology.

Early vs. late disease stages

Manipulations of the complement system in experimental models have permitted the investigation of the role of the complement components in AD. Recent *in vitro* and *in vivo* data have highlighted a neuroprotective role of C1q. A direct positive effect against Aβ fibrillar and oligomeric-induced neuronal death in primary cortical neurons was demonstrated (Pisalyaput and Tenner, 2008; Benoit et al., 2013). *In vivo* studies using AD transgenic mouse models (one expressing the mutant form of human amyloid precursor protein, hAPP and a second expressing mutated Tau and/or presenilin 1) have been used to understand the role of complement system in AD pathology. In these studies, during the early stages of the disease, C1q induced a potent cascade of neuroprotective gene expression via the activation of the transcription factor cAMP response element-binding protein (CREB) and by increasing the expression of downstream pro-survival effectors (low density lipoprotein receptor-related protein 1B—LRP1B and G protein-coupled receptor 6—GPR6) (Benoit et al., 2013). Conversely, at later stages of AD progression, during Aβ accumulation, C1q-/- AD mice showed a significant decreased microglial activation (50–60%) surrounding the Aβ plaques accompanied by elevated expression of neuronal markers with subsequent protective effect on neuronal integrity (Fonseca et al., 2004b). Taken together, these data are suggestive of a protective role for C1q in the early stages of AD, prior to Aβ deposition, converting to a pathogenic role in association with toxic events over time in the more chronic phases of the disease (late stages).

Similar to C1q, increased C3 CSF levels in advanced AD patients (Finehout et al., 2005; Wang et al., 2011; Daborg et al., 2012) and C3 brain expression in aged AD transgenic mice (Wyss-Coray et al., 2002; Zhou et al., 2008; Reichwald et al., 2009) have been reported. The effects of experimental manipulation of C3 on Aβ deposition, neuronal damage and activation of inflammatory cells have been investigated by multiple approaches at more chronic stages of AD pathology. Transgenic AD mice (over-expressing hAPP and TGF-β) were found to have elevated C3 brain levels associated with reduced Aβ accumulation (Wyss-Coray et al., 2002). Inhibition of C3 convertase formation by the transgenic expression of the sCrry gene, leading to loss of opsonizing effect of C3b, was also shown to result in 2 to 3-fold increase of Aβ accumulation and subsequent neurodegeneration (Wyss-Coray et al., 2002). Subsequently, C3-/- transgenic AD mice showed an age-associated increase in cerebral Aβ deposition and neuronal loss compared with C3-sufficient AD mice (Maier et al., 2008). It is known that C3 products may act as chemoattractant factors for microglial cells involved in the clearance of Aβ protein deposits and C3 deficiency/inhibition has been shown to consistently impair monocyte/macrophage phagocytic capability, likely contributing to Aβ protein accumulation (Maier et al., 2008). These studies demonstrate that the absence/inhibition of the central complement component C3, accelerates AD-like Aβ plaque pathology with aging once plaque pathogenesis is underway and suggest that complement C3 may play an important role in maintaining tissue homeostasis (vide infra). The mechanism(s) underlying the biological importance of increased expression of C3 protein observed both in AD humans and mice at delayed stages remains unclear and may represent an attempt to protect the brain via C3 up-regulation rather than a byproduct of neuronal damage (Maier et al., 2008).

In contrast to the data available on C3, data concerning TP products consistently suggest that they exert detrimental effects during the pathological progression of AD (Yao et al., 1990). In AD patients, an increase in the terminal components (C9 and C5b-9) have been reported only in severe AD (Zanjani et al., 2005; Loeffler et al., 2008). During plaque accumulation, the receptors for C5a (C5aR) have been shown to increase and colocalize with neurofibrillary tangles in human AD brains (Fonseca et al., 2013). C5aR has been reported to be expressed in astrocytes and microglia and to be up-regulated during neurodegeneration (Woodruff et al., 2010). *In vitro*, the combination of Aβ-protein and C5a activated monocytes/microglial cells induced an increase in proinflammatory cytokines (O'Barr et al., 2001), supporting the hypothesis that Aβ and C5a together can induce a chronic microglia-mediated focal inflammatory response in a synergistic manner. *In vivo*, an age- and disease-associated up-regulation of C5aR on microglia in the proximity of Aβ plaques has been reported in transgenic AD mice (Ager et al., 2010). Inhibition of C5a using a C5aR antagonist, induced a decrease in Aβ plaque burden and microglial activation with a concomitant increase in cognitive performance in transgenic AD mice (Fonseca et al., 2009). This effect does not appear to be mediated by the modulation of C1q and/or C3, which remain unaffected after treatment, but by the selective inhibition of deleterious C5a–C5aR signaling (Ager et al., 2010). Thus, the inhibition of the complement TP during AD progression leads to a substantial improvement in behavioral and histopathological outcome in AD mice, suggesting that pharmacological manipulation of this pathway may be a novel strategy to treat neurodegeneration.

Little is known concerning the involvement of LP in AD. Studies showing lower MBL levels in CSF of AD patients when compared to controls (Lanzrein et al., 1998), together with more recent evidence that MBL deficiency in humans is associated with AD risk (Sjölander et al., 2013), underscore the need for further studies to better characterize the role of this pathway in AD pathogenesis and progression.

Thus, AD represents an excellent paradigm to explore the differential role of specific complement factors in relation to time and degree of neuropathological injury. The available data indicate that the complement system plays a dual role in AD pathogenesis and progression. Beneficial effects of complement activation occur during the early stages of AD (Fonseca et al., 2004b; Pisalyaput and Tenner, 2008; Benoit et al., 2013), possibly contributing to Aβ plaques clearance by microglia through complement-dependent opsonization (mediated by C1q, C3b) (Alexander et al., 2008). Conversely, during the more chronic phases of AD progression, complement activation appears to transition to a deleterious role, contributing to neurotoxicity with subsequent exacerbation of the inflammatory reaction at the site of injury (Alexander et al., 2008).

PARKINSON'S DISEASE AND AMYOTROPHIC LATERAL SCLEROSIS

Evidence also exists for complement involvement in PD and ALS. In PD patients, increased complement activation (through formation of C5b-9), has been identified in Lewy bodies (LBs, intraneuronal fibrillar aggregates containing a high concentration of α-synuclein) and in oligodendroglia in the substantia nigra, as well as in serum and CSF of patients with either sporadic or familial PD (McGeer and McGeer, 2004; Goldknopf et al., 2006; Wang et al., 2011; Depboylu et al., 2011a; More et al., 2013). Similar to what has been observed in PD, increased complement components in serum (C3c, C3d, FH), in CSF (C4d) (Tsuboi and Yamada, 1994; Goldknopf et al., 2006), as well as in affected postmortem spinal cord tissue (C1q/C2/C4/C3/MAC) have been reported in ALS patients (Grewal et al., 1999; Sta et al., 2011). In experimental rodent models of ALS pathology (one expressing ALS-causing mutations in superoxide dismutase SOD1 and a second engineered to be deficient in the low molecular weight neurofilament- NFL subunit protein) similar findings have also been reported in spinal cord (Lobsiger et al., 2007; Woodruff et al., 2008; Humayun et al., 2009; Takeuchi et al., 2010; Heurich et al., 2011; Lee et al., 2013) and along peripheral nerves (Chiu et al., 2009). Increased expression of C1q reported in brain tissue from humans and mouse models of both PD (Depboylu et al., 2011a,b) and ALS (Lobsiger et al., 2007; Heurich et al., 2011; Sta et al., 2011) highlights the potential involvement of C1q in neurodegenerative processes via microglial-mediated synaptic elimination. The lack of effect of C1q gene deletion on onset and disease progression in either PD mice (Depboylu et al., 2011b), or SOD1 mutant mice complicates our understanding of the role of C1q in these conditions (Lobsiger et al., 2013) and the exact role of CP in PD and ALS pathogenesis and progression remains poorly understood.

No additional data are available concerning the possible role of other complement proteins in PD. In ALS, however, the role of C3 (Lobsiger et al., 2013) and C4 (Chiu et al., 2009) using gene deletion techniques has been studied in SOD1 mutant mice showing no major effect on outcome. Alternatively, recent evidence suggests that the C5 downstream protein may be a key mediator of complement-mediated neurotoxicity in ALS models. Studies in transgenic SOD1 mutant rats and NFL knock-out mice have reproducibly shown an up-regulation of the major proinflammatory C5aR during disease progression (Woodruff et al., 2008; Humayun et al., 2009). Furthermore, chronic administration of C5aR antagonist in transgenic SOD1 mutant rats was reported to exert beneficial effects on neuronal survival during disease progression (Woodruff et al., 2008). These results indicate that, under stress, local complement signaling might therefore promote damage and motor neuron death in ALS.

THE COMPLEMENT SYSTEM IN HOMEOSTASIS, PLASTICITY AND REGENERATION

Growing evidence highlights that the versatile functions of the complement system extend far beyond those of immune surveillance and the elimination/neutralization of pathogens and altered host cells. Indeed, recent evidence point to an active involvement of complement in lipid metabolism, angiogenesis, tissue remodeling and maintenance in the CNS (Veerhuis et al., 2003; Ricklin et al., 2010; Rutkowski et al., 2010; Stephan et al., 2012).

SYNAPTIC REMODELING

Plasticity and remodeling of new synaptic circuits characterize the early stages of brain development (Stephan et al., 2012). Molecular and cellular mechanisms underlying synapse refinement during development have been studied using the retinogeniculate system. Early in development, axons from retinal ganglion cells (RGCs) form transient functional synaptic connections with neurons of dorsal lateral geniculate nucleus (dLGN). Subsequently, during the first 2 weeks of post-natal development, the retinogeniculate system circuit is subjected to precise sculpting through the pruning of any overlapping or redundant transient connections and the strengthening of the remaining ones (Hooks and Chen, 2006). The failure of this mechanism results in uncorrected eye-segregation and visual deficits. During this period of synaptic refinement, a close interaction/interplay amongst complement proteins, immature astrocytes and neurons has been revealed to occur. In the postnatal retinogeniculate system, TGF-β released by immature astrocytes, induces in RGCs the up-regulation of C1q which is transported from cell bodies along axons to the dLGN, where it is released to bind transient synapses. C1q is therefore believed to contribute to synapse elimination through direct connection tagging (Eggleton et al., 2000) or through C3b formation (Bialas and Stevens, 2013) that, in turn, opsonizes the target synapses. The contribution of C1q and C3b to synaptogenesis and synaptic remodeling is also supported by their punctate colocalization with pre and postsynaptic markers during normal retinogeniculate development (Stevens et al., 2007). However, the mechanism that drives the opsonization process of synapses destined to be pruned is not fully understood. Two different mechanisms, both claiming a central role of complement opsonin (C1q and C3b) and microglial interplay (Schafer et al., 2012), have been suggested: (1) C1q and C3b, via an unknown selection strategy, only tag the overlapping and weaker synapses, thereby inducing their elimination by phagocytic microglia (Stevens et al., 2007), or (2) C1q and C3b tag all synapses but the more active or stronger ones are, in turn, able to express specific membrane-bound complement inhibitors which confer selective protection against microglial phagocytosis (Kim and Song, 2006; Kim et al., 2008; Stephan et al., 2012). In addition, resident microglia are not only involved in active phagocytosis of tagged synapses but may participate to synaptic modeling through the secretion of C1q. To this end, increased concentrations of C1q have been shown to be present in microglia during the postnatal period that coincides with the peak of synaptic refinement (Fiske and Brunjes, 2000). The involvement of C1q and C3 fragments in brain sculpting is likewise supported by studies in knock-out animals who display an incorrect eye-specific segregation, due to overlapping RGC projections and overabundant excitatory connectivity in the cortex, resulting from defective synapse elimination (Stevens et al., 2007; Chu et al., 2010; Stephan et al., 2012). However, the phenotype of C1q-/- and C3-/- mice also shows residual synapse refinement, suggesting that other molecules may participate in this process, including both major histocompatibility complex I (MHC-I) and neuronal pentraxins (Corriveau et al., 1998; Huh et al., 2000; Bjartmar et al., 2006; Datwani et al., 2009). These findings show that complement proteins are important in cooperating with other pathways to regulate normal synaptic circuit development.

While complement activation and its interaction with microglial cells appear necessary for brain wiring during the postnatal period, recent evidence indicate that when this developmental program becomes aberrant in the immature brain or is recapitulated during adulthood molecular cascades related to neurodegenerative processes may be initiated (Stephan et al., 2012). For example, during the postnatal period, the inappropriate activation of the complement cascade causes profound synapse elimination that leads to neuropsychiatric diseases, such as autism or schizophrenia (Patterson, 2011). Defects in pruning have also been reported to be associated with the development of epilepsy (Chu et al., 2010) or glaucoma (Howell et al., 2011) where C1q and C3 are pathologically up-regulated and cause destabilization of neuronal circuits (see Stephan et al., 2012).

COMPLEMENT-MEDIATED EFFECTS ON CELLULAR WASTE REMOVAL

One of the main "housekeeping" functions of the complement cascade involves the removal of apoptotic cells and the scavenging of cellular debris and immune complexes. Senescent or defective cells typically undergo apoptosis via a non-inflammatory cell death. Normally, apoptotic cell bodies are rapidly removed to avoid the unwanted over-activation of immunological processes, since failure to clear or scavenge dead cells may induce an exaggerated inflammatory reaction against other tissues (Savill et al., 2002; Cole et al., 2006). Apoptosis induces membrane phospholipid and ionic charge changes leading to deposition of innate system effectors (Flierman and Daha, 2007). As for the brain, *in vitro* studies have shown that C1q binds to neuronal apoptotic cells and activates the CP with subsequent production of opsonizing fragments (C3b and C4b), responsible for apoptotic cell phagocytosis (Cole et al., 2006). Furthermore, biochemical studies have demonstrated that C1q is able to bind IgM, serum amyloid P component (SAP), CRP and pentraxin-3 (PTX3), suggesting their involvement in C1q- mediated apoptotic cell removal (Kishore et al., 2004). The relevance of C1q in the physiological clearance of apoptotic cells has been studied in C1q-/- mice who displayed an impaired elimination of immune complexes and susceptibility to autoimmune disease (Mitchell et al., 2002).

The overall role of phagocytosis is complex and depends on the context. When occurring on the target cell dying by some means such as apoptosis it is believed to be a beneficial activity, preventing the release of damaging and/or proinflammatory intracellular components (referred to as "secondary phagocytosis", Neher et al., 2011, 2012). However, under certain conditions, such as acute brain injury, complement overactivation may induce microglial cells to phagocyte also viable neurons, thus executing their death (referred to as "primary phagocytosis") (Neher et al., 2011, 2012).

After injury such phagocytic activity may result from exposure of eat-me signals (C3b, C4b and C5b) on otherwise viable neurons as a result of subtoxic and reversible insults, thus contributing to injury amplification.

COMPLEMENT-MEDIATED EFFECTS ON MATURE BRAIN CELL SURVIVAL AND ON NEUROGENESIS

In vitro studies have shown pro-survival effects of C1q in mature brain cells, under normal conditions. Specifically, rat neuronal cell cultures treated with C1q showed prolonged cell survival associated with higher number of neuronal processes when compared to untreated cells (Pisalyaput and Tenner, 2008). These pro-survival effects of C1q may be due to an up-regulation of cholesterol metabolism and cytoskeleton-related gene expression and to an increase of nerve growth factor (NGF) and neurotrophin-3 protein levels (Benoit and Tenner, 2011). Indirect evidence for a pro-survival action of C3a and C5a have also been presented and C3a and C5a treatment of astrocytes and microglial cell cultures has been shown to up-regulate NGF, suggesting a common pro-survival pathway in the CNS under normal conditions (Heese et al., 1998). Under neurodegenerative conditions, a protective role of C1q and C3 in preserving tissue homeostasis during AD progression has been reported (vide supra).

Complement proteins have been shown to be involved in migration and maturation of stem cells in the CNS under physiological conditions. Neural stem and progenitor cells (NPCs) have been reported to express C3aR and C5aR (Rahpeymai et al., 2006). *In vitro* studies have demonstrated that treatment of NPCs with C3a facilitates their migration and maturation without affecting proliferation (Shinjyo et al., 2009). In addition, it has been reported that mice treated with a C3aR antagonist display reduced neurogenesis in different brain areas, including the subventricular zone (SVZ), hippocampal dentate gyrus and olfactory bulb. Overall, these findings indicate that cellular signaling via C3a positively regulates basal neurogenesis (Rahpeymai et al., 2006).

Complement seems to be involved also in brain injury-induced neurogenesis. After transient ischemia, C3-/- mice showed a significant reduction (by 24%) in neurogenesis (doublecortin positive cells) in the SVZ compared to ischemic WT mice at 7 days after insult. Moreover, the reduction in neurogenesis was independent of either microglia activation or reactive gliosis that remained unaffected in C3-/- compared to WT mice (Rahpeymai et al., 2006). Further evidence suggesting a contribution of C3a to CNS neurogenesis comes from the literature concerning experimental neonatal brain ischemia. Ischemic neonatal mice treated with C3a exhibited improved memory function at 41 days and this effect was abolished in C3aR-/- neonatal mice (Järlestedt et al., 2013). As discussed previously, a large body of evidence has been generated demonstrating the detrimental effects of several complement-activated products after acute brain injury. While these findings suggest a contribution of C3a to ischemia-induced neurogenesis, it should be emphasized that C3 is not a unique/major neurogenic factor since consistent and residual neurogenesis remains after C3 removal. Continued investigation addressing the temporal role of the complement system in mediating neurogenesis in the injured brain is warranted to elucidate how the delicate balance between complement-dependent neurotoxicity and its potential neurogenic effects can be modulated to promote neuroprotection.

CONCLUDING REMARKS

Far beyond the view of the complement as a supplementary molecule needed for bacterial lysis, the available data show that the complement cascade is involved in several aspects of brain development, homeostasis, injury and regeneration. The versatility of this cascade in participating in diverse processes in the nervous system under both physiological and pathological conditions appears to be dependent on a fine balance within an intricate network of effectors, receptors and regulators. When the critical factors involved with this system are finely regulated, they participate in the maintenance of brain homeostasis. Conversely, deregulation between activators and regulators leads to aberrant complement activation with subsequent exacerbation of inflammation and worsening of the damage induced by brain injury and neurodegenerative diseases. Importantly, evidence that targeting selective steps of this cascade leads to amelioration of brain injury strongly support the concept of the complement system as an important therapeutic target in brain injury and disease.

ACKNOWLEDGMENTS

The authors would like to thank Dr. Tracy K. McIntosh for carefully editing the manuscript. Financial support was provided by Fondazione Cariplo (grant number 2012-0590). Dr. Orsini was funded by a fellowship in memory of Amalia Ghezzi.

REFERENCES

Ager, R. R., Fonseca, M. I., Chu, S.-H., Sanderson, S. D., Taylor, S. M., Woodruff, T. M., et al. (2010). Microglial C5aR (CD88) expression correlates with amyloid-beta deposition in murine models of Alzheimer's disease. *J. Neurochem.* 113, 389–401. doi: 10.1111/j.1471-4159.2010.06595.x

Akita, N., Nakase, H., Kaido, T., Kanemoto, Y., and Sakaki, T. (2003). Protective effect of C1 esterase inhibitor on reperfusion injury in the rat middle cerebral artery occlusion model. *Neurosurgery* 52, 395–400; discussion 400–401. doi: 10.1227/01.neu.0000043710.61233.b4

Alexander, J. J., Anderson, A. J., Barnum, S. R., Stevens, B., and Tenner, A. J. (2008). The complement cascade: Yin-Yang in neuroinflammation—neuro-protection and -degeneration. *J. Neurochem.* 107, 1169–1187. doi: 10.1111/j.1471-4159.2008.05668.x

Amara, U., Flierl, M. A., Rittirsch, D., Klos, A., Chen, H., Acker, B., et al. (2010). Molecular intercommunication between the complement and coagulation systems. *J. Immunol.* 185, 5628–5636. doi: 10.4049/jimmunol.0903678

Arumugam, T. V., Tang, S.-C., Lathia, J. D., Cheng, A., Mughal, M. R., Chigurupati, S., et al. (2007). Intravenous immunoglobulin (IVIG) protects the brain against experimental stroke by preventing complement-mediated neuronal cell death. *Proc. Natl. Acad. Sci. U S A* 104, 14104–14109. doi: 10.1073/pnas.0700506104

Arumugam, T. V., Woodruff, T. M., Lathia, J. D., Selvaraj, P. K., Mattson, M. P., and Taylor, S. M. (2009). Neuroprotection in stroke by complement inhibition and immunoglobulin therapy. *Neuroscience* 158, 1074–1089. doi: 10.1016/j.neuroscience.2008.07.015

Atkinson, C., Zhu, H., Qiao, F., Varela, J. C., Yu, J., Song, H., et al. (2006). Complement-dependent P-selectin expression and injury following ischemic stroke. *J. Immunol.* 177, 7266–7274. doi: 10.4049/jimmunol.177.10.7266

Barnum, S. R., Ames, R. S., Maycox, P. R., Hadingham, S. J., Meakin, J., Harrison, D., et al. (2002). Expression of the complement C3a and C5a receptors after permanent focal ischemia: an alternative interpretation. *Glia* 38, 169–173. doi: 10.1002/glia.10069

Bellander, B. M., Singhrao, S. K., Ohlsson, M., Mattsson, P., and Svensson, M. (2001). Complement activation in the human brain after traumatic head injury. *J. Neurotrauma* 18, 1295–1311. doi: 10.1089/08977150152725605

Bellavance, M.-A., and Rivest, S. (2012). The neuroendocrine control of the innate immune system in health and brain diseases. *Immunol. Rev.* 248, 36–55. doi: 10.1111/j.1600-065x.2012.01129.x

Benoit, M. E., Hernandez, M. X., Dinh, M. L., Benavente, F., Vasquez, O., and Tenner, A. J. (2013). C1q-induced LRP1B and GPR6 proteins expressed early in Alzheimer disease mouse models, are essential for the C1q-mediated protection against amyloid-β neurotoxicity. *J. Biol. Chem.* 288, 654–665. doi: 10.1074/jbc.M112.400168

Benoit, M. E., and Tenner, A. J. (2011). Complement protein C1q-mediated neuroprotection is correlated with regulation of neuronal gene and microRNA expression. *J. Neurosci.* 31, 3459–3469. doi: 10.1523/JNEUROSCI.3932-10.2011

Bialas, A. R., and Stevens, B. (2013). TGF-β signaling regulates neuronal C1q expression and developmental synaptic refinement. *Nat. Neurosci.* 16, 1773–1782. doi: 10.1038/nn.3560

Bjartmar, L., Huberman, A. D., Ullian, E. M., Rentería, R. C., Liu, X., Xu, W., et al. (2006). Neuronal pentraxins mediate synaptic refinement in the developing visual system. *J. Neurosci.* 26, 6269–6281. doi: 10.1523/jneurosci.4212-05.2006

Bossi, F., Bulla, R., and Tedesco, F. (2008). Endothelial cells are a target of both complement and kinin system. *Int. Immunopharmacol.* 8, 143–147. doi: 10.1016/j.intimp.2007.08.006

Bossi, F., Fischetti, F., Pellis, V., Bulla, R., Ferrero, E., Mollnes, T. E., et al. (2004). Platelet-activating factor and kinin-dependent vascular leakage as a novel functional activity of the soluble terminal complement complex. *J. Immunol.* 173, 6921–6927. doi: 10.4049/jimmunol.173.11.6921

Bossi, F., Peerschke, E. I., Ghebrehiwet, B., and Tedesco, F. (2011). Cross-talk between the complement and the kinin system in vascular permeability. *Immunol. Lett.* 140, 7–13. doi: 10.1016/j.imlet.2011.06.006

Brennan, F. H., Anderson, A. J., Taylor, S. M., Woodruff, T. M., and Ruitenberg, M. J. (2012). Complement activation in the injured central nervous system: another dual-edged sword? *J. Neuroinflammation* 9:137. doi: 10.1186/1742-2094-9-137

Buchner, H. (1981). Centr Bakteriol Parasitenk. *Zur. Nomenkl. Schutzenden Eiweisskorper* 10, 699–701.

Burke, J. F., Stulc, J. L., Skolarus, L. E., Sears, E. D., Zahuranec, D. B., and Morgenstern, L. B. (2013). Traumatic brain injury may be an independent risk factor for stroke. *Neurology* 81, 33–39. doi: 10.1212/WNL.0b013e318297eecf

Castellano, G., Melchiorre, R., Loverre, A., Ditonno, P., Montinaro, V., Rossini, M., et al. (2010). Therapeutic targeting of classical and lectin pathways of complement protects from ischemia-reperfusion-induced renal damage. *Am. J. Pathol.* 176, 1648–1659. doi: 10.2353/ajpath.2010.090276

Cervera, A., Planas, A. M., Justicia, C., Urra, X., Jensenius, J. C., Torres, F., et al. (2010). Genetically-defined deficiency of mannose-binding lectin is associated with protection after experimental stroke in mice and outcome in human stroke. *PLoS One* 5:e8433. doi: 10.1371/journal.pone.0008433

Chamorro, Á., Meisel, A., Planas, A. M., Urra, X., van de Beek, D., and Veltkamp, R. (2012). The immunology of acute stroke. *Nat. Rev. Neurol.* 8, 401–410. doi: 10.1038/nrneurol.2012.98

Chiu, I. M., Phatnani, H., Kuligowski, M., Tapia, J. C., Carrasco, M. A., Zhang, M., et al. (2009). Activation of innate and humoral immunity in the peripheral nervous system of ALS transgenic mice. *Proc. Natl. Acad. Sci. U S A* 106, 20960–20965. doi: 10.1073/pnas.0911405106

Chu, Y., Jin, X., Parada, I., Pesic, A., Stevens, B., Barres, B., et al. (2010). Enhanced synaptic connectivity and epilepsy in C1q knockout mice. *Proc. Natl. Acad. Sci. U S A* 107, 7975–7980. doi: 10.1073/pnas.0913449107

Cole, D. S., Hughes, T. R., Gasque, P., and Morgan, B. P. (2006). Complement regulator loss on apoptotic neuronal cells causes increased complement activation and promotes both phagocytosis and cell lysis. *Mol. Immunol.* 43, 1953–1964. doi: 10.1016/j.molimm.2005.11.015

Collard, C. D., Montalto, M. C., Reenstra, W. R., Buras, J. A., and Stahl, G. L. (2001). Endothelial oxidative stress activates the lectin complement pathway: role of cytokeratin 1. *Am. J. Pathol.* 159, 1045–1054. doi: 10.1016/s0002-9440(10)61779-8

Collard, C. D., Väkevä, A., Morrissey, M. A., Agah, A., Rollins, S. A., Reenstra, W. R., et al. (2000). Complement activation after oxidative stress: role of the lectin complement pathway. *Am. J. Pathol.* 156, 1549–1556. doi: 10.1016/S0002-9440(10)65026-2

Corbyn, Z. (2014). Stroke: a growing global burden. *Nature* 510, S2–S3. doi: 10.1038/510S2a

Corriveau, C. C., Madara, P. J., Van Dervort, A. L., Tropea, M. M., Wesley, R. A., and Danner, R. L. (1998). Effects of nitric oxide on chemotaxis and endotoxin-induced interleukin-8 production in human neutrophils. *J. Infect. Dis.* 177, 116–126. doi: 10.1086/513829

Daborg, J., Andreasson, U., Pekna, M., Lautner, R., Hanse, E., Minthon, L., et al. (2012). Cerebrospinal fluid levels of complement proteins C3, C4 and CR1 in Alzheimer's disease. *J. Neural Transm.* 119, 789–797. doi: 10.1007/s00702-012-0797-8

Datwani, A., McConnell, M. J., Kanold, P. O., Micheva, K. D., Busse, B., Shamloo, M., et al. (2009). Classical MHCI molecules regulate retinogeniculate refinement and limit ocular dominance plasticity. *Neuron* 64, 463–470. doi: 10.1016/j.neuron.2009.10.015

Davis, A. E., Lu, F., and Mejia, P. (2010). C1 inhibitor, a multi-functional serine protease inhibitor. *Thromb. Haemost.* 104, 886–893. doi: 10.1160/TH10-01-0073

de la Rosa, X., Cervera, A., Kristoffersen, A. K., Valdés, C. P., Varma, H. M., Justicia, C., et al. (2014). Mannose-binding lectin promotes local microvascular thrombosis after transient brain ischemia in mice. *Stroke* 45, 1453–1459. doi: 10.1161/STROKEAHA.113.004111

Depboylu, C., Schäfer, M. K.-H., Arias-Carrión, O., Oertel, W. H., Weihe, E., and Höglinger, G. U. (2011a). Possible involvement of complement factor C1q in the clearance of extracellular neuromelanin from the substantia nigra in Parkinson disease. *J. Neuropathol. Exp. Neurol.* 70, 125–132. doi: 10.1097/NEN.0b013e31820805b9

Depboylu, C., Schorlemmer, K., Klietz, M., Oertel, W. H., Weihe, E., Höglinger, G. U., et al. (2011b). Upregulation of microglial C1q expression has no effects on nigrostriatal dopaminergic injury in the MPTP mouse model of Parkinson disease. *J. Neuroimmunol.* 236, 39–46. doi: 10.1016/j.jneuroim.2011.05.006

De Simoni, M. G., Rossi, E., Storini, C., Pizzimenti, S., Echart, C., and Bergamaschini, L. (2004). The powerful neuroprotective action of C1-inhibitor on brain ischemia-reperfusion injury does not require C1q. *Am. J. Pathol.* 164, 1857–1863. doi: 10.1016/s0002-9440(10)63744-3

De Simoni, M. G., Storini, C., Barba, M., Catapano, L., Arabia, A. M., Rossi, E., et al. (2003). Neuroprotection by complement (C1) inhibitor in mouse transient brain ischemia. *J. Cereb. Blood Flow Metab.* 23, 232–239. doi: 10.1097/00004647-200302000-00010

Dobó, J., Schroeder, V., Jenny, L., Cervenak, L., Závodszky, P., and Gál, P. (2014). Multiple roles of complement MASP-1 at the interface of innate immune response and coagulation. *Mol. Immunol.* 61, 69–78. doi: 10.1016/j.molimm.2014.05.013

Ducruet, A. F., Hassid, B. G., Mack, W. J., Sosunov, S. A., Otten, M. L., Fusco, D. J., et al. (2008). C3a receptor modulation of granulocyte infiltration after murine focal cerebral ischemia is reperfusion dependent. *J. Cereb. Blood Flow Metab.* 28, 1048–1058. doi: 10.1038/sj.jcbfm.9600608

Eggleton, P., Tenner, A. J., and Reid, K. B. (2000). C1q receptors. *Clin. Exp. Immunol.* 120, 406–412. doi: 10.1046/j.1365-2249.2000.01218.x

Ehrlich, P., and Morgenroth, J. (1899). Zur Theorie der Lysenwirkung [in German]. *Berl. Klin. Wschr.* 36, 6–9.

Ehrnthaller, C., Ignatius, A., Gebhard, F., and Huber-Lang, M. (2011). New insights of an old defense system: structure, function and clinical relevance of the complement system. *Mol. Med.* 17, 317–329. doi: 10.2119/molmed.2010.00149

Elvington, A., Atkinson, C., Zhu, H., Yu, J., Takahashi, K., Stahl, G. L., et al. (2012). The alternative complement pathway propagates inflammation and injury in murine ischemic stroke. *J. Immunol.* 189, 4640–4647. doi: 10.4049/jimmunol.1201904

Figueroa, E., Gordon, L. E., Feldhoff, P. W., and Lassiter, H. A. (2005). The administration of cobra venom factor reduces post-ischemic cerebral injury in adult and neonatal rats. *Neurosci. Lett.* 380, 48–53. doi: 10.1016/j.neulet.2005.01.027

Finehout, E. J., Franck, Z., and Lee, K. H. (2005). Complement protein isoforms in CSF as possible biomarkers for neurodegenerative disease. *Dis. Markers* 21, 93–101. doi: 10.1155/2005/806573

Fiske, B. K., and Brunjes, P. C. (2000). Microglial activation in the developing rat olfactory bulb. *Neuroscience* 96, 807–815. doi: 10.1016/s0306-4522(99)00601-6

Flierman, R., and Daha, M. R. (2007). The clearance of apoptotic cells by complement. *Immunobiology* 212, 363–370. doi: 10.1016/j.imbio.2006.11.005

Fluiter, K., Opperhuizen, A. L., Morgan, B. P., Baas, F., and Ramaglia, V. (2014). Inhibition of the membrane attack complex of the complement system reduces secondary neuroaxonal loss and promotes neurologic recovery after traumatic brain injury in mice. *J. Immunol.* 192, 2339–2348. doi: 10.4049/jimmunol.1302793

Fonseca, M. I., Ager, R. R., Chu, S.-H., Yazan, O., Sanderson, S. D., LaFerla, F. M., et al. (2009). Treatment with a C5aR antagonist decreases pathology and enhances behavioral performance in murine models of Alzheimer's disease. *J. Immunol.* 183, 1375–1383. doi: 10.4049/jimmunol.0901005

Fonseca, M. I., Kawas, C. H., Troncoso, J. C., and Tenner, A. J. (2004a). Neuronal localization of C1q in preclinical Alzheimer's disease. *Neurobiol. Dis.* 15, 40–46. doi: 10.1016/j.nbd.2003.09.004

Fonseca, M. I., McGuire, S. O., Counts, S. E., and Tenner, A. J. (2013). Complement activation fragment C5a receptors, CD88 and C5L2, are associated with neurofibrillary pathology. *J. Neuroinflammation* 10:25. doi: 10.1186/1742-2094-10-25

Fonseca, M. I., Zhou, J., Botto, M., and Tenner, A. J. (2004b). Absence of C1q leads to less neuropathology in transgenic mouse models of Alzheimer's disease. *J. Neurosci.* 24, 6457–6465. doi: 10.1523/jneurosci.0901-04.2004

Füst, G., Munthe-Fog, L., Illes, Z., Széplaki, G., Molnar, T., Pusch, G., et al. (2011). Low ficolin-3 levels in early follow-up serum samples are associated with the severity and unfavorable outcome of acute ischemic stroke. *J. Neuroinflammation* 8:185. doi: 10.1186/1742-2094-8-185

Gasque, P., Dean, Y. D., McGreal, E. P., VanBeek, J., and Morgan, B. P. (2000). Complement components of the innate immune system in health and disease in the CNS. *Immunopharmacology* 49, 171–186. doi: 10.1016/s0162-3109(00)80302-1

Gesuete, R., Storini, C., Fantin, A., Stravalaci, M., Zanier, E. R., Orsini, F., et al. (2009). Recombinant C1 inhibitor in brain ischemic injury. *Ann. Neurol.* 66, 332–342. doi: 10.1002/ana.21740

Goldknopf, I. L., Sheta, E. A., Bryson, J., Folsom, B., Wilson, C., Duty, J., et al. (2006). Complement C3c and related protein biomarkers in amyotrophic lateral sclerosis and Parkinson's disease. *Biochem. Biophys. Res. Commun.* 342, 1034–1039. doi: 10.1016/j.bbrc.2006.02.051

Grewal, R. P., Morgan, T. E., and Finch, C. E. (1999). C1qB and clusterin mRNA increase in association with neurodegeneration in sporadic amyotrophic lateral sclerosis. *Neurosci. Lett.* 271, 65–67. doi: 10.1016/s0304-3940(99)00496-6

Harhausen, D., Khojasteh, U., Stahel, P. F., Morgan, B. P., Nietfeld, W., Dirnagl, U., et al. (2010). Membrane attack complex inhibitor CD59a protects against focal cerebral ischemia in mice. *J. Neuroinflammation* 7:15. doi: 10.1186/1742-2094-7-15

Heese, K., Hock, C., and Otten, U. (1998). Inflammatory signals induce neurotrophin expression in human microglial cells. *J. Neurochem.* 70, 699–707. doi: 10.1046/j.1471-4159.1998.70020699.x

Heimann, A., Takeshima, T., Horstick, G., and Kempski, O. (1999). C1-esterase inhibitor reduces infarct volume after cortical vein occlusion. *Brain Res.* 838, 210–213. doi: 10.1016/s0006-8993(99)01740-0

Heurich, B., El Idrissi, N. B., Donev, R. M., Petri, S., Claus, P., Neal, J., et al. (2011). Complement upregulation and activation on motor neurons and neuromuscular junction in the SOD1 G93A mouse model of familial amyotrophic lateral sclerosis. *J. Neuroimmunol.* 235, 104–109. doi: 10.1016/j.jneuroim.2011.03.011

Heydenreich, N., Nolte, M. W., Göb, E., Langhauser, F., Hofmeister, M., Kraft, P., et al. (2012). C1-inhibitor protects from brain ischemia-reperfusion injury by combined antiinflammatory and antithrombotic mechanisms. *Stroke* 43, 2457–2467. doi: 10.1161/STROKEAHA.112.660340

Hill, J. H., and Ward, P. A. (1971). The phlogistic role of C3 leukotactic fragments in myocardial infarcts of rats. *J. Exp. Med.* 133, 885–900. doi: 10.1084/jem.133.4.885

Hooks, B. M., and Chen, C. (2006). Distinct roles for spontaneous and visual activity in remodeling of the retinogeniculate synapse. *Neuron* 52, 281–291. doi: 10.1016/j.neuron.2006.07.007

Howell, G. R., Macalinao, D. G., Sousa, G. L., Walden, M., Soto, I., Kneeland, S. C., et al. (2011). Molecular clustering identifies complement and endothelin induction as early events in a mouse model of glaucoma. *J. Clin. Invest.* 121, 1429–1444. doi: 10.1172/JCI44646

Huber-Lang, M., Sarma, J. V., Zetoune, F. S., Rittirsch, D., Neff, T. A., McGuire, S. R., et al. (2006). Generation of C5a in the absence of C3: a new complement activation pathway. *Nat. Med.* 12, 682–687. doi: 10.1038/nm1419

Hugo, J., and Ganguli, M. (2014). Dementia and cognitive impairment: epidemiology, diagnosis and treatment. *Clin. Geriatr. Med.* 30, 421–442. doi: 10.1016/j.cger.2014.04.001

Huh, G. S., Boulanger, L. M., Du, H., Riquelme, P. A., Brotz, T. M., and Shatz, C. J. (2000). Functional requirement for class I MHC in CNS development and plasticity. *Science* 290, 2155–2159. doi: 10.1126/science.290.5499.2155

Humayun, S., Gohar, M., Volkening, K., Moisse, K., Leystra-Lantz, C., Mepham, J., et al. (2009). The complement factor C5a receptor is upregulated in NFL-/- mouse motor neurons. *J. Neuroimmunol.* 210, 52–62. doi: 10.1016/j.jneuroim.2009.01.028

Hummelshoj, T., Fog, L. M., Madsen, H. O., Sim, R. B., and Garred, P. (2008). Comparative study of the human ficolins reveals unique features of Ficolin-3 (Hakata antigen). *Mol. Immunol.* 45, 1623–1632. doi: 10.1016/j.molimm.2007.10.006

Jani, P. K., Kajdácsi, E., Megyeri, M., Dobó, J., Doleschall, Z., Futosi, K., et al. (2014). MASP-1 induces a unique cytokine pattern in endothelial cells: a novel link between complement system and neutrophil granulocytes. *PLoS One* 9:e87104. doi: 10.1371/journal.pone.0087104

Järlestedt, K., Rousset, C. I., Ståhlberg, A., Sourkova, H., Atkins, A. L., Thornton, C., et al. (2013). Receptor for complement peptide C3a: a therapeutic target for neonatal hypoxic-ischemic brain injury. *FASEB J.* 27, 3797–3804. doi: 10.1096/fj.13-230011

Jiang, H., Burdick, D., Glabe, C. G., Cotman, C. W., and Tenner, A. J. (1994). beta-Amyloid activates complement by binding to a specific region of the collagen-like domain of the C1q A chain. *J. Immunol.* 152, 5050–5059.

Kaczorowski, S. L., Schiding, J. K., Toth, C. A., and Kochanek, P. M. (1995). Effect of soluble complement receptor-1 on neutrophil accumulation after traumatic brain injury in rats. *J. Cereb. Blood Flow Metab.* 15, 860–864. doi: 10.1038/jcbfm.1995.107

Kerr, F. K., Thomas, A. R., Wijeyewickrema, L. C., Whisstock, J. C., Boyd, S. E., Kaiserman, D., et al. (2008). Elucidation of the substrate specificity of the MASP-2 protease of the lectin complement pathway and identification of the enzyme as a major physiological target of the serpin, C1-inhibitor. *Mol. Immunol.* 45, 670–677. doi: 10.1016/j.molimm.2007.07.008

Kim, G. H., Mocco, J., Hahn, D. K., Kellner, C. P., Komotar, R. J., Ducruet, A. F., et al. (2008). Protective effect of C5a receptor inhibition after murine reperfused stroke. *Neurosurgery* 63, 122–125; discussion 125–126. doi: 10.1227/01.NEU.0000335079.70222.8D

Kim, D. D., and Song, W.-C. (2006). Membrane complement regulatory proteins. *Clin. Immunol.* 118, 127–136. doi: 10.1016/j.clim.2005.10.014

Kishore, U., Ghai, R., Greenhough, T. J., Shrive, A. K., Bonifati, D. M., Gadjeva, M. G., et al. (2004). Structural and functional anatomy of the globular domain of complement protein C1q. *Immunol. Lett.* 95, 113–128. doi: 10.1016/j.imlet.2004.06.015

Kjaer, T. R., Thiel, S., and Andersen, G. R. (2013). Toward a structure-based comprehension of the lectin pathway of complement. *Mol. Immunol.* 56, 413–422. doi: 10.1016/j.molimm.2013.05.007

Kossmann, T., Stahel, P. F., Morganti-Kossmann, M. C., Jones, J. L., and Barnum, S. R. (1997). Elevated levels of the complement components C3 and factor B in ventricular cerebrospinal fluid of patients with traumatic brain injury. *J. Neuroimmunol.* 73, 63–69. doi: 10.1016/s0165-5728(96)00164-6

Lanzrein, A. S., Jobst, K. A., Thiel, S., Jensenius, J. C., Sim, R. B., Perry, V. H., et al. (1998). Mannan-binding lectin in human serum, cerebrospinal fluid and brain tissue and its role in Alzheimer's disease. *Neuroreport* 9, 1491–1495. doi: 10.1097/00001756-199805110-00045

Lassiter, H. A., Feldhoff, R. C., Dabhia, N., Parker, J. C., and Feldhoff, P. W. (2001). Complement inhibition does not reduce post-hypoxic-ischemic cerebral injury in 21-day-old rats. *Neurosci. Lett.* 302, 37–40. doi: 10.1016/s0304-3940(01)01653-6

Lee, J. D., Kamaruzaman, N. A., Fung, J. N. T., Taylor, S. M., Turner, B. J., Atkin, J. D., et al. (2013). Dysregulation of the complement cascade in the hSOD1G93A transgenic mouse model of amyotrophic lateral sclerosis. *J. Neuroinflammation* 10:119. doi: 10.1186/1742-2094-10-119

Leinhase, I., Rozanski, M., Harhausen, D., Thurman, J. M., Schmidt, O. I., Hossini, A. M., et al. (2007). Inhibition of the alternative complement activation pathway in traumatic brain injury by a monoclonal anti-factor B antibody: a randomized placebo-controlled study in mice. *J. Neuroinflammation* 4:13. doi: 10.1186/1742-2094-4-13

Leinhase, I., Schmidt, O. I., Thurman, J. M., Hossini, A. M., Rozanski, M., Taha, M. E., et al. (2006). Pharmacological complement inhibition at the C3 convertase level promotes neuronal survival, neuroprotective intracerebral gene expression and neurological outcome after traumatic brain injury. *Exp. Neurol.* 199, 454–464. doi: 10.1016/j.expneurol.2006.01.033

Lew, S. M., Gross, C. E., Bednar, M. M., Russell, S. J., Fuller, S. P., Ellenberger, C. L., et al. (1999). Complement depletion does not reduce brain injury in a rabbit model of thromboembolic stroke. *Brain Res. Bull.* 48, 325–331. doi: 10.1016/s0361-9230(99)00004-0

Lindsberg, P. J., Ohman, J., Lehto, T., Karjalainen-Lindsberg, M. L., Paetau, A., Wuorimaa, T., et al. (1996). Complement activation in the central nervous system following blood-brain barrier damage in man. *Ann. Neurol.* 40, 587–596. doi: 10.1002/ana.410400408

Lingsma, H. F., Roozenbeek, B., Steyerberg, E. W., Murray, G. D., and Maas, A. I. R. (2010). Early prognosis in traumatic brain injury: from prophecies to predictions. *Lancet Neurol.* 9, 543–554. doi: 10.1016/S1474-4422(10)70065-X

Lister, K. J., James, W. G., and Hickey, M. J. (2007). Immune complexes mediate rapid alterations in microvascular permeability: roles for neutrophils, complement and platelets. *Microcirculation* 14, 709–722. doi: 10.1080/10739680701404879

Liu, Z. M., Zhu, S. M., Qin, X. J., Cheng, Z. D., Liu, M. Y., Zhang, H. M., et al. (2010). Silencing of C5a receptor gene with siRNA for protection from Gram-negative bacterial lipopolysaccharide-induced vascular permeability. *Mol. Immunol.* 47, 1325–1333. doi: 10.1016/j.molimm.2009.11.001

Lobsiger, C. S., Boillée, S., and Cleveland, D. W. (2007). Toxicity from different SOD1 mutants dysregulates the complement system and the neuronal regenerative response in ALS motor neurons. *Proc. Natl. Acad. Sci. U S A* 104, 7319–7326. doi: 10.1073/pnas.0702230104

Lobsiger, C. S., Boillée, S., Pozniak, C., Khan, A. M., McAlonis-Downes, M., Lewcock, J. W., et al. (2013). C1q induction and global complement pathway activation do not contribute to ALS toxicity in mutant SOD1 mice. *Proc. Natl. Acad. Sci. U S A* 110, E4385–E4392. doi: 10.1073/pnas.1318309110

Loeffler, D. A., Camp, D. M., and Bennett, D. A. (2008). Plaque complement activation and cognitive loss in Alzheimer's disease. *J. Neuroinflammation* 5:9. doi: 10.1186/1742-2094-5-9

Longhi, L., Orsini, F., De Blasio, D., Fumagalli, S., Ortolano, F., Locatelli, M., et al. (2014). Mannose-binding lectin is expressed after clinical and experimental traumatic brain injury and its deletion is protective*. *Crit. Care Med.* 42, 1910–1918. doi: 10.1097/CCM.0000000000000399

Longhi, L., Perego, C., Ortolano, F., Zanier, E. R., Bianchi, P., Stocchetti, N., et al. (2009). C1-inhibitor attenuates neurobehavioral deficits and reduces contusion volume after controlled cortical impact brain injury in mice. *Crit. Care Med.* 37, 659–665. doi: 10.1097/CCM.0B013e318195998a

Lozada, C., Levin, R. I., Huie, M., Hirschhorn, R., Naime, D., Whitlow, M., et al. (1995). Identification of C1q as the heat-labile serum cofactor required for immune complexes to stimulate endothelial expression of the adhesion molecules E-selectin and intercellular and vascular cell adhesion molecules 1. *Proc. Natl. Acad. Sci. U S A* 92, 8378–8382. doi: 10.1073/pnas.92.18.8378

Mack, W. J., Sughrue, M. E., Ducruet, A. F., Mocco, J., Sosunov, S. A., Hassid, B. G., et al. (2006). Temporal pattern of C1q deposition after transient focal cerebral ischemia. *J. Neurosci. Res.* 83, 883–889. doi: 10.1002/jnr.20775

Maier, M., Peng, Y., Jiang, L., Seabrook, T. J., Carroll, M. C., and Lemere, C. A. (2008). Complement C3 deficiency leads to accelerated amyloid beta plaque deposition and neurodegeneration and modulation of the microglia/macrophage phenotype in amyloid precursor protein transgenic mice. *J. Neurosci.* 28, 6333–6341. doi: 10.1523/JNEUROSCI.0829-08.2008

Markiewski, M. M., Nilsson, B., Ekdahl, K. N., Mollnes, T. E., and Lambris, J. D. (2007). Complement and coagulation: strangers or partners in crime? *Trends Immunol.* 28, 184–192. doi: 10.1016/j.it.2007.02.006

McGeer, P. L., and McGeer, E. G. (2004). Inflammation and neurodegeneration in Parkinson's disease. *Parkinsonism Relat. Disord.* 10(Suppl. 1), S3–S7. doi: 10.1016/j.parkreldis.2004.01.005

McMullen, M. E., Hart, M. L., Walsh, M. C., Buras, J., Takahashi, K., and Stahl, G. L. (2006). Mannose-binding lectin binds IgM to activate the lectin complement pathway in vitro and in vivo. *Immunobiology* 211, 759–766. doi: 10.1016/j.imbio.2006.06.011

Megyeri, M., Makó, V., Beinrohr, L., Doleschall, Z., Prohászka, Z., Cervenak, L., et al. (2009). Complement protease MASP-1 activates human endothelial cells: PAR4 activation is a link between complement and endothelial function. *J. Immunol.* 183, 3409–3416. doi: 10.4049/jimmunol.0900879

Meraz-Ríos, M. A., Toral-Rios, D., Franco-Bocanegra, D., Villeda-Hernández, J., and Campos-Peña, V. (2013). Inflammatory process in Alzheimer's disease. *Front. Integr. Neurosci.* 7:59. doi: 10.3389/fnint.2013.00059

Mitchell, D. A., Pickering, M. C., Warren, J., Fossati-Jimack, L., Cortes-Hernandez, J., Cook, H. T., et al. (2002). C1q deficiency and autoimmunity: the effects of genetic background on disease expression. *J. Immunol.* 168, 2538–2543. doi: 10.4049/jimmunol.168.5.2538

Mocco, J., Mack, W. J., Ducruet, A. F., Sosunov, S. A., Sughrue, M. E., Hassid, B. G., et al. (2006a). Complement component C3 mediates inflammatory injury following focal cerebral ischemia. *Circ. Res.* 99, 209–217. doi: 10.1161/01.res.0000232544.90675.42

Mocco, J., Wilson, D. A., Komotar, R. J., Sughrue, M. E., Coates, K., Sacco, R. L., et al. (2006b). Alterations in plasma complement levels after human ischemic stroke. *Neurosurgery* 59, 28–33; discussion 28–33. doi: 10.1227/01.neu.0000219221.14280.65

Møller-Kristensen, M., Wang, W., Ruseva, M., Thiel, S., Nielsen, S., Takahashi, K., et al. (2005). Mannan-binding lectin recognizes structures on ischaemic reperfused mouse kidneys and is implicated in tissue injury. *Scand. J. Immunol.* 61, 426–434. doi: 10.1111/j.1365-3083.2005.01591.x

Monsinjon, T., Gasque, P., Chan, P., Ischenko, A., Brady, J. J., and Fontaine, M. C. (2003). Regulation by complement C3a and C5a anaphylatoxins of cytokine production in human umbilical vein endothelial cells. *FASEB J.* 17, 1003–1014. doi: 10.1096/fj.02-0737com

More, S. V., Kumar, H., Kim, I. S., Song, S.-Y., and Choi, D.-K. (2013). Cellular and molecular mediators of neuroinflammation in the pathogenesis of Parkinson's disease. *Mediators Inflamm.* 2013:952375. doi: 10.1155/2013/952375

Morgan, B. P. (1990). *Complement: Clinical Aspects and Relevance to Disease.* UK: Academic Press.

Morgan, B. P., and Gasque, P. (1997). Extrahepatic complement biosynthesis: where, when and why? *Clin. Exp. Immunol.* 107, 1–7. doi: 10.1046/j.1365-2249.1997.d01-890.x

Neher, J. J., Neniskyte, U., and Brown, G. C. (2012). Primary phagocytosis of neurons by inflamed microglia: potential roles in neurodegeneration. *Front. Pharmacol.* 3:27. doi: 10.3389/fphar.2012.00027

Neher, J. J., Neniskyte, U., Zhao, J.-W., Bal-Price, A., Tolkovsky, A. M., and Brown, G. C. (2011). Inhibition of microglial phagocytosis is sufficient to prevent inflammatory neuronal death. *J. Immunol.* 186, 4973–4983. doi: 10.4049/jimmunol.1003600

Nesargikar, P. N., Spiller, B., and Chavez, R. (2012). The complement system: history, pathways, cascade and inhibitors. *Eur. J. Microbiol. Immunol. (Bp)* 2, 103–111. doi: 10.1556/EuJMI.2.2012.2.2

O'Barr, S. A., Caguioa, J., Gruol, D., Perkins, G., Ember, J. A., Hugli, T., et al. (2001). Neuronal expression of a functional receptor for the C5a complement activation fragment. *J. Immunol.* 166, 4154–4162. doi: 10.4049/jimmunol.166.6.4154

Oroszlán, M., Daha, M. R., Cervenak, L., Prohászka, Z., Füst, G., and Roos, A. (2007). MBL and C1q compete for interaction with human endothelial cells. *Mol. Immunol.* 44, 1150–1158. doi: 10.1016/j.molimm.2006.06.015

Orsini, F., Villa, P., Parrella, S., Zangari, R., Zanier, E. R., Gesuete, R., et al. (2012). Targeting mannose-binding lectin confers long-lasting protection with a surprisingly wide therapeutic window in cerebral ischemia. *Circulation* 126, 1484–1494. doi: 10.1161/CIRCULATIONAHA.112.103051

Osthoff, M., Katan, M., Fluri, F., Schuetz, P., Bingisser, R., Kappos, L., et al. (2011). Mannose-binding lectin deficiency is associated with smaller infarction size and favorable outcome in ischemic stroke patients. *PLoS One* 6:e21338. doi: 10.1371/journal.pone.0021338

Patterson, P. H. (2011). Maternal infection and immune involvement in autism. *Trends Mol. Med.* 17, 389–394. doi: 10.1016/j.molmed.2011.03.001

Pavlov, V. I., Skjoedt, M.-O., Siow Tan, Y., Rosbjerg, A., Garred, P., and Stahl, G. L. (2012). Endogenous and natural complement inhibitor attenuates myocardial injury and arterial thrombogenesis. *Circulation* 126, 2227–2235. doi: 10.1161/CIRCULATIONAHA.112.123968

Pavlovski, D., Thundyil, J., Monk, P. N., Wetsel, R. A., Taylor, S. M., and Woodruff, T. M. (2012). Generation of complement component C5a by ischemic neurons promotes neuronal apoptosis. *FASEB J.* 26, 3680–3690. doi: 10.1096/fj.11-202382

Pedersen, E. D., Løberg, E. M., Vege, E., Daha, M. R., Maehlen, J., and Mollnes, T. E. (2009). In situ deposition of complement in human acute brain ischaemia. *Scand. J. Immunol.* 69, 555–562. doi: 10.1111/j.1365-3083.2009.02253.x

Pedersen, E. D., Waje-Andreassen, U., Vedeler, C. A., Aamodt, G., and Mollnes, T. E. (2004). Systemic complement activation following human acute ischaemic stroke. *Clin. Exp. Immunol.* 137, 117–122. doi: 10.1111/j.1365-2249.2004.02489.x

Pisalyaput, K., and Tenner, A. J. (2008). Complement component C1q inhibits beta-amyloid- and serum amyloid P-induced neurotoxicity via caspase- and calpain-independent mechanisms. *J. Neurochem.* 104, 696–707. doi: 10.1111/j.1471-4159.2007.05012.x

Rahpeymai, Y., Hietala, M. A., Wilhelmsson, U., Fotheringham, A., Davies, I., Nilsson, A.-K., et al. (2006). Complement: a novel factor in basal and ischemia-induced neurogenesis. *EMBO J.* 25, 1364–1374. doi: 10.1038/sj.emboj.7601004

Rancan, M., Morganti-Kossmann, M. C., Barnum, S. R., Saft, S., Schmidt, O. I., Ertel, W., et al. (2003). Central nervous system-targeted complement inhibition mediates neuroprotection after closed head injury in transgenic mice. *J. Cereb. Blood Flow Metab.* 23, 1070–1074. doi: 10.1097/01.wcb.0000084250.20114.2c

Reichwald, J., Danner, S., Wiederhold, K.-H., and Staufenbiel, M. (2009). Expression of complement system components during aging and amyloid deposition in APP transgenic mice. *J. Neuroinflammation* 6:35. doi: 10.1186/1742-2094-6-35

Ricklin, D., Hajishengallis, G., Yang, K., and Lambris, J. D. (2010). Complement: a key system for immune surveillance and homeostasis. *Nat. Immunol.* 11, 785–797. doi: 10.1038/ni.1923

Ricklin, D., and Lambris, J. D. (2007). Complement-targeted therapeutics. *Nat. Biotechnol.* 25, 1265–1275. doi: 10.1038/nbt1342

Rogers, J., Cooper, N. R., Webster, S., Schultz, J., McGeer, P. L., Styren, S. D., et al. (1992). Complement activation by beta-amyloid in Alzheimer disease. *Proc. Natl. Acad. Sci. U S A* 89, 10016–10020. doi: 10.1073/pnas.89.21.10016

Rutkowski, M. J., Sughrue, M. E., Kane, A. J., Ahn, B. J., Fang, S., and Parsa, A. T. (2010). The complement cascade as a mediator of tissue growth and regeneration. *Inflamm. Res.* 59, 897–905. doi: 10.1007/s00011-010-0220-6

Savill, J., Dransfield, I., Gregory, C., and Haslett, C. (2002). A blast from the past: clearance of apoptotic cells regulates immune responses. *Nat. Rev. Immunol.* 2, 965–975. doi: 10.1038/nri957

Schafer, D. P., Lehrman, E. K., Kautzman, A. G., Koyama, R., Mardinly, A. R., Yamasaki, R., et al. (2012). Microglia sculpt postnatal neural circuits in an activity and complement-dependent manner. *Neuron* 74, 691–705. doi: 10.1016/j.neuron.2012.03.026

Schäfer, M. K., Schwaeble, W. J., Post, C., Salvati, P., Calabresi, M., Sim, R. B., et al. (2000). Complement C1q is dramatically up-regulated in brain microglia in response to transient global cerebral ischemia. *J. Immunol.* 164, 5446–5452. doi: 10.4049/jimmunol.164.10.5446

Schraufstatter, I. U., Trieu, K., Sikora, L., Sriramarao, P., and DiScipio, R. (2002). Complement c3a and c5a induce different signal transduction cascades in endothelial cells. *J. Immunol.* 169, 2102–2110. doi: 10.4049/jimmunol.169.4.2102

Sewell, D. L., Nacewicz, B., Liu, F., Macvilay, S., Erdei, A., Lambris, J. D., et al. (2004). Complement C3 and C5 play critical roles in traumatic brain cryoinjury: blocking effects on neutrophil extravasation by C5a receptor antagonist. *J. Neuroimmunol.* 155, 55–63. doi: 10.1016/j.jneuroim.2004.06.003

Shen, Y., Lue, L., Yang, L., Roher, A., Kuo, Y., Strohmeyer, R., et al. (2001). Complement activation by neurofibrillary tangles in Alzheimer's disease. *Neurosci. Lett.* 305, 165–168. doi: 10.1016/s0304-3940(01)01842-0

Shinjyo, N., Ståhlberg, A., Dragunow, M., Pekny, M., and Pekna, M. (2009). Complement-derived anaphylatoxin C3a regulates in vitro differentiation and migration of neural progenitor cells. *Stem Cells* 27, 2824–2832. doi: 10.1002/stem.225

Singhrao, S. K., Neal, J. W., Rushmere, N. K., Morgan, B. P., and Gasque, P. (2000). Spontaneous classical pathway activation and deficiency of membrane regulators render human neurons susceptible to complement lysis. *Am. J. Pathol.* 157, 905–918. doi: 10.1016/s0002-9440(10)64604-4

Sjölander, A., Minthon, L., Nuytinck, L., Vanmechelen, E., Blennow, K., and Nilsson, S. (2013). Functional mannose-binding lectin haplotype variants are associated with Alzheimer's disease. *J. Alzheimers Dis.* 35, 121–127. doi: 10.3233/JAD-122044

Sta, M., Sylva-Steenland, R. M. R., Casula, M., de Jong, J. M. B. V., Troost, D., Aronica, E., et al. (2011). Innate and adaptive immunity in amyotrophic lateral sclerosis: evidence of complement activation. *Neurobiol. Dis.* 42, 211–220. doi: 10.1016/j.nbd.2011.01.002

Stahel, P. F., Flierl, M. A., Morgan, B. P., Persigehl, I., Stoll, C., Conrad, C., et al. (2009). Absence of the complement regulatory molecule CD59a leads to exacerbated neuropathology after traumatic brain injury in mice. *J. Neuroinflammation* 6:2. doi: 10.1186/1742-2094-6-2

Stahel, P. F., Morganti-Kossmann, M. C., Perez, D., Redaelli, C., Gloor, B., Trentz, O., et al. (2001). Intrathecal levels of complement-derived soluble membrane attack complex (sC5b-9) correlate with blood-brain barrier dysfunction in patients with traumatic brain injury. *J. Neurotrauma* 18, 773–781. doi: 10.1089/089771501316919139

Stephan, A. H., Barres, B. A., and Stevens, B. (2012). The complement system: an unexpected role in synaptic pruning during development and disease. *Annu. Rev. Neurosci.* 35, 369–389. doi: 10.1146/annurev-neuro-061010-113810

Stephan, A. H., Madison, D. V., Mateos, J. M., Fraser, D. A., Lovelett, E. A., Coutellier, L., et al. (2013). A dramatic increase of C1q protein in the CNS during normal aging. *J. Neurosci.* 33, 13460–13474. doi: 10.1523/JNEUROSCI.1333-13.2013

Stevens, B., Allen, N. J., Vazquez, L. E., Howell, G. R., Christopherson, K. S., Nouri, N., et al. (2007). The classical complement cascade mediates CNS synapse elimination. *Cell* 131, 1164–1178. doi: 10.1016/j.cell.2007.10.036

Stokowska, A., Olsson, S., Holmegaard, L., Jood, K., Blomstrand, C., Jern, C., et al. (2013). Cardioembolic and small vessel disease stroke show differences in associations between systemic C3 levels and outcome. *PLoS One* 8:e72133. doi: 10.1371/journal.pone.0072133

Stoltzner, S. E., Grenfell, T. J., Mori, C., Wisniewski, K. E., Wisniewski, T. M., Selkoe, D. J., et al. (2000). Temporal accrual of complement proteins in amyloid plaques in down's syndrome with Alzheimer's disease. *Am. J. Pathol.* 156, 489–499. doi: 10.1016/S0002-9440(10)64753-0

Storini, C., Rossi, E., Marrella, V., Distaso, M., Veerhuis, R., Vergani, C., et al. (2005). C1-inhibitor protects against brain ischemia-reperfusion injury via inhibition of cell recruitment and inflammation. *Neurobiol. Dis.* 19, 10–17. doi: 10.1016/j.nbd.2004.11.001

Széplaki, G., Szegedi, R., Hirschberg, K., Gombos, T., Varga, L., Karádi, I., et al. (2009). Strong complement activation after acute ischemic stroke is associated with unfavorable outcomes. *Atherosclerosis* 204, 315–320. doi: 10.1016/j.atherosclerosis.2008.07.044

Takeuchi, S., Fujiwara, N., Ido, A., Oono, M., Takeuchi, Y., Tateno, M., et al. (2010). Induction of protective immunity by vaccination with wild-type apo superoxide dismutase 1 in mutant SOD1 transgenic mice. *J. Neuropathol. Exp. Neurol.* 69, 1044–1056. doi: 10.1097/NEN.0B013e3181f4a90a

Tedesco, F., Pausa, M., Nardon, E., Introna, M., Mantovani, A., and Dobrina, A. (1997). The cytolytically inactive terminal complement complex activates endothelial cells to express adhesion molecules and tissue factor procoagulant activity. *J. Exp. Med.* 185, 1619–1627. doi: 10.1084/jem.185.9.1619

Ten, V. S., Sosunov, S. A., Mazer, S. P., Stark, R. I., Caspersen, C., Sughrue, M. E., et al. (2005). C1q-deficiency is neuroprotective against hypoxic-ischemic brain injury in neonatal mice. *Stroke* 36, 2244–2250. doi: 10.1161/01.str.0000182237.20807.d0

Tsuboi, Y., and Yamada, T. (1994). Increased concentration of C4d complement protein in CSF in amyotrophic lateral sclerosis. *J. Neurol. Neurosurg. Psychiatry* 57, 859–861. doi: 10.1136/jnnp.57.7.859

Van Beek, J., Bernaudin, M., Petit, E., Gasque, P., Nouvelot, A., MacKenzie, E. T., et al. (2000). Expression of receptors for complement anaphylatoxins C3a and C5a following permanent focal cerebral ischemia in the mouse. *Exp. Neurol.* 161, 373–382. doi: 10.1006/exnr.1999.7273

van den Berg, R. H., Faber-Krol, M. C., Sim, R. B., and Daha, M. R. (1998). The first subcomponent of complement, C1q, triggers the production of IL-8, IL-6 and monocyte chemoattractant peptide-1 by human umbilical vein endothelial cells. *J. Immunol.* 161, 6924–6930.

Vasthare, U. S., Barone, F. C., Sarau, H. M., Rosenwasser, R. H., DiMartino, M., Young, W. F., et al. (1998). Complement depletion improves neurological function in cerebral ischemia. *Brain Res. Bull.* 45, 413–419. doi: 10.1016/s0361-9230(97)00408-5

Veerhuis, R., Nielsen, H. M., and Tenner, A. J. (2011). Complement in the brain. *Mol. Immunol.* 48, 1592–1603. doi: 10.1016/j.molimm.2011.04.003

Veerhuis, R., Van Breemen, M. J., Hoozemans, J. M., Morbin, M., Ouladhadj, J., Tagliavini, F., et al. (2003). Amyloid beta plaque-associated proteins C1q and SAP enhance the Abeta1–42 peptide-induced cytokine secretion by adult human microglia in vitro. *Acta Neuropathol.* 105, 135–144. doi: 10.1007/s00401-002-0624-7

Wagner, E., and Frank, M. M. (2010). Therapeutic potential of complement modulation. *Nat. Rev. Drug Discov.* 9, 43–56. doi: 10.1038/nrd3011

Wang, Y., Hancock, A. M., Bradner, J., Chung, K. A., Quinn, J. F., Peskind, E. R., et al. (2011). Complement 3 and factor h in human cerebrospinal fluid in Parkinson's disease, Alzheimer's disease and multiple-system atrophy. *Am. J. Pathol.* 178, 1509–1516. doi: 10.1016/j.ajpath.2011.01.006

Wang, Y., Li, Y., Dalle Lucca, S. L., Simovic, M., Tsokos, G. C., and Dalle Lucca, J. J. (2010). Decay accelerating factor (CD55) protects neuronal cells from chemical hypoxia-induced injury. *J. Neuroinflammation* 7:24. doi: 10.1186/1742-2094-7-24

Webster, S. D., Galvan, M. D., Ferran, E., Garzon-Rodriguez, W., Glabe, C. G., and Tenner, A. J. (2001). Antibody-mediated phagocytosis of the amyloid beta-peptide in microglia is differentially modulated by C1q. *J. Immunol.* 166, 7496–7503. doi: 10.4049/jimmunol.166.12.7496

Woodruff, T. M., Ager, R. R., Tenner, A. J., Noakes, P. G., and Taylor, S. M. (2010). The role of the complement system and the activation fragment C5a in the central nervous system. *Neuromolecular Med.* 12, 179–192. doi: 10.1007/s12017-009-8085-y

Woodruff, T. M., Costantini, K. J., Crane, J. W., Atkin, J. D., Monk, P. N., Taylor, S. M., et al. (2008). The complement factor C5a contributes to pathology in a rat model of amyotrophic lateral sclerosis. *J. Immunol.* 181, 8727–8734. doi: 10.4049/jimmunol.181.12.8727

Wyss-Coray, T., Yan, F., Lin, A. H.-T., Lambris, J. D., Alexander, J. J., Quigg, R. J., et al. (2002). Prominent neurodegeneration and increased plaque formation in complement-inhibited Alzheimer's mice. *Proc. Natl. Acad. Sci. U S A* 99, 10837–10842. doi: 10.1073/pnas.162350199

Yager, P. H., You, Z., Qin, T., Kim, H.-H., Takahashi, K., Ezekowitz, A. B., et al. (2008). Mannose binding lectin gene deficiency increases susceptibility to traumatic brain injury in mice. *J. Cereb. Blood Flow Metab.* 28, 1030–1039. doi: 10.1038/sj.jcbfm.9600605

Yao, J., Harvath, L., Gilbert, D. L., and Colton, C. A. (1990). Chemotaxis by a CNS macrophage, the microglia. *J. Neurosci. Res.* 27, 36–42. doi: 10.1002/jnr.490270106

Yasojima, K., Schwab, C., McGeer, E. G., and McGeer, P. L. (1999). Up-regulated production and activation of the complement system in Alzheimer's disease brain. *Am. J. Pathol.* 154, 927–936. doi: 10.1016/s0002-9440(10)65340-0

Yin, W., Ghebrehiwet, B., Weksler, B., and Peerschke, E. I. (2007). Classical pathway complement activation on human endothelial cells. *Mol. Immunol.* 44, 2228–2234. doi: 10.1016/j.molimm.2006.11.012

You, Z., Yang, J., Takahashi, K., Yager, P. H., Kim, H.-H., Qin, T., et al. (2007). Reduced tissue damage and improved recovery of motor function after traumatic brain injury in mice deficient in complement component C4. *J. Cereb. Blood Flow Metab.* 27, 1954–1964. doi: 10.1038/sj.jcbfm.9600497

Zanier, E. R., Zangari, R., Munthe-Fog, L., Hein, E., Zoerle, T., Conte, V., et al. (2014). Ficolin-3-mediated lectin complement pathway activation in patients with subarachnoid hemorrhage. *Neurology* 82, 126–134. doi: 10.1212/WNL.0000000000000020

Zanjani, H., Finch, C. E., Kemper, C., Atkinson, J., McKeel, D., Morris, J. C., et al. (2005). Complement activation in very early Alzheimer disease. *Alzheimer Dis. Assoc. Disord.* 19, 55–66. doi: 10.1097/01.wad.0000165506.60370.94

Zhou, J., Fonseca, M. I., Pisalyaput, K., and Tenner, A. J. (2008). Complement C3 and C4 expression in C1q sufficient and deficient mouse models of Alzheimer's disease. *J. Neurochem.* 106, 2080–2092. doi: 10.1111/j.1471-4159.2008.05558.x

Ziccardi, R. J. (1981). Activation of the early components of the classical complement pathway under physiologic conditions. *J. Immunol.* 126, 1769–1773.

8

Different immunological mechanisms govern protection from experimental stroke in young and older mice with recombinant TCR ligand therapy

Abby L. Dotson[1,2†], Wenbin Zhu[3†], Nicole Libal[3], Nabil J. Alkayed[2,3,4] and Halina Offner[1,2,3]*

[1] Neuroimmunology Research, VA Medical Center, Portland, OR, USA
[2] Department of Neurology, Oregon Health and Science University, Portland, OR, USA
[3] Department of Anesthesiology and Perioperative Medicine, Oregon Health and Science University, Portland, OR, USA
[4] Knight Cardiovascular Institute, Oregon Health and Science University, Portland, OR, USA

***Correspondence:**
Halina Offner, Neuroimmunology Research, R&D-31, Portland Veterans Affairs Medical Center, 3710 SW US Veterans Hospital Rd., Portland, OR 97239, USA
e-mail: offnerva@ohsu.edu

† These authors have contributed equally to this work.

Stroke is a leading cause of death and disability in the United States. The lack of clinical success in stroke therapies can be attributed, in part, to inadequate basic research on aging rodents. The current study demonstrates that recombinant TCR ligand therapy uses different immunological mechanisms to protect young and older mice from experimental stroke. In young mice, RTL1000 therapy inhibited splenocyte efflux while reducing frequency of T cells and macrophages in the spleen. Older mice treated with RTL1000 exhibited a significant reduction in inflammatory cells in the brain and inhibition of splenic atrophy. Our data suggest age specific differences in immune response to stroke that allow unique targeting of stroke immunotherapies.

Keywords: experimental stroke, aging, RTL1000, therapy, immune response, neuroinflammation

INTRODUCTION

Stroke is a leading cause of death and disability in the United States. It is now increasingly evident that the immune response plays an important role in neurodegeneration following stroke. Splenic activation after stroke leads to an efflux of immune cells into the blood that subsequently target the brain, activate microglial cells and exacerbate the evolving brain infarct (Offner et al., 2006a,b; Seifert et al., 2012a,b). T cells are thought to be among the major contributors in post-ischemic immune response. T cells infiltrate the brain, perpetuate inflammatory conditions and contribute to increased neuronal damage following stroke (Shichita et al., 2009; Gronberg et al., 2013). Additionally, T cell knockout mice exhibit reduced infarct volume (Yilmaz et al., 2006).

Given their significant involvement in the pathogenesis of stroke, T cells are a crucial target for stroke therapy. Recombinant T-cell receptor ligand (RTL) molecules consist of the $\alpha1$ and $\beta1$ domains of MHC class II molecules expressed as a single polypeptide with or without antigenic amino terminal extensions (Burrows et al., 1999; Vandenbark et al., 2003). RTLs are partial agonists that deviate autoreactive T cells to become non-pathogenic (Burrows et al., 2001; Wang et al., 2003). Previous work done by our lab has shown that RTL could treat both experimental autoimmune encephalomyelitis (EAE) and experimental stroke in mice (Burrows et al., 1998, 2001; Vandenbark et al., 2003; Huan et al., 2004; Subramanian et al., 2009; Akiyoshi et al., 2011; Dziennis et al., 2011; Benedek et al., 2014). RTL1000 is comprised of an HLA-DR2 moiety linked to human MOG-35-55 peptide (Offner et al., 2011) and has been shown to reduce infarct size when young humanized DR2 mice were treated following experimental stroke (Akiyoshi et al., 2011; Pan et al., 2014; Zhu et al., 2014).

With the potential success of RTL as a stroke therapy it becomes imperative to not only characterize the effects of RTL on the inflammatory response following stroke but to also test the RTL therapy in older mice during experimental stroke. The increased risk for stroke with age along with the substantially growing aging population will lead to an additional 3.4 million people affected by stroke by the year 2030 compared to 2012 (Ovbiagele et al., 2013). Despite the unavoidable and increasing financial burden of post-stroke care, many experimental stroke therapies have been abandoned due to their failure in the clinical setting (O'Collins et al., 2006). The inability of stroke therapy to be translated from bench to clinical success can be attributed, in part, to the lack of aging rodents used in basic research (Liu and McCullough, 2011). By examining the effects of RTL therapy on experimental stroke in both young and older mice we can more accurately determine the mechanism of therapy and predict its translation to clinical use.

Abbreviations: RTL, recombinant T-cell receptor ligand; MCAO, middle cerebral artery occlusion; Treg, regulatory T cell; MHC, Major Histocompatibility Complex; HLA, Human leukocyte antigen; MOG, myelin oligodendrocyte glycoprotein; LDF, Laser Doppler flowmetry; PHA, Phytohemagglutinin; PMA, Phorbol myristate acetate.

MATERIALS AND METHODS

ETHICS STATEMENT

The study was conducted in accordance with National Institutes of Health guidelines for the use of experimental animals, and the protocols were approved by Animal Care and Use Committee at Oregon Health & Science University and the Portland Veteran Affairs Medical Center.

ANIMALS

All experiments used age-matched, sexually mature (20–25 g) male HLA-DRB1*1502 (DR2-Tg) mice produced by Dr. Chella David (Gonzalez-Gay et al., 1996). The mice were housed and bred at the Veterans Affairs Medical Center and studies were conducted at Oregon Health and Science University.

RTL1000 CONSTRUCTION AND PRODUCTION

RTL molecules consist of the $\alpha 1$ and $\beta 1$ domains of major histocompatibility complex (MHC) II molecules and are expressed as a single polypeptide with or without antigenic amino terminal extensions (Burrows et al., 1999). RTL1000 ($\beta 1 \alpha 1$[5D substituted] domains of HLA-DR2 linked to human [h]MOG-35-55 peptide [MEVGWYRPPFSRVVHLYRNGK]) was constructed de novo or by sequential site-directed mutagenesis of previous constructs (Sinha et al., 2007). Protein purification was carried out as previously described (Burrows et al., 1999).

TREATMENT WITH RTL1000

Mice were randomized to receive 0.1 mL (100 μg) RTL1000 or 0.1 mL vehicle (5% dextrose in Tris-HCl, pH 8.5) by subcutaneous injection 4 h after the onset of reperfusion followed by doses at 24, 48, and 72 h of reperfusion for a total of four treatments each of RTL1000 or Vehicle. Both RTL1000 and vehicle treated mice were euthanized at the 96 h time-point after MCAO for further examination of tissues and cells.

TRANSIENT MIDDLE CEREBRAL ARTERY OCCLUSION

Transient focal cerebral ischemia was induced in male DR2-Tg mice for 1 h by reversible right MCAO under isoflurane anesthesia followed by 96 h of reperfusion as described previously (Zhang et al., 2008). Head and body temperature were controlled at 36.5 ± 0.5°C throughout MCAO surgery with warm water pads and a heating lamp. Occlusion and reperfusion were verified in each animal by laser Doppler flowmetry (LDF) (Model DRT4, Moor Instruments Ltd., Oxford, England). The common carotid artery was exposed and the external carotid artery was ligated and cauterized. Unilateral MCAO was accomplished by inserting a 6-0 nylon monofilament surgical suture (ETHICON, Inc., Somerville, NJ, USA) with a heat-rounded and silicone-coated (Xantopren comfort light, Heraeus, Germany) tip into the internal carotid artery via the external carotid artery stump. Adequacy of MCAO was confirmed by monitoring cortical blood flow at the onset of the occlusion with a LDF probe affixed to the skull. Animals were excluded if mean intra-ischemic LDF was greater than 30% pre-ischemic baseline. At 1 h of occlusion, the occluding filament was withdrawn to allow for reperfusion. Mice were then allowed to recover from anesthesia and survived for 96 h following initiation of reperfusion.

DETERMINATION OF INFARCT SIZE

The brains were harvested after 96 h of reperfusion and sliced into four 2-mm-thick coronal sections for staining with 1.2% 2,3,5-triphenyltetrazolium chloride (TTC; Sigma, St. Louis, MO, USA) in saline as described previously (Hurn et al., 2007). The 2-mm brain sections were incubated in 1.2% TTC for 15 min at 37°C, and then fixed in 10% formalin for 24 h. Infarction volume was measured using digital imaging and image analysis software (Systat, Inc., Point Richmond, CA, USA). To control for edema, infarct volume (cortex, striatum, and hemisphere) was determined by subtraction of the ipsilateral non-infarcted regional volume from the contralateral regional volume. This value was then divided by the contralateral regional volume and multiplied by 100 to yield regional infarction volume as a percent of the contralateral region.

LEUKOCYTE ISOLATION FROM BRAIN AND SPLEEN

Spleens from individual MCAO-treated mice were removed and a single-cell suspension was prepared by passing the tissue through a 100 μm nylon mesh (BD Falcon, Bedford, MA). The cells were washed using RPMI 1640 and the red blood cells lysed using 1× red blood cell lysis buffer (eBioscience, Inc., San Diego, CA) and incubated for 1 min. The cells were then washed with RPMI 1640, counted on a Cellometer Auto T4 cell counter (Nexcelom, Lawrence, MA), and resuspended in staining medium [PBS containing 0.1% NaN3 and 1% bovine serum albumin (Sigma, IL)] for flow cytometry. The brain was divided into the ischemic (right) and non-ischemic (left) hemispheres, digested for 60 min with 1 mg/ml Type IV collagenase (Sigma Aldrich, St. Louis, MO) and DNase I (50 mg/ml, Roche Diagnostics, Indianapolis, IN) at 37°C with intermittent shaking. Samples were mixed with a 1 ml pipette every 15 min. The suspension was washed 1× in RPMI, resuspended in 80% Percoll overlayed with 40% Percoll, and centrifuged for 30 min at 1600 RPM. The cells were then washed twice with RPMI 1640 and resuspended in staining medium for flow cytometry.

ANALYSIS OF CELL POPULATIONS BY FLOW CYTOMETRY

All antibodies were purchased (BD Biosciences, San Jose, CA or eBioscience, Inc., San Diego, CA) as published. Four-color (FITC, PE, APC, and PerCP) fluorescence flow cytometry analyses were performed to determine the phenotypes of splenocytes and brain cells. One million cells were washed with staining medium, blocked with Anti-mouse CD16/CD32 Mouse BD Fc Block™ (BD Biosciences, San Jose) for 15 min at 4°C and then incubated with combinations of the following monoclonal antibodies: CD11b (MAC-1), CD45 (Ly-5), CD3 (145-2C11), CD11c (HL-3), CD19 (1D3), CD4 (GK1.5), CD8 (53-6.7), Ly6C (AL-21), Ly6G (RB6-8C5), CD122 (TM-β1), CD44 (IM7), CCR5 (HM-CCR5), and CD69 (H1.2F3) for 20 min at 4°C. 7-AAD was added to identify dead cells. CD4+ regulatory T cells were identified using Foxp3 (FJK-16s) and accompanying Fixation/Permeabilization reagents as per manufacturer's instructions (eBioscience, Inc., San Diego, CA). Isotype matched mAb served as a negative control. Data were collected with BD Accuri™ C6 software on a BD Accuri™ C6 (BD Biosciences, San Jose, CA).

CYTOKINE DETERMINATION BY INTRACELLULAR CYTOKINE FLOW CYTOMETRY ANALYSIS

Splenocytes from individual mice were cultured at 2×10^6 cells/well in a 24-well culture plate in stimulation medium (RPMI, 1% sodium pyruvate, 1% L-glutamine, 0.4% 2-β-mercaptoethanol, 2% FBS) with PMA (50 ng/ml), ionomycin (500 ng/ml), and brefeldin A (1 ul/mL) (all reagents from Sigma-Aldrich, St. Louis, MO) for 4 h. Cells were blocked, surface stained (see Section Analysis of Cell Populations by Flow Cytometry), and then fixed and permeabilized using a Cytofix/Cytoperm kit (BD Biosciences), according to manufacturer's instructions. Fixed cells were washed with 1× permeablization buffer (BD Biosciences) and stained with antibodies to IFNγ, TNFα, IL-10, IL-17, or IL-21. Isotype matched mAbs served as negative controls to establish background cytokine staining levels. Data were collected with BD Accuri™ C6 software on a BD Accuri™ C6 (BD Biosciences, San Jose, CA).

STATISTICAL ANALYSIS

Data are presented as mean ± s.e.m. Differences in cortical, striatal, and total (hemispheric) infarct size data was analyzed by Two-Way ANOVA, with one factor being brain region and the other factor treatment group. Spleen and brain cell counts and percentages of cellular subtypes for FACS analysis were analyzed by Student's t-test. Statistical significance was $p < 0.05$. Statistical analyses were performed using Prism (GraphPad, La Jolla, CA).

RESULTS

RTL1000 REDUCES INFARCT VOLUME IN YOUNG AND OLDER MICE

Eight week HLA-DR2 mice exhibited a significant reduction in infarct volume with RTL compared to vehicle (**Figures 1A,B**). Representative TTC-stained cerebral sections illustrate reduction in infarct in mice that received RTL after MCAO compared to vehicle in young mice (**Figure 1A**). Cortical infarct volume was reduced from 46.4 ± 1.7% to 28 ± 3.7% and striatal infarct volume decreased from 60.1 ± 5.9% to 34.7 ± 6.1% when mice were given RTL following MCAO (**Figure 1B**). Total hemispheric infarct volume was also significantly reduced from 31.8 ± 2.1% to 19.1 ± 2.4% with RTL (**Figure 1B**). Similarly, infarct volume was significantly decreased in 16-month-old mice given RTL compared to vehicle (**Figures 1C,D**). Representative TTC-stained cerebral sections illustrate reduction in infarct in older mice that received RTL after MCAO compared to vehicle (**Figure 1C**). Cortical and striatal infarct volume went from 40.1 ± 1.6% to 20.7 ± 2.8% and 67.5 ± 3.9% to 47.7 ± 4.0% respectively, when RTL was administered after MCAO (**Figure 1D**). Total hemispheric infarct was also significantly reduced from 26.2 ± 1.2% to 16.0 ± 1.3% with RTL (**Figure 1D**). The mortality rate of MCAO in both treatment groups was less in young mice compared to older mice while RTL reduced mortality in older mice only (**Table 1**). Together, these data reveal that RTL1000 improves stroke outcome in both young and older mice.

RTL1000 REDUCES ACTIVATED AND INFILTRATING CELLS IN THE ISCHEMIC HEMISPHERE OF 16 MONTH BUT NOT 8-WEEK-OLD MICE

We wanted to decipher the mechanism of protection with RTL1000 in young and older mice following MCAO by examining brain infiltrating immune and inflammatory cells. Cells were isolated from the ischemic hemisphere 96 h after MCAO, phenotyped and counted (**Table 2**). The percent of activated microglia and/or infiltrating monocytes/macrophages (CD11b+CD45^{hi}) in the ischemic hemisphere after MCAO was reduced in both 8-week- and 16-month-old mice treated with RTL (**Figure 2A**). Absolute number of activated microglia/monocytes was also significantly reduced in the 16-month-old mice that received RTL and there was a trend reduction in young mice that received RTL ($p = 0.068$) (**Figure 2B**). Ischemic hemispheres of 16-month-old mice that received RTL after MCAO also exhibited a significant reduction in absolute CD3+ T cells and CD11c+ dendritic cells compared to vehicle (**Figures 2C,D**). Young mice exhibited a trend reduction in number of T cells in the ischemic hemisphere with RTL ($p = 0.064$) but did not have a significantly reduced number of dendritic cells after treatment with RTL compared to vehicle (**Figures 2C,D**). The number of infiltrating B cells in the ischemic hemisphere following MCAO with or without RTL did not display significance difference in either young or older mice (**Figure 2E**). Additionally, total infiltrating cells and cell death were not affected by RTL treatment in either age group (**Figures 2F,G**). Control (non-ischemic) hemispheres did not exhibit an increase in inflammatory parameters (data not shown). These data suggest that RTL1000 may reduce infarct volume following stroke using different mechanisms between young and older mice.

SPLENIC ATROPHY IS PREVENTED WITH RTL1000

To determine other possible mechanisms of RTL1000 protection following stroke, we examined immune parameters in the periphery. The spleen is known to have a major impact on stroke. Our lab and others have established that splenic atrophy occurs following stroke, releasing splenocytes into systemic circulation and exacerbating neurodegeneration (Offner et al., 2006b; Seifert et al., 2012a). Spleens were harvested 96 h after MCAO and splenocytes were counted and evaluated for viability (**Table 3**). RTL treatment significantly inhibited splenic atrophy in both 8-week- and 16-month-old mice (**Figure 3A**). Splenocyte number correlated inversely with cell death in young mice as determined by 7-AAD staining. Young mice treated with RTL exhibited a significant decrease in splenocyte death compared to vehicle while older mice showed no change in 7-AAD positive cells between the treatments (**Figure 3B**).

RTL1000 PRIMARILY AFFECTS PERIPHERAL IMMUNE SUBSETS IN YOUNGER MICE

We also characterized immune cell phenotypes within the spleens of young and old mice, with and without RTL treatment following MCAO (**Table 4**). We found a significant reduction in the frequency of CD4+ T cells with RTL treatment in both young and old mice (**Figure 4A**). RTL treatment also significantly reduced the percent of CD8+ T cells, CD3+ total T cells, and CD11b+ myeloid cells in young mice only (**Figures 4B–D**). Furthermore, only the Ly6C+, not Ly6G+, subset of CD11b cells were reduced with RTL in young mice indicating that the reduction of total CD11b cells was due to a reduction in monocytes/macrophages not CD11b+ neutrophils (**Figure 4E**, **Table 4**). The percent of CD19+ B cells in the spleens of young RTL treated mice following

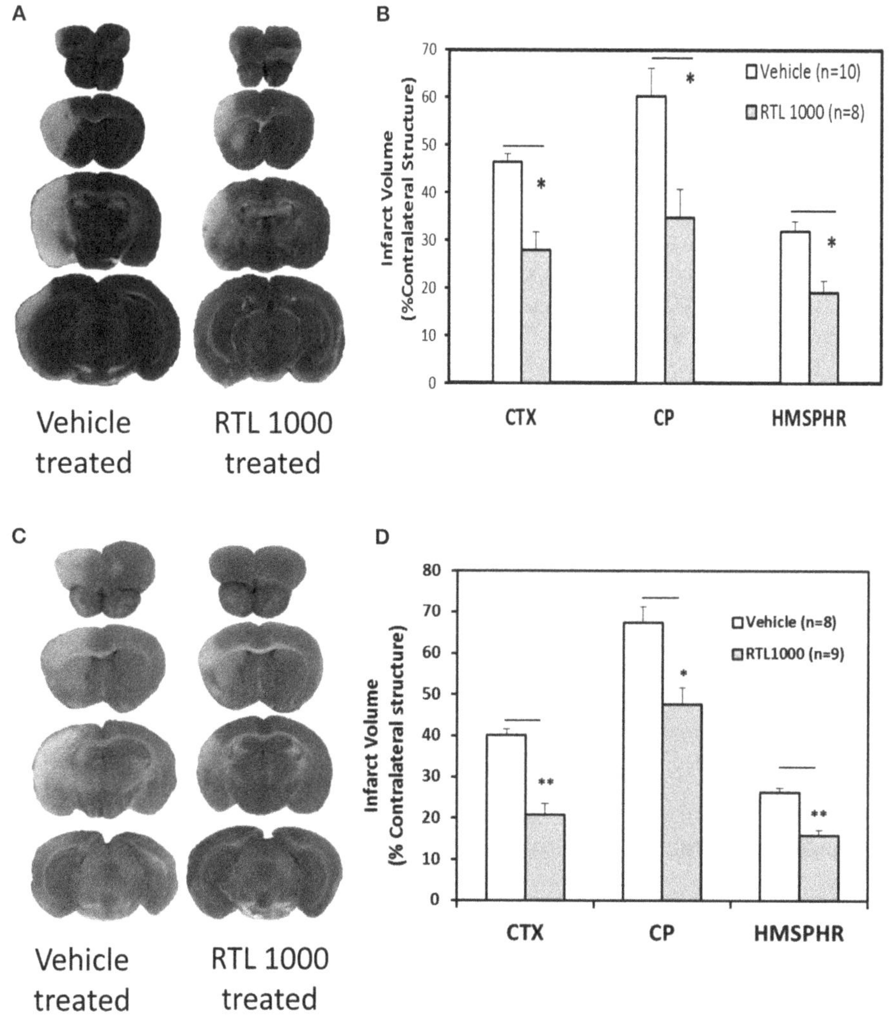

FIGURE 1 | RTL1000 reduces infarct volume in young and older mice. Transient MCAO (60 min) male mice were treated with 100 μl vehicle or 100 μg RTL1000 given S.C. at 4, 24, 48, and 72 h after MCAO. Brains were harvested 96 h after MCAO and brain slices were stained with 2,3,5-triphenyltetrazolium chloride (TTC) **(A,C)**. Infarct volumes were measured as percentage of contralateral structure in young **(B)** and older mice **(D)**. * Indicates $p < 0.05$ and ** indicates $p < 0.01$ compared with vehicle group by Two-Way ANOVA.

Table 1 | Mortality and success rate of MCAO.

	Animal numbers underwent MCAO	Number of animals died after MCAO	Number of animals excluded for SAH	Number of animals excluded for other reasons	Final animal numbers
Vehicle (8 week)	13	3 (23%)	0	0	10
RTL1000 (8 week)	12	3 (25%)	0	1 (Massive cerebral hemorrhage)	8
Vehicle (16 month)	18	8 (44.4%)	2	0	8
RTL1000 (16 month)	15	5 (33.3%)	0	1 (LDF > 30%)	9

MCAO was significantly greater compared to vehicle (**Figure 4F**). Collectively, in young mice RTL treatment reduces the percent of T cells and monocytes/macrophages, both of which are known to contribute to neurodegeneration following stroke (Campanella et al., 2002; Yilmaz et al., 2006), while increasing potentially protective B cells (Bodhankar et al., 2014). The data also demonstrate that RTL significantly impacts multiple subsets of splenocytes in young mice while having much less impact on the splenocytes of older mice after MCAO, supporting the hypothesis that RTL1000 targets different immune pathways in younger and older mice.

PERIPHERAL IMMUNE PROPERTIES CHANGE WITH AGE FOLLOWING STROKE

In addition to the differential effects of RTL on immune subsets after MCAO between the age groups, we also observed baseline immunological discrepancies in the periphery of young and

Table 2 | Ischemic (right) hemisphere.

Cell type	8-week-old mice		16-month-old mice	
	Vehicle	RTL1000	Vehicle	RTL1000
Total cell number	$3.4 \times 10^5 \pm 7.4 \times 10^4$	$2.7 \times 10^5 \pm 3.0 \times 10^4$	$6.0 \times 10^5 \pm 8.6 \times 10^{4\#}$	$5.4 \times 10^5 \pm 6.3 \times 10^{4\#}$
7AAD+	$2.4 \times 10^4 \pm 3451$	$2.0 \times 10^4 \pm 2671$	$3.8 \times 10^4 \pm 3395^{\#}$	$2.7 \times 10^4 \pm 3674$
CD11b+ CD45^{hi}	$6.9 \times 10^4 \pm 1.5 \times 104$	$3.3 \times 10^4 \pm 5135$	$6.4 \times 10^4 \pm 8554$	$1.7 \times 10^4 \pm 5891^{**}$
CD3+ T cells	2769 ± 591	1375 ± 107	3109 ± 624	$1188 \pm 457^{*}$
CD11c+ DC	$4.1 \times 10^4 \pm 9840$	$2.6 \times 10^4 \pm 6420$	$2.6 \times 10^4 \pm 5916$	$5073 \pm 1017^{*\#}$
CD19+ B cells	6149 ± 1526	3754 ± 734	7471 ± 719	5679 ± 508

** indicates significance compare to vehicle $^{*}p \leq 0.05$; $^{**}p \leq 0.01$.*
\# indicates significance compared to 8-week-old mice $^{\#}p \leq 0.05$.

older mice. The frequency of CD3+ total T cells and CD4+ helper T cells were significantly greater in 8-week-old vehicle and RTL treated mice following MCAO than in 16-month-old vehicle and RTL treated mice, respectively (**Figures 4A,C**). CD8+ T cells were significantly greater in younger MCAO vehicle mice compared older MCAO vehicle mice (**Figure 4B**). Total CD11b cells and CD11b+Ly6C+ monocyte/macrophage subset were both significantly higher in the spleens of young mice that received vehicle after MCAO vs. their older counterparts (**Figures 4D,E**). Additionally, the frequency of CD19+ B cells was significantly less in the spleen following MCAO in both vehicle and RTL treated younger mice than older mice. Innate differences in the peripheral immune composition between 8-week- and 16-month-old mice following MCAO may give insight into the different possible targets of RTL1000 following stroke.

SPLENIC CD4+ REGULATORY T CELLS INCREASE WITH AGE IN MCAO MICE WHILE CD8+ REGULATORY T CELLS ARE INCREASED BY RTL1000 TREATMENT

CD4+ regulatory T cells are upregulated following stroke (Offner et al., 2006b) and CD8+ regulatory T cells are known to suppress CD4+ and CD8+ T cell proliferation and IFNγ production by secreting IL-10 (Rifa'i et al., 2008). Therefore, we wanted to characterize regulatory populations in the spleen to determine their role in the periphery following stroke (**Table 5**). We saw no difference in CD4+ regulatory T cells (CD4+Foxp3+) in young or older mice treated with or without RTL after stroke (**Figure 5A**). However, there was a significant increase in regulatory CD4+ T cells following MCAO in older compared to younger RTL treated mice and the same trend ($p = 0.0675$) is seen with the vehicle mice (**Figure 5A**). Regulatory CD8+ T cells (CD122+IL-10+) were significantly increased in the spleens of young mice treated with RTL after MCAO but not in older mice (**Figure 5B**).

T CELLS IN THE SPLEEN OF YOUNGER MICE INCREASE ACTIVATION MARKER CD69 WHILE OLDER MICE DISPLAY ELEVATED CD44 EXPRESSION FOLLOWING MCAO

In addition to identifying the frequency of different immune subsets in the spleen, functionality of those subsets following stroke and RTL1000 treatment was also examined. CD69 is the earliest activation-inducible cell surface molecule and is involved in cell signaling and lymphocyte proliferation (Serra et al., 1996). CD44 is an adhesion receptor on T cells that is upregulated following initial activation and remains highly expressed on effector and memory T cells (Baaten et al., 2012). No significant differences were seen in CD69 or CD44 expression on T cells between vehicle and RTL treatment in either mouse group with the exception of an increase of CD44 with RTL treatment on CD4+ T cells T cells in young mice (**Figures 6A–D**). There was, however, a significant or trend increase in CD69 expression on CD4 and CD8 T cells in young mice compared to older mice (**Figures 6A,B**). Furthermore, CD44 was significantly increased on splenic CD4 and CD8 T cells from older mice after MCAO compared to younger mice (**Figures 6C,D**). We hypothesize that T cells in the younger mice are able to become activated efficiently, thus the increased CD69 expression after MCAO, yet elevated frequencies of effector/memory T cells observed in older mice lead to a sustained greater number of T cells with high CD44 expression. An examination of migration marker and chemokine receptor CCR5 indicated no change in expression after MCAO between vehicle and RTL treatment or age groups (**Table 6**).

INFLAMMATORY CYTOKINES ARE ELEVATED IN SPLEENS FROM OLDER MICE AFTER MCAO

Inflammatory cytokines play an integral role in the effector functions of the immune response. Spleen derived IFNγ directly contributes to neurodegeneration related to stroke (Yilmaz et al., 2006; Seifert et al., 2012b). TNFα, IL-17, and IL-21 have also have also been linked to stroke progression (Barone et al., 1997; Li et al., 2001; Pan and Kastin, 2007; Gelderblom et al., 2012; Swardfager et al., 2013; Clarkson et al., 2014). We found no significance difference in the frequency of specific immune cells secreting IFNγ, TNFα, IL-17, or IL-21 between vehicle and RTL treated mice with either young or old MCAO mice (**Table 7**). IL-21 production by splenic CD4+ T cells was significantly greater in older mice compared to younger mice following MCAO for the RTL treated group only and there was no difference in IL-17 production between the two age groups with either vehicle or treatment (**Table 7**). IFNγ producing CD4+ and CD8+ T cells were significantly greater in the spleens of older mice than younger mice following MCAO (**Figures 7A,C,D**). Similarly, TNFα positive CD4+ and CD11b+ cells were also increased in the spleens of older mice than younger mice (**Figures 7B,E,F**). We believe that 96 h post-MCAO may be a window of time where memory and

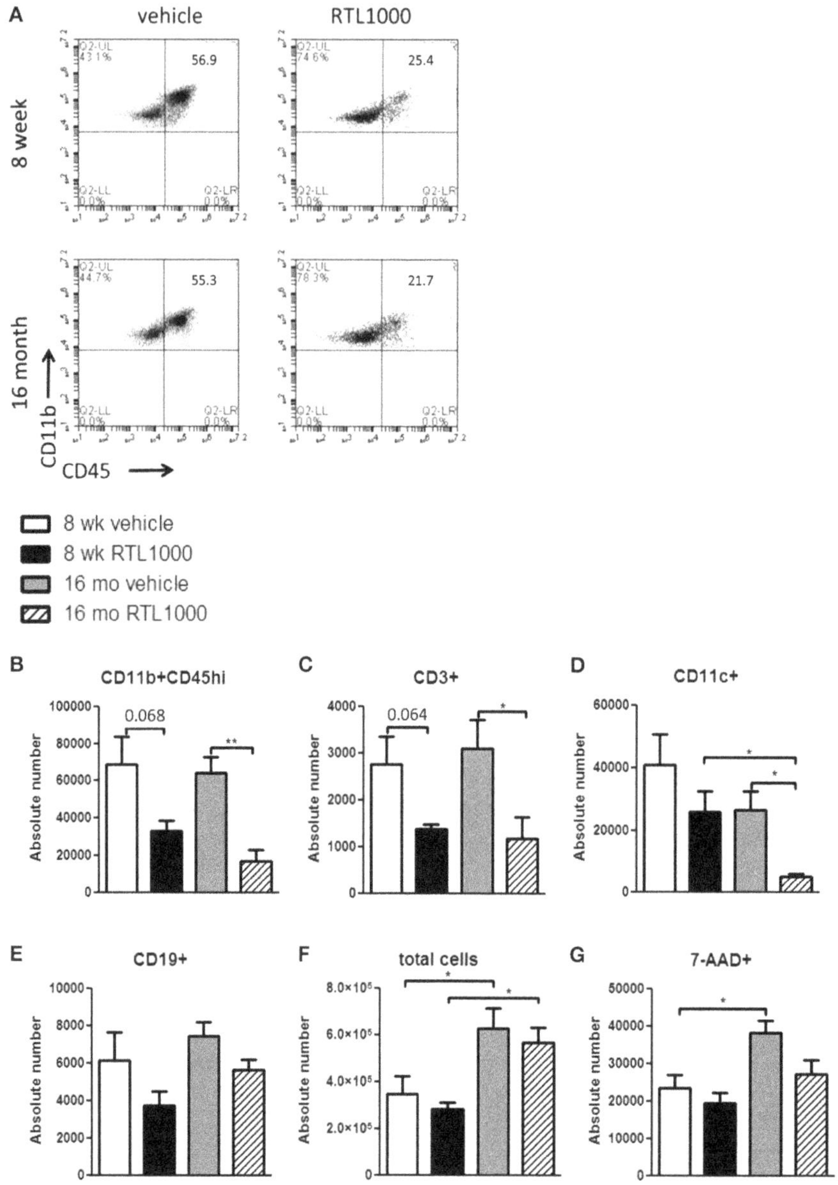

FIGURE 2 | RTL1000 reduces activated and infiltrating cells in the ischemic hemisphere of 16 month but not 8-week-old mice. Brains from young or older male mice were harvested 96 h after MCAO. Leukocytes were isolated from the ischemic hemisphere and phenotyped by flow cytometry. Representative flow cytometry dot plots of activated microglia/monocytes **(A)**. Absolute number of each cell phenotype was calculated using phenotype percent and total cell numbers. CD11b+CD45^{hi} activated microglia/monocytes **(B)**, CD3+ T cells **(C)**, CD11c+ dendritic cells **(D)** and CD19+ B cells **(E)** in the ischemic hemisphere were determined. Total cell number was calculated by multiplying cells per microliter run through the flow cytometer by the total sample volume **(F)**. Cells were analyzed for death by 7-AAD **(G)**. Values represent mean numbers (±s.e.m.) of indicated cell subsets from 5 to 6 young mice per treatment group, from 2 to 3 separate experiments and 4 older mice per group, from 2 separate experiments each. * Indicates $p < 0.05$ and ** indicates $p < 0.01$ compared with vehicle group by *t*-test.

effector immune cells which are quick to reactivate have accumulated in older mice, thus leading to immediate and amplified cytokine production compared to the higher frequency of naïve cells in young mice.

DISCUSSION

In the next few decades nearly 4% of the population will be affected by stroke (Ovbiagele et al., 2013) leading to increase in stroke-related mortality and disability and an even greater need for stroke therapies. Furthermore, understanding how the body responds to stroke as we age is equally as imperative. Previous work done by our lab and others has outlined the contributing immunological factors that influence neurodegeneration following stroke. In young male mice, MCAO induces peripheral immune pro-inflammatory activation that triggers immune cell efflux from the spleen into circulation, some of which go on

Table 3 | Splenocyte number and viability.

	8-week-old mice		16-month-old mice	
	Vehicle	**RTL1000**	**Vehicle**	**RTL1000**
Splenocyte number	$1.9 \times 10^7 \pm 5.5 \times 10^6$	$4.2 \times 10^7 \pm 5.6 \times 10^6$*	$2.6 \times 10^7 \pm 3.8 \times 10^6$	$4.2 \times 10^7 \pm 4.1 \times 10^6$**
Cell death %	11.3 ± 0.8	5.3 ± 1.36**	9.2 ± 1.28	9.2 ± 1.63

** indicates significance compare to vehicle *$p \leq 0.05$ **$p \leq 0.01$.*

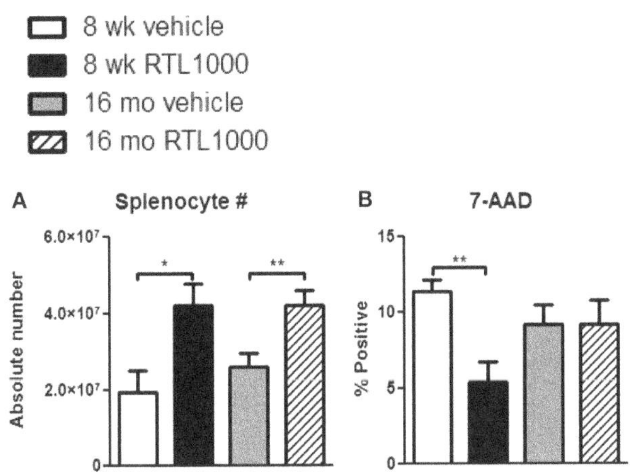

FIGURE 3 | Splenic atrophy is prevented with RTL1000. Spleens were harvested 96 h after MCAO. Splenocytes were isolated and counted by a Cellometer T4 and total splenocyte number was calculated **(A)**. Values represent mean numbers (±s.e.m.) of 6 young vehicle, 5 young RTL, 12 older vehicle, and 13 older RTL mice. Splenocyte death was determined by 7-AAD fluorescence **(B)**. Values represent mean numbers (±s.e.m.) of 5 young mice from each treatment group, 6 older vehicle and 9 older RTL mice. * Indicates $p < 0.05$ and ** indicates $p < 0.01$ compared with vehicle group by *t*-test.

Table 4 | Cell types in the spleen.

	8-week-old mice		16-month-old mice	
Cell type	**Vehicle**	**RTL1000**	**Vehicle**	**RTL1000**
Total CD3+ T cells	34.2 ± 1.6	27.7 ± 1.8*	21.0 ± 2.1##	18.4 ± 0.7###
CD4+ T cells	18.7 ± 1.2	15.1 ± 0.6*	12.8 ± 0.8##	9.8 ± 0.3**###
CD8+ T cells	13.9 ± 0.9	9.9 ± 1.2*	10.0 ± 1.0#	10.0 ± 0.9
CD11b+ myeloid cells	4.9 ± 0.4	3.6 ± 0.4*	3.2 ± 0.2##	3.5 ± 0.2
CD11b+Ly6G+ neutrophils	4.9 ± 0.4	3.8 ± 0.5	4.7 ± 0.3	4.3 ± 0.3
CD11b+Ly6C+ monocytes	3.5 ± 0.3	2.2 ± 0.4*	2.6 ± 0.3#	2.9 ± 0.2
CD11c+ dendritic cells	1.6 ± 0.1	1.8 ± 0.2	1.3 ± 0.1	1.9 ± 0.2
CD19+ B cells	42.8 ± 2.7	53.7 ± 2.0*	59.0 ± 1.5##	62.3 ± 1.5##

** indicates significance compare to vehicle *$p \leq 0.05$; **$p \leq 0.01$.*

 # indicates significance compared to 8-week-old mice #$p \leq 0.05$; ##$p \leq 0.01$; ###$p \leq 0.001$.

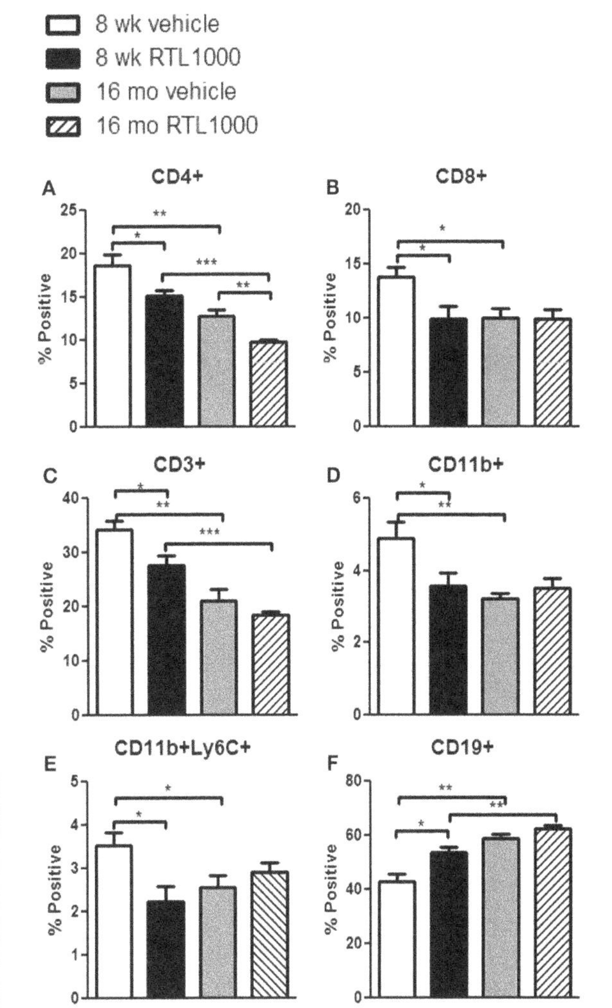

FIGURE 4 | The effect of RTL1000 on peripheral immune subsets in younger vs. older mice. Spleens were harvested 96 h after MCAO and immunophenotyped by flow cytometry. The frequency of CD4+ T cells **(A)**, CD8+ T cells **(B)**, CD3+ T cells **(C)**, CD11b+ monocytes/neutrophils **(D)**, CD11b+Ly6C+ monocytes/macrophages **(E)**, and CD19+ B cells **(F)** were determined. Values represent mean numbers (±s.e.m.) of 5 young mice from each treatment group, 4–6 older vehicle and 9 older RTL mice. * Indicates $p < 0.05$, ** indicates $p < 0.01$, and *** indicates $p < 0.001$ compared with vehicle group by *t*-test.

to target the brain (Offner et al., 2006a,b; Seifert et al., 2012a). Despite the over 1000 neuroprotectants that have been successful in preclinical studies and more than 100 clinical trials initiated, there has been an astounding failure in translation of those neuroprotectants to successful stroke therapies in humans (Turner et al., 2013). One contributing factor to the lack of success in clinical stroke therapy is the underrepresentation of older mice in therapy based research to more accurately represent the age of most humans afflicted by stroke.

Table 5 | Regulatory cells in the spleen.

Cell type	8-week-old mice		16-month-old mice	
	Vehicle	RTL1000	Vehicle	RTL1000
CD4+Foxp3+	15.42 ± 2.0	16.12 ± 0.8	21.63 ± 2.0	20.2 ± 1.4#
CD8+CD122+ IL-10+	3.9 ± 0.4	5.2 ± 0.4*	4.2 ± 0.2	3.4 ± 0.8

** indicates significance compare to vehicle *$p \leq 0.05$.*
 # indicates significance compared to 8-week-old mice #$p \leq 0.05$.

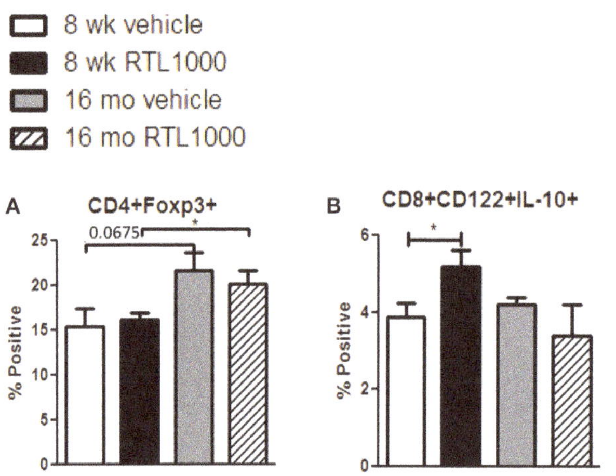

FIGURE 5 | Splenic CD4+ regulatory T cells increase with age in MCAO mice while CD8+ regulatory T cells are increased by RTL1000 treatment. Spleens were harvested 96 h after MCAO and immunophenotyped by flow cytometry. CD4+ regulatory T cells were gated on CD4+ positive splenocytes and determined by Foxp3 expression compared to isotype **(A)**. Values represent mean numbers (±s.e.m.) of 5 young mice from each treatment group, 4 older vehicle and 7 older RTL mice. CD8+ regulatory T cells were gated on the CD8+CD122+ subset and determined by IL-10 expression compared to isotype **(B)**. Values represent mean numbers (±s.e.m.) of 5 young mice from each treatment group, 3 older vehicle and 5 older RTL mice. * indicates $p < 0.05$.

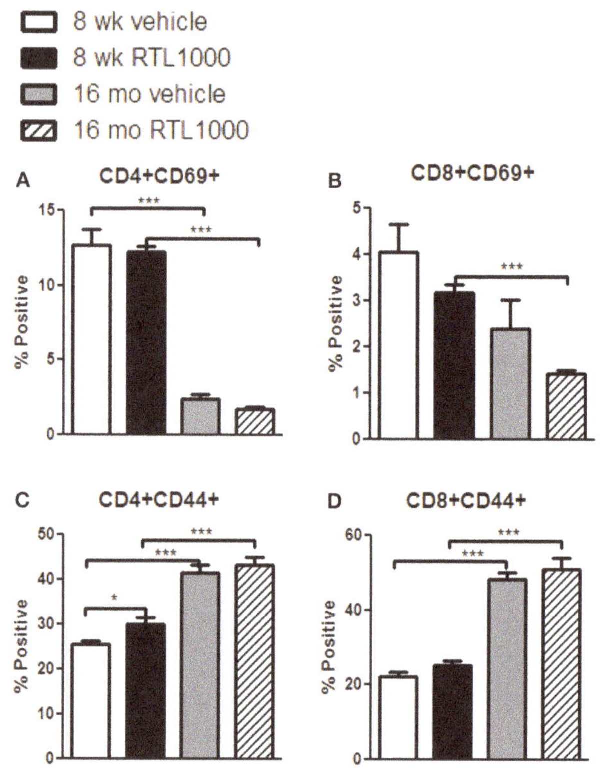

FIGURE 6 | T cells in the spleen of younger mice increase activation marker CD69 while older mice display elevated CD44 expression following MCAO. Spleens were harvested 96 h after MCAO. Early T cell activation was determined by gating on CD4+ **(A)** or CD8+ **(B)** subsets and measuring expression of early activation marker, CD69. Effector/central memory was determined by gating on CD4+ **(C)** or CD8+ **(D)** subsets and measuring expression of CD44. Values represent mean numbers (±s.e.m.) of 5 young mice from each treatment group, 7 older vehicle and 9 older RTL mice. * indicates $p < 0.05$ and *** indicates $p < 0.001$ compared with vehicle group by *t*-test.

RTL therapy has been shown by our lab to be a promising neuroprotectant therapy for stroke in young male mice (Akiyoshi et al., 2011; Dziennis et al., 2011). Here we report that RTL1000 similarly reduced infarct volume in older and younger HLA-DR2 male mice when administered after the onset of MCAO. RTL1000 also reduced the mortality rate of MCAO in older mice. Cerebral ischemia induces activation of resident microglia and an influx of peripheral leukocytes into the brain (Huang et al., 2006). In older mice, RTL treatment significantly reduced the absolute number of activated monocytes/microglia, T cells, and dendritic cells in the ischemic hemisphere following MCAO. Although these cell numbers were also reduced with RTL in young mice after MCAO, the differences remained insignificant. RTL did not affect ischemic total infiltrating cell number or cell death, yet both were greater in older mice compared to younger mice after MCAO indicating possible differences in how young and older individuals respond to stroke.

The peripheral inflammatory response to stroke has been extensively studied and can give crucial insight into the mechanisms of neuroprotection of stroke therapy. One of the hallmarks of the immune response to stroke is splenic atrophy (Offner et al., 2006b). RTL1000 therapy restored total splenocyte numbers in young and older mice after MCAO compared to vehicle indicating a therapy based prevention of splenic atrophy in both age groups. There is an inverse correlation of percent cell death and total cell number in the spleen of young mice. The same trend of increased splenocyte death following MCAO was also observed in young male C57BL/6 mice by our lab (Offner et al., 2006b). RTL therapy did not, however, reduce splenocyte death in older mice compared to vehicle. These data suggest that RTL therapy prevents splenic atrophy by preventing cell death and likely by inhibiting splenocyte migration in young mice while only preventing splenocyte migration in older mice.

Previous work published by our lab revealed that in addition to a total reduction of cell numbers in the spleen, MCAO also contributes to a shift in the frequencies of the different immune subsets that comprise the spleen (Offner et al., 2006b).

Table 6 | Activation/migration markers on T cells.

Cell type/Marker	8-week-old mice		16-month-old mice	
	Vehicle	RTL1000	Vehicle	RTL1000
CD4+CD69+	12.7 ± 1.1	12.3 ± 0.4	2.4 ± 0.4###	1.8 ± 0.1###
CD8+CD69+	4.1 ± 0.6	3.2 ± 0.2	2.4 ± 0.6	1.4 ± 0.1###
CD4+CD44+	25.5 ± 0.8	30.1 ± 1.5*	41.5 ± 1.7###	43.3 ± 1.9###
CD8+CD44+	22.3 ± 1.3	25.1 ± 1.3	48.5 ± 1.7###	51.0 ± 3.0###
CD3+CCR5+	8.5 ± 1.3	9.3 ± 0.4	8.6 ± 1.3	8.4 ± 0.4

** indicates significance compare to vehicle *$p \leq 0.05$.*
 # indicates significance compared to 8-week-old mice ###$p \leq 0.001$.

Table 7 | Cytokine production.

Cell type/Cytokine	8-week-old mice		16-month-old mice	
	Vehicle	RTL1000	Vehicle	RTL1000
CD4+IFNγ+	4.8 ± 0.7	5.6 ± 0.3	10.2 ± 1.7#	9.5 ± 1.6#
CD8+IFNγ+	6.0 ± 1.2	7.0 ± 0.4	21.7 ± 1.5###	22.1 ± 5.1#
CD4+TNFα+	7.2 ± 2.1	6.9 ± 1.4	30.7 ± 1.9###	33.1 ± 3.2###
CD11b+TNFα+	7.0 ± 0.6	7.1 ± 0.5	33.1 ± 2.6###	39.4 ± 1.4###
CD4+IL-17+	1.3 ± 0.1	1.8 ± 0.2	1.6 ± 0.6	1.7 ± 0.4
CD4+IL-21+	1.8 ± 0.3	1.6 ± 0.2	3.5 ± 1.2	3.0 ± 0.5#

 # indicates significance compared to 8-week-old mice #$p \leq 0.05$; ###$p \leq 0.001$.

Specifically, we saw a significant increase in CD4+, CD8+, and CD3+ T cells and a significant decrease of B cells in the spleens of C57BL/6 mice 96 h after MCAO compared to sham (Offner et al., 2006b). RTL treatment significantly decreased the frequency of CD4+, CD8+, and CD3+ T cells and increased B cells in the spleen of young mice following MCAO suggesting that in young mice, RTL treatment counteracts changes in immune cell subsets that occur in the spleen after stroke. In addition to stroke induced changes in T and B cell frequencies in the spleen, RTL treatment led to a modest but significant reduction in monocytes/macrophages in young mice. Circulating monocytes and macrophages are recruited to the ischemic brain 3–7 days after stroke where they contribute to neurodegeneration and recruitment of additional pathogenic immune cells (Chiba and Umegaki, 2013). Since we do not observe a recruitment of activated monocytes/macrophages into the ischemic brain of RTL treated young mice after MCAO, we can hypothesize that the reduction of monocytes/macrophages in the spleen is due to inhibition of activation-induced cell expansion and not cellular migration out of the spleen.

The changes in splenocyte subsets between RTL treated and vehicle control mice were not the only remarkable differences observed in the spleen 96 h after MCAO. In fact, of the six immune subsets that were significantly affected by RTL treatment after MCAO in young mice, CD4+ T cells were the only cell group that were also significantly reduced with older, RTL treated MCAO mice compared to vehicle. Additionally, major differences were observed in peripheral immune cell frequencies after stroke in young vs. older control mice. CD4+, CD8+, and CD3+ T cells, total CD11b+ and CD11b+Ly6C+ monocytes/macrophages were all significantly reduced in the older control MCAO mice compared to the young control mice. RTL treated groups followed the same pattern for CD4+ and CD3+ T cells. CD19+ B cells were significantly elevated in both the control and RTL groups of older mice following MCAO compared to young mice. Such notable disparities in peripheral immune frequencies continue to confirm that younger and older mice respond to stroke and RTL treatment following stroke through different immunological mechanisms.

The frequency of CD4+ Foxp3+ regulatory cells in the spleen increases after MCAO (Offner et al., 2006b) although there are contradicting data on whether CD4+ regulatory T cells diminish or exacerbate stroke related neuronal damage (Schabitz, 2013; Xu et al., 2013). Recent studies have reported that CD4+ Tregs play a protective role against damage following stroke (Liesz et al., 2009; Planas and Chamorro, 2009; Li et al., 2013), while others demonstrate Tregs as harmful promoters of neurodegeneration (Kleinschnitz et al., 2013a; Kleinschnitz and Wiendl, 2013b) or find that Tregs do not influence stroke (Ren et al., 2011; Gu et al., 2012; Stubbe et al., 2013). The conflicting reports of CD4+ Tregs and stroke thus far indicate that there is still much unknown about the regulation of the immune response after stroke and even less known about Treg response to stroke in older subjects. In our study RTL did not affect the frequency of CD4+Foxp3+ Tregs in either older or younger mice. There was, however, a trending increase ($p = 0.0675$) in Tregs in older vehicle vs. younger vehicle mice and a significant increase in RTL treated mice compared to younger RTL mice. The increase in spleen derived Tregs after MCAO in older mice agrees with multiple reports of Treg increase with age contributing to immune senescence (Sharma et al., 2006; Rosenkranz et al., 2007; Lages et al., 2008; Williams-Bey et al., 2011; Raynor et al., 2012). There are far fewer reports on the effect of regulatory CD8+ T cells during and after stroke. CD8+ Tregs co-express CD122 and kill/suppress effector cells via perforin and immunosuppressive cytokines, such as IL-10 (Wang and Alexander, 2009). IL-10 producing CD8+CD122+ Tregs have been directly correlated with a decrease in infarct after MCAO (Banerjee et al., 2013; Bodhankar et al., 2013). CD8+CD122+IL-10+ cells were significantly greater in the periphery of young RTL treated mice but not older RTL treated mice compared to their vehicle counterparts. Although infarct sizes were significantly less with RTL treatment of both age groups, only older mice had a significant reduction in activated microglia/monocytes, T cells, and dendritic cells compared to vehicle. We speculate that CD8+ regulatory cells from the periphery of RTL treated older mice had already migrated to the brain, thus reducing activated immune cells in the ischemic hemisphere, while remaining in the spleen of younger RTL treated mice.

CD69 is the earliest inducible cell surface antigen expressed with T cell activation. Although we observed no change in CD69 expression in mice that received RTL treatment after MCAO, there were significantly less CD69+ T cells from older mice after MCAO. In humans, aged subjects have a lower proportion of recently activated CD69+ T cells compared to younger controls and fail to upregulate CD69 expression following stimulation through CD3, PHA or PMA/Ionomycin as effectively as younger

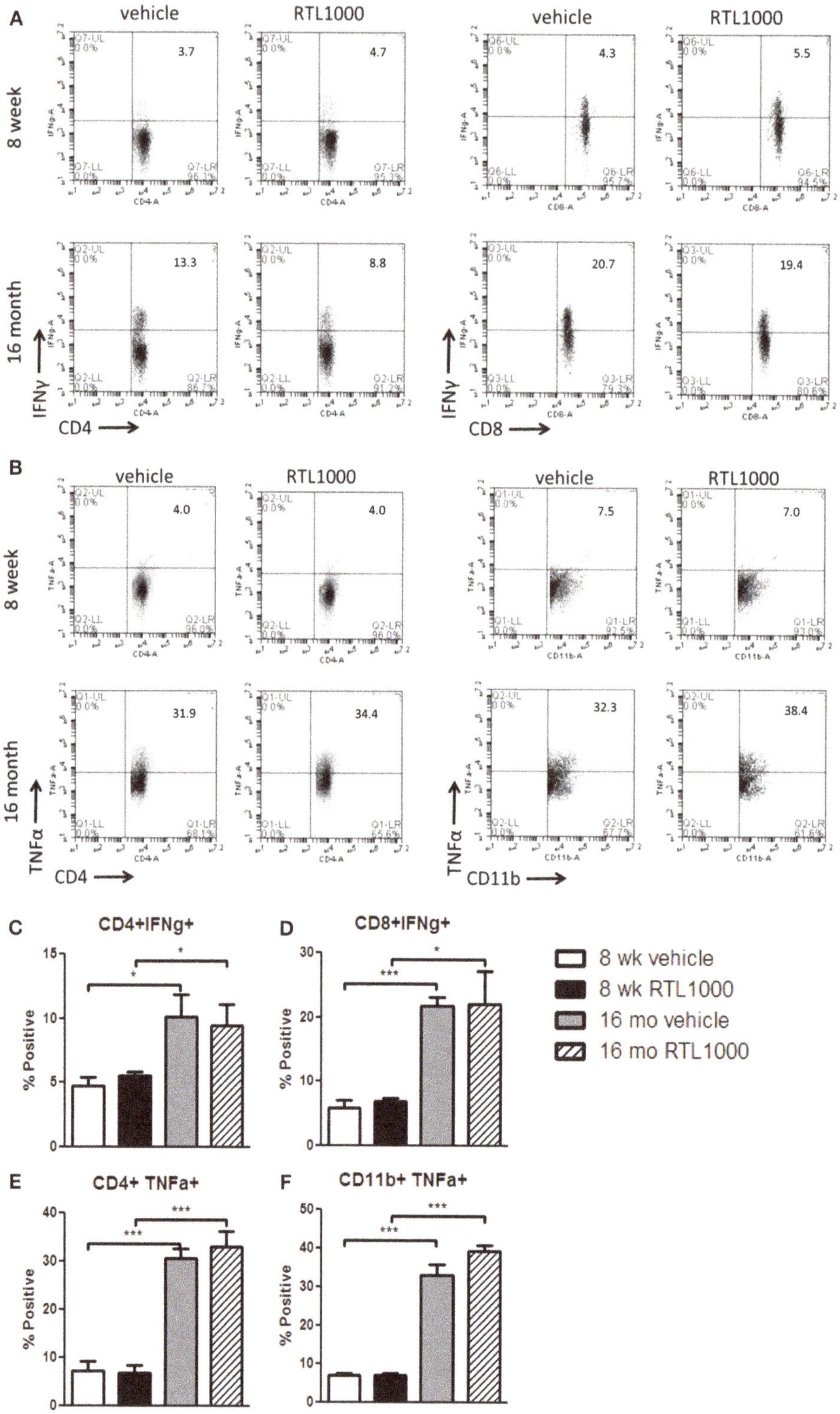

FIGURE 7 | Inflammatory cytokines are elevated in spleens from older mice after MCAO. Spleens were harvested 96 h after MCAO. Representative flow cytometry dot plots of IFNγ **(A)** and TNFα **(B)** producing immune subsets. IFNγ production was determined by gating on CD4+ **(C)** or CD8+ **(D)** subsets and measuring IFNγ positive cells compared to isotype. TNFα production was determined by gating on CD4+ **(E)** or CD11b+ **(F)** subsets and measuring TNFα positive cells compared to isotype. Values represent mean numbers (±s.e.m.) of 5 young mice from each treatment group, 3 older vehicle and 5 older RTL mice. * Indicates $p < 0.05$ and *** indicates $p < 0.001$ compared with vehicle group by *t*-test.

controls (Serra et al., 1996; Schindowski et al., 2002). Therefore, the discrepancy in CD69 expression between older and younger mice can be attributed to age related immune senescence in T cell activation. CD44 is a widely expressed adhesion receptor that becomes upregulated and maintained on T cells after antigen specific activation. CD44 is commonly associated with the effector memory and central memory T cell populations and has numerous functions. We were surprised to see an elevated level of CD44 on CD4+ T cells from younger mice that had received RTL treatment after MCAO. Although commonly known for its role in promoting the immune response, cell migration and T cell proliferation, CD44 is also involved in various regulatory mechanisms such as maintaining functional Tregs and cell survival (Baaten et al., 2010). CD44 has also been shown to be involved in limiting and resolving inflammation (Johnson and Ruffell, 2009). We speculate the increase in CD44 on CD4+ T cells from younger mice that received RTL after MCAO could be linked to a regulatory role that assisted in the decrease of neuroinflammation and splenic atrophy. The percent of CD44+ and memory T cells increases with age (Barrat et al., 1995; Naylor et al., 2005); therefore the significantly greater CD44 expressing CD4 and CD8 T cells in the spleen of older vehicle or RTL treated mice after MCAO is likely indicative of a larger effector and central memory population.

Inflammatory cytokines are well-known to play a destructive role in brain inflammation following stroke. Spleen derived IFNγ is directly linked to neurodegeneration (Seifert et al., 2012b) and TNFα promotes inflammation and leukocyte infiltration into the brain, thus increasing infarct size (Feuerstein et al., 1994; Barone et al., 1997). The neuroprotection observed with RTL therapy in both young and older mice cannot be attributed to a change in peripheral cytokine secretion as demonstrated in **Figure 7**. Interestingly, with both treatment and vehicle, IFNγ or TNFα production by CD4+ and CD8+ T cells or CD4+ T cells and CD11b+ macrophages, respectively, was significantly greater in older mice compared to young mice after MCAO. Both IFNγ and TNFα production increase with age in CD4+/CD8+ T cells and mononuclear cells, respectively (Fagiolo et al., 1993; Bandres et al., 2000; Yen et al., 2000). The abundant amount of memory cells in older compared to younger individuals, which we also observed, requires less secondary stimulus for activation and cytokine secretion and is hypothesized to be partially responsible for the cytokine elevation with age. Although the increase in IFNγ and TNFα in the older mice did not lead to an increase of infarct size compared with young mice, there were significantly greater total cells and cell death in the ischemic hemisphere of 16-month-old mice.

To summarize, the current study demonstrates that treatment with RTL1000 following MCAO significantly reduces infarct volume in 16-month-old mice similar to 8-week-old mice. However, the mechanism of neuroprotection is different between older and younger mice. RTL1000 significantly reduced infiltrating leukocytes in the brain of older mice while significantly reducing cell death and altering the frequency of specific splenocyte subsets in young mice. RTL1000 also inhibited splenic atrophy in both age groups. Additionally, there were major differences in splenocyte activation and cytokine secretion between younger and older mice in response to stroke. In conclusion, age-specific differences in the immune response to stroke resulted in RTL protection from experimental stroke through peripheral-based immune regulation in young mice and inflammatory tissue-specific protection of older mice.

ACKNOWLEDGMENTS

The authors wish to thank Gail Kent for assistance with manuscript submission. This work was supported by NIH Grants # NS065515-02A1 (STTR) and by the Department of Veterans Affairs, Veterans Health Administration, Office of Research and Development, Biomedical Laboratory Research and Development. The contents do not represent the views of the Department of Veterans Affairs or the United States Government. Dr. Offner discloses US patent #8,491,913 B2 for the use of recombinant molecules in treatment of stroke.

REFERENCES

Akiyoshi, K., Dziennis, S., Palmateer, J., Ren, X., Vandenbark, A. A., Offner, H., et al. (2011). Recombinant T cell receptor ligands improve outcome after experimental cerebral ischemia. *Transl. Stroke Res.* 2, 404–410. doi: 10.1007/s12975-011-0085-1

Baaten, B. J., Li, C. R., and Bradley, L. M. (2010). Multifaceted regulation of T cells by CD44. *Commun. Integr. Biol.* 3, 508–512. doi: 10.4161/cib.3.6.13495

Baaten, B. J., Tinoco, R., Chen, A. T., and Bradley, L. M. (2012). Regulation of antigen-experienced T cells: lessons from the quintessential memory marker CD44. *Front. Immunol.* 3:23. doi: 10.3389/fimmu.2012.00023

Bandres, E., Merino, J., Vazquez, B., Inoges, S., Moreno, C., Subira, M. L., et al. (2000). The increase of IFN-gamma production through aging correlates with the expanded CD8(+high)CD28(-)CD57(+) subpopulation. *Clin. Immunol.* 96, 230–235. doi: 10.1006/clim.2000.4894

Banerjee, A., Wang, J., Bodhankar, S., Vandenbark, A. A., Murphy, S. J., and Offner, H. (2013). Phenotypic changes in immune cell subsets reflect increased infarct volume in male vs. female mice. *Transl. Stroke Res.* 4, 554–563. doi: 10.1007/s12975-013-0268-z

Barone, F. C., Arvin, B., White, R. F., Miller, A., Webb, C. L., Willette, R. N., et al. (1997). Tumor necrosis factor-alpha. A mediator of focal ischemic brain injury. *Stroke* 28, 1233–1244. doi: 10.1161/01.STR.28.6.1233

Barrat, F., Haegel, H., Louise, A., Vincent-Naulleau, S., Boulouis, H. J., Neway, T., et al. (1995). Quantitative and qualitative changes in CD44 and MEL-14 expression by T cells in C57BL/6 mice during aging. *Res. Immunol.* 146, 23–34. doi: 10.1016/0923-2494(96)80237-9

Benedek, G., Zhu, W., Libal, N., Casper, A., Yu, X., Meza-Romero, R., et al. (2014). A novel HLA-DRalpha1-MOG-35-55 construct treats experimental stroke. *Metab. Brain Dis.* 29, 37–45. doi: 10.1007/s11011-013-9440-0

Bodhankar, S., Chen, Y., Vandenbark, A. A., Murphy, S. J., and Offner, H. (2013). PD-L1 enhances CNS inflammation and infarct volume following experimental stroke in mice in opposition to PD-1. *J. Neuroinflammation* 10:111. doi: 10.1186/1742-2094-10-111

Bodhankar, S., Chen, Y., Vandenbark, A. A., Murphy, S. J., and Offner, H. (2014). Treatment of experimental stroke with IL-10-producing B-cells reduces infarct size and peripheral and CNS inflammation in wild-type B-cell-sufficient mice. *Metab. Brain Dis.* 29, 59–73. doi: 10.1007/s11011-013-9474-3

Burrows, G., Chang, J. W., Bächinger, H. P., Bourdette, D. N., Offner, H., and Vandenbark, A. A. (1999). Design, engineering and production of functional single-chain T cell receptor ligands. *Protein Eng.* 12, 771–778. doi: 10.1093/protein/12.9.771

Burrows, G. G., Bebo, B. F. Jr., Adlard, K. L., Vandenbark, A. A., and Offner, H. (1998). Two-domain MHC class II molecules form stable complexes with myelin basic protein 69-89 peptide that detect and inhibit rat encephalitogenic T cells and treat experimental autoimmune encephalomyelitis. *J. Immunol.* 161, 5987–5996.

Burrows, G. G., Chou, Y. K., Wang, C., Chang, J. W., Finn, T. P., Culbertson, N. E., et al. (2001). Rudimentary TCR signaling triggers default IL-10 secretion by human Th1 cells. *J. Immunol.* 167, 4386–4395. doi: 10.4049/jimmunol.167.8.4386

Campanella, M., Sciorati, C., Tarozzo, G., and Beltramo, M. (2002). Flow cytometric analysis of inflammatory cells in ischemic rat brain. *Stroke* 33, 586–592. doi: 10.1161/hs0202.103399

Chiba, T., and Umegaki, K. (2013). Pivotal roles of monocytes/macrophages in stroke. *Mediat. Inflamm.* 2013:759103. doi: 10.1155/2013/759103

Clarkson, B. D., Ling, C., Shi, Y., Harris, M. G., Rayasam, A., Sun, D., et al. (2014). T cell-derived interleukin (IL)-21 promotes brain injury following stroke in mice. *J. Exp. Med.* 211, 595–604. doi: 10.1084/jem.20131377

Dziennis, S., Mader, S., Akiyoshi, K., Ren, X., Ayala, P., Burrows, G. G., et al. (2011). Therapy with recombinant T-cell receptor ligand reduces infarct size and infiltrating inflammatory cells in brain after middle cerebral artery occlusion in mice. *Metab. Brain Dis.* 26, 123–133. doi: 10.1007/s11011-011-9241-2

Fagiolo, U., Cossarizza, A., Scala, E., Fanales-Belasio, E., Ortolani, C., Cozzi, E., et al. (1993). Increased cytokine production in mononuclear cells of healthy elderly people. *Eur. J. Immunol.* 23, 2375–2378. doi: 10.1002/eji.1830230950

Feuerstein, G. Z., Liu, T., and Barone, F. C. (1994). Cytokines, inflammation, and brain injury: role of tumor necrosis factor-alpha. *Cerebrovasc. Brain Metab. Rev.* 6, 341–360.

Gelderblom, M., Weymar, A., Bernreuther, C., Velden, J., Arunachalam, P., Steinbach, K., et al. (2012). Neutralization of the IL-17 axis diminishes neutrophil invasion and protects from ischemic stroke. *Blood* 120, 3793–3802. doi: 10.1182/blood-2012-02-412726

Gonzalez-Gay, M. A., Zanelli, E., Khare, S. D., Krco, C. J., Zhou, P., Inoko, H., et al. (1996). Human leukocyte antigen-DRB1*1502 (DR2Dw12) transgene reduces incidence and severity of arthritis in mice. *Hum. Immunol.* 50, 54–60. doi: 10.1016/0198-8859(96)00123-1

Gronberg, N. V., Johansen, F. F., Kristiansen, U., and Hasseldam, H. (2013). Leukocyte infiltration in experimental stroke. *J. Neuroinflammation* 10:115. doi: 10.1186/1742-2094-10-115

Gu, L., Xiong, X., Zhang, H., Xu, B., Steinberg, G. K., and Zhao, H. (2012). Distinctive effects of T cell subsets in neuronal injury induced by cocultured splenocytes *in vitro* and by *in vivo* stroke in mice. *Stroke* 43, 1941–1946. doi: 10.1161/STROKEAHA.112.656611

Huan, J., Subramanian, S., Jones, R., Rich, C., Link, J., Mooney, J., et al. (2004). Monomeric recombinant TCR ligand reduces relapse rate and severity of experimental autoimmune encephalomyelitis in SJL/J mice through cytokine switch. *J. Immunol.* 172, 4556–4566. doi: 10.4049/jimmunol.172.7.4556

Huang, J., Upadhyay, U. M., and Tamargo, R. J. (2006). Inflammation in stroke and focal cerebral ischemia. *Surg. Neurol.* 66, 232–245. doi: 10.1016/j.surneu.2005.12.028

Hurn, P. D., Subramanian, S., Parker, S. M., Afentoulis, M. E., Kaler, L. J., Vandenbark, A. A., et al. (2007). T- and B-cell-deficient mice with experimental stroke have reduced lesion size and inflammation. *J. Cereb. Blood Flow Metab.* 27, 1798–1805. doi: 10.1038/sj.jcbfm.9600482

Johnson, P., and Ruffell, B. (2009). CD44 and its role in inflammation and inflammatory diseases. *Inflamm. Allergy Drug Targets* 8, 208–220. doi: 10.2174/18715 2809788680994

Kleinschnitz, C., Kraft, P., Dreykluft, A., Hagedorn, I., Gobel, K., Schuhmann, M. K., et al. (2013a). Regulatory T cells are strong promoters of acute ischemic stroke in mice by inducing dysfunction of the cerebral microvasculature. *Blood* 121, 679–691. doi: 10.1182/blood-2012-04-426734

Kleinschnitz, C., and Wiendl, H. (2013b). Con: regulatory T cells are protective in ischemic stroke. *Stroke* 44, e87–e88. doi: 10.1161/STROKEAHA.113.001268

Lages, C. S., Suffia, I., Velilla, P. A., Huang, B., Warshaw, G., Hildeman, D. A., et al. (2008). Functional regulatory T cells accumulate in aged hosts and promote chronic infectious disease reactivation. *J. Immunol.* 181, 1835–1848. doi: 10.4049/jimmunol.181.3.1835

Li, H. L., Kostulas, N., Huang, Y. M., Xiao, B. G., Van Der Meide, P., Kostulas, V., et al. (2001). IL-17 and IFN-gamma mRNA expression is increased in the brain and systemically after permanent middle cerebral artery occlusion in the rat. *J. Neuroimmunol.* 116, 5–14. doi: 10.1016/S0165-5728(01)00264-8

Li, P., Gan, Y., Sun, B. L., Zhang, F., Lu, B., Gao, Y., et al. (2013). Adoptive regulatory T-cell therapy protects against cerebral ischemia. *Ann. Neurol.* 74, 458–471. doi: 10.1002/ana.23815

Liesz, A., Suri-Payer, E., Veltkamp, C., Doerr, H., Sommer, C., Rivest, S., et al. (2009). Regulatory T cells are key cerebroprotective immunomodulators in acute experimental stroke. *Nat. Med.* 15, 192–199. doi: 10.1038/nm.1927

Liu, F., and McCullough, L. D. (2011). Middle cerebral artery occlusion model in rodents: methods and potential pitfalls. *J. Biomed. Biotechnol.* 2011:464701. doi: 10.1155/2011/464701

Naylor, K., Li, G., Vallejo, A. N., Lee, W. W., Koetz, K., Bryl, E., et al. (2005). The influence of age on T cell generation and TCR diversity. *J. Immunol.* 174, 7446–7452. doi: 10.4049/jimmunol.174.11.7446

O'Collins, V. E., Macleod, M. R., Donnan, G. A., Horky, L. L., Van Der Worp, B. H., and Howells, D. W. (2006). 1,026 experimental treatments in acute stroke. *Ann. Neurol.* 59, 467–477. doi: 10.1002/ana.20741

Offner, H., Sinha, S., Burrows, G. G., Ferro, A. J., and Vandenbark, A. A. (2011). RTL therapy for multiple sclerosis: a Phase I clinical study. *J. Neuroimmunol.* 231, 7–14. doi: 10.1016/j.jneuroim.2010.09.013

Offner, H., Subramanian, S., Parker, S. M., Afentoulis, M. E., Vandenbark, A. A., and Hurn, P. D. (2006a). Experimental stroke induces massive, rapid activation of the peripheral immune system. *J. Cereb. Blood Flow Metab.* 26, 654–665. doi: 10.1038/sj.jcbfm.9600217

Offner, H., Subramanian, S., Parker, S. M., Wang, C., Afentoulis, M. E., Lewis, A., et al. (2006b). Splenic atrophy in experimental stroke is accompanied by increased regulatory T cells and circulating macrophages. *J. Immunol.* 176, 6523–6531. doi: 10.4049/jimmunol.176.11.6523

Ovbiagele, B., Goldstein, L. B., Higashida, R. T., Howard, V. J., Johnston, S. C., Khavjou, O. A., et al. (2013). Forecasting the future of stroke in the United States: a policy statement from the American Heart Association and American Stroke Association. *Stroke* 44, 2361–2375. doi: 10.1161/STR.0b013e31829734f2

Pan, J., Palmateer, J., Schallert, T., Hart, M., Pandya, A., Vandenbark, A. A., et al. (2014). Novel humanized recombinant T cell receptor ligands protect the female brain after experimental stroke. *Transl. Stroke Res.* 5, 577–585. doi: 10.1007/s12975-014-0345-y

Pan, W., and Kastin, A. J. (2007). Tumor necrosis factor and stroke: role of the blood-brain barrier. *Prog. Neurobiol.* 83, 363–374. doi: 10.1016/j.pneurobio.2007.07.008

Planas, A. M., and Chamorro, A. (2009). Regulatory T cells protect the brain after stroke. *Nat. Med.* 15, 138–139. doi: 10.1038/nm0209-138

Raynor, J., Lages, C. S., Shehata, H., Hildeman, D. A., and Chougnet, C. A. (2012). Homeostasis and function of regulatory T cells in aging. *Curr. Opin. Immunol.* 24, 482–487. doi: 10.1016/j.coi.2012.04.005

Ren, X., Akiyoshi, K., Vandenbark, A. A., Hurn, P. D., and Offner, H. (2011). CD4+FoxP3+ regulatory T-cells in cerebral ischemic stroke. *Metab. Brain Dis.* 26, 87–90. doi: 10.1007/s11011-010-9226-6

Rifa'i, M., Shi, Z., Zhang, S. Y., Lee, Y. H., Shiku, H., Isobe, K., et al. (2008). CD8+CD122+ regulatory T cells recognize activated T cells via conventional MHC class I-alphabetaTCR interaction and become IL-10-producing active regulatory cells. *Int. Immunol.* 20, 937–947. doi: 10.1093/intimm/dxn052

Rosenkranz, D., Weyer, S., Tolosa, E., Gaenslen, A., Berg, D., Leyhe, T., et al. (2007). Higher frequency of regulatory T cells in the elderly and increased suppressive activity in neurodegeneration. *J. Neuroimmunol.* 188, 117–127. doi: 10.1016/j.jneuroim.2007.05.011

Schabitz, W. R. (2013). Regulatory T cells in ischemic stroke: helpful or hazardous? *Stroke* 44, e84. doi: 10.1161/STROKEAHA.113.002228

Schindowski, K., Frohlich, L., Maurer, K., Muller, W. E., and Eckert, A. (2002). Age-related impairment of human T lymphocytes' activation: specific differences between CD4(+) and CD8(+) subsets. *Mech. Ageing Dev.* 123, 375–390. doi: 10.1016/S0047-6374(01)00396-7

Seifert, H. A., Hall, A. A., Chapman, C. B., Collier, L. A., Willing, A. E., and Pennypacker, K. R. (2012a). A transient decrease in spleen size following stroke corresponds to splenocyte release into systemic circulation. *J. Neuroimmune Pharmacol.* 7, 1017–1024. doi: 10.1007/s11481-012-9406-8

Seifert, H. A., Leonardo, C. C., Hall, A. A., Rowe, D. D., Collier, L. A., Benkovic, S. A., et al. (2012b). The spleen contributes to stroke induced neurodegeneration through interferon gamma signaling. *Metab. Brain Dis.* 27, 131–141. doi: 10.1007/s11011-012-9283-0

Serra, J. A., Fernandez-Gutierrez, B., Hernandez-Garcia, C., Vidan, M., Banares, A., Ribera, J. M., et al. (1996). Early T-cell activation in elderly humans. *Age Ageing* 25, 470–478. doi: 10.1093/ageing/25.6.470

Sharma, S., Dominguez, A. L., and Lustgarten, J. (2006). High accumulation of T regulatory cells prevents the activation of immune responses in aged animals. *J. Immunol.* 177, 8348–8355. doi: 10.4049/jimmunol.177.12.8348

Shichita, T., Sugiyama, Y., Ooboshi, H., Sugimori, H., Nakagawa, R., Takada, I., et al. (2009). Pivotal role of cerebral interleukin-17-producing gammadeltaT cells in the delayed phase of ischemic brain injury. *Nat. Med.* 15, 946–950. doi: 10.1038/nm.1999

Sinha, S., Subramanian, S., Proctor, T. M., Kaler, L. J., Grafe, M., Dahan, R., et al. (2007). A promising therapeutic approach for multiple sclerosis: recombinant T-cell receptor ligands modulate experimental autoimmune encephalomyelitis by reducing interleukin-17 production and inhibiting migration of encephalitogenic cells into the CNS. *J. Neurosci.* 27, 12531–12539. doi: 10.1523/JNEUROSCI.3599-07.2007

Stubbe, T., Ebner, F., Richter, D., Engel, O., Klehmet, J., Royl, G., et al. (2013). Regulatory T cells accumulate and proliferate in the ischemic hemisphere for up to 30 days after MCAO. *J. Cereb. Blood Flow Metab.* 33, 37–47. doi: 10.1038/jcbfm.2012.128

Subramanian, S., Zhang, B., Kosaka, Y., Burrows, G. G., Grafe, M. R., Vandenbark, A. A., et al. (2009). Recombinant T cell receptor ligand treats experimental stroke. *Stroke* 40, 2539–2545. doi: 10.1161/STROKEAHA.108.543991

Swardfager, W., Winer, D. A., Herrmann, N., Winer, S., and Lanctot, K. L. (2013). Interleukin-17 in post-stroke neurodegeneration. *Neurosci. Biobehav. Rev.* 37, 436–447. doi: 10.1016/j.neubiorev.2013.01.021

Turner, R. C., Lucke-Wold, B., Lucke-Wold, N., Elliott, A. S., Logsdon, A. F., Rosen, C. L., et al. (2013). Neuroprotection for ischemic stroke: moving past shortcomings and identifying promising directions. *Int. J. Mol. Sci.* 14, 1890–1917. doi: 10.3390/ijms14011890

Vandenbark, A. A., Rich, C., M. J., Zamora, A., W. C., Huan, J., Fugger, L., Offner, H., et al. (2003). Recombinant TCR ligand induces tolerance to myelin oligodendrocyte glycoprotein 35-55 peptide and reverses clinical and histological signs of chronic experimental autoimmune encephalomyelitis in HLA-DR2 transgenic mice. *J. Immunol.* 171, 127–133. doi: 10.4049/jimmunol.171.1.127

Wang, C., Mooney, J. L., Meza-Romero, R., Chou, Y. K., Huan, J., Vandenbark, A. A., et al. (2003). Recombinant TCR ligand induces early TCR signaling and a unique pattern of downstream activation. *J. Immunol.* 171, 1934–1940. doi: 10.4049/jimmunol.171.4.1934

Wang, Y. M., and Alexander, S. I. (2009). CD8 regulatory T cells: what's old is now new. *Immunol. Cell Biol.* 87, 192–193. doi: 10.1038/icb.2009.8

Williams-Bey, Y., Jiang, J., and Murasko, D. M. (2011). Expansion of regulatory T cells in aged mice following influenza infection. *Mech. Ageing Dev.* 132, 163–170. doi: 10.1016/j.mad.2011.03.001

Xu, X., Li, M., and Jiang, Y. (2013). The paradox role of regulatory T cells in ischemic stroke. *Sci. World J.* 2013:174373. doi: 10.1155/2013/174373

Yen, C. J., Lin, S. L., Huang, K. T., and Lin, R. H. (2000). Age-associated changes in interferon-gamma and interleukin-4 secretion by purified human CD4+ and CD8+ T cells. *J. Biomed. Sci.* 7, 317–321. doi: 10.1007/BF02253251

Yilmaz, G., Arumugam, T. V., Stokes, K. Y., and Granger, D. N. (2006). Role of T lymphocytes and interferon-gamma in ischemic stroke. *Circulation* 113, 2105–2112. doi: 10.1161/CIRCULATIONAHA.105.593046

Zhang, W., Otsuka, T., Sugo, N., Ardeshiri, A., Alhadid, Y. K., Iliff, J. J., et al. (2008). Soluble epoxide hydrolase gene deletion is protective against experimental cerebral ischemia. *Stroke* 39, 2073–2078. doi: 10.1161/STROKEAHA.107.508325

Zhu, W., Libal, N. L., Casper, A., Bodhankar, S., Offner, H., and Alkayed, N. J. (2014). Recombinant T cell receptor ligand treatment improves neurological outcome in the presence of tissue plasminogen activator in experimental ischemic stroke. *Transl. Stroke Res.* 5, 612–617. doi: 10.1007/s12975-014-0348-8

9

Role of mitochondria ROS generation in ethanol-induced NLRP3 inflammasome activation and cell death in astroglial cells

Silvia Alfonso-Loeches[†], Juan R. Ureña-Peralta[†], Maria José Morillo-Bargues, Jorge Oliver-De La Cruz and Consuelo Guerri*

Molecular and Cellular Pathology of Alcohol Laboratory, Prince Felipe Research Center, Valencia, Spain

Correspondence:
Consuelo Guerri, Molecular and Cellular Pathology of Alcohol Laboratory, Prince Felipe Research Center, C/Eduardo Primo Yúfera 3, Valencia 46012, Spain
e-mail: cguerri@cipf.es

[†] Silvia Alfonso-Loeches and Juan R. Ureña-Peralta have contributed equally to this work.

Toll-like receptors (TLRs) and NOD-like receptors (NLRs) are innate immunity sensors that provide an early/effective response to pathogenic or injury conditions. We have reported that ethanol-induced TLR4 activation triggers signaling inflammatory responses in glial cells, causing neuroinflammation and brain damage. However, it is uncertain if ethanol is able to activate NLRs/inflammasome in astroglial cells, which is the mechanism of activation, and whether there is crosstalk between both immune sensors in glial cells. Here we show that chronic ethanol treatment increases the co-localization of caspase-1 with GFAP$^+$ cells, and up-regulates IL-1β and IL-18 in the frontal medial cortex in WT, but not in TLR4 knockout mice. We further show that cultured cortical astrocytes expressed several inflammasomes (NLRP3, AIM2, NLRP1, and IPAF), although NLRP3 mRNA is the predominant form. Ethanol, as ATP and LPS treatments, up-regulates NLRP3 expression, and causes caspase-1 cleavage and the release of IL-1β and IL-18 in astrocytes supernatant. Ethanol-induced NLRP3/caspase-1 activation is mediated by mitochondrial (m) reactive oxygen species (ROS) generation because when using a specific mitochondria ROS scavenger, the mito-TEMPO (500 μM) or NLRP3 blocking peptide (4 μg/ml) or a specific caspase-1 inhibitor, Z-YVAD-FMK (10 μM), abrogates mROS release and reduces the up-regulation of IL-1β and IL-18 induced by ethanol or LPS or ATP. Confocal microscopy studies further confirm that ethanol, ATP or LPS promotes NLRP3/caspase-1 complex recruitment within the mitochondria to promote cell death by caspase-1-mediated pyroptosis, which accounts for ≈73% of total cell death (≈22%) and the remaining (≈25%) die by caspase-3-dependent apoptosis. Suppression of the TLR4 function abrogates most ethanol effects on NLRP3 activation and reduces cell death. These findings suggest that NLRP3 participates, in ethanol-induced neuroinflammation and highlight the NLRP3/TLR4 crosstalk in ethanol-induced brain injury.

Keywords: ethanol, astrocytes, TLR4, NLRP3-inflammasome, ROS, pyroptosis, IL-β, apoptosis

INTRODUCTION

Inflammation in the central nervous system (CNS), or neuroinflammation, is a key component of many neurological and neurodegenerative disorders characterized by lymphocyte/macrophage infiltration, glial activation, enhanced cytokine/chemokine production, demyelination and axonal loss (Sospedra and Martin, 2005; Pittock and Lucchinetti, 2007). The neuroinflammatory process is initiated by several receptors of the innate immune system, which recognize a diverse range of microbial and damage signals, coordinate protection and repair mechanisms.

Toll-like receptors (TLRs) and nucleotide-binding oligomerization domain (NOD)-like receptors (NLRs) are two major forms of innate immune sensors which provide immediate responses against pathogenic invasion, tissue injury and stress conditions. Both the TLRs and NLRs families of receptors are activated through the recognition of both conserved microbial structures, called pathogen-associated molecular patterns (PAMPs) and damage-associated molecular patterns (DAMPs). However, unlike membrane-bound TLRs that sense PAMPs or DAMPs on the cell surface or within endosomes, NLRs recognize microbial molecules or DAMPs in the host cytosol. Activation of these receptors induces the recruitment of innate immune cells, which initiates tissue repair processing and adaptive immune activation. Abnormalities in any of these innate sensor-mediated processes may cause excessive inflammation due to either hyper-responsive innate immune signaling or sustained compensatory adaptive immune activation.

NOD-like receptors family members, NLRP1, NLRP3, NLRC4, and AIM2 (a member of the PYHIN protein family), have been identified as being capable of forming inflammasomes, multiprotein complexes that activate caspase-1, which leads to the processing and secretion of pro-inflammatory cytokines interleukin-1β (IL-1β) and IL-18. Among NLRs, NLRP3 is currently the most fully described inflammasome. It consists of the NLRP3 scaffold, adaptor ASC (apoptosis-associated speck-like protein containing a CARD) and caspase-1. Nevertheless, the molecular and cellular mechanisms of NLRP3 activation remain unclear. Different mechanisms have been postulated, such as lysosomal damage (Hornung and Latz, 2010), potassium leakage (Arlehamn et al., 2010), and reactive oxygen species (ROS) formation (Schroder et al., 2010; Shimada et al., 2012a). Recent studies support the role of mitochondrial adaptors (Subramanian et al., 2013), mitochondria calcium fluxes (Triantafilou et al., 2013) and ROS formation (Zhou et al., 2011; Shimada et al., 2012b) in inflammasome activation.

NOD-like receptors P3 is activated upon exposure to whole pathogens, but also by a number of host-derived danger signals, which are indicative of not only tissue injury (DAMPs), but also environmental irritants (Schroder and Tschopp, 2010). Mutation of NLRP3 is responsible for rare autoinflammatory diseases, collectively referred to as cryopyrin-associated periodic syndromes (CAPS; Neven et al., 2004; Ting and Davis, 2005; Jha and Ting, 2009), characterized by the hyperactivation of the inflammasome complex and increased IL-1β (Neven et al., 2004; Goldbach-Mansky et al., 2006). In addition, there is emerging evidence for the participation of the NLRP3 inflammasome as a sensor of metabolic stress (i.e., De Nardo and Latz, 2011), demyelination, and it is also involved in some neurodegenerative disorders such as the multiple sclerosis model (Jha et al., 2010) and Alzheimer's disease (Heneka et al., 2013; Sheedy et al., 2013; Tan et al., 2013).

Alcohol is a neurotoxic compound and its abuse can induce brain damage and neurodegeneration. We have demonstrated that ethanol is capable of activating TLR4/IL-1RI receptors in astroglial and microglial cells to trigger TLR4 signaling and to produce cytokines induction (IL-1β, TNF-α, IL-6) and inflammatory mediators (iNOS, COX-2), which can lead to neuroinflammation and brain injury. Elimination of the TLR4 function abolishes most neuroinflammation and neural death (Alfonso-Loeches et al., 2010). Our recent studies have further demonstrated that neuroinflammation induced by ethanol abuse in mice is associated with demyelination and disruptions in the myelin structure and that these alterations are, in part, dependent on TLR4 signaling (Alfonso-Loeches et al., 2012).

Crosstalk between TLRs and NLRs in the secretion of mature IL-1β during microbial infection has been reported (Kahlenberg et al., 2005; Becker and O'Neill, 2007; Mariathasan and Monack, 2007), although it is unknown whether this crosstalk occurs in brain damage and demyelination. A recent study shows that ethanol activates NLRP3 inflammasome in the brain (Lippai et al., 2013). However, the cellular and molecular mechanisms of ethanol-induced inflammasome activation in the brain and glial cells, and the interactions of TLRs and NLRs, are presently unknown. Here we present evidence for NLRP3 expression in astrocytes and that by stimulating mitochondria ROS (mROS) generation, ethanol, ATP or LPS triggers NLRP3/caspase-1 activation and the production of IL-1β and IL-18 in astrocytes. These findings further demonstrate that ethanol promotes NLRP3/caspase-1 co-localization within mitochondria to trigger pyroptosis and a small proportion of apoptosis. Elimination of the TLR4 function reduces the damaging actions of ethanol on NLRP3 inflammasome activation in astroglial cells in both primary culture and cerebral cortex *in vivo*, suggesting that TLR4 plays a key role in ethanol-induced NLRP3 activation, neuroinflammation and brain damage.

MATERIAL AND METHODS

MICE AND ETHANOL TREATMENT

Female C57BL/6 WT (Harlan Ibérica S.L., Barcelona) and TLR4 *knockout* (TLR4-KO) mice (C57BL/6 background, kindly provided by Dr. S. Akira, Osaka University, Japan) were used. Animals were kept under controlled light and dark conditions (12/12 h) at a temperature of 23°C and at 60% humidity. All the animal experiments were carried out in accordance with the guidelines set out in European Communities Council Directive (86/609/ECC) and Spanish Royal Decree 1201/2005. The experimental procedures were approved by the *Ethical Committee of Animal Experimentation of the Prince Felipe Research Center* (Protocol numbers 08-0060 and 08-0099) and were in accordance with the recommendations in the ARRIVE Guidelines for the care and use of experimental animals.

For chronic ethanol treatment, 40 (10 animals/group) 7-week-old C57BL/6 (WT/TLR4$^{+/+}$) and TLR4-KO mice weighing 18–20 g were housed (four animals/cage), and were maintained with water (WT and TLR4-KO control) or water containing 10% (v/v) ethanol, and were placed on a solid diet *ad libitum* for 5 months.

BRAIN TISSUE PREPARATION

Mice were deeply anesthetized by an intraperitoneal injection with sodium penthobarbital (60 mg/kg) and fentanyl (0.05 mg/kg) for analgesia. Animals were then transcardially perfused with 0.9% saline containing heparin (2 U/ml), immediately followed by 4% paraformaldehyde (PF) in 0.1 M phosphate buffer, pH 7.4, for tissue fixation to be post-fixed overnight at 4°C in 4% PF and stored in 30% sucrose solution at 4°C for cryoprotection. Coronal brain sections (40 μm) were obtained with a cryostat (Microm HM 505E) and were collected on polysine^{TM} glass slides (Menzel-Gläser, Thermo Scientific, Germany).

Some mice were killed by cervical dislocation; brains were removed, dissected using the mouse brain atlas coordinates (Franklin and Paxinos, 1997), and immediately snap-frozen in liquid nitrogen until used in the Western blot, RT-PCR, caspase-1 enzymatic activity and cytokines determination analyses.

IMMUNOFLUORESCENCE

*(i) Double co-localization of caspase-1 and GFAP in cortical astrocytes**: cortical brain sections were defrosted for 30 min and incubated with 0.25% Triton in PBS solution for 10 min. Sections were blocked for 1 h/RT with 10% normal goat serum in TBS/T (0.1%) and were incubated overnight at 4°C with the following primary antibodies; anti-caspase-1 (1/50, Santa Cruz) and anti-GFAP (1/400, Sigma–Aldrich) following incubation with the respective Alexa-fluor-conjugated secondary antibodies (1/500, Invitrogen, Molecular Probes). Nuclei were stained with DAPI. Negative controls were performed by replacing the respective primary antibodies with IgG isotype control and concentration-matched irrelevant antibodies (**Figure 1F**). Sections were mounted onto glass slides with Dako Fluorescent Mounting medium (Dako North America Inc., CA, USA). All the images were analyzed with the ImageJ 1.42 software (NIH). We determined fluorescence intensity of three different animals per group by randomly taking four medial-frontal-cortex sections for each one. At least 800–1000 cells were counted per experimental condition. *(ii) Double*

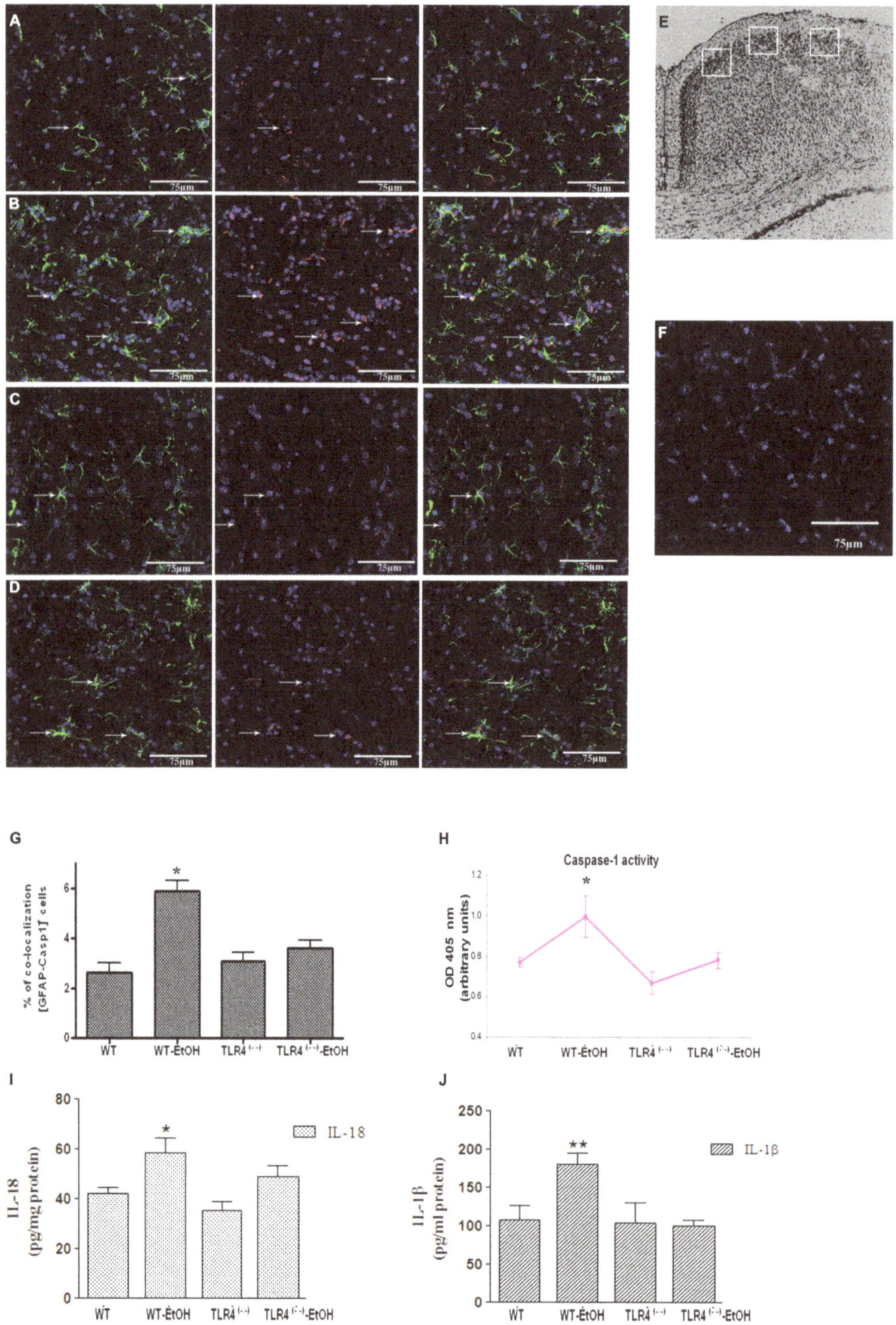

FIGURE 1 | Chronic ethanol intake increases caspase-1 activity in cortical astroglial cells of TLR4 mice. (A–D) Confocal images illustrate the co-localization of caspase-1 (red) with GFAP (green) in the cortex area **(E)** of TLR4$^{+/+}$ **(A,B)** and TLR4$^{-/-}$ **(C,D)** mice (arrows indicate co-localization of the Casp-1 and GFAP-positive cells). **(F)** Confocal negative controls, in the absence of primary antibodies. We used four independent biological replicates from each experimental condition. Scale bar: 75 μm. **(G)** The quantitative analysis shows the percentage of the increased number of Casp-1/GFAP-positive co-localized cells in the cortices of ethanol-treated WT mice in relation to the untreated control mice. Non-significant changes were observed for the treated/untreated TLR4$^{-/-}$ (TLR4-KO) mice. **(H)** Caspase-1 enzymatic activity was determined in the brain cortex. **(I,J)** The analysis of the IL-1β and IL-18 cytokines in the cortical homogenates of TLR4 mice was conducted by ELISA. Values represent the [mean ± SEM] of at least six to eight individual experiments. $*p < 0.05$, $**p < 0.01$ (Mann–Whitney *U* non-parametric test or a Student's *t*-test).

*labeling of NLRP3-inflammasome and GFAP in cultured astrocytes**. Treated/untreated astroglial cells were previously incubated with 0.25% Triton in PBS solution for 10 min for cellular permeabilization. Cells were then blocked for 1 h at room temperature with 10% normal goat serum in TBS/T (0.1%), and were incubated overnight at 4°C with the following primary antibodies; anti-NLRP3 (1/150, AdipoGen) and anti-GFAP (1/400, Sigma–Aldrich), following incubation with the respective Alexa-fluor-conjugated secondary antibodies (1/500, Invitrogen, Molecular Probes). Nuclei were stained with DAPI. All the negative controls were also performed as described above *(i)*. Cells were mounted onto glass slides with Dako Fluorescent Mounting medium (Dako North America Inc., CA, USA), and confocal images were analyzed with the ImageJ 1.42 software (NIH). All the confocal images were acquired using the same settings, while fluorescence distribution was acquired with a Leica TCS-SP2-AOBA confocal laser-scanning microscope (Leica Microsystems, Heidelberg GmbH, Mannheim, Germany) using the 10× Plan-HCX PL APO CS10 and the 40× Plan-HCX PL APO CS40 × 1.25 oil objectives. All the confocal images were acquired with the same settings and the fluorescence distributions were analyzed by the Leica Confocal Software "Leica Lite," version 2.61.

CASPASE-1 ASSAY ACTIVITY

Caspase-1 activity was measured by the Colorimetric Assay Kit (Abcam). This assay allows the detection of chromophore *p*-nitroanilide (*p*NA) after cleavage from labeled substrate YVAD-*p*NA, performed following the manufacturer's instructions. *p*NA light emission was quantified by a spectrophotometer at 405 nm. The comparison of the absorbance of *p*NA from treated vs. untreated controls allowed the determination of the fold increase in caspase-1 activity.

PRIMARY CULTURE OF ASTROCYTES AND TREATMENTS

Primary cultured astrocytes of mice cortices (WT or TLR4-KO) from newborn pups were prepared and characterized as previously described (Minana et al., 2000). Cells were plated on 60-mm diameter plates in Dulbecco's modified Eagle's medium (DMEM, Gibco Invitrogen Corporation, Barcelona) containing 20% FBS, supplemented with L-glutamine (1%), glucose (1%), fungizone (1%), and antibiotics (1%). Cultures were grown in a humidified atmosphere of 5% CO_2/95% air at 37°C. After 1 week of culture, FBS was reduced to 10%, and the medium was changed twice a week. Cells were grown to confluence and were used after 12 days in culture. The purity of astrocytes was assessed by immunofluorescence using: anti-glial fibrillary acidic protein (anti-GFAP, astrocyte marker, Sigma-Aldrich, Madrid, Spain), anti-CD11b (microglial marker, Serotec, Bionova, Madrid, Spain), anti-myelin basic protein (MBP, olygodendroglial marker, Sigma–Aldrich, Madrid, Spain) and anti-microtubule-associated protein 2 (MAP-2, neuronal marker, Sigma–Aldrich, Madrid, Spain). Astrocyte cultures were found to be at least 98% GFAP-positive and 2% CD11b-positive.

To assess the effect of ethanol (EtOH; 10 or 50 mM), lipopolysaccharide (LPS; 50 ng/ml) or ATP (5 mM), these compounds were added to DMEM in the absence of serum, but in the presence of 1 mg/ml bovine serum albumin. After 24 h of LPS, ATP or ethanol treatments, cells were harvested by trypsinization, centrifuged and used for specific determinations. The medium was used for cytokine determination.

In some experiments, astrocytes were incubated with a medium containing Z-YVAD-FMK (10 μM), a potent cell permeable and irreversible caspase-1 inhibitor (ICE; Parajuli et al., 2013; Tseng et al., 2013) or with Z-VAD-FMK (20 μM), a pan-caspase inhibitor (Dostert et al., 2009) or NLRP3 blocking peptide (bp; 4 μg/ml; Abcam) or Mito-TEMPO (500 μM), a ROS scavenger, for 30 or 60 min (for Mito-TEMPO) before and during ethanol (50 mM), or with ATP (5 mM) or LPS (50 ng/ml) treatments. Caspase-1 enzymatic activity, ROS release, IL-1β and IL-18 cytokines were determined in cells after 24 h treatments. Sterile toxin-free culture materials were used for all the experiments. In addition, the possible contamination of ethanol with LPS was determined by using the chromogenic limulus amebocyte lysate test, following the manufacturer's instructions (Lonza Verviers SPRL). The endotoxin content in ethanol solution was 2.98×10^3 pg/ml, which is far below the concentration required to induce astroglial activation under our assay conditions, as previously described (Alfonso-Loeches et al., 2010).

FLUORESCENCE-ACTIVATED CELL SORTING (FACS)

MitoSOX™ red mitochondrial superoxide indicator

To evaluate superoxide production by mitochondria, the MitoSOX™ Red reagent (1.25 μM, Molecular Probes) was used in live cells, a fluorogenic dye specifically targeted to mitochondria in live cells. This reagent is readily oxidized by superoxide, but not by other ROS- or reactive nitrogen species (RNS)-generating systems. Oxidation of MitoSOX™ Red reagent by superoxide produces red fluorescence. For these experiments, astrocytes were incubated for 24 h with different treatments; ethanol (10, 50 mM), LPS (50 ng/ml), ATP (5 mM) or rotenone (25 μM) as the positive controls, and with inhibitors Z-YVAD-FMK (Calbiochem) or NLRP3 bp or Mito-TEMPO. Then cells were further incubated with MitoSOX™ (1.25 μM) for 30 min at 25°C in the darkness. Cell samples were acquired with a Cytomics FC500 flow cytometer (Beckman-Coulter, USA) equipped with 488 and 635 nm lasers detectors for forward scatter (FS) and side scatter (SS). We defined the cell population with the FS and SS parameters, MitoSOX Red was excited by laser at 488 nm, and its fluorescence emission was collected at 620 nm. In order to perform the analysis in live cells, a gate in the dot plot FS vs. SS was used, where cell debris was gated out for the analysis. We also used the LIVE/DEAD® Fixable Near-IR Dead Cell Stain Kit (Molecular Probes) to determine the viability of cells, and only the live cell population was used for the analysis. Data were represented as the [mean ± SEM], showing the percentage of gated mean intensity of MitoSOX fluorescence expressed as a percentage when comparing untreated or DMSO vehicle control-cells with MitoSOX positive-cells.

AN IN CELL ANALYZER FOR CELLULAR DEATH DETECTION

The six-well plated cultured cells were incubated with the red caspase-1 detection probe, 660-YVAD-FMK (FLICA) following the manufacturer's instructions (ImmunoChemistry Technologies, USA). Cells were washed with 4°C PBS before adding the

500 μl Annexin-binding buffer containing 2.5 μl of Annexin-V fluorescein isothiocyanate (FITC) and Hoechst (5 μg/ml) for 30 min of incubation. Finally, we added 1 μl propidium iodide (PI) solution for a further 5-min incubation in the dark. The stained samples were imaged live in an In Cell Analyzer 1000 high-content analysis system (GE Healthcare Life Sciences) equipped with a CCD camera and a 10×/0.45 NA objective. The 51008 polychroic mirror set was used in conjunction with the following excitation (×) and emission (m) filter combinations: 405/20×, 535/50m for Hoechst 33342, 475/20×, 535/50 m for Annexin-V FITC, 475/20×, 620/60 m for PI and 620/60×, 700/75 m for FLICA 660-YVAD-FMK. For the analysis, we defined a segmentation based on nuclei staining with Hoechst 33342. Then we established four groups in order to classify five populations: (1) Live cells were defined as negative cells for PI and normal staining with Hoechst 33342; (2) Apoptotic cells were defined as negative cells for PI and nuclei with increased staining with Hoechst 33342 (due to DNA condensation); (3) Necrotic cells were defined as positive for PI and negative for FLICA 660-YVAD-FMK staining; (4) pyroptotic cells were defined as double positive for PI and FLICA 660-YVAD-FMK. Twenty fields were acquired for each well. Four different experiments were performed and approximately 2000–10,000 cells were analyzed per experimental condition. The analysis was performed in the In Cell Analyzer 1000 Workstation software using the Multi Target Analysis Module.

MITOTRACKER LIVE CELLS STAINING AND CO-LOCALIZATION STUDIES IN ASTROGLIAL CELLS

The astrocytes in primary culture were incubated for 10 min at 37°C with the MitoTracker® Red CMXRos probe (50 nM, Molecular Probes, USA). This probe passively allows diffusion across the plasma membrane and is accumulated in active mitochondria. Cells were then treated with an aldehyde-based fixative, 3.7% of paraformaldehyde to allow further sample processing. For the co-localization studies, the cells stained with MitoTracker were immunostained with NLRP3 and with caspase-1 activity labeling. For this end, cells were incubated for 10 min in PBS containing 0.1% Triton X-100, rinsed off with PBS (1×) and blocked for 1 h/RT with 10% normal goat serum in TBS/T (0.1%). After blocking, sections were incubated with the mouse monoclonal anti-NLRP3 (1/150, AdipoGEN) followed by Alexa fluor 405 (1/500, Molecular Probes). Then sections were incubated with caspase-1 fluorescence activity using the FAM-FLICA™ Caspase-1 assay kit (ImmunoChemistry Technologies, USA). For this labeling, cells were incubated for 1 h at RT with the fluorescent FAM-YVAD-FMK FLICA reagent following the manufacturer's instructions (ImmunoChemistry Technologies, USA). The reagent becomes covalently coupled to the active enzyme and is retained within the cell, while the unbound FAM-YVAD-FMK FLICA reagent diffuses out of the cell and is washed away. The remaining green fluorescent signal is a direct measure of active caspase-1 enzyme activity. All the negative controls were performed by replacing the respective primary antibodies with isotype and concentration-matched irrelevant antibodies.

Sections were mounted onto glass slides with FluorSave Reagent (Calbiochem, USA). All the images were acquired using the same settings under a Leica TCS-SP2-AOBA confocal laser-scanning microscope (Leica Microsystems, Heidelberg GmbH, Mannheim, Germany) employing the 63× N.A. 1.4 oil objective. All the confocal images were acquired with the same settings and fluorescence distribution was analyzed by the Leica Confocal Software "Leica Lite," version 2.61. Graphs represent the number of cellular co-localizations expressed as a percentage (%) of mitochondria co-localized with the NLRP3 receptor or the NLRP3 receptor with caspase-1 activity after the different treatments had been applied.

CYTOKINES DETECTION

The supernatant medium from the 24 h-treated astrocytes and lysates from the brain cortices were used for cytokine determinations. Brain tissue was homogenized in cold lysis buffer (1% NP-40, 20 mM Tris-HCl, pH 8, 130 mM NaCl, 10 mM NaF, 10 μg/ml aprotinin, 10 mg/ml leupeptin, 10 μM DTT, 1 mM Na_3VO_4 and 1 mM PMSF; 250 mg tissue/0.5 ml). Lysis samples were kept on ice for 30 min and were centrifuged at maximum speed for 15 min, and the supernatant was collected for protein and cytokines determination. Protein was determined by the Bradford Assay (Bio-Rad, Hercules, CA, USA). The cytokine levels of IL-18 and IL-1β were measured using the enzyme-linked immunosorbent assay (ELISA) kits (Bender MedSystems GmbH, Austria) following the manufacturer's instructions.

WESTERN BLOT ANALYSIS

The protein extracts from the cortex and cultured astrocytes were homogenized in 250 mg tissue/0.5 ml cold lysis buffer (see above). Then they were kept on ice for 30 min, centrifuged at maximum speed for 15 min, and the supernatant was collected to determine the proteins levels using the Bradford Assay (Bio-Rad, Hercules, CA, USA). Lysates were separated by SDS-PAGE gels and were transferred to PVDF membranes following standard techniques. Membranes were blocked with 5% non-fat dried milk in TBS containing 0.1% Tween-20 (TBS-T). Next they were then incubated overnight with the following primary antibodies: anti-NLRP3 (1 μg/ml, Abcam), anti-caspase-1 (1/100, Santa Cruz Biotechnology); anti-pro-caspase-1 (1/200, Abcam); anti-Apaf-1 (1 μg/ml, Millipore Bioscience Research Reagents); anti-caspase-3 (1:500) and anti-caspase-9 (1:1000, Cell Signaling).

Some membranes were stripped for 1 h at 60°C in an SDS solution (2% SDS, 0.85% 2-ME, and 65 mM Tris-HCl, pH 6.8, and were washed and incubated with anti-GAPDH (1/3000, Chemicon) for 2 h as a loading control. The intensity of the bands was quantified with the image analysis program, α-Ease FC, version α Imager 2200 (Alpha Innotech Corporation).

ASC OLIGOMERIZATION ASSAY

Apoptosis-associated speck-like protein containing a CARD pyroptosome were performed following the procedure of (Fernandes-Alnemri and Alnemri, 2008) with minor modifications. Thus, astrocytes were seeded in 50-mm diameter plates (1×10^6 cells per well) and treated with different stimuli. Cells were pelleted by centrifugation and resuspended in 0.5 ml of ice-cold buffer containing PBS/Triton 0.5%, and lysed by shearing 10 times. Cell lysates were then centrifuged at 8000 × *g* for 15 min at 4°C, and the resultant pellets were washed twice with PBS and resuspended in 200 μl of PBS. The resuspended pellets, were then cross-linked with fresh disuccinimidyl suberate (DSS; 2 mM) for 30 min at room temperature, and pelleted by centrifugation at 8000 × *g* for 15 min. The cross-linked pellets were resuspended in 30 μl of SDS sample buffer, separated using 12% SDS-PAGE and immunoblotted employing anti-mouse ASC antibodies. The dimer band was quantified by densitometry.

CO-IMMUNOPRECIPITATION OF NLRP3 AND CASPASE-1

Pre-cleared cell lysates were used for the co-immunoprecipitation (Co-IP) analysis using a Pierce Co-IP kit (Thermo Scientific Pierce) and following the manufacturer's instructions. This kit provides covalent antibody immobilization onto an insoluble agarose support, and then incubated with a cell lysate containing the target protein. We use the purify mouse anti-NLRP3 antibody (10 μg, AdipoGEn) to immunoprecipitate the antigen (bait protein, IB) which bind the interacting protein (prey protein, IP) caspase-1 (1/100, Santa Cruz). Upon elution the immune complexes, the samples were resolved with 15% SDS-PAGE and transferred to PVDF membranes (Bio-Rad) for immunoblotting. The mouse IgG was used as a negative control.

LACTATE DEHYDROGENASE (LDH) ACTIVITY

The release of LDH in the culture supernatant of astrocytes was measured using the colorimetric Cyto-Tox 96 Non-radioactive Assay (Promega) following the manufacturer's instructions. This assay is a coupled enzymatic assay, which results in the conversion of a tetrazolium salt into a formazan product which, in turn, is proportional to the number of lysed cells. We used triton X-100 as a positive control. The LDH value was expressed as the percentage of total LDH activity, according to the following equation: %LDH release rate = 100 × [(Experimental − Effector Spontaneous − Target Spontaneous)/(Target Maximum − Target Spontaneous)].

TERMINAL DEOXYNUCLEOTIDYL TRANSFERASE dUTP NICK END LABELING (TUNEL)

To assess cellular apoptosis (programmed cell death), we used the *in Situ* Cell Death Detection Kit (Roche), Fluorescein. In brief, coverslips with adherent cells were fixed and permeabilized (see Immunofluorescence) following incubation in a nucleotide mixture containing fluorescein-dUTP and TdT (terminal transferase), according to the manufacturer's instructions. Cell nuclei were detected by incubation with DAPI. Micrographs were digitally recorded with a Leica DM6000 FS fluorescence microscope. TUNEL-positive cells appeared green, whereas TUNEL-negative nuclei appeared blue. Negative controls were incubated without TdT. The percentage of TUNEL-positive cells *vs.* TUNEL-negative cells was quantified for each experimental condition.

RNA ISOLATION, REVERSE TRANSCRIPTION PCR AND QUANTIFICATION OF mRNA LEVELS

RNA was extracted from the cortex brain area using Trizol according to the manufacturer's instructions (Sigma). RNA was measured in a NanoDrop ND-1000 Spectrophotometer (260/280 nm ratio). First-strand cDNA synthesis was performed with the *Transcriptor First Strand cDNA Synthesis Kit* (Roche Applied Biosystems) using 2000 ng of total RNA according to the manufacturer's instructions. The RT-PCR reactions contained *LightCycler 480 SYBR Green I Master (2×*; Roche Applied Science), 5 μM forward and reverse primers, and 1 μl of cDNA. RT-PCR was performed in a LightCycler® *480 System* (Roche). The amplification efficiency (E) of the primers was calculated from the plot of the Cq values against the cDNA input according to the equation $E = [10(-1/\text{slope})]$. The relative expression ratio of a target/reference gene was calculated according to the Pfaffl equation (Pfaffl, 2001). The sequence of both the forward and reverse primers used in this study is detailed in **Table 1**. Housekeeping cyclophilin A (PPIA) was used as an internal control. Fluorescence was recorded in the annealing/elongation step in each cycle. A melting curve analysis was performed at the end of each PCR to check the specificity of the primers.

STATISTICAL ANALYSIS

Data were analyzed using a Mann–Whitney *U* non-parametric test or one-way ANOVA followed by a Dunnett's Multiple Comparison or a Student's *t*-test (SPSS program, version 17.0). Differences at a value of $p < 0.05$ were considered statistically significant

RESULTS

ETHANOL ACTIVATES THE NLRP3 INFLAMMASOME-COMPLEX FORMATION IN ASTROGLIAL CELLS FROM CEREBRAL CORTEX AND PRIMARY CULTURE

Glial cells are important players in the immune response in the CNS (Farina et al., 2007). Our previous studies demonstrated that ethanol activates TLR4 signaling in astrocytes (Blanco et al., 2005; Alfonso-Loeches et al., 2010). We therefore wondered if ethanol was also capable of activating the inflammasome in astroglial cells to contribute to ethanol-induced neuroinflammation. To answer this question, we first evaluated whether ethanol treatment promotes caspase-1 activation and the release of interleukins IL-1β and IL-18 in both cerebral cortex (Ctx) area (**Figure 1E**) and in cortical astroglial cells (**Figure 2C**). The biochemical and immunohistochemical analyses revealed that chronic ethanol treatment increases the co-localization of caspase-1 with GFAP-positive cells (**Figures 1B,G**) and up-regulates the total caspase-1 activity levels (**Figure 1H**) in the cerebral Ctx of WT mice when

Table 1 | Gene primer sequences.

Gene	Sequences	cDNA size	T_m
NLRP3-F	*GGGCTTCTGCACCCGGACTG*	328	65°
NLRP3-R	*GGTGGTCCTGCTTCCACGCC*	328	65°
AIM2-F	*GTCACCAGTTCCTCAGTTGTG*	259	60°
AIM2-R	*TGTCTCCTTCCTCGCACTTT*	259	60°
NLRP1-F	*TCTCAGTGCCCAGGTGATTA*	151	60°
NLRP1-R	*TTGTCTCTGCTGCTTGAATGA*	151	60°
IPAF-F	*AAGGATGAAGGGCTGAAGGT*	159	60°
IPAF-R	*CGAAACTTGTAGGCTGACCA*	159	60°

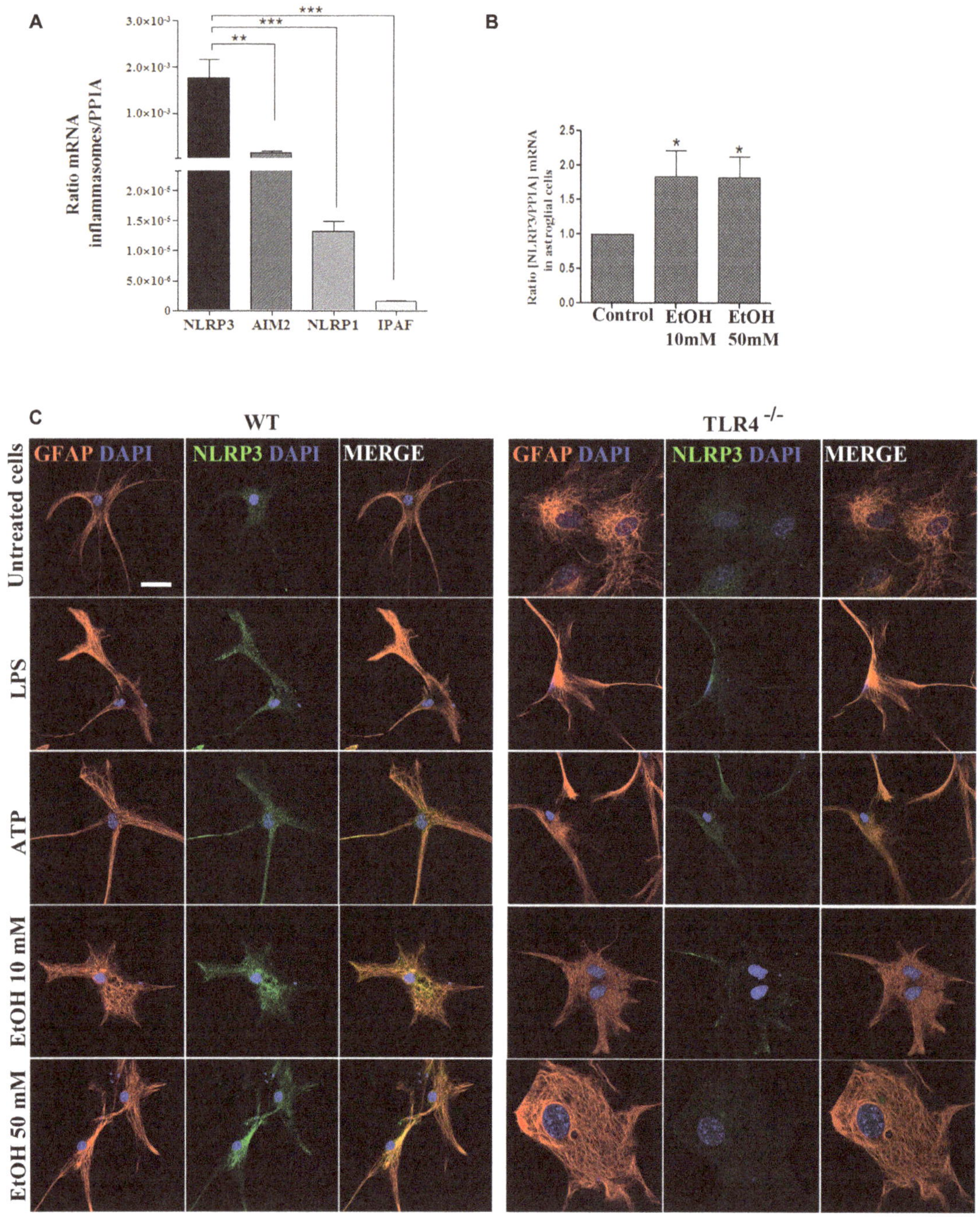

FIGURE 2 | Astrocytes in primary culture expresses high levels of NLRP3 mRNA. (A) mRNA expression of NLRP3, AIM2, NLRP1, and IPAF inflammasomes in cultured astrocytes evaluated by RT-PCR. **(B)** Ethanol treatment (10 and 50 mM) for 24 h up-regulates the NLRP3 mRNA levels in the cultured astrocytes from TLR4 mice. We used $n = 5–7$ independent experiments and ratios were normalized with the PPIA housekeeping gene. Bars represent the [mean ± SEM]. $*p < 0.05$, $**p < 0.01$, $***p < 0.001$ (Mann–Whitney *U* non-parametric test or a Student's *t*-test). **(C)** Immunofluorescence of NLRP3 (green) and GFAP- (red) co-localization in the astrocytes from TLR4 and TLR4-knockout mice. Scale bar 20 μm.

compared with untreated animals (**Figures 1A,G**). We also determined interleukins IL-1β and IL-18 in the Ctx of the WT and TLR4-KO mice treated with or without ethanol for 5 months. **Figures 1I,J** shows that ethanol treatment up-regulates the levels of IL-1β and IL-18 in the Ctx of the WT mice. Conversely, the same ethanol treatment neither increased caspase-1 activation (**Figures 1C,D,G,H**) nor the levels of IL-1β and IL-18 (**Figures 1I,J**) in the Ctx of TLR4-KO mice.

To gain further insight into how ethanol affects inflammasome activation and which type of inflammasome was activated in astroglial cells, we used highly enriched astrocytes in primary culture, and the gene expression of different inflammasomes were assessed. An RT-PCR analysis revealed (**Figure 2A**) that although inflammasomes NLRP3, AIM2, NLRP1, and IPAF are expressed in astrocytes; the NLRP3 mRNA level was higher than the other inflammasomes, and the ethanol treatment (10 and 50 mM) was capable of up-regulating the NLRP3 mRNA levels (**Figure 2B**). The immunofluorescence studies also revealed that the NLRP3 protein expression is expressed in the cytosol of GFAP$^+$ cells (**Figure 2C**), although higher NLRP3 expression are noted in WT astrocytes treated with LPS, ATP or ethanol (10, 50 mM).

The assembly of the NLRP3 inflammasome complex required adaptor protein ASC and its oligomerization to bring the receptor and zymogen pro-caspase-1 into close proximity, which led to caspase-1 activation, and to the cleavage of pro-IL-1β and pro-IL-18 into their active cytokine and pyroptotic cell death (Fernandes-Alnemri et al., 2007). Therefore, in order to evaluate if ethanol, in comparison with other inflammasome stimuli, was capable of inducing ASC oligomerization, the cleavage of caspase-1 and the production of IL-1β and IL-18, astrocytes were treated with LPS, ATP (a positive control of NLRP3 activation) and ethanol (10, 50 mM). **Figure 3** shows that ethanol and the LPS or ATP treatment promoted: (i) up-regulation of NLRP3; (ii) caspase-1 activation, as evidenced by the appearance of the 10 kDa active caspase-1-clevage peptide (**Figure 3A**); (iii) ASC oligomerization, as demonstrated by the notably presence of ASC dimers and some trimers (Fernandes-Alnemri and Alnemri, 2008; **Figure 3B**); (iv) the association between caspase-1 cleavage and NLRP3, as demonstrated by the Co-IP of both proteins with the appearance of the active p20/p10 caspase-1 in treated-astrocytes (**Figure 3C**); and (v) the production of pro-inflammatory cytokines IL-1β and IL-18 (**Figure 3D**). If we consider that ASC is an adaptor protein required for the activation of both NLRP3 inflammasome and caspase-1 (Fernandes-Alnemri et al., 2007), the results indicate that by inducing NLRP3 inflammasome complex activation and ASC-pyroptosome formation, ethanol was capable of inducing the innate immune response. Our results further suggest that activation of NLRP3/caspase-1 is associated with the TLR4 function since the astrocytes from TLR4-KO mice presented no response or a minimal one to different stimuli, including alcohol, on NLRP3 inflammasome activation (**Figures 3A–D**).

ETHANOL-INDUCED MITOCHONDRIAL ROS FORMATION TRIGGERS NLRP3 INFLAMMASOME COMPLEX ACTIVATION

One of the mechanisms by which NLRP3 inflammasome can be activated is ROS generation (Tschopp and Schroder, 2010), and mROS formation seems particularly critical for NLRP3 activation (Zhou et al., 2011). We therefore explored the potential role of ethanol-induced mROS in NLRP3 inflammasome activation. To assess superoxide production by mitochondria in cultured astrocytes, we used the MitoSOX^{TM} Red reagent in live cells, a fluorogenic dye that specifically targets mitochondria in live cells, and a flow cytometry analysis. For these experiments, astrocytes were treated with ethanol (10 and 50 mM), LPS and ATP for 24 h in the presence or absence of Mito-TEMPO [a mitochondria (m) ROS scavenger] or a Z-YVAD-FMK (specific caspase-1 inhibitor) or z-VAD-FMK (inhibitor of caspase proteases) or a NLRP3 bp. Then mROS production was measured. The results indicate that treating WT astrocytes with ATP or LPS or ethanol (10 mM or 50 mM) markedly induced mROS production (**Figure 4A**). Notably, the mROS production induced by ethanol (10 and 50 mM) or LPS or ATP was significantly abrogated by Mito-TEMPO, z-YVAD-FMK, or Z-VAD-FMK by the presence of NLRP3 bp (**Figure 4A**). Strikingly, small, but non-significant, changes were noted in the TLR4-KO astrocytes incubated with ATP, or LPS or ethanol (**Figure 4B**). These results suggest that mROS generation induced by ATP or LPS or ethanol mediates NLRP3/caspase-1 inflammasome activation. Our findings also suggest crosstalk between TLR4 and NLRP3 inflammasome.

To confirm the above results, we measured the levels of IL-1β and IL-18 in the medium of astrocytes incubated for 24 h with ATP or LPS or ethanol (10 and 50 mM), in the presence or absence of Mito-TEMPO or z-YVAD-FMK or Z-VAD-FMK or NLRP3 bp. According to the above results, ATP or LPS or ethanol (10 and 50 mM) treatment induces the production of IL-1β and IL-18 in the astrocytes supernatant, while the presence of Mito-TEMPO or z-YVAD-FMK or Z-VAD-FMK or NLRP3 bp abolishes most of the cytokine released in the cell medium (**Figures 5A,B**). However, the results presented in **Figure 5** illustrate that while both Z-YVAD-FMK and z-VAD-FMK were more efficient than NLRP3 bp or Mito-TEMPO in inhibiting IL-18 in all the treatments, the caspase-1 inhibitor did not completely abolish the release of IL-1β induced by ATP or LPS or ethanol, suggesting that this cytokine may be produced by other mechanisms (Hanamsagar et al., 2012). No significant variations in the levels of IL-1β or IL-18 were noted in the TLR4-KO astrocytes treated with ATP, LPS or even ethanol (**Figures 5A,B**).

INFLAMMASOME STIMULATION INDUCES CASPASE-1 AND NLRP3 RECRUITMENT WITHIN THE MITOCHONDRIA IN ASTROCYTES

Previous studies have shown that NLRP3 is located at the endoplasmic reticulum (ER) in the steady state and that it translocates to the mitochondria-associated ER membranes following stimulation (Zhou et al., 2011). Therefore, in order to gain further insights into ethanol-induced NLRP3 inflammasome activation, we used confocal microscopy to assess the location of NLRP3 under basal and stimulated conditions. We noted that under basal conditions, NLRP3 was located at the cytoplasm, but not within mitochondria (**Figure 6A**). We were unable to detect caspase-1 under the steady-state conditions. However, stimulation of astrocytes with ATP, LPS or ethanol (10 mM) led to the recruitment of caspase-1 and NLRP3 within mitochondria, as demonstrated by the overlap of caspase-1 and NLRP3 in the mitochondria (mitotracker staining). Strikingly, ATP and ethanol stimulation promoted higher caspase-1 levels within mitochondria than LPS. Inhibiting caspase-1 with Z-VAD-FMK (**Figure 6B**) or mROS with Mito-TEMPO (**Figure 6C**) mostly abolished NLRP3/caspase1 recruitment within mitochondria.

It is noteworthy that ATP, LPS, or ethanol (10 mM) did not promote NLRP3/caspase-1 activation and recruitment into the mitochondria in TLR4-KO astrocytes (**Figure 6**). Immunofluorescence studies with pro-caspase-1 and NLRP3 in untreated

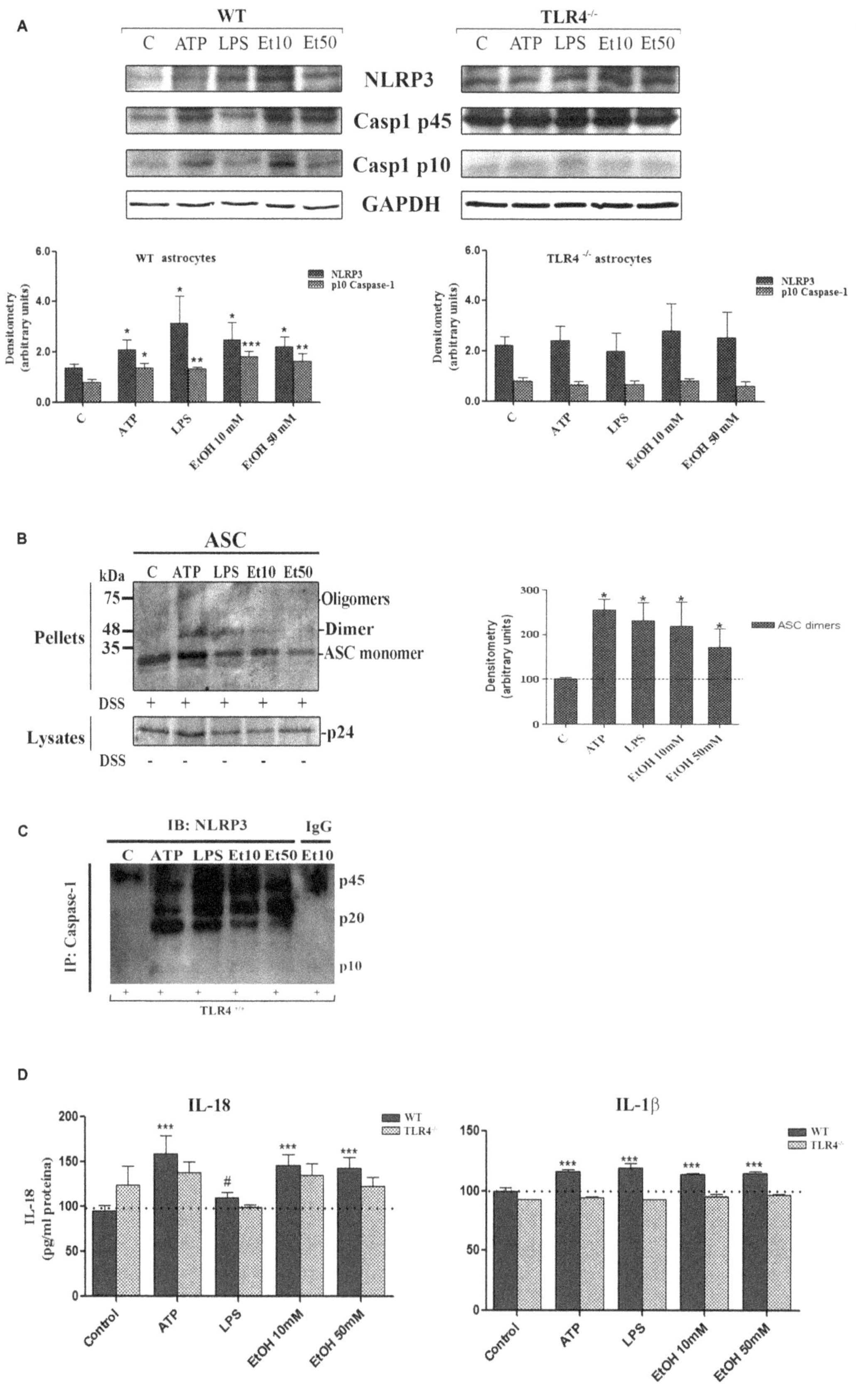

FIGURE 3 | Continued

FIGURE 3 | Continued
Ethanol treatment activates the NLRP3 inflammasome complex in cultured astrocytes from TLR4-WT mice. (A) Western blot analysis shows the NLRP3 and p10/caspase-1 active cleavage (the initiator caspase in pyroptosis) protein levels in the LPS-, ATP-, and ethanol- (10 and 50 mM) treated astrocytes. **(B)** We show ASC oligomerization and quantification of the ASC dimer by densitometry. Cells were lysed, pelleted by centrifugation and incubated with DSS for 30 min. The cross-linked pellets were resuspended in SDS sample buffer, and proteins were separated using 12% SDS-PAGE and Western blotted with anti-mouse ASC antibodies as described under Section "Material and Methods." The presence of dimers and trimers was observed in the ATP-, LPS-, or ethanol-treated astrocytes correlating with a significative up-regulation of ASC dimers. **(C)** Cell lysates were collected and co-immunoprecipitated with the NLRP3 Ab (IP), and the immune complexes were detected by Western blot with Caspase-1 (IB). We show the presence of the p45 caspase-1 precursor and the active p20/p10 Caspase-1 in treated/untreated astrocytes. The mouse IgG was used as a negative control. **(D)** ELISA measured determined the IL-1β and IL-18 levels in the supernatant of the astrocytes treated with LPS, ATP and ethanol (10 and 50 mM) after 24 h. Non-significant differences were observed between the treated or non-treated TLR4-KO astrocytes. Values represent the mean ± SEM of 3–9 individual experiments. $^{\#}p < 0.06$, $^{*}p < 0.05$, $^{**}p < 0.01$, $^{***}p < 0.001$ (Mann–Whitney *U* non-parametric test or a Student's *t*-test).

astrocytes and those treated with ATP, LPS and ethanol (10 mM) from WT and TLR4-KO mice also demonstrated that while stimulation with ATP, LPS or ethanol reduces the pro-caspase-1 levels and increases NLRP3 expression (**Figure 2**) and its co-localization in the WT cell cytoplasm, no changes in these parameters were observed in untreated or treated TLR4-KO astrocytes. In short, the results suggest that the by triggering pro-IL-1β production (Gross et al., 2011), TLR4 acts as a priming signal which, along with ROS production (second signal), promotes NLRP3 inflammasome activation. Lack of TLR4 signaling (TLR4-KO) was able to abolish the production of not only pro-IL-1, but also of other cytokines which might target to the mitochondria to initiate mROS production.

ETHANOL-INDUCED NLRP3 INFLAMMASOME ACTIVATION TRIGGERS PYROPTOSIS AND APOPTOSIS

Inflammasome-dependent caspase-1 activity has been shown to cause a rapid inflammatory form of cell death called pyroptosis, in which cytoplasmic content and pro-inflammatory cytokines, including IL-1β and IL-18, are released (Miao et al., 2011). However, apoptosis can also be induced by mitochondria stress and NLRP3 activation (Morizot, 2012), and our previous studies have indicated that ethanol can cause activation of caspase-3-dependent apoptosis and necrosis in the cerebral cortex (Alfonso-Loeches et al., 2010). Therefore, in order to evaluate whether ethanol-induced TLR4-dependent mitochondrial ROS production and NLRP3 activation promote pyroptosis and/or apoptosis, treated and untreated astrocytes were labeled with different staining and then, the proportion of those cells that died by apoptosis, necrosis or pyroptosis were evaluated using an In Cell Analyzer. As shown in **Figure 7A**, treatment of the astrocytes with ATP or LPS or ethanol 10 mM or ethanol 50 mM promotes 10.2, 15, 15.9, and 9.5% of pyroptosis (PI^{+} and FLICA 660-YVAD-FMK^{+} cells), respectively, when compared with untreated control cells.

Pyroptosis was also evaluated by measuring the levels of LDH release upon the different treatments. The results in **Figure 7B** illustrate that either ethanol or ATP treatments induces the release of cytoplasmic LDH in the cell medium. In all cases, pyroptosis was abrogated by Z-YVAD-FMK (a caspase-1 inhibitor) or Z-VAD-FMK or Mito-TEMPO treatments (**Figures 7A,B**). Notably, ATP, LPS or ethanol also induced a slight, yet significant increase in apoptosis (PI^{-} cells and increased staining with Hoechst 33342 due to DNA condensation). Thus, the percentage of apoptosis was 3.2, 3.3, 2.9, and 3.3% upon treatment with ATP, LPS or ethanol (10 and 50 mM), respectively (**Figure 7A**). No significant or minimal changes in pyroptosis or apoptosis were observed in treated TLR4-KO astrocytes.

Although apoptosis represents a small proportion of cell death induced by NLRP3 inflammasome activation, recent evidence has indicated that mitochondria stress can also lead to inflammation, NLRP3 activation and cell death by apoptosis (Morizot, 2012). We therefore evaluated the role of mitochondria ROS production and apoptosome formation by assessing the levels of Apaf-1 and active peptide caspase-9/caspase-3 in the astrocytes stimulated with ATP and ethanol. As shown in **Figure 8A**, both ATP and ethanol (10 mM and 50 mM) increase the levels of Apaf-1 and the active (cleaved) forms of caspase-9 and caspase-3 to trigger apoptosis, as confirmed by the TUNEL assay (**Figure 8B**). These results suggest that ethanol-induced NLRP3 inflammasome activation can trigger mainly pyroptosis, but may also induce apoptosis.

DISCUSSION

Innate immune activation can occur in the nervous system in response to infections and/or tissue damage (Lampron et al., 2013). Two main receptors and signaling pathways are involved in this response, membrane receptors TLRs and cytoplasm sensors NLRPs, which regulate caspase-1 activity through inflammasome formation. Activation of TLRs has been shown to participate in brain infection and neurodegenerative disorders (Hanamsagar et al., 2012). However, less information is available on the role of inflammasome in brain damage and neuroinflammation, and the cellular source of inflammasome activation during brain infection or injury is lacking. In this study, we show that astrocytes express various inflammasomes, although NRLP3 expression is higher. We further demonstrate that ethanol as well as ATP or LPS, triggers the recruitment of NLRP3 and active caspase-1 within mitochondria by inducing mROS formation, which promotes the production of IL-1β and IL-18. The present findings also reveal crosstalk between TLR4 and the NLRP3 inflammasome complex since the elimination of the TLR4 function markedly reduces ethanol- or ATP-induced NLRP3 inflammasome activation and cytokines production.

NLRP3 is an intracellular protein complex composed of NLRP3, ASC, and pro-caspase-1, and it serves as a platform to activate pro-inflammatory cytokines IL-1β and IL-18 (Schroder et al., 2010). Recent structural studies have revealed the importance of ASC^{PYD}/ASC^{PYD} and $NLRP3^{PYD}/ASC^{PYD}$ interactions during inflammasome activation (Lu et al., 2014). NLRP3 can be activated by pathogens and by a wide range of cytosolic DAMPs, including ATP, potassium efflux, alum, uric acid

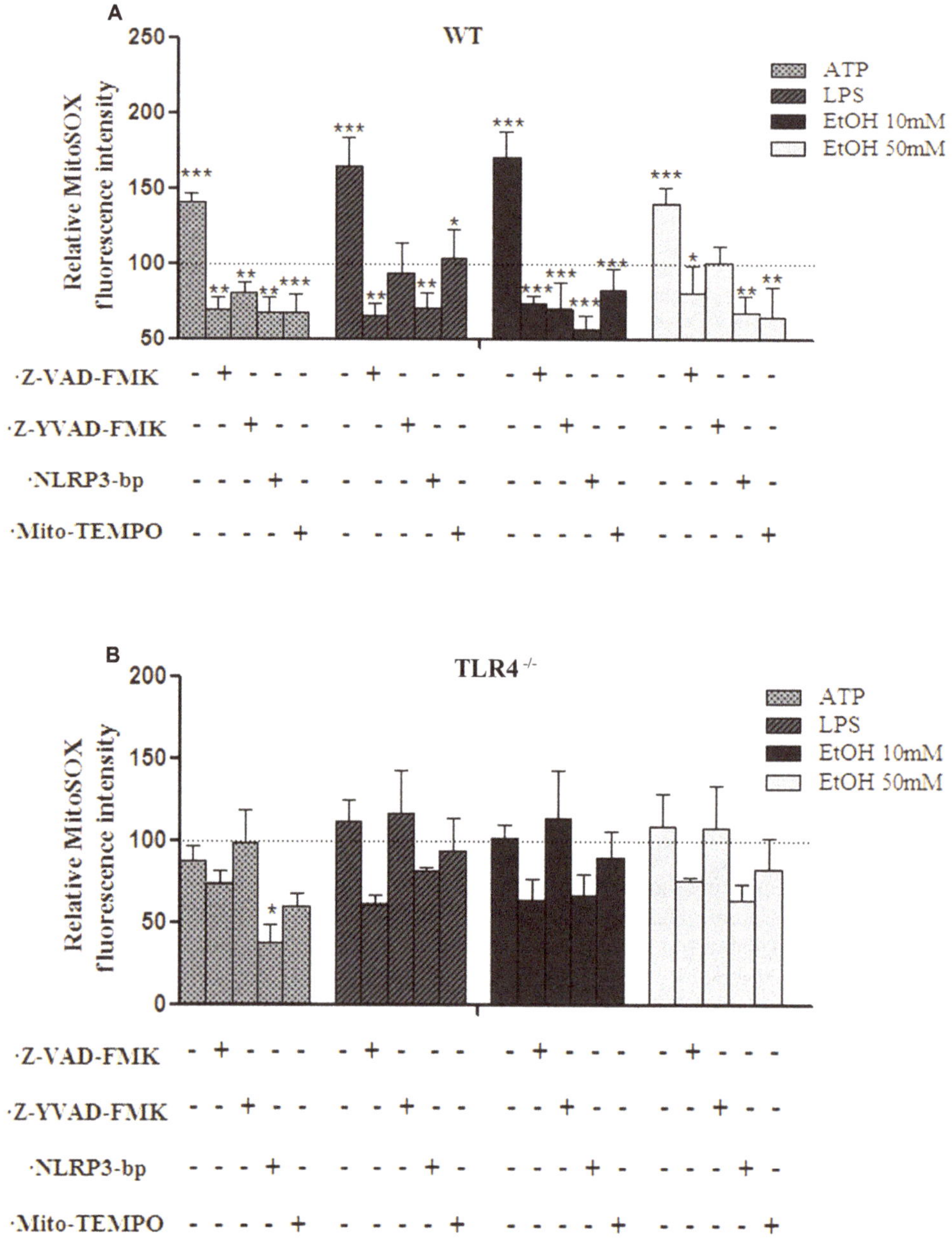

FIGURE 4 | The ethanol-induced mitochondria ROS production level measured by MitoSOX Red fluorescence intensity. (A) A flow cytometry analysis shows that the ATP or LPS or ethanol (10 and 50 mM) treatments increased mROS generation in the WT astrocytes. Incubation with Z-YVAD-FMK, Z-VAD-FMK, the NLRP3 blocking peptide or Mito-TEMPO before and during treatments notably reduces mROS generation activation in WT astrocytes. **(B)** No significant changes in mROS generation were observed in the TLR4-KO-astrocytes incubated with the same inhibitors and treatments as used in the TLR4-astrocytes. Bars represent the (mean ± SEM) of 4–12 individual experiments. $*p < 0.05$, $**p < 0.01$, $***p < 0.001$ (one-way ANOVA followed by a Dunnett's Multiple Comparison Test or a Student's *t*-test).

crystals and amyloid β (Jin and Flavell, 2010; Schroder et al., 2010) and is also involved in the pathogenesis of metabolic diseases, brain disorders, such as Alzheimer's disease (Heneka et al., 2013), autoimmune encephalomyelitis (EAE), and it also contributes to ethanol-induced neuroinflammation in the cerebellum of ethanol-treated mice (Lippai et al., 2013). Although the cellular and molecular mechanisms of ethanol-induced inflammasome activation in the brain remain to be defined, we herein provide evidence that cultured astrocytes express NLRP3 and are capable of promoting ASC oligomerization to allow the recruitment of NLRP3 and caspase-1 activation (Lu et al., 2014) along with the production of IL-1β and IL-18 in response to ethanol, ATP or LPS. Inhibition of caspase-1 by Z-YVAD-FMK abolishes the production of IL-1β and IL18, suggesting the role of caspase-1 in NLRP3 activation and cytokine production.

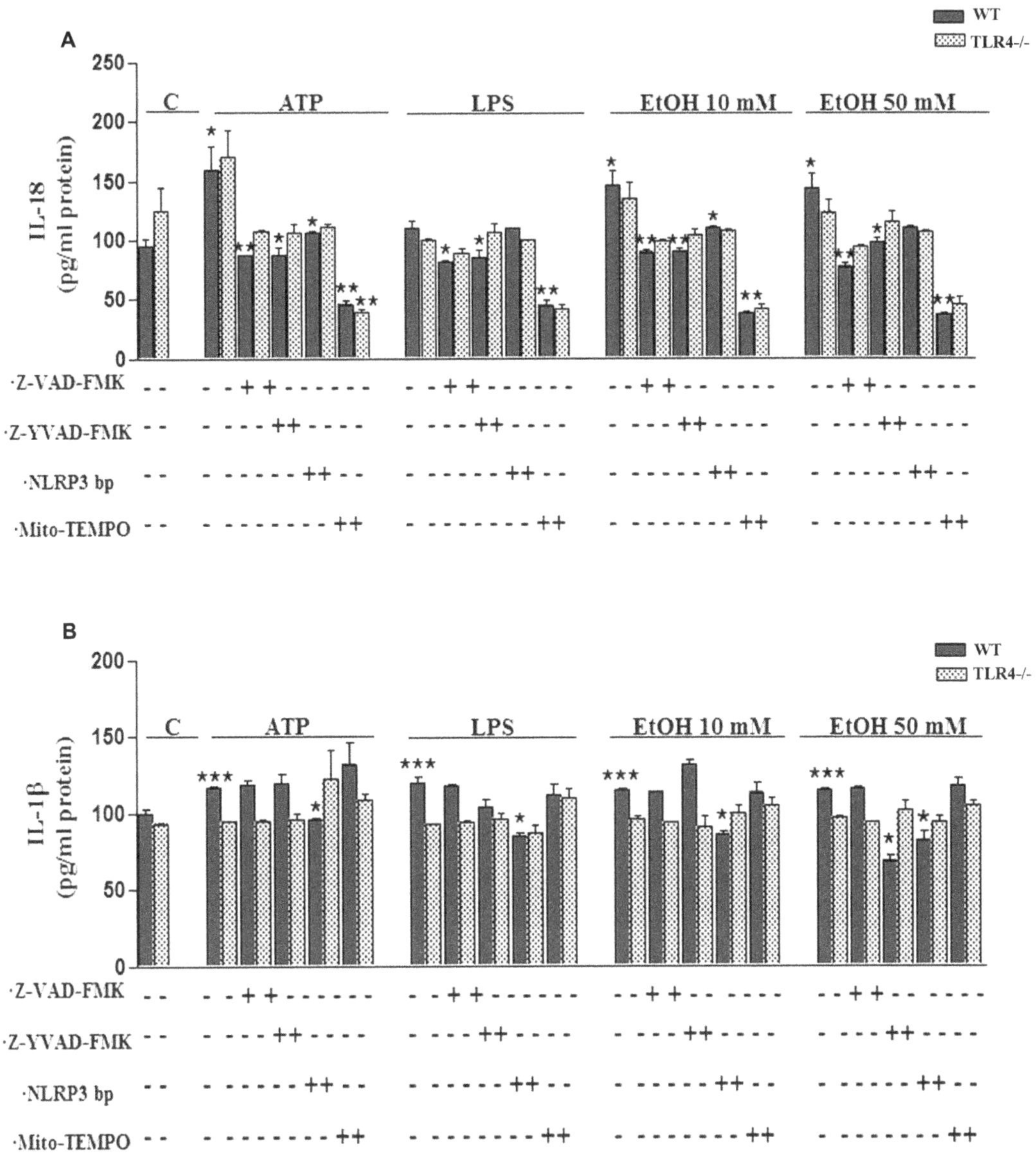

FIGURE 5 | Ethanol enhances the production of IL-18 and IL-1β in WT astroglial cells. (A,B) Graphs represent the levels of IL-18 **(A)** and IL-1β **(B)** measured in the supernatant medium of the WT and TLR4-KO astrocytes treated with ATP, LPS or ethanol (10 and 50 mM) for 24 h. Incubation with Z-YVAD-FMK, Z-VAD-FMK, the NLRP3 blocking peptide or Mito-TEMPO, along with the different treatments, reduces, or even abolishes, the up-regulation of the cytokine release. No changes in the levels of cytokines were noted in the supernatant medium for the TLR4-KO-astrocytes for any of the treatments and inhibitors used, except for the Mito-TEMPO treatment at the IL-18 released levels. Bars represent the (mean ± SEM) expressed as a percentage (%) of 6–10 individual experiments. $^{*}p < 0.05$, $^{**}p < 0.01$, $^{***}p < 0.001$ (two-way ANOVA with *post hoc* Bonferroni's correction).

Notably, while microglia appear to be the main player in NLRP3 inflammasome activation in the brain (Hanamsagar et al., 2012), recent studies have independently demonstrated that rat or human astrocytes express NLRP3 (Tezel et al., 2012) and NLRP2 (Minkiewicz et al., 2013) and are able to activate NLRP3 in response to DAMPs. Our *in vivo* immunohistochemical studies further support that *in vivo* ethanol treatment increases NLRP3 inflammasome activation in GFAP^{+} astroglial cells along with the production of IL-1β and IL-18 in WT mice cerebral cortex. According to these results, prior work from our laboratory has shown that ethanol promotes IL-1β production in both astrocytes (Blanco et al., 2005; Alfonso-Loeches et al., 2010) and microglia (Fernandez-Lizarbe et al., 2009) in culture, as well as in the cerebral cortex of ethanol-treated mice (Alfonso-Loeches et al., 2010).

Activation of the NLRP3 inflammasome by diverse stimuli usually requires two signals (Gross et al., 2011): the first signal, or priming signal is usually induced by TLRs/LPS signaling which triggers pro-IL-1β; and a second signal, induced by a diverse array of stimuli (e.g., ROS, ion membrane perturbations, ATP, etc.) and different mechanisms (Martinon, 2007; Petrilli et al., 2007; Qu et al., 2007). Recent evidence supported the critical role of mROS generation in NLRP3 activation (Nakahira et al., 2011;

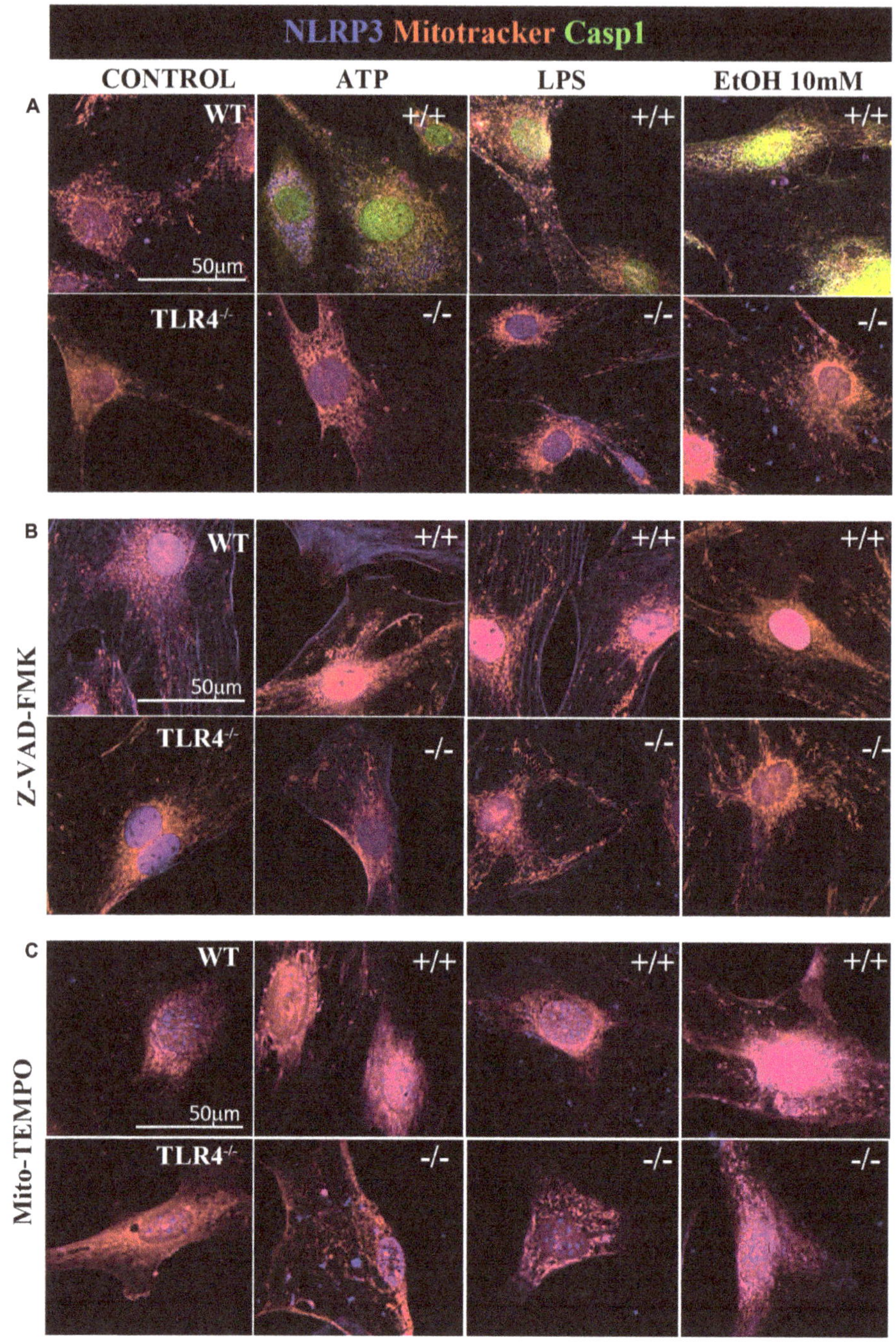

FIGURE 6 | Confocal images of NLRP3/caspase-1 co-localization within mitochondria of the astrocytes treated with ethanol, ATP, or LPS. Microphotographs show that the ATP, LPS, or ethanol (10 mM) treatments promote the co-localization of NLRP3 inflammasome (blue) with active caspase-1 (green) within mitochondria (red) in the WT-astrocytes when compared with the untreated control astrocytes **(A)**. Astrocytes treated with Z-VAD-FMK **(B)** and with Mito-TEMPO **(C)** treatments do not induce caspase-1 activation in both WT and TLR4-KO astrocytes. We performed at least three independent experiments under each experimental condition. Representative pictures are presented.

Shimada et al., 2012b). According to these findings, here we show that ethanol, similarly to other NLRP3 activators like ATP or LPS (Sutterwala et al., 2006), is capable of inducing mROS generation in astrocytes by triggering NLRP3 inflammasome activation, along with active caspase-1 maturation and the production of IL-1β and IL-18. The role of mROS in NLRP3 inflammasome activation has been supported by data demonstrating that blocking mROS or NLRP3, or the inhibition of caspase-1, abrogates both mROS generation and the up-regulation of IL-1β and IL-18 induced by ATP, LPS or ethanol. Indeed, previous studies demonstrate that

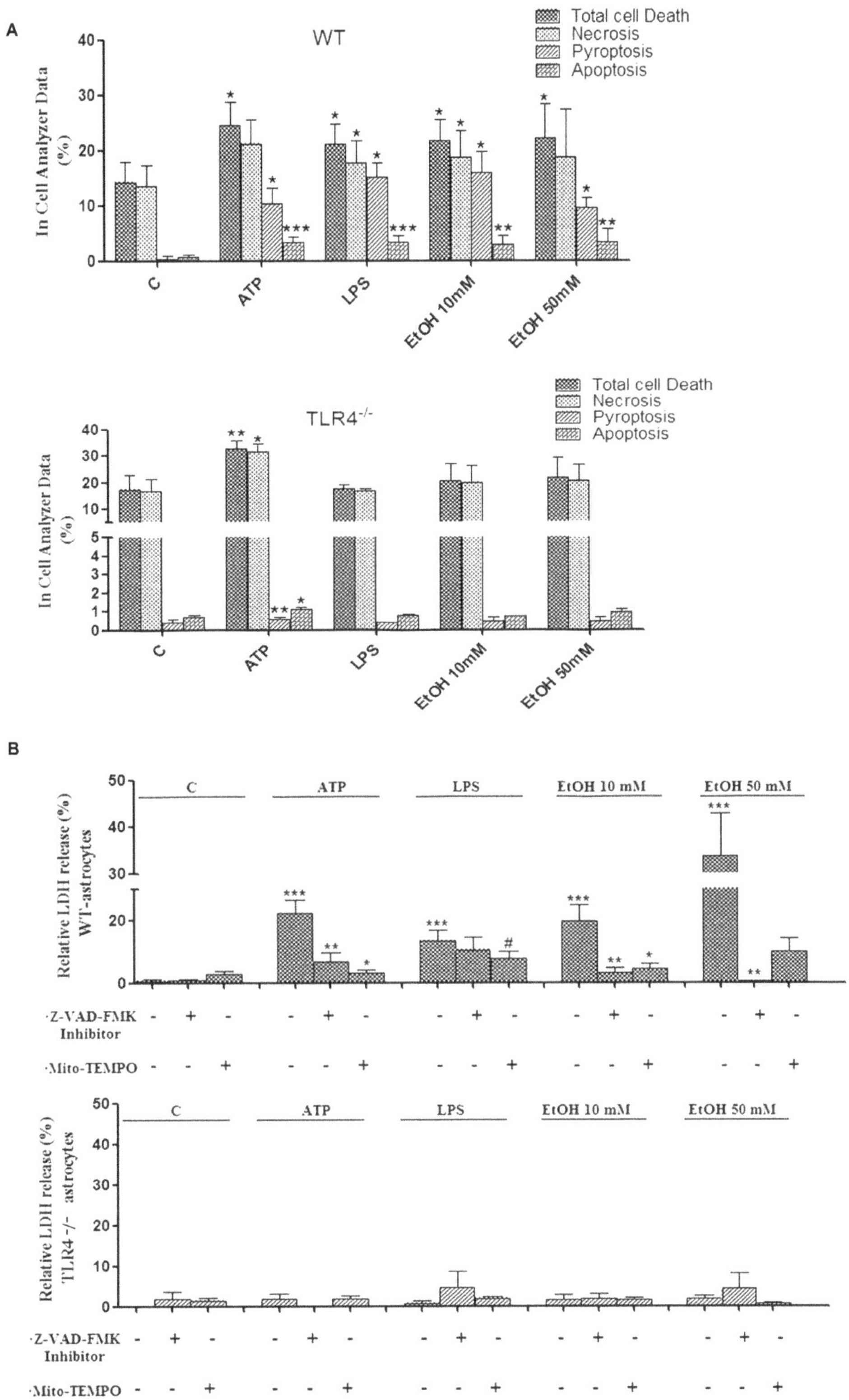

FIGURE 7 | Activation of the NLRP3 inflammasome complex triggers pyroptosis and apoptosis in ethanol-induced astroglial cells. (A) Bars show the percentage of cell dead by pyroptosis, necrosis and apoptosis in astrocytes treated for 24 h with ATP, LPS, and ethanol (10 and 50 mM) evaluated by an In Cell Analyzer. Approximately 1000–5000 cells were analyzed/experimental condition. Bars represent the (mean ± SD). **(B)** LDH activity in the supernatant astrocytes was measured with different treatments. Bars represent the (mean ± SEM) of at least 6–10 individual experiments. $^{*}p < 0.05$, $^{**}p < 0.01$ (Mann–Whitney *U* non-parametric test).

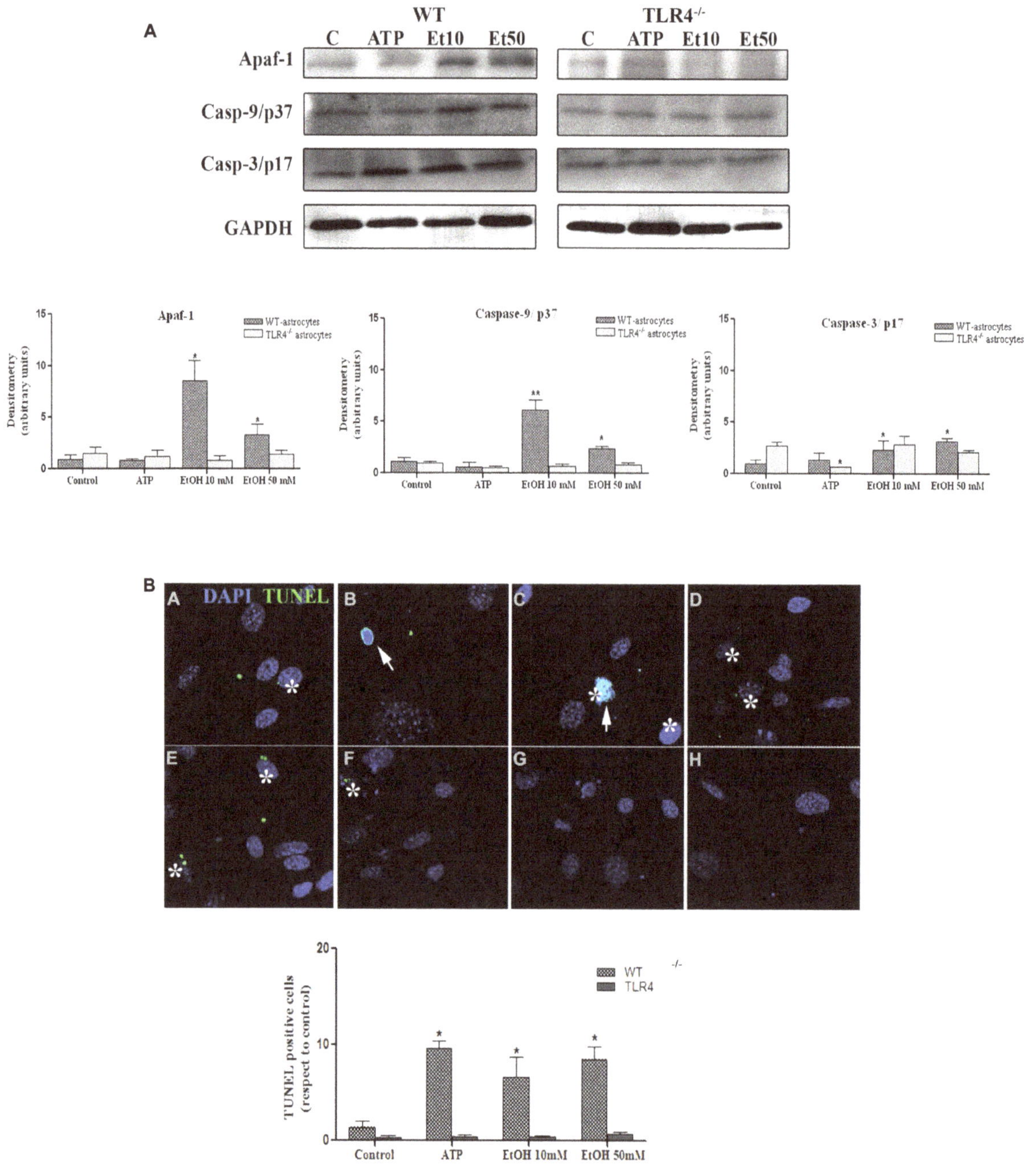

FIGURE 8 | Ethanol can also induce the apoptosome formation in astrocytes. (A) The Western blot analyses of Apaf-1, the active fragments from caspase-9 (37 kDa) and caspase-3 (17 kDa), in the astrocytes treated with ATP (5 μM) or ethanol (10 and 50 mM). Bars represent the (mean ± SEM) of at least 6–10 individual experiments. $*p < 0.05$, $**p < 0.01$ (Mann–Whitney *U* non-parametric test or a Student's *t*-test). **(B)** The percentage of apoptosis in the astrocytes incubated with ATP or ethanol (10 mM, 50 mM) for 24 h was assessed by a TUNEL assay in the WT and TLR4-KO astrocytes. Scale bar: 20 μm. Arrowheads show different apoptotic processes, blebbing and nuclei condensation. Asterisk show positive TUNEL cells. Bars represent the (mean ± SEM) of three individual experiments. $*p < 0.05$, $**p < 0.01$ (two-way ANOVA with *post hoc* Bonferroni's correction).

ethanol-induced mROS generation participate in ethanol toxicity in both astrocytes (Gonzalez et al., 2007) and liver (Manzo-Avalos and Saavedra-Molina, 2010).

Cell death is ultimately caused by cellular innate immune response elicited by the inflammasome activation. We show that the activation of NLRP3 by either ATP, LPS or ethanol mainly triggers pyroptosis a caspase-1-dependent inflammatory form of programmed cells in which dying cells release their cytoplasmic content, including cytokines, into the extracellular space. Nevertheless, ethanol or ATP by inducing mitochondrial stress and mROS production, can also trigger apoptosis by activating Apaf-1, caspase-9, and caspase-3, and the apoptosome complex (Morizot, 2012). It is noteworthy that inflammasomes and apoptosomes are two mechanisms of the immune cells by which compromised cells are eliminated and share many similarities in their regulatory response to cellular stress (Latz et al., 2013). Yet whether these two mechanisms act independently or are linked, and whether their individual contributions depend on the intensity and type of cell stimuli (e.g., bacteria, virus, DAMPs; Doitsh et al., 2014), are uncertain (Latz et al., 2013). Nevertheless, *in vivo* evidence from the immunohistochemical data reported herein (**Figure 1**) and our previous studies support the *in vitro* finding since we observed that chronic ethanol treatment increases IL-1β levels and induces both apoptosis and caspase-3 activation, as well as necrosis, in the WT mice but not in the TLR4-KO mice cerebral cortex (Alfonso-Loeches et al., 2010).

Indeed, the present findings also support the role of TLR4 signaling in ethanol-induced NLRP3 activation, since the elimination of the TLR4 function in astrocytes abolishes ethanol- or ATP-induced NLRP3 activation. As commented above, a crosstalk between TLRs and inflammasome (Hanamsagar et al., 2012) has been reported. Activation of TLRs and the production of pro-IL-1β is the priming step for NLRP3 activation (Gross et al., 2011). Then, a second signal, induced by a diverse stimuli (e.g., ROS, ion membrane perturbations, ATP, etc.), promotes ASC-inflammasome oligomerization, caspase-1 activation, followed by the maturation and secretion of IL-1β and IL-18. A recent report has suggested that NLRP3 is activated by a two-step, deubiquitination mechanism initiated by TLRs signaling and mROS and that it is further potentiated by ATP, events which might explain how NLRP3 is activated by diverse danger signals (Juliana et al., 2012). Therefore, the lack of TLR4 function in TLR4-KO astrocytes not only eliminates the priming signal, as production of pro-IL-1β, but also the production of cytokines and free radicals-mediated by TLR4 signaling. These later events could, sensitize the mitochondria to induce ROS production and consequently NLRP3 activation and cell death by pyroptosis and apoptosis. Accordingly, recent evidence has demonstrated that TLR4 signaling induce mitochondria ROS production, contributing to the gastric cancer progression (Yuan et al., 2013). The functional role of TLR4 in the inflammasome activation is further supported by the demonstration that TLR4 deficiency not only protects ethanol-induced NLRP3 inflammasome activation and the induction of cytokines, but also attenuates the increased in ethanol-induced IL-1β production in the cerebellum (Lippai et al., 2013). We also noted that *in vivo* ethanol treatment abolishes the induction of IL-18 and IL-1β production in the cerebral cortex of TLR4-KO mice.

The role of TLR4 in ethanol-induced neuroinflammation and brain damage has been clearly demonstrated. Our previous studies have shown that by interacting with membrane microdomains "lipid rafts" in glial cells, ethanol can induce TLR4 dimerization and signaling to trigger the release of cytokines and inflammatory mediators (Blanco et al., 2005, 2008; Fernandez-Lizarbe et al., 2009). By using small interfering RNA (siRNA) or cells from TLR4-deficient mice (TLR4-KO), knockdown TLR4, abolish MAPK and NFk-B signaling pathways and the release of inflammatory mediators in glial cells (Fernandez-Lizarbe et al., 2009; Alfonso-Loeches et al., 2010). The *in vivo* relevance of these findings is evidenced by the demonstration that while chronic ethanol intake causes neuroinflammation, gliosis, demyelination and cell death (apoptosis and necrosis) in the cerebral cortex, TLR4-KO mice are protected against ethanol-induced brain inflammatory mediators, cell death and brain injury (Alfonso-Loeches et al., 2010, 2012). The present findings further support the role of TLR4 in ethanol-induced NLRP3 inflammasome activation and IL-1β and IL-18 production in glial cells, events that contribute to ethanol-induced neuroinflammation. To support our results, a recent study has demonstrated that ethanol-impaired neurogenesis is associated with induction of IL-1β and with inflammasome NALP1 and NALP3 activation in both neurons and astrocytes, and that these events can be blocked with both the IL-1β receptor and antagonist rIL-1Ra (Zou and Crews, 2012). Similarly, the intracranial administration of IL-1Ra prevents alcohol-induced inflammasome activation and the up-regulation of IL-1β and TNF-α in the cerebellum of ethanol-treated mice (Lippai et al., 2013). These results indicate the importance of ethanol-induced inflammasome activation and IL-1β production in the neuroinflammatory effects of ethanol.

CONCLUSION

Taken together, our results demonstrate for the first time that, by promoting mROS generation, ethanol induces NLRP3/caspase-1 activation to trigger IL-1β/IL-18 production and cell death by pyroptosis and apoptosis, events that could contribute to neuroinflammation and brain damage induced by ethanol abuse. We further show crosstalk between NLRP3 and TLR4 since the elimination of TLR4 markedly diminishes ethanol actions on NLRP3 inflammasome activation and the production of the inflammatory cytokines IL-1β/IL-18. Our findings suggest that inflammasome activation may represent a new target in ethanol-induced neuroinflammation, and they support the potential role of IL-1Ra in the treatment of the neuropathological changes associated with alcohol abuse.

AUTHOR CONTRIBUTIONS

Consuelo Guerri, Silvia Alfonso-Loeches, and Juan R. Ureña-Peralta conceived and designed the experiments. Silvia Alfonso-Loeches, Juan R. Ureña-Peralta, Maria José Morillo-Bargues, and Jorge Oliver-De La Cruz performed the experiments. Silvia Alfonso-Loeches and Juan R. Ureña-Peralta analyzed the data. Consuelo Guerri contributed reagents/material/ analysis tools. Consuelo Guerri, Silvia Alfonso-Loeches, and Juan R. Ureña-Peralta wrote the paper.

ACKNOWLEDGMENTS

We are thankful to Dr. S. Akira who provided us with the TLR4 knockout mice. In addition, we thank the Confocal and Cytometry Services from the Prince Felipe Research Center. This work has been supported by grants from the Ministry of Science and Innovation (SAF-2009-07503), the Spanish Ministry of Economy and Competitiveness (SAF-2012-33747), the Spanish Ministry of Health, the Carlos III Institute, FEDER funds (RTA-Network

RD12-0028-007), ERAB (EA 13 08) and Generalitat Valenciana-Consellería de Educación: PROMETEO/2009/072, GV.

REFERENCES

Alfonso-Loeches, S., Pascual-Lucas, M., Blanco, A. M., Sanchez-Vera, I., and Guerri, C. (2010). Pivotal role of TLR4 receptors in alcohol-induced neuroinflammation and brain damage. *J. Neurosci.* 30, 8285–8295. doi: 10.1523/JNEUROSCI.0976-10.2010

Alfonso-Loeches, S., Pascual, M., Gomez-Pinedo, U., Pascual-Lucas, M., Renau-Piqueras, J., and Guerri, C. (2012). Toll-like receptor 4 participates in the myelin disruptions associated with chronic alcohol abuse. *Glia* 60, 948–964. doi: 10.1002/glia.22327

Arlehamn, C. S., Petrilli, V., Gross, O., Tschopp, J., and Evans, T. J. (2010). The role of potassium in inflammasome activation by bacteria. *J. Biol. Chem.* 285, 10508–10518. doi: 10.1074/jbc.M109.067298

Becker, C. E., and O'Neill, L. A. (2007). Inflammasomes in inflammatory disorders: the role of TLRs and their interactions with NLRs. *Semin. Immunopathol.* 29, 239–248. doi: 10.1007/s00281-007-0081-4

Blanco, A. M., Perez-Arago, A., Fernandez-Lizarbe, S., and Guerri, C. (2008). Ethanol mimics ligand-mediated activation and endocytosis of IL-1RI/TLR4 receptors via lipid rafts caveolae in astroglial cells. *J. Neurochem.* 106, 625–639. doi: 10.1111/j.1471-4159.2008.05425.x

Blanco, A. M., Valles, S. L., Pascual, M., and Guerri, C. (2005). Involvement of TLR4/type I IL-1 receptor signaling in the induction of inflammatory mediators and cell death induced by ethanol in cultured astrocytes. *J. Immunol.* 175, 6893–6899. doi: 10.4049/jimmunol.175.10.6893

De Nardo, D., and Latz, E. (2011). NLRP3 inflammasomes link inflammation and metabolic disease. *Trends Immunol.* 32, 373–379. doi: 10.1016/j.it.2011.05.004

Doitsh, G., Galloway, N. L., Geng, X., Yang, Z., Monroe, K. M., Zepeda, O., et al. (2014). Cell death by pyroptosis drives CD4 T-cell depletion in HIV-1 infection. *Nature* 505, 509–514. doi: 10.1038/nature12940

Dostert, C., Guarda, G., Romero, J. F., Menu, P., Gross, O., Tardivel, A., et al. (2009). Malarial hemozoin is a Nalp3 inflammasome activating danger signal. *PLoS ONE* 4:e6510. doi: 10.1371/journal.pone.0006510

Farina, C., Aloisi, F., and Meinl, E. (2007). Astrocytes are active players in cerebral innate immunity. *Trends Immunol.* 28, 138–145. doi: 10.1016/j.it.2007.01.005

Fernandes-Alnemri, T., and Alnemri, E. S. (2008). Assembly, purification, and assay of the activity of the ASC pyroptosome. *Methods Enzymol.* 442, 251–270. doi: 10.1016/S0076-6879(08)01413-4

Fernandes-Alnemri, T., Wu, J., Yu, J. W., Datta, P., Miller, B., Jankowski, W., et al. (2007). The pyroptosome: a supramolecular assembly of ASC dimers mediating inflammatory cell death via caspase-1 activation. *Cell Death Differ.* 14, 1590–1604. doi: 10.1038/sj.cdd.4402194

Fernandez-Lizarbe, S., Pascual, M., and Guerri, C. (2009). Critical role of TLR4 response in the activation of microglia induced by ethanol. *J. Immunol.* 183, 4733–4744. doi: 10.4049/jimmunol.0803590

Franklin, K. B. J., and Paxinos, G. (1997). *The Mouse Brain in Stereotaxic Coordinates.* San Diego: Academic Press.

Goldbach-Mansky, R., Dailey, N. J., Canna, S. W., Gelabert, A., Jones, J., Rubin, B. I., et al. (2006). Neonatal-onset multisystem inflammatory disease responsive to interleukin-1β inhibition. *N. Engl. J. Med.* 355, 581–592. doi: 10.1056/NEJMoa055137

Gonzalez, A., Pariente, J. A., and Salido, G. M. (2007). Ethanol stimulates ROS generation by mitochondria through Ca^{2+} mobilization and increases GFAP content in rat hippocampal astrocytes. *Brain Res.* 1178, 28–37. doi: 10.1016/j.brainres.2007.08.040

Gross, O., Thomas, C. J., Guarda, G., and Tschopp, J. (2011). The inflammasome: an integrated view. *Immunol. Rev.* 243, 136–151. doi: 10.1111/j.1600-065X.2011.01046.x

Hanamsagar, R., Torres, V., and Kielian, T. (2012). Inflammasome activation and IL-1β/IL-18 processing are influenced by distinct pathways in microglia. *J. Neurochem.* 119, 736–748. doi: 10.1111/j.1471-4159.2011.07481.x

Heneka, M. T., Kummer, M. P., Stutz, A., Delekate, A., Schwartz, S., Vieira-Saecker, A., et al. (2013). NLRP3 is activated in Alzheimer's disease and contributes to pathology in APP/PS1 mice. *Nature* 493, 674–678. doi: 10.1038/nature11729

Hornung, V., and Latz, E. (2010). Critical functions of priming and lysosomal damage for NLRP3 activation. *Eur. J. Immunol.* 40, 620–623. doi: 10.1002/eji.200940185

Jha, S., Srivastava, S. Y., Brickey, W. J., Iocca, H., Toews, A., Morrison, J. P., et al. (2010). The inflammasome sensor, NLRP3, regulates CNS inflammation and demyelination via caspase-1 and interleukin-18. *J. Neurosci.* 30, 15811–15820. doi: 10.1523/JNEUROSCI.4088-10.2010

Jha, S., and Ting, J. P. (2009). Inflammasome-associated nucleotide-binding domain, leucine-rich repeat proteins and inflammatory diseases. *J. Immunol.* 183, 7623–7629. doi: 10.4049/jimmunol.0902425

Jin, C., and Flavell, R. A. (2010). Molecular mechanism of NLRP3 inflammasome activation. *J. Clin. Immunol.* 30, 628–631. doi: 10.1007/s10875-010-9440-3

Juliana, C., Fernandes-Alnemri, T., Kang, S., Farias, A., Qin, F., and Alnemri, E. S. (2012). Non-transcriptional priming and deubiquitination regulate NLRP3 inflammasome activation. *J. Biol. Chem.* 287, 36617–36622. doi: 10.1074/jbc.M112.407130

Kahlenberg, J. M., Lundberg, K. C., Kertesy, S. B., Qu, Y., and Dubyak, G. R. (2005). Potentiation of caspase-1 activation by the P2X7 receptor is dependent on TLR signals and requires NF-kappaB-driven protein synthesis. *J. Immunol.* 175, 7611–7622. doi: 10.4049/jimmunol.175.11.7611

Lampron, A., Elali, A., and Rivest, S. (2013). Innate immunity in the CNS: redefining the relationship between the CNS and Its environment. *Neuron* 78, 214–232. doi: 10.1016/j.neuron.2013.04.005

Latz, E., Xiao, T. S., and Stutz, A. (2013). Activation and regulation of the inflammasomes. *Nat. Rev. Immunol.* 13, 397–411. doi: 10.1038/nri3452

Lippai, D., Bala, S., Csak, T., Kurt-Jones, E. A., and Szabo, G. (2013). Chronic alcohol-induced microRNA-155 contributes to neuroinflammation in a TLR4-dependent manner in mice. *PLoS ONE* 8:e70945. doi: 10.1371/journal.pone.0070945

Lu, A., Magupalli, V. G., Ruan, J., Yin, Q., Atianand, M. K., Vos, M. R., et al. (2014). Unified polymerization mechanism for the assembly of ASC-dependent inflammasomes. *Cell* 156, 1193–1206. doi: 10.1016/j.cell.2014.02.008

Manzo-Avalos, S., and Saavedra-Molina, A. (2010). Cellular and mitochondrial effects of alcohol consumption. *Int. J. Environ. Res. Public Health* 7, 4281–4304. doi: 10.3390/ijerph7124281

Mariathasan, S., and Monack, D. M. (2007). Inflammasome adaptors and sensors: intracellular regulators of infection and inflammation. *Nat. Rev. Immunol.* 7, 31–40. doi: 10.1038/nri1997

Martinon, F. (2007). Orchestration of pathogen recognition by inflammasome diversity: variations on a common theme. *Eur. J. Immunol.* 37, 3003–3006. doi: 10.1002/eji.200737871

Miao, E. A., Rajan, J. V., and Aderem, A. (2011). Caspase-1-induced pyroptotic cell death. *Immunol. Rev.* 243, 206–214. doi: 10.1111/j.1600-065X.2011.01044.x

Minana, R., Climent, E., Barettino, D., Segui, J. M., Renau-Piqueras, J., and Guerri, C. (2000). Alcohol exposure alters the expression pattern of neural cell adhesion molecules during brain development. *J. Neurochem.* 75, 954–964. doi: 10.1046/j.1471-4159.2000.0750954.x

Minkiewicz, J., de Rivero Vaccari, J. P., and Keane, R. W. (2013). Human astrocytes express a novel NLRP2 inflammasome. *Glia* 61, 1113–1121. doi: 10.1002/glia.22499

Morizot, B. (2012). Chance: from metaphysical principle to explanatory concept. The idea of uncertainty in a natural history of knowledge. *Prog. Biophys. Mol. Biol.* 110, 54–60. doi: 10.1016/j.pbiomolbio.2012.04.007

Nakahira, K., Haspel, J. A., Rathinam, V. A., Lee, S. J., Dolinay, T., Lam, H. C., et al. (2011). Autophagy proteins regulate innate immune responses by inhibiting the release of mitochondrial DNA mediated by the NALP3 inflammasome. *Nat. Immunol.* 12, 222–230. doi: 10.1038/ni.1980

Neven, B., Callebaut, I., Prieur, A. M., Feldmann, J., Bodemer, C., Lepore, L., et al. (2004). Molecular basis of the spectral expression of CIAS1 mutations associated with phagocytic cell-mediated autoinflammatory disorders CINCA/NOMID, MWS, and FCU. *Blood* 103, 2809–2815. doi: 10.1182/blood-2003-07-2531

Parajuli, B., Sonobe, Y., Horiuchi, H., Takeuchi, H., Mizuno, T., and Suzumura, A. (2013). Oligomeric amyloid β induces IL-1β processing via production of ROS: implication in Alzheimer's disease. *Cell Death Dis.* 4:e975. doi: 10.1038/cddis.2013.503

Petrilli, V., Dostert, C., Muruve, D. A., and Tschopp, J. (2007). The inflammasome: a danger sensing complex triggering innate immunity. *Curr. Opin. Immunol.* 19, 615–622. doi: 10.1016/j.coi.2007.09.002

Pfaffl, M. W. (2001). A new mathematical model for relative quantification in real-time RT-PCR. *Nucleic Acids Res.* 29:e45. doi: 10.1093/nar/29.9.e45

Pittock, S. J., and Lucchinetti, C. F. (2007). The pathology of MS: new insights and potential clinical applications. *Neurologist* 13, 45–56. doi: 10.1097/01.nrl.0000253065.31662.37

Qu, Y., Franchi, L., Nunez, G., and Dubyak, G. R. (2007). Nonclassical IL-1 β secretion stimulated by P2X7 receptors is dependent on inflammasome activation and correlated with exosome release in murine macrophages. *J. Immunol.* 179, 1913–1925. doi: 10.4049/jimmunol.179.3.1913

Schroder, K., and Tschopp, J. (2010). The inflammasomes. *Cell* 140, 821–832. doi: 10.1016/j.cell.2010.01.040

Schroder, K., Zhou, R., and Tschopp, J. (2010). The NLRP3 inflammasome: a sensor for metabolic danger? *Science* 327, 296–300. doi: 10.1126/science.1184003

Sheedy, F. J., Grebe, A., Rayner, K. J., Kalantari, P., Ramkhelawon, B., Carpenter, S. B., et al. (2013). CD36 coordinates NLRP3 inflammasome activation by facilitating intracellular nucleation of soluble ligands into particulate ligands in sterile inflammation. *Nat. Immunol.* 14, 812–820. doi: 10.1038/ni.2639

Shimada, K., Crother, T. R., and Arditi, M. (2012a). Innate immune responses to Chlamydia pneumoniae infection: role of TLRs, NLRs, and the inflammasome. *Microbes Infect.* 14, 1301–1307. doi: 10.1016/j.micinf.2012.08.004

Shimada, K., Crother, T. R., Karlin, J., Dagvadorj, J., Chiba, N., Chen, S., et al. (2012b). Oxidized mitochondrial DNA activates the NLRP3 inflammasome during apoptosis. *Immunity* 36, 401–414. doi: 10.1016/j.immuni.2012.01.009

Sospedra, M., and Martin, R. (2005). Antigen-specific therapies in multiple sclerosis. *Int. Rev. Immunol.* 24, 393–413. doi: 10.1080/08830180500371256

Subramanian, N., Natarajan, K., Clatworthy, M. R., Wang, Z., and Germain, R. N. (2013). The adaptor MAVS promotes NLRP3 mitochondrial localization and inflammasome activation. *Cell* 153, 348–361. doi: 10.1016/j.cell.2013.02.054

Sutterwala, F. S., Ogura, Y., Szczepanik, M., Lara-Tejero, M., Lichtenberger, G. S., Grant, E. P., et al. (2006). Critical role for NALP3/CIAS1/Cryopyrin in innate and adaptive immunity through its regulation of caspase-1. *Immunity* 24, 317–327. doi: 10.1016/j.immuni.2006.02.004

Tan, M. S., Yu, J. T., Jiang, T., Zhu, X. C., and Tan, L. (2013). The NLRP3 inflammasome in Alzheimer's disease. *Mol. Neurobiol.* 48, 875–882. doi: 10.1007/s12035-013-8475-x

Tezel, G., Yang, X., Luo, C., Cai, J., and Powell, D. W. (2012). An astrocyte-specific proteomic approach to inflammatory responses in experimental rat glaucoma. *Invest. Ophthalmol. Vis. Sci.* 53, 4220–4233. doi: 10.1167/iovs.11-9101

Ting, J. P., and Davis, B. K. (2005). CATERPILLER: a novel gene family important in immunity, cell death, and diseases. *Annu. Rev. Immunol.* 23, 387–414. doi: 10.1146/annurev.immunol.23.021704.115616

Triantafilou, K., Hughes, T. R., Triantafilou, M., and Morgan, B. P. (2013). The complement membrane attack complex triggers intracellular Ca^{2+} fluxes leading to NLRP3 inflammasome activation. *J. Cell Sci.* 126, 2903–2913. doi: 10.1242/jcs.124388

Tschopp, J., and Schroder, K. (2010). NLRP3 inflammasome activation: the convergence of multiple signalling pathways on ROS production? *Nat. Rev. Immunol.* 10, 210–215. doi: 10.1038/nri2725

Tseng, W. A., Thein, T., Kinnunen, K., Lashkari, K., Gregory, M. S., D'Amore, P. A., et al. (2013). NLRP3 inflammasome activation in retinal pigment epithelial cells by lysosomal destabilization: implications for age-related macular degeneration. *Invest. Ophthalmol. Vis. Sci.* 54, 110–120. doi: 10.1167/iovs.12-10655

Yuan, X., Zhou, Y., Wang, W., Li, J., Xie, G., Zhao, Y., et al. (2013). Activation of TLR4 signaling promotes gastric cancer progression by inducing mitochondrial ROS production. *Cell Death Dis.* 4:e794. doi: 10.1038/cddis.2013.334

Zhou, R., Yazdi, A. S., Menu, P., and Tschopp, J. (2011). A role for mitochondria in NLRP3 inflammasome activation. *Nature* 469, 221–225. doi: 10.1038/nature09663

Zou, J., and Crews, F. T. (2012). Inflammasome-IL-1β signaling mediates ethanol inhibition of hippocampal neurogenesis. *Front. Neurosci.* 6:77. doi: 10.3389/fnins.2012.00077

10

Nanobodies as modulators of inflammation: potential applications for acute brain injury

Björn Rissiek[1]*, Friedrich Koch-Nolte[2] and Tim Magnus[1]

[1] Department of Neurology, University Medical Center Hamburg-Eppendorf, Hamburg, Germany
[2] Department of Immunology, University Medical Center Hamburg-Eppendorf, Hamburg, Germany

Correspondence:
Björn Rissiek, Department of Neurology, University Medical Center Hamburg-Eppendorf, Martinistraße 52, 20246 Hamburg, Germany
e-mail: b.rissiek@uke.de

Nanobodies are single domain antibodies derived from llama heavy-chain only antibodies (HCAbs). They represent a new generation of biologicals with unique properties: nanobodies show excellent tissue distribution, high temperature and pH stability, are easy to produce recombinantly and can readily be converted into different formats such as Fc-fusion proteins or hetero-dimers. Moreover, nanobodies have the unique ability to bind molecular clefts, such as the active site of enzymes, thereby interfering with the function of the target protein. Over the last decade, numerous nanobodies have been developed against proteins involved in inflammation with the aim to modulate their immune functions. Here, we give an overview about recently developed nanobodies that target immunological pathways linked to neuroinflammation. Furthermore, we highlight strategies to modify nanobodies so that they can overcome the blood brain barrier and serve as highly specific therapeutics for acute inflammatory brain injury.

Keywords: nanobodies, single domain antibodies, VHH, blood-brain barrier, neuroinflammation

FROM LLAMA HEAVY-CHAIN-ONLY ANTIBODIES TO SINGLE DOMAIN NANOBODIES

Mammalian immunoglobulins are composed of two heavy and two light chains which together form the antigen-binding paratope. In 1993, the group of Raymond Hamers demonstrated the existence of a new type of immunoglobulin in the serum of camels (*Camelus dromedarius*). These antibodies consist of heavy-chain dimers devoid of light chains, which brought them the name "heavy-chain-only antibodies" (HCAbs; Hamers-Casterman et al., 1993). These HCAbs are present in all members of the camelid family and account for 30 to 75% of circulating immunoglobulins (Hamers-Casterman et al., 1993; Sundberg and Mariuzza, 2002; Blanc et al., 2009; Muyldermans, 2013).

Structurally, the heavy-chains of HCAbs are composed of the antigen-binding variable domain (VHH) followed by a hinge region and two constant domains (CH2 and CH3), whereas the CH1 domain known from conventional antibodies is missing (**Figure 1A**; Hamers-Casterman et al., 1993). Apart from their unusual architecture, HCAbs also differ from conventional antibodies in their antigen recognition: VH and VL of conventional antibodies usually form a concave or flat shaped paratope suited for the binding of small molecules, peptides, or large antigens (Sundberg and Mariuzza, 2002; Blanc et al., 2009; Muyldermans, 2013). The paratope formed by a VHH domain, however, shows a convex shape and, therefore, enables the binding to molecular cavities or clefts, e.g., the active site of enzymes. Many enzyme-specific VHH domains thereby act as antagonists (**Figure 1B**). This unique feature could be attributed to the long complementarity determining region 3 (CDR3) of the VHH domain which is able to form finger-like extensions (De Genst et al., 2006).

With approximately 15 kDa VHHs are the smallest naturally occurring antigen-binding protein domains. The name "nanobodies" was coined to reflect the small size of VHHs as recombinant proteins (Muyldermans, 2013). In order to generate nanobodies from HCAbs, llamas are immunized and boosted with the desired antigen. After the last boost, B cells are collected from peripheral blood to isolate mRNA, which is transcribed into cDNA. The gene region encoding for the VHH domain can be amplified via PCR and cloned into a phagemid vector. This strategy generates phages that express one particular nanobody clone on their surface and, at the same time, carry the DNA sequence encoding for this specific nanobody. Applying the phage display technology finally allows the selection of nanobody clones against the desired antigen (Clackson et al., 1991). Taken together, this approach allows the selection of target-specific nanobodies and, simultaneosly, delivers the DNA sequence coding for the selected nanobodies which then can be further used for recombinant expression (Wesolowski et al., 2009).

Most generated nanobodies are stable at high temperatures, low and high pH, and other stringent conditions (Arbabi Ghahroudi et al., 1997; Dumoulin et al., 2002). Additionally, phage display selection can be performed under harsh conditions, e.g., the presence of detergents to improve the selection of more resistant clones. If applied *in vivo*, nanobodies display low toxicity and immunogenicity due to their small size, their relatively high sequence identity to human VH, and to their rapid clearance from the periphery via the kidney (Hamers-Casterman et al., 1993; Muyldermans, 2013). To increase the *in vivo* half-life

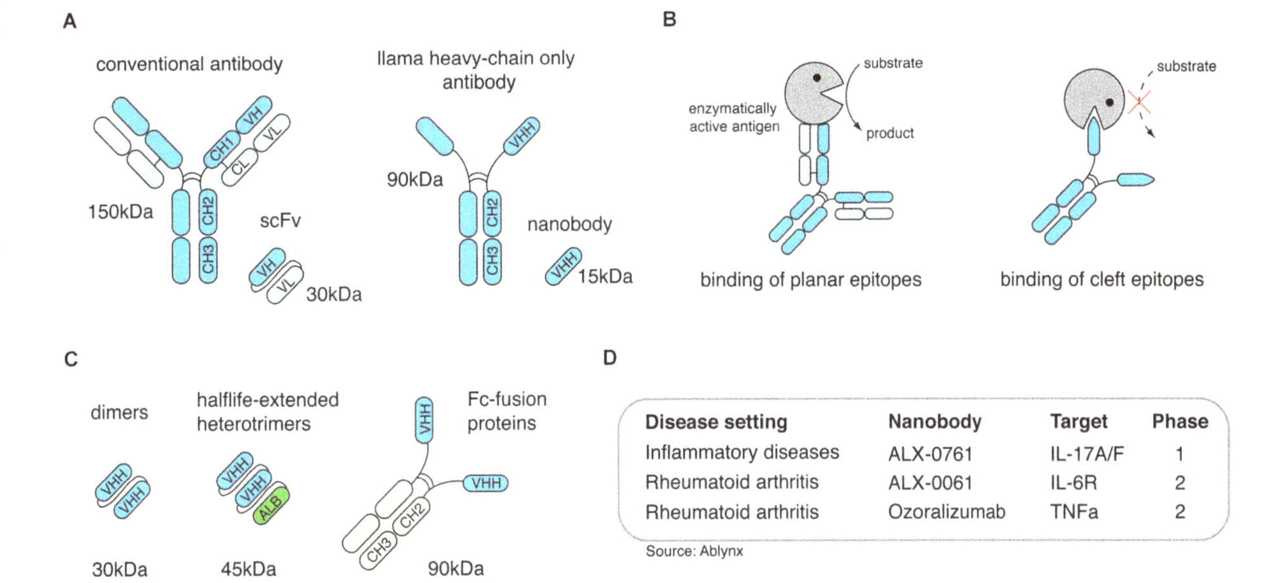

Disease setting	Nanobody	Target	Phase
Inflammatory diseases	ALX-0761	IL-17A/F	1
Rheumatoid arthritis	ALX-0061	IL-6R	2
Rheumatoid arthritis	Ozoralizumab	TNFa	2

FIGURE 1 | Nanobodies are single-domain antibodies derived from llama heavy-chain-only antibodies. (A) Conventional antibodies from mammals are composed of two heavy- and two light chains, camelidae additionally express antibodies devoid of ligh chains, so called heavy-chain only antibodies. **(B)** Heavy-chain-only antibodies can bind to molecular crevices thereby blocking the active site of enzymes. **(C)** Nanobodies derived from heavy-chain-only antibodies can be engineered as dimers, half-life-extended heterotrimers containing an anti-albumin nanobody or as dimeric Fc-fusionprotein. **(D)** Anti-inflammatory nanobodies are currently evaluated in clinical trials.

nanobodies can be reformatted (converted into other formats by genetic engineering), e.g., to homodimers, heterotrimers containing an anti-serum-albumin nanobody (Sundberg and Mariuzza, 2002; Coppieters et al., 2006; Tijink et al., 2008; Blanc et al., 2009; Muyldermans, 2013) or nanobody-Fc-fusion proteins (**Figure 1C**). Thereby, nanobodies can be tailored for the desired *in vivo* application, e.g., small monomers for short-term *in vivo* imaging or half life-extended nanobodies for long-term therapeutic treatment (Hamers-Casterman et al., 1993; Hassanzadeh-Ghassabeh et al., 2013). The potential to antagonize targeted antigens, the high stability, the low toxicity and the possibility to tailor them for *in vivo* applications makes nanobodies a promising new generation of therapeutic proteins. To date, several anti-inflammatory nanobodies are in clinical trials (**Figure 1D**), and more than 700 persons have received nanobodies in clinical trials without any adverse off-target side effects (Van Bockstaele et al., 2009; Williams, 2013).

NANOBODIES AS MODULATORS OF IMMUNE CELLS AND INFLAMMATION

In order to fight infectious diseases, numerous nanobodies have been generated against bacterial and viral antigens to prevent or ameliorate pathogenicity (Sundberg and Mariuzza, 2002; Blanc et al., 2009; Wesolowski et al., 2009; Muyldermans, 2013). More recently, key players of immunological pathways have come into focus as targets for nanobodies in order to modulate immune responses. This has resulted in the generation of nanobodies directed against Fc-receptors (FcR), chemokine receptors, chemokines, cytokines, and ecto-enzymes. These nanobodies often show high target specificities and are able to modulate the function of their target in an agonistic or antagonistic fashion.

NANOBODIES DIRECTED AGAINST Fc-RECEPTORS

Fc receptors are expressed on the cell surface of diverse immune cells and are able to bind the Fc portion of antibodies thereby conducting either stimulatory or inhibitory signals, depending on the Fc receptor class (De Genst et al., 2006; Nimmerjahn and Ravetch, 2007). In 2008, Behar et al. described the isolation of Fc-γ-RIII-specific nanobodies from a llama immune library (Behar et al., 2008; Muyldermans, 2013). The selected nanobodies (C21 and C28) showed specific binding to both, Fc-γ-RIIIB and Fc-γ-RIIIA, and no binding to Fc-γ-RI or Fc-γ-RII. Binding of the Fc-part of an antibody to the Fc-γ-RIII on NK cells conducts an activating signal leading to the release of the proinflammatory cytokine interferon gamma (IFNγ). Binding of nanobodies C21 and C28 in an agonistic fashion to Fc-γ-RIIIA on human NK cells induced the expression of IFNγ (Clackson et al., 1991; Behar et al., 2008). In later studies, these nanobodies were used to generate Fab-like bispecific antibodies containing one nanobody directed against the Fc-γ-RIIIA and one directed against the carcinoembryogenic antigen (CEA; Behar et al., 2009; Wesolowski et al., 2009). By this strategy, the agonistic anti-Fc-γ-RIIIA nanobodies could be targeted to CEA^+-tumor cells where they activate NK cells *in situ* inducing the lysis of the tumor cells. Further, injection of these bispecific constructs reduced the tumor growth in immunodeficient mice xenografted with CEA^+-tumor cells when co-administered with human peripheral blood mononuclear cells (PBMCs; Arbabi Ghahroudi et al., 1997; Dumoulin et al., 2002; Rozan et al., 2013). It has to be evaluated whether FcR targeting nanobodies could also be applied as therapeutics for acute brain injury. A study using Fc-γ-R deficient mice showed a reduced infarct size compared to WT animals which could be linked to decreased microglia activation (Komine-Kobayashi et al., 2004).

NANOBODIES DIRECTED AGAINST CHEMOKINE RECEPTORS AND CHEMOKINES

The generation of functional monoclonal antibodies against G-protein coupled receptors (GPCRs) such as chemokine receptors is notoriously difficult. With their unique binding features, nanobodies display a promising alternative for the generation of functional biologics to modulate chemokine receptor function, e.g., to inhibit immune cell migration to inflammatory sites. In 2010, the group of Martine Smit reported the generation of two nanobodies that specifically target the chemokine receptor CXCR4 (Jähnichen et al., 2010). Nanobodies 238D2 and 238D4 showed potent competitive inhibition of CXCL12 binding to CXCR4. When injected into monkeys, anti-CXCR4 nanobodies induced the mobilization of hematopoetic stem cells by disrupting the CXCR4/CXCL12 axis contributing to the residence of hematopoetic stem cells in the bone marrow. In 2013, the same group reported the generation of antagonistic nanobodies targeting CXCR7. Injected into mice, these nanobodies showed beneficial effects in an *in vivo* xenograft model of head and neck cancer (Maussang et al., 2013). Simultaneously, the same group published a panel of nanobodies specifically targeting CCL2, CCL5, CXCL11 and CXCL12. Binding of nanobodies to CXCL11 and CXCL12 inhibited chemokine receptor binding and thereby preventing chemokine receptor activation induced cell migration *in vitro* (Blanchetot et al., 2013). Since diverse chemokines and their receptors are known to contribute to the migration of immune cells to the brain after brain damage (Amantea et al., 2009), the nanobodies described above might be a promising therapeutic alternative for the treatment of acute brain injury.

NANOBODIES DIRECTED AGAINST CYTOKINES

Targeting and neutralization of proinflammatory cytokines by monoclonal antibodies is a promising strategy for the treatment of inflammatory diseases (Kopf et al., 2010). Tumor necrosis factor α (TNFα) was the first cytokine functionally targeted by nanobodies (TR2 = anti-human TNFα, MT1 = anti-mouse TNFα). Expressed as bivalent molecules TR2-TR2 nanobodies showed a slightly higher neutralizing capacity than the TNFα neutralizing biologicals infliximab, adalimumab and etanercept (Coppieters et al., 2006). Further, heterotrimeric nanobodies (MT1-MT1-AR1) consisting of two MT1 and one serum albumin-binding nanobody (AR1) showed excellent therapeutic effects in the collagen-induced arthritis mouse model (Coppieters et al., 2006). Another study evaluating the therapeutic potential of bivalent TNFα nanobodies in a mouse model of chronic colitis impressively demonstrated the versatility of the nanobody technology: genetically engineered *Lactococcus lactis* secreting MT1-MT1 bivalent anti-TNFα nanobodies profoundly reduced gut inflammation when daily administered by gavage (Vandenbroucke et al., 2010). Apart from neutralizing cytokines nanobodies can be used to "guide" cytokines to their desired target cells. In a proof-of-concept study Garcin et al. (2014) demonstrated that the toxicity of type I interferons, when applied *in vivo*, could be markedly reduced by genetically engineering fusion proteins of mutated IFNα2 with lower receptor affinities and nanobodies targeting programmed cell death 1 ligand 2 (PD-L2; Garcin et al., 2014). When injected into mice these fusion proteins preferentially induced IFNα2-mediated STAT1 phosphorylation in PD-L2 expressing cells in peritoneum and spleen, illustrating that nanobodies are valuable tools for "activity-by-targeting" based therapeutic approaches. For the treatment of acute brain injury, the nanobody-based neutralization of proinflammatory cytokines such as TNFα could be a promising approach to minimize inflammation-related further loss of brain tissue. Conversely, it is conceivable that nanobodies could be used to guide modified anti-inflammatory cytokines such as interleukin-10 to sites of brain inflammation to suppress inflammatory responses *in situ*.

NANOBODIES DIRECTED AGAINST ECTO-ENZYMES

The first cell surface resident ecto-enzyme targeted by nanobodies was murine ADP-ribosyltransferase C2 (ARTC2; Koch-Nolte et al., 2007; Menzel et al., 2013). ARTC2 is expressed on the cell surface of T cells and covalently attaches the ADP-ribose group of its substrate nicotinamide adenin dinucleotide (NAD) to arginine residues of several cell surface proteins. One well-characterized target of ARTC2 is the ATP-gated P2X7 ion channel. ADP-ribosylation of P2X7 on T cells induces channel opening and influx of calcium ions. Prolonged activation by ADP-ribosylation causes shedding of cell surface proteins such as CD62L and CD27, externalization of phosphatidylserin und ultimately cell death (Seman et al., 2003). Analyses of T cell subpopulations revealed different sensitivities to NAD-mediated cell death, with regulatory T cells (Tregs) and natural killer T cells (NKT cells) being highly susceptible (Hubert et al., 2010; Rissiek et al., 2014b). Antagonizing ARTC2 with nanobody s+16a prevents ADP-ribosylation of P2X7 *in vitro* and *in vivo*. In a proof-of-principle study Scheuplein et al. showed that injection of s+16a as Fc-fusion protein restores an otherwise naturally NAD-depleted NKT cell population in diabetogenic NOD-CD38ko mice (Scheuplein et al., 2010). When activated *in vivo* by injection of α-galactosylceramide, s+16a-restored NKT cells were capable of inhibiting the development of type 1 diabetes. A further study showed that injection of s+16a prevented ARTC2/P2X7 mediated cell death of highly susceptible Tregs and NKT cells during *in vitro* assays and adoptive transfer experiments, revealing the potential of s+16a as valuable tool for research and as potential therapeutic agent (Rissiek et al., 2014a). It has been shown that P2X7 activation is detrimental for the outcome of ischemic stroke (Arbeloa et al., 2012). Further, genetic deletion of the NAD-degrading ecto-enzyme CD38 in mice exacerbates ischemic damage (Choe et al., 2011), which might provide ARTC2 with an increased access to its substrate NAD. Therefore, s+16a could be used to clarify the role of the ARTC2/P2X7 axis during acute brain damage.

MODIFYING NANOBODIES TO CROSS THE BLOOD-BRAIN BARRIER

The therapeutic application of nanobodies has been tested in diverse mouse models of inflammation. However, therapeutic applications of biologics in neuroinflammatory diseases face an important biological barrier. The obstacle for effective delivery of therapeutic drugs, especially antibodies, is the blood brain barrier, which is only permeable for lipophilic molecules of up to 400 kDa of size (Pardridge, 2012). The delivery of conventional antibodies to the brain is especially tedious because of Fc-receptor mediated efflux to the blood (Cooper et al., 2013). Therefore, nanobodies lacking an Fc-part represent a promising alternative to brain targeting monoclonal antibodies. Indeed, several groups have tested different strategies to deploy nanobodies as brain-drug deliverers or as bonafide brain-targeting drugs (**Figure 2**).

Muruganadam et al. described in 2002 the selection of a nanobody (FC5) that transmigrates across human blood-brain-barrier endothelium *in vitro* (Muruganandam et al., 2002). Later, the same group suggested that FC5 binds a putative α(2,3)-sialoglycoprotein receptor and is transcytosed via clathrin vesicles (Abulrob et al., 2005). In a therapeutic experimental setup using the Hargreaves model of inflammatory pain, it was shown that FC5 conjugated with opioid peptide Dal could be deployed as drug delivery shuttle *in vivo* to induce a significant analgesic response in contrast to unconjugated Dal peptide (Farrington et al., 2014). Other approaches utilize receptor-mediated transcytosis for brain targeting. A recently published study showed that a fusionprotein of a peptide derived from apolipoprotein E (ApoE) and a model therapeutic protein (α-L-iduronidase) could be transferred to the brain via binding to the LDL receptor (LRP) expressed on cells of the blood-brain barrier (Wang et al., 2013). Furthermore, the transferrin receptor and the insulin receptor have also been exploited for receptor-mediated transcytosis of small molecule drugs and therapeutic proteins (Boado et al., 2012; Xiao and Gan, 2013). These studies indicate that nanobodies binding these receptors and triggering transcytosis could be a promising alternative to ligand-based delivery of drugs to the brain.

A study by Pierre Lafaye's group (Li et al., 2012) reported that nanobodies with a high isoelectric point (pI) spontaneously cross the blood brain barrier. Such nanobodies not only gained access to the brain but were even found to penetrate cells and bind to intracellular proteins. In a mouse study, the nanobody E9 (pI = 9.4) directed against glial fibrillary acidic protein (GFAP) crossed the BBB after injection via the tail vein and was able to bind to intracellularly expressed GFAP in astrocytes. Conjugation of fluorescent proteins to nanobody E9 (generating a "fluobody") allowed *in vivo* labeling of astrocytes, however, only if the basic pI was preserved. One possible limitation of this approach is that fairly large amounts (2 mg) of nanobody had to be injected to obtain the desired effect. However, combining this approach—adjusting the pI to a basic level—with other approaches could possibly show beneficial effects. Indeed, the FC5 nanobody described above also has a basic pI (9.2) which might contribute to or facility transcytosis into the brain parenchyma

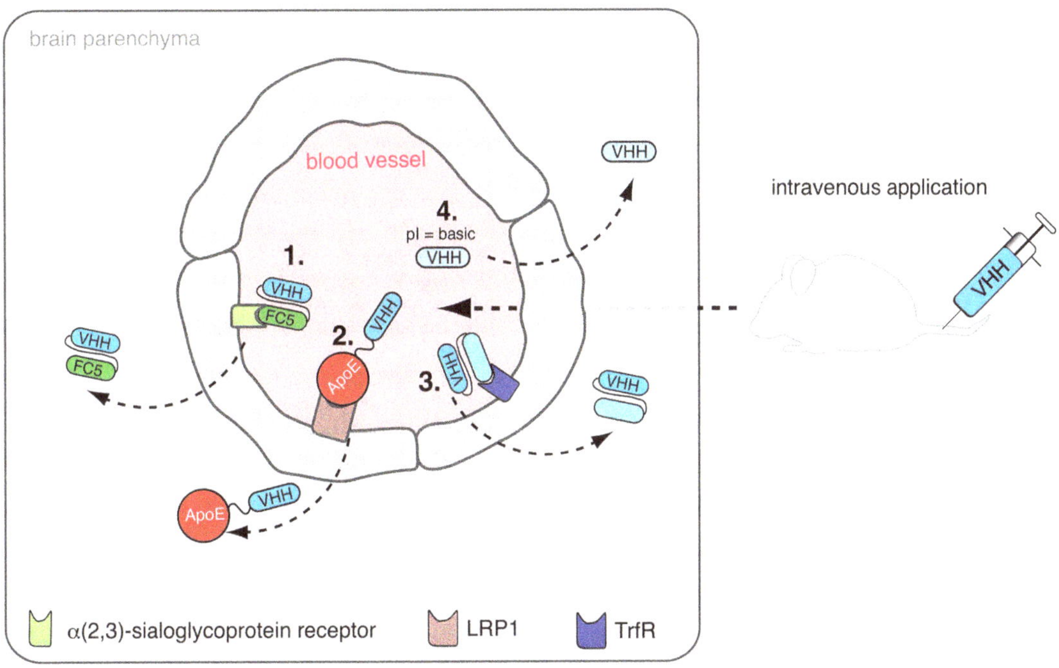

FIGURE 2 | Delivery of nanobodies to the brain. The blood-brain-barrier (BBB) hampers the delivery of intravenously injected nanobodies (VHH) to the brain. To overcome this, diverse strategies are being developed: **(1)** Nanobody FC5, binding to a putative α(2,3)-sialoglycoprotein receptor, can potentially be used as shuttling-nanobody to deliver other therapeutic proteins e.g., nanobodies to the brain. **(2)** Apolipoprotein E (ApoE) binds to low density lipoprotein receptor-related protein 1 (LRP1) inducing transcytosis, which can be exploited as shuttle for therapeutic nanobodies. **(3)** In a similare fashion, other receptors triggering transcytosis across the BBB such as the transferrin receptor (TrfR) could be targeted for the transfer of therapeutic nanobodies. **(4)** Finally, shifting the isoelectric point (pI) of therapeutic nanobodies to a basic level facilitates crossing of the BBB by these nanobodies.

(Farrington and Sisk, 2013). Further studies are needed to determine whether therapeutic nanobodies against inflammatory target proteins can be shuttled to the brain, e.g., by fusion to FC5 and by adjusting their pI with the aim of treating neuroinflammatory disease.

IMPLICATION OF NANOBODIES TO TREAT ACUTE BRAIN INFLAMMATION

After acute brain damage, e.g., ischemic stroke or trauma, the release of danger associated molecular pattern (DAMPs) from necrotic cells activates resident microglia, leading to the production of proinflammatory mediators such as cytokines and chemokines attracting other immune cells (Amantea et al., 2009; Iadecola and Anrather, 2011). Preventing local inflammation could be a means to prevent further loss of brain tissue. High mobility group box 1 (HMGB1) and nucleotide DAMPs such as adenosinetriphosphate (ATP) are released during cerebral ischemia (Magnus et al., 2012). Antibody-mediated neutralization of HMGB1 or antagonism of its receptor (receptor for advanced glycation end products, RAGE) markedly reduced the infarct size in a mouse ischemia/reperfusion model middle cerebral artery occlusion (MCAO; Muhammad et al., 2008). The ATP receptor P2X7, which mediates inflammasome formation and cell death (Bartlett et al., 2014), was antagonized with small molecule inhibitors in a mouse model of transient focal ischemia, again resulting in a reduction of infarct size (Arbeloa et al., 2012). Both pathways, HMGB1/RAGE and ATP/P2X7, display promising targets for nanobody-mediated antagonism. However, release of DAMPs occurs shortly after the ischemic insult and before the breakdown of the BBB (Muhammad et al., 2008; Cisneros-Mejorado et al., 2014), requiring the generation of nanobodies that are able to cross the BBB applying the strategies described above. Currently, nanobodies directed against the P2X7 receptor are under development (Laeremans et al., 2010).

An approach to control ischemia-related brain inflammation is to prevent migration of immune cells to the penumbra of ischemic lesions. Two independent studies demonstrated that blockade of the CXCL12/CXCR4 axis improved the functional outcome after stroke by attenuating post-ischemic inflammation (Huang et al., 2013; Ruscher et al., 2013). CXCL12-CXCR4 blockade was conducted using the small molecule inhibitor AMD3100. Since nanobodies against CXCL12 and CXCR4 have been generated (Jähnichen et al., 2010; Maussang et al., 2013), it may be worthwhile to evaluate their potential in ischemia/reperfusion animal models. To restrict the blockade of CXCR4 to infiltrating proinflammatory cells one could apply the "activity-by-targeting" strategy described above for IFNα2-guiding nanobodies. This could be useful in order to allow the CXCR4-dependend migration of cells important for brain recovery after stroke such as mesenchymal stem cells (Tsai et al., 2011). Furthermore, blockade of other chemokine receptors such as CXCR1 and CXCR2 by small molecule inhibitor Reparixin also reduces infiltration of proinflammatory neutrophiles and improves the motoric recovery after stroke (Sousa et al., 2013). Therefore, generation and application of nanobodies directed against CXCR1 and CXCR2 may represent one further strategy to ameliorate consequences of cerebral ischemia and beyond.

CONCLUSIONS

Nanobodies have been shown to be versatile and efficient biologicals suitable for therapy of inflammatory diseases. Due to their unique structure, nanobodies have the potential to modulate the function of cell surface and secreted proteins in an agonistic or antagonistic fashion. They can be genetically engineered to extend their half-life *in vivo* and, shown in a proof-of-concept study, to serve as shuttles for the delivery of therapeutic agents across the BBB. Future studies will have to show whether this strategy could also be applied to deliver therapeutic nanobodies to the brain to ameliorate the consequences of neuroinflammation.

ACKNOWLEDGMENTS

We thank Dr. Anne Rissiek for critical reading of the manuscript. This work was supported by the ERA-NET NEURON research grant (NanoStroke) to Tim Magnus and Friedrich Koch-Nolte and a publication grant from NEUROWIND e.V. to Björn Rissiek.

REFERENCES

Abulrob, A., Sprong, H., Van Bergen en Henegouwen, P., and Stanimirovic, D. (2005). The blood-brain barrier transmigrating single domain antibody: mechanisms of transport and antigenic epitopes in human brain endothelial cells. *J. Neurochem.* 95, 1201–1214. doi: 10.1111/j.1471-4159.2005.03463.x

Amantea, D., Nappi, G., Bernardi, G., Bagetta, G., and Corasaniti, M. T. (2009). Post-ischemic brain damage: pathophysiology and role of inflammatory mediators. *FEBS J.* 276, 13–26. doi: 10.1111/j.1742-4658.2008.06766.x

Arbabi Ghahroudi, M., Desmyter, A., Wyns, L., Hamers, R., and Muyldermans, S. (1997). Selection and identification of single domain antibody fragments from camel heavy-chain antibodies. *FEBS Lett.* 414, 521–526. doi: 10.1016/s0014-5793(97)01062-4

Arbeloa, J., Pérez-Samartín, A., Gottlieb, M., and Matute, C. (2012). P2X7 receptor blockade prevents ATP excitotoxicity in neurons and reduces brain damage after ischemia. *Neurobiol. Dis.* 45, 954–961. doi: 10.1016/j.nbd.2011.12.014

Bartlett, R., Stokes, L., and Sluyter, R. (2014). The P2X7 receptor channel: recent developments and the use of P2X7 antagonists in models of disease. *Pharmacol. Rev.* 66, 638–675. doi: 10.1124/pr.113.008003

Behar, G., Chames, P., Teulon, I., Cornillon, A., Alshoukr, F., Roquet, F., et al. (2009). Llama single-domain antibodies directed against nonconventional epitopes of tumor-associated carcinoembryonic antigen absent from nonspecific cross-reacting antigen. *FEBS J.* 276, 3881–3893. doi: 10.1111/j.1742-4658.2009.07101.x

Behar, G., Sibéril, S., Groulet, A., Chames, P., Pugnière, M., Boix, C., et al. (2008). Isolation and characterization of anti-FcgammaRIII (CD16) llama single-domain antibodies that activate natural killer cells. *Protein Eng. Des. Sel.* 21, 1–10. doi: 10.1093/protein/gzm064

Blanc, M. R., Anouassi, A., Abed, M. A., Tsikis, G., Canepa, S., Labas, V., et al. (2009). A one-step exclusion-binding procedure for the purification of functional heavy-chain and mammalian-type γ-globulins from camelid sera. *Biotechnol. Appl. Biochem.* 54, 207–212. doi: 10.1042/ba20090208

Blanchetot, C., Verzijl, D., Mujić-Delić, A., Bosch, L., Rem, L., Leurs, R., et al. (2013). Neutralizing nanobodies targeting diverse chemokines effectively inhibit chemokine function. *J. Biol. Chem.* 288, 25173–25182. doi: 10.1074/jbc.m113.467969

Boado, R. J., Hui, E. K.-W., Lu, J. Z., and Pardridge, W. M. (2012). Glycemic control and chronic dosing of rhesus monkeys with a fusion protein of iduronidase and a monoclonal antibody against the human insulin receptor. *Drug Metab. Dispos.* 40, 2021–2025. doi: 10.1124/dmd.112.046375

Choe, C.-U., Lardong, K., Gelderblom, M., Ludewig, P., Leypoldt, F., Koch-Nolte, F., et al. (2011). CD38 exacerbates focal cytokine production, postischemic inflammation and brain injury after focal cerebral ischemia. *PLoS One* 6:e19046. doi: 10.1371/journal.pone.0019046

Cisneros-Mejorado, A., Pérez-Samartín, A., Gottlieb, M., and Matute, C. (2014). ATP signaling in brain: release, excitotoxicity and potential therapeutic targets. *Cell. Mol. Neurobiol.* doi: 10.1007/s10571-014-0092-3. [Epub ahead of print].

Clackson, T., Hoogenboom, H. R., Griffiths, A. D., and Winter, G. (1991). Making antibody fragments using phage display libraries. *Nature* 352, 624–628. doi: 10.1038/352624a0

Cooper, P. R., Ciambrone, G. J., Kliwinski, C. M., Maze, E., Johnson, L., Li, Q., et al. (2013). Efflux of monoclonal antibodies from rat brain by neonatal Fc receptor, FcRn. *Brain Res.* 1534, 13–21. doi: 10.1016/j.brainres.2013.08.035

Coppieters, K., Dreier, T., Silence, K., de Haard, H., Lauwereys, M., Casteels, P., et al. (2006). Formatted anti-tumor necrosis factor alpha VHH proteins derived from camelids show superior potency and targeting to inflamed joints in a murine model of collagen-induced arthritis. *Arthritis Rheum.* 54, 1856–1866. doi: 10.1002/art.21827

De Genst, E., Silence, K., Decanniere, K., Conrath, K., Loris, R., Kinne, J., et al. (2006). Molecular basis for the preferential cleft recognition by dromedary heavy-chain antibodies. *Proc. Natl. Acad. Sci. U S A* 103, 4586–4591. doi: 10.1073/pnas.0505379103

Dumoulin, M., Conrath, K., Van Meirhaeghe, A., Meersman, F., Heremans, K., Frenken, L. G. J., et al. (2002). Single-domain antibody fragments with high conformational stability. *Protein Sci.* 11, 500–515. doi: 10.1110/ps.34602

Farrington, G. K., Caram-Salas, N., Haqqani, A. S., Brunette, E., Eldredge, J., Pepinsky, B., et al. (2014). A novel platform for engineering blood-brain barrier-crossing bispecific biologics. *FASEB J.* doi: 10.1096/fj.14-253369. [Epub ahead of print].

Farrington, G. K., and Sisk, W. (2013). Enhancement of transport of therapeutic molecules across the blood brain barrier. *Patent*

Garcin, G., Paul, F., Staufenbiel, M., Bordat, Y., Van der Heyden, J., Wilmes, S., et al. (2014). High efficiency cell-specific targeting of cytokine activity. *Nat. Commun.* 5:3016. doi: 10.1038/ncomms4016

Hamers-Casterman, C., Atarhouch, T., Muyldermans, S., Robinson, G., Hamers, C., Songa, E. B., et al. (1993). Naturally occurring antibodies devoid of light chains. *Nature* 363, 446–448. doi: 10.1038/363446a0

Hassanzadeh-Ghassabeh, G., Devoogdt, N., De Pauw, P., Vincke, C., and Muyldermans, S. (2013). Nanobodies and their potential applications. *Nanomedicine (Lond)* 8, 1013–1026. doi: 10.2217/nnm.13.86

Huang, J., Li, Y., Tang, Y., Tang, G., Yang, G.-Y., and Wang, Y. (2013). CXCR4 antagonist AMD3100 protects blood-brain barrier integrity and reduces inflammatory response after focal ischemia in mice. *Stroke* 44, 190–197. doi: 10.1161/strokeaha.112.670299

Hubert, S., Rissiek, B., Klages, K., Huehn, J., Sparwasser, T., Haag, F., et al. (2010). Extracellular NAD+ shapes the Foxp3+ regulatory T cell compartment through the ART2–P2X7 pathway. *J. Exp. Med.* 207, 2561–2568. doi: 10.1084/jem.20091154

Iadecola, C., and Anrather, J. (2011). The immunology of stroke: from mechanisms to translation. *Nat. Med.* 17, 796–808. doi: 10.1038/nm.2399

Jähnichen, S., Blanchetot, C., Maussang, D., Gonzalez-Pajuelo, M., Chow, K. Y., Bosch, L., et al. (2010). CXCR4 nanobodies (VHH-based single variable domains) potently inhibit chemotaxis and HIV-1 replication and mobilize stem cells. *Proc. Natl. Acad. Sci. U S A* 107, 20565–20570. doi: 10.1073/pnas.1012865107

Koch-Nolte, F., Reyelt, J., Schössow, B., Schwarz, N., Scheuplein, F., Rothenburg, S., et al. (2007). Single domain antibodies from llama effectively and specifically block T cell ecto-ADP-ribosyltransferase ART2.2 in vivo. *FASEB J.* 21, 3490–3498. doi: 10.1096/fj.07-8661com

Komine-Kobayashi, M., Chou, N., Mochizuki, H., Nakao, A., Mizuno, Y., and Urabe, T. (2004). Dual role of Fcgamma receptor in transient focal cerebral ischemia in mice. *Stroke* 35, 958–963. doi: 10.1161/01.str.0000120321.30916.8e

Kopf, M., Bachmann, M. F., and Marsland, B. J. (2010). Averting inflammation by targeting the cytokine environment. *Nat. Rev. Drug Discov.* 9, 703–718. doi: 10.1038/nrd2805

Laeremans, T., Stortelers, C., Koch-Nolte, F., Gonzalez, M., Assuncao, J., and van Rompaey, P. (2010). Genetic immunization for producing immunoglobulins against cell-associated antigens such as p2x7, cxcr7 or cxcr4. *Patent*

Li, T., Bourgeois, J. P., Celli, S., Glacial, F., Le Sourd, A. M., Mecheri, S., et al. (2012). Cell-penetrating anti-GFAP VHH and corresponding fluorescent fusion protein VHH-GFP spontaneously cross the blood-brain barrier and specifically recognize astrocytes: application to brain imaging. *FASEB J.* 26, 3969–3979. doi: 10.1096/fj.11-201384

Magnus, T., Wiendl, H., and Kleinschnitz, C. (2012). Immune mechanisms of stroke. *Curr. Opin. Neurol.* 25, 334–340. doi: 10.1097/WCO.0b013e328352ede6

Maussang, D., Mujić-Delić, A., Descamps, F. J., Stortelers, C., Vanlandschoot, P., Stigter-van Walsum, M., et al. (2013). Llama-derived single variable domains (nanobodies) directed against chemokine receptor CXCR7 reduce head and neck cancer cell growth in vivo. *J. Biol. Chem.* 288, 29562–29572. doi: 10.1074/jbc.m113.498436

Menzel, S., Rissiek, B., Haag, F., Goldbaum, F. A., and Koch-Nolte, F. (2013). The art of blocking ADP-ribosyltransferases (ARTs): nanobodies as experimental and therapeutic tools to block mammalian and toxin ARTs. *FEBS J.* 280, 3543–3550. doi: 10.1111/febs.12313

Muhammad, S., Barakat, W., Stoyanov, S., Murikinati, S., Yang, H., Tracey, K. J., et al. (2008). The HMGB1 receptor RAGE mediates ischemic brain damage. *J. Neurosci.* 28, 12023–12031. doi: 10.1523/JNEUROSCI.2435-08.2008

Muruganandam, A., Tanha, J., Narang, S., and Stanimirovic, D. (2002). Selection of phage-displayed llama single-domain antibodies that transmigrate across human blood-brain barrier endothelium. *FASEB J.* 16, 240–242. doi: 10.1096/fj.01-0343fje

Muyldermans, S. (2013). Nanobodies: natural single-domain antibodies. *Annu. Rev. Biochem.* 82, 775–797. doi: 10.1146/annurev-biochem-063011-092449

Nimmerjahn, F., and Ravetch, J. V. (2007). Fc-receptors as regulators of immunity. *Adv. Immunol.* 96, 179–204. doi: 10.1016/s0065-2776(07)96005-8

Pardridge, W. M. (2012). Drug transport across the blood-brain barrier. *J. Cereb. Blood Flow Metab.* 32, 1959–1972. doi: 10.1038/jcbfm.2012.126

Rissiek, B., Danquah, W., Haag, F., and Koch-Nolte, F. (2014a). Technical Advance: a new cell preparation strategy that greatly improves the yield of vital and functional Tregs and NKT cells. *J. Leukoc. Biol.* 95, 543–549. doi: 10.1189/jlb.0713407

Rissiek, B., Haag, F., Boyer, O., Koch-Nolte, F., and Adriouch, S. (2014b). ADP-Ribosylation of P2X7: a matter of life and death for regulatory T cells and natural killer T cells. *Curr. Top. Microbiol. Immunol.* doi: 10.1007/82_2014_420. [Epub ahead of print].

Rozan, C., Cornillon, A., Pétiard, C., Chartier, M., Behar, G., Boix, C., et al. (2013). Single-domain antibody-based and linker-free bispecific antibodies targeting FcγRIII induce potent antitumor activity without recruiting regulatory T cells. *Mol. Cancer Ther.* 12, 1481–1491. doi: 10.1158/1535-7163.mct-12-1012

Ruscher, K., Kuric, E., Liu, Y., Walter, H. L., Issazadeh-Navikas, S., Englund, E., et al. (2013). Inhibition of CXCL12 signaling attenuates the postischemic immune response and improves functional recovery after stroke. *J. Cereb. Blood Flow Metab.* 33, 1225–1234. doi: 10.1038/jcbfm.2013.71

Scheuplein, F., Rissiek, B., Driver, J. P., Chen, Y.-G., Koch-Nolte, F., and Serreze, D. V. (2010). A recombinant heavy chain antibody approach blocks ART2 mediated deletion of an iNKT cell population that upon activation inhibits autoimmune diabetes. *J. Autoimmun.* 34, 145–154. doi: 10.1016/j.jaut.2009.08.012

Seman, M., Adriouch, S., Scheuplein, F., Krebs, C., Freese, D., Glowacki, G., et al. (2003). NAD-induced T cell death: ADP-ribosylation of cell surface proteins by ART2 activates the cytolytic P2X7 purinoceptor. *Immunity* 19, 571–582. doi: 10.1016/S1074-7613(03)00266-8

Sousa, L. F. D. C., Coelho, F. M., Rodrigues, D. H., Campos, A. C., Barcelos, L. D. S., Teixeira, M. M., et al. (2013). Blockade of CXCR1/2 chemokine receptors protects against brain damage in ischemic stroke in mice. *Clinics (Sao Paulo)* 68, 391–394. doi: 10.6061/clinics/2013(03)oa17

Sundberg, E. J., and Mariuzza, R. A. (2002). Molecular recognition in antibody-antigen complexes. *Adv. Protein Chem.* 61, 119–160. doi: 10.1016/s0065-3233(02)61004-6

Tijink, B. M., Laeremans, T., Budde, M., Stigter-van Walsum, M., Dreier, T., de Haard, H. J., et al. (2008). Improved tumor targeting of anti-epidermal growth factor receptor Nanobodies through albumin binding: taking advantage of modular Nanobody technology. *Mol. Cancer Ther.* 7, 2288–2297. doi: 10.1158/1535-7163.mct-07-2384

Tsai, L.-K., Wang, Z., Munasinghe, J., Leng, Y., Leeds, P., and Chuang, D.-M. (2011). Mesenchymal stem cells primed with valproate and lithium robustly migrate to infarcted regions and facilitate recovery in a stroke model. *Stroke* 42, 2932–2939. doi: 10.1161/strokeaha.110.612788

Van Bockstaele, F., Holz, J. B., and Revets, H. (2009). The development of nanobodies for therapeutic applications. *Curr. Opin. Investig. Drugs* 10, 1212–1224.

Vandenbroucke, K., de Haard, H., Beirnaert, E., Dreier, T., Lauwereys, M., Huyck, L., et al. (2010). Orally administered L. lactis secreting an anti-TNF Nanobody demonstrate efficacy in chronic colitis. *Mucosal Immunol.* 3, 49–56. doi: 10.1038/mi.2009.116

Wang, D., El-Amouri, S. S., Dai, M., Kuan, C.-Y., Hui, D. Y., Brady, R. O., et al. (2013). Engineering a lysosomal enzyme with a derivative of receptor-binding domain of apoE enables delivery across the blood-brain barrier. *Proc. Natl. Acad. Sci. U S A* 110, 2999–3004. doi: 10.1073/pnas.1222742110

Wesolowski, J., Alzogaray, V., Reyelt, J., Unger, M., Juarez, K., Urrutia, M., et al. (2009). Single domain antibodies: promising experimental and therapeutic tools in infection and immunity. *Med. Microbiol. Immunol.* 198, 157–174. doi: 10.1007/s00430-009-0116-7

Williams, S. C. P. (2013). Small nanobody drugs win big backing from pharma. *Nat. Med.* 19, 1355–1356. doi: 10.1038/nm1113-1355

Xiao, G., and Gan, L.-S. (2013). Receptor-mediated endocytosis and brain delivery of therapeutic biologics. *Int. J. Cell Biol.* 2013:703545. doi: 10.1155/2013/703545

11

Antigen-specific immune reactions to ischemic stroke

Xabier Urra[1,2], Francesc Miró[2], Angel Chamorro[1,2] and Anna M. Planas[2,3]*

[1] *Functional Unit of Cerebrovascular Diseases, Hospital Clínic, Barcelona, Spain*
[2] *August Pi i Sunyer Biomedical Research Institute (IDIBAPS), Barcelona, Spain*
[3] *Department of Brain Ischemia and Neurodegeneration, Instituto de Investigaciones Biomédicas de Barcelona (IIBB), Consejo Superior de Investigaciones Científicas (CSIC), Barcelona, Spain*

Correspondence:
Anna M. Planas, Department of Brain Ischemia and Neurodegeneration, Instituto de Investigaciones Biomédicas de Barcelona (IIBB), Consejo Superior de Investigaciones Científicas (CSIC), Rosselló 161 Planta 6, Barcelona E-08036, Spain
e-mail: anna.planas@iibb.csic.es

Brain proteins are detected in the cerebrospinal fluid (CSF) and blood of stroke patients and their concentration is related to the extent of brain damage. Antibodies against brain antigens develop after stroke, suggesting a humoral immune response to the brain injury. Furthermore, induced immune tolerance is beneficial in animal models of cerebral ischemia. The presence of circulating T cells sensitized against brain antigens, and antigen presenting cells (APCs) carrying brain antigens in draining lymphoid tissue of stroke patients support the notion that stroke might induce antigen-specific immune responses. After stroke, brain proteins that are normally hidden from the periphery, inflammatory mediators, and danger signals can exit the brain through several efflux routes. They can reach the blood after leaking out of the damaged blood-brain barrier (BBB) or following the drainage of interstitial fluid to the dural venous sinus, or reach the cervical lymph nodes through the nasal lymphatics following CSF drainage along the arachnoid sheaths of nerves across the nasal submucosa. The route and mode of access of brain antigens to lymphoid tissue could influence the type of response. Central and peripheral tolerance prevents autoimmunity, but the actual mechanisms of tolerance to brain antigens released into the periphery in the presence of inflammation, danger signals, and APCs, are not fully characterized. Stroke does not systematically trigger autoimmunity, but under certain circumstances, such as pronounced systemic inflammation or infection, autoreactive T cells could escape the tolerance controls. Further investigation is needed to elucidate whether antigen-specific immune events could underlie neurological complications impairing recovery from stroke.

Keywords: stroke, antigens, autoimmunity, tolerance, brain, lymphoid tissue

INTRODUCTION

Ischemic stroke induces acute brain damage and cell death. The lack of sufficient energy to maintain the membrane potential of the cells causes necrosis. Necrosis, in contrast to apoptosis or other forms of cell death, promotes a strong inflammatory response after the intracellular content spills into the extracellular environment. Stroke fuels a sterile local and systemic inflammatory response with the release of danger signals or damage-associated molecular patterns from the injured tissue (Iadecola and Anrather, 2011), which could in turn stimulate a pro-thrombotic cascade, as well as activate the innate and adaptive arms of the immune system, with still poorly understood consequences. Inflammation is necessary to clear the dead cells and cell debris but it needs to be tightly regulated to avoid excessive release of neurotoxic mediators, damage to the blood-brain barrier (BBB), and cause uncontrolled activation of the immune system. Cytokines, chemokines and adhesion molecules participate in the recruitment of peripheral leukocytes that are attracted to the injury site (Gelderblom et al., 2009). Extracellular proteolytic enzymes are rapidly activated degrading the extracellular matrix and activating pro-zymogens that cleave proteins, all in preparation for further tissue remodeling (Yang et al., 2013). These proteolytic processes can expose otherwise hidden epitopes that can act as danger signals, release pro-inflammatory mediators, and damage the BBB. Inflammatory mediators cause indirect activation of antigen-presenting cells (APCs) driving T cell proliferation and clonal expansion, but indirectly activated APCs cannot support differentiation of CD4+ T cells into Th1 effectors *in vivo* (Spörri and Reis e Sousa, 2005). Therefore, inflammation allows APCs to sense danger but direct danger signal recognition is necessary to better identify the quality of the danger (Spörri and Reis e Sousa, 2005). Danger signals activate pattern-recognition receptors, such as toll-like receptors (TLR), inducing full maturation of APCs (Janeway and Medzhitov, 1999). Although microglia and macrophages can present antigen, dendritic cells (DCs) are the professional APCs, and they are found in the brain after stroke (Felger et al., 2010). Dendritic cells capture antigen mainly in its immature stage and then undergo maturation enabling them to efficiently present antigen by increasing the expression of MHC II and co-stimulatory molecules, and producing cytokines that stimulate T cells (Steinman and Nussenzweig, 2002). For efficient naïve T cell stimulation, peripheral antigen-loaded DCs migrate toward tissue-draining lymph nodes. However, it is currently unknown whether stroke-induced brain DCs migrate to the cervical lymph nodes due to the absence of direct lymphatic connection. Also, soluble proteins and protein fragments normally confined to brain cells or trapped in the extracellular matrix could reach the periphery through the leaky BBB or through the drainage pathways of interstitial fluid and cerebrospinal fluid (CSF; Cserr et al., 1992; Weller et al., 2009; Carare et al., 2014), as we will describe below. Once in the periphery, brain proteins could be taken up by APCs, processed, and presented to T cells in lymphoid tissue.

Brain antigens were found in draining lymphoid tissue of stroke patients (Planas et al., 2012) and mice (van Zwam et al., 2009), suggesting that antigen-specific immune reactions could take place after stroke. This possibility does not necessarily imply that an immune attack to the brain would be expected after stroke. There are indeed powerful mechanisms to control autoimmunity ensuring tolerance (Hogquist et al., 2005), and regulatory mechanisms operate in stroke (Liesz et al., 2009). However, tolerance can be breached under certain circumstances and several lines of evidence support that inflammation and/or infection can facilitate autoimmune reactions in experimental animal models of brain ischemia (Becker et al., 2005; Gee et al., 2009; Zierath et al., 2010) and in human stroke (Becker et al., 2011). While this concept is not new and some previous reviews have addressed related issues (e.g., Becker, 2009, 2012; Vogelgesang and Dressel, 2011; Vogelgesang et al., 2014), we will discuss the phenomenon of induction of tolerance in experimental stroke, the presence of autoantibodies in stroke patients, the presence of antigen-specific T cells in stroked animals and humans, in the context of antigen presentation, and we will address the possible relevance of such phenomena in medium or long-term stroke outcome.

The effects we will be referring to in this manuscript involve an adaptive immune response that is different from the damaging effects of T cells found in the very acute phase of stroke. Acute deleterious effects of T cells were perceived through the protection detected in lymphocyte-deficient mice after cerebral ischemia/reperfusion, and the capacity to reverse this phenomenon by adoptive transfer of T cells (Yilmaz et al., 2006; Hurn et al., 2007; Kleinschnitz et al., 2010). The acutely detrimental T-cell-mediated actions are mediated, at least in part, by impairment of the brain microcirculation through leukocyte adhesion to brain vessel walls (Yilmaz et al., 2006) promoting secondary microthrombosis (Kleinschnitz et al., 2010, 2013). Early detrimental effects of innate natural killer (NK) lymphocytes have also been reported in brain ischemia (Gan et al., 2014). These very acute lymphocyte effects contribute to the innate immune response to stroke (Magnus et al., 2012) but are not antigen specific and will not be addressed in this review.

BRAIN PROTEIN RELEASE TO THE PERIPHERY IN ISCHEMIC STROKE

After cerebral ischemia, metabolites of the ischemic molecular cascade and CNS proteins are released to the periphery, putatively enabling the generation of autoimmune responses against brain-specific antigens (Iadecola and Anrather, 2011; Chamorro et al., 2012). Protein markers of cerebral damage, including myelin basic protein (MBP), neuron-specific enolase (NSE), S100β, and glial fibrillary acidic protein (GFAP), are found in CSF and serum after stroke. Moreover, the concentration of these proteins is related to the severity of the neurological deficits (Jauch et al., 2006) and the extent of the brain lesion on neuroimaging in humans (Jauch et al., 2006) and experimental animals (Gelderblom et al., 2013). High levels of MBP and S100β are also predictive of poor functional recovery (Strand et al., 1984; Missler et al., 1997; Herrmann et al., 2000; Jauch et al., 2006). Brain antigens are not only found in the CSF and serum but also in lymphoid tissue of stroke patients (Planas et al., 2012; Gómez-Choco et al., 2014) where they can be presented by APCs and could trigger autoimmune or tolerogenic immune responses.

AUTOANTIBODIES

The presence of IgG immunoglobulin bands in the CSF of stroke patients was reported a long time ago (Roström and Link, 1981), suggesting that the release of brain antigens could be followed by intrathecal B-cell responses. Other researchers have confirmed the presence of specific IgG, IgM and IgA autoantibodies in the CSF (Prüss et al., 2012), and this is often accompanied by pleocytosis and altered albumin quotients of CSF/serum indicating BBB dysfunction. Overall, these findings suggest local activation of the immune system and possibly a pathogenic role of specific autoantibodies in stroke patients. Autoantibodies were also reported in serum. For example, anti-neurofilament antibodies were elevated after stroke, while antibodies against a ubiquitous antigen, cardiolipin, did not increase, again suggesting that brain antigens exposed in stroke are able to initiate an specific antibody response (Bornstein et al., 2001). Antibodies against the NR2A/2B subtype of N-methyl-D-aspartate (NMDA) receptor in serum are also more frequent in patients with transient ischemic attack (TIA) and acute ischemic stroke compared to non-stroke patients (patients admitted with suspected stroke but who had a non-stroke diagnosis at discharge) or healthy controls (Weissman et al., 2011), with high sensitivity, specificity, and predictive values (Dambinova et al., 2003). The presence of these autoantibodies may harbinger an increased risk of stroke as identification of anti-NMDA antibodies in patients before cardiopulmonary bypass surgery was associated with the development of neurological deficits and stroke (Bokesch et al., 2006). Patients with TIA and with ischemic stroke had similar titers of antibodies to NR2A/2B, suggesting that minor ischemic insults, and even subclinical lesions, may be sufficient to activate immunity (Dambinova et al., 2003). It is possible that the loss of BBB integrity is critical to allow autoantibodies to exert pathological effects, since to some extent the presence of autoantibodies is also seen in healthy subjects (Hammer et al., 2013).

Antibody-producing B cells, although not numerous in lesions, contribute to anti-atherosclerotic activity, perhaps as a result of specific antibodies against plaque antigens, binding of antibodies to inhibitory Fc receptors, or cytokines produced by B cells. Spleen B cells are particularly effective inhibitors of atherosclerosis (Caligiuri et al., 2002), possibly because certain natural antibodies produced by some of these cells recognize phosphorylcholine, a molecule present in oxidized LDL, apoptotic cell membranes, and the cell wall of *Streptococcus pneumoniae*. These antibodies may contribute to the elimination of oxidized LDL and dead cells, as well as to the defense against pneumococcal infections. Interestingly, persons who have undergone splenectomy have increased susceptibility not only to pneumococcal infections but also to coronary artery diseases (Sherer and Shoenfeld, 2006). However in experimental animals, intrastriatal, but not systemic, administration of splenic CD19+ B-cells reduced infarct volume in B-cell deficient mice (Chen et al., 2012) suggesting that B-cells exert protective effects against ischemic brain injury. In human studies we found a positive association between the number of circulating CD19+ B cells and good functional outcome after stroke (Urra et al., 2009a). Therefore, the role of B cell responses and antibody production in stroke outcome is still far from being fully understood. Whether circulating autoantibodies impair long-term functional outcome after stroke has not been demonstrated so far but it is plausible that they could exert pathogenic effects if they reached the brain under particular situations where the functionality of BBB was perturbed.

ANATOMIC PATHS THAT BRAIN PROTEINS CAN FOLLOW TO REACH THE PERIPHERY

Brain components could reach the lymphoid tissue either through the blood after crossing the leaky BBB, through interstitial fluid drainage to the blood or to the cervical lymph nodes, or after their local capture by migrating APCs (**Figure 1**). Understanding the route of access of brain proteins to the lymphoid tissue is not solely an anatomic issue, because depending on the way and form of entry to the lymphoid tissue, brain proteins/peptides will be encountered by different immune cells in different environments that may strongly influence the subsequent type of response, as we will discuss below.

Increased BBB permeability is a characteristic of stroke that could facilitate the leakage of brain proteins or protein fragments to the bloodstream. Proteolytic enzymes activated after stroke damage structural BBB components and cause BBB breakdown (Yang and Rosenberg, 2011). Neutrophils contain high levels of metalloproteinases (MMPs), such as MMP-9, and other destructive proteolytic enzymes, normally prepared to fight microbes, and contribute to the proteolytic activity after brain ischemia (Justicia et al., 2003; Gidday et al., 2005). Exposure of the neurovascular unit to such proteolytic activity cleaves tight junction proteins and damages the basement membranes, eventually causing BBB breakdown in acute stroke (Cunningham et al., 2005; Ludewig et al., 2013; Yang et al., 2013). However, BBB dysfunction may involve different degrees of cellular, structural, and molecular changes ranging from transient reversible dysfunction to more long-lasting alterations. Results obtained with different methods assessing BBB permeability support that there must be different grades of BBB dysfunction after brain ischemia (Nagaraja et al., 2008). The extent and nature of such alterations might exert some selectivity in the actual leakage of CNS protein components to the circulation, based on their size and other physical or biochemical features.

Besides exiting the brain through the leaky BBB, brain molecules can reach the periphery through the anatomic paths that allow for direct interstitial fluid drainage by bulk flow to the blood or to the lymphatics (Cserr et al., 1992; Weller et al., 1992; Abbott, 2004). The physical connection circuitry out of the brain towards the immune system enables draining of CSF into the lymphatics (Cserr et al., 1992; Weller et al., 1992). Interstitial extracellular fluid from the brain tissue drains to the CSF through perivascular spaces surrounding brain arterioles, but not venules (Arbel-Ornath et al., 2013; Carare et al., 2014). Perivascular spaces are connected to the subarachnoid space, allowing for fluid drainage to the venous blood through the arachnoid villi located at the dural venous sinuses (Cserr et al., 1992; Ransohoff et al., 2003). In addition, fluid from the subarachnoid space drains directionally to the cervical lymph nodes (Cserr et al., 1992; Zhang et al., 1992; Carare et al., 2014). Olfactory nerves are ensheated by arachnoid membranes allowing the drainage of CSF to the nasal mucosa through the cribiform plate, reaching nasal lymphatics, and from there, the CSF drains to the cervical lymph nodes (Harling-Berg et al., 1989; Cserr et al., 1992). An example of the functional relevance of this pathway is that the cervical lymph nodes are involved in the systemic humoral immune response to antigen infused into rat cerebrospinal fluid (Harling-Berg et al., 1989). Impairment of drainage of interstitial fluid out of the brain is believed to play a crucial role in the failure to adequately eliminate amyloid-β from the brain promoting its accumulation in the arterial walls in the elderly, and more prominently in patients with cerebral amyloid angiopathy (Weller et al., 2008; Hawkes et al., 2011, 2014; Arbel-Ornath et al., 2013). Since the force driving perivascular drainage is attributed to arterial vessel pulsations, it is not surprising that fluid drainage was found to be obstructed in an experimental model of focal brain ischemia induced by photothrombosis (Arbel-Ornath et al., 2013). This finding implies that stroke could impair the possible transfer of brain antigens from the interstitial fluid of the ischemic tissue to the CSF, but might not necessarily prevent the transfer connection from CSF to the cervical lymph nodes. In any case, ischemia-induced bulk-flow alterations might reverse, at least in part, at reperfusion.

Besides the possible exit of brain antigen from the brain tissue in a soluble form through the pathways indicated above (**Figure 1**), antigen can also be taken up locally in the brain by APCs. Dendritic cells (CD11c+) expressing MHC II and co-stimulatory molecules are found in the ischemic tissue (Felger et al., 2010) suggesting that they can present antigen. Migrating DCs traffic from peripheral tissues to their nearest lymph nodes through a process orchestrated by CCR7 in response to chemokines CCL19 and CCL20 (Förster et al., 1999), but other pathways could also be implicated such as sphingosine-1-phosphate (S1P) signaling (Czeloth et al., 2005) or the MHC II invariant chain (CD74) (Faure-André et al., 2008). Since the brain lacks lymphatic vessels, it is currently unknown whether mature DCs carrying antigen can migrate from the injured brain tissue to the peripheral lymphoid tissue. It was reported that cells from the brain could reach the deep cervical lymph nodes through the nasal submucosa (Cserr et al., 1992), supporting that cells in the subarachnoid space might be able to reach the draining lymph nodes. This possibility would imply that APCs could follow chemoattractant gradients along the anatomic

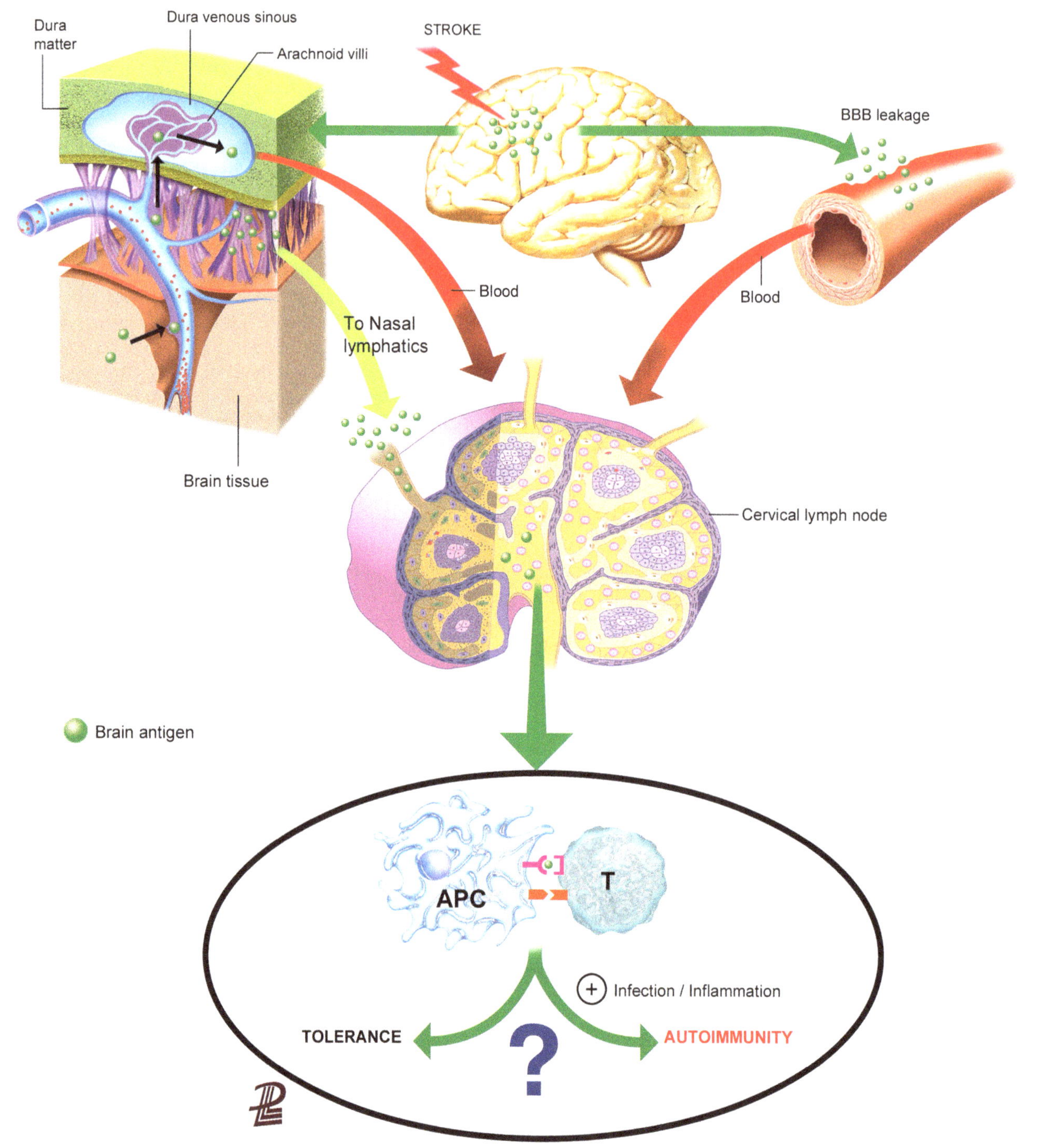

FIGURE 1 | Routes for the presentation of brain antigens in the lymphoid tissue. Brain antigens can reach regional lymphoid tissue through various routes after stroke. Ischemic stroke increases BBB permeability that can allow the leakage of proteins or peptides into the blood. Soluble proteins/peptides in brain interstitial fluid can reach the CSF through perivascular spaces and flow to the venous blood through the arachnoid villi or drain from the CSF may also drain along the arachnoid sheaths of the olfactory nerves towards the regional lymphatics. Although brain antigens are depicted as traveling in a soluble form in the figure, it is also possible that peptides were internalized, processed and presented by APCs in the brain, and that they reached regional lymph nodes through migrating APCs. Antigen presentation in the lymph nodes will usually induce tolerance to self-antigens, but under some circumstances that favor an inflammatory milieu presentation of brain antigens may result in activation of autorreactive T cells.

connections between the CSF and the cervical lymph nodes playing a natural role in the process of brain immunosurveillance. A study injecting DCs into the brain parenchyma showed little migration from their site of injection and cells did not reach the cervical lymph nodes, while intra-CSF-injected DCs did, and they preferentially targeted B-cell follicles rather than T-cell-rich areas suggesting that they favored humoral responses rather than cellular immunity (Hatterer et al., 2006). Efflux of solutes injected into the interstitial fluid of the brain was found to take place along basement membranes in the walls of capillaries and arteries (Carare et al., 2008). These basement membranes are very narrow, about 100 nm-thick, and therefore in normal conditions this pathway does not seem to be large enough to allow the trafficking of cells (Carare et al., 2008, 2014). Therefore, further studies are needed to find out whether and how mature APCs exit the brain to reach the peripheral lymphoid tissue after stroke.

ANTIGEN PRESENTATION: IMMUNITY VS. TOLERANCE

We identified in human stroke an increased presence of brain-derived antigens in migrating DCs and macrophages in lymphoid tissue located within the draining pathways of the CNS (Planas et al., 2012). This finding extends previous observations accrued in the cervical lymph nodes of rodents with ischemic brain damage or autoimmune disease, and in patients with multiple sclerosis (de Vos et al., 2002). These studies raise the issue of whether APCs in lymph nodes can present brain antigens to T cells after acute brain damage, and whether they can induce immune reactions that will either exacerbate the brain injury or promote mechanisms of T-cell tolerance. Central tolerance ensures, through negative selection, the elimination of most T cells recognizing self-antigens in the thymus. This process is complemented with peripheral tolerance that guarantees tolerization of autoreactive T cells and involves the action of peripheral APCs (Steinman and Nussenzweig, 2002). Cytoplasmic endogenous peptides are processed mostly through the proteasome, loaded into MHC class I in the endoplasmic reticulum, and shuttled to the cell membrane through the secretory pathway for presentation by MHC I in all cells, allowing recognition by CD8+ cytotoxic lymphocytes (Hulpke and Tampé, 2013). In contrast, exogenous peptides are presented through MHC class II after capture by APCs through endocytosis, including pinocytosis, phagocytosis, and receptor-mediated endocytosis (Wilson and Villadangos, 2005). Antigen presentation through MHC II elicits responses in CD4+ T helper (Th) cells. The exception to this role is cross-presentation of exogenous antigens by APCs through MHC I. This process occurs when exogenous peptides from the cell environment reach the cytoplasm, are presented through MHC I, and activate CD8+ T cells (Heath and Carbone, 2001; Joffre et al., 2012).

Presentation of exogenous proteins by APCs through MHC II, and also through cross-presentation, is essential for T cell priming against invading pathogens and for the induction of tolerance to self-tissue-specific proteins. Immune tolerance to self-antigens is based on the regulation of autoreactive lymphocytes by several mechanisms including deletion, clonal anergy, or suppression by regulatory T cells (Tregs) and other regulatory cells (Goodnow et al., 2005), and is dependent on the features of the interactions between T cells and APCs (Heath and Carbone, 2001). Dendritic cells are tolerogenic according to their maturation and functional status and are able to delete or silence autoreactive T cells and facilitate the development of Tregs (Rescigno, 2010; Ganguly et al., 2013), which play critical roles in controlling autoimmunity (Sakaguchi et al., 2001). Endogenous Tregs increase after experimental brain ischemia (Offner et al., 2006), and they proliferate and accumulate in the ischemic tissue up to 30 days after middle cerebral artery occlusion (MCAO; Stubbe et al., 2013). Regulatory T cells are involved in suppressing potentially harmful immune responses in stroke through the production of interleukin 10 (IL-10; Liesz et al., 2009), although some studies found no differences in the neurological outcome of stroke after depleting CD25(+) Tregs (Stubbe et al., 2013). Enhancing the immunosuppressive function of Tregs with histone deacetylase inhibitors was reported to reduce ischemic brain damage (Liesz et al., 2013). Immunotherapies with Tregs are currently under investigation to promote immune tolerance in various diseases (Singer et al., 2014). However, the effects of exogenous Treg administration in experimental brain ischemia are controversial, with some studies reporting protective actions (Li et al., 2013a,b), and other studies finding damaging effects related to the non-antigen specific impairment of the microcirculation (Kleinschnitz et al., 2013), as attributed to other T cells (Kleinschnitz et al., 2010). Regulatory B cells (Bregs) also produce IL-10 and TGF-β and exert immunomodulatory functions contributing to the maintenance of self-tolerance (Vadasz et al., 2013). Interleukin 10 producing Bregs were found to exert protection in experimental brain ischemia in mice, and Breg administration increased Treg numbers and the expression of the co-inhibitory receptor programmed death (PD)-1 (CD279) (Ren et al., 2011a; Bodhankar et al., 2013a).

The pathway of antigen access to the draining lymphoid tissue might influence the type of immune response since immature DCs that are resident in the lymph nodes efficiently take up, process and present antigen to induce tolerance (Inaba et al., 1997). Soluble brain peptides traveling through afferent lymphatic vessels to lymph nodes could be taken up by APCs or could be degraded extracellularly since immature DCs secrete proteases able to generate antigens that are eventually loaded on surface MHC II molecules (Santambrogio et al., 1999). Therefore, brain proteins or peptides reaching the lymphoid tissue in a soluble form could be internalized by resident macrophages or by immature DCs following prior extracellular degradation. We did not detect brain-derived antigens in lymphoid tissue resident DCs after stroke, but the brain-antigen loaded APCs were compatible with macrophages and migratory DCs (Planas et al., 2012). Antigen presentation by macrophages or DCs seems to be dependent on the form of antigen delivery to the cells, possibly due to different cell-type dependent internalization mechanisms. Dendritic cells preferentially internalize protein fragments whereas native proteins are better taken up by macrophages after receptor-mediated internalization or phagocytosis of apoptotic cells (Tsark et al., 2002). Dendritic cells are more efficient APCs than macrophages since they process antigen through a mechanism better preserving epitopes for T cell activation (Savina et al., 2006), whereas macrophages induce a very strong lysosomal acidification for protein degradation and display a different repertoire of lysosome proteases than DCs (Burster et al., 2005). Interestingly, we observed contacts between brain-antigen immunoreactive APCs and lymphoid resident DCs (Planas et al., 2012), which suggested the possibility of cargo exchange between these cells. It has been reported that antigens can be transferred from migrating APCs to lymph node-resident DCs for presentation and priming of cytotoxic lymphocytes (Allan et al., 2006). Cell-to-cell antigen transfer can be mediated through gap junctions (Neijssen et al., 2005). A recent study showed connexin 43 gap junction-mediated transfer of antigen from macrophages to CD103+ DCs, and the involvement of this process in the establishment of oral tolerance (Mazzini et al., 2014). Another pathway of possible antigen transfer between cells is via exosomes, i.e., externalized endosomal vesicles secreted by different cell types including DC and B cells. Exosomes are formed by direct fusion of membranes of the MHC II-enriched compartment with plasma membrane containing co-stimulatory molecules such as CD86 (Raposo et al., 1996; Denzer et al., 2000; Harvey et al., 2007). These vesicles are transferred from cell-to-cell by adherence to the cell surface rather than by membrane fusion (Denzer et al., 2000). The expected response to antigen transfer mediated by gap junctions or by exosomes would be different since the latter carry co-stimulatory molecules. It is unknown whether any of these mechanisms could support the transfer of brain antigen from macrophages or migrating DCs to resident DCs in the lymph node after stroke, and whether such processes could be involved in tolerization.

The maintenance of peripheral tolerance involves cross-presentation (Belz et al., 2002). CD8+ T cells recognizing self-antigen with high affinity are eliminated in the peripheral lymph nodes, and this process is termed cross-tolerance (Redmond and Sherman, 2005). Myelin-specific CD8+-T-cells play a pathogenic role in experimental models of multiple sclerosis (Huseby et al., 2001). Cross-presentation requires that the internalized Ag in the endosomal compartment access the cytosol. This process is regulated in diverse ways by chaperone proteins of the heat-shock family (HSPs) that prevent protein aggregation and misfolding (Srivastava, 2002). Heat-shock proteins mediate the transfer of antigenic peptides from the endosome compartment to the cytosol facilitating cross-presentation in immature DCs (Todryk et al., 1999), which then interact with cytotoxic T cells in an antigen-dependent fashion (Noessner et al., 2002; Binder and Srivastava, 2005). Also, HSPs undergo receptor-mediated endocytosis in DCs (Arnold-Schild et al., 1999), and induce maturation and migration of DCs (Binder et al., 2000). HSP-70 is not normally expressed in the brain under physiological conditions but is highly induced after ischemia (Planas et al., 1997; de la Rosa et al., 2013). HSP-70 is released from necrotic cells to the extracellular space (Todryk et al., 1999), and it can reach the bloodstream (Campisi and Fleshner, 2003). Because of the immunological properties of HSPs, the high induction of HSP-70 in the ischemic brain, and the presence of HSP-70 in the blood, led us to deduce that APCs in peripheral lymphoid tissue might carry HSP-70 after stroke. Indeed, we found that stroke patients showed higher immunoreactivity to HSP-70 and more HSP-70 immunoreactive APCs in lymphoid tissue than the controls, and that stronger presence of HSP-70 in lymphoid tissue was associated with smaller infarctions and better functional outcome (Gómez-Choco et al., 2014). Although a causal relationship between the presence of HSP-70 in the lymphoid tissue and the better outcome of the patients was not proved, it is feasible that the immunoregulatory properties of HSP-70 could modulate autoimmune responses after stroke. In other situations, HSP-70 has been implicated in the development of autoimmunity by promoting inflammatory responses, enhancing DC antigen presentation, and cytotoxic lymphocyte function (Millar et al., 2003) and it is involved in direct chaperoning of antigens into DCs (Todryk et al., 1999). While other HSP proteins, such as HSP-90, facilitate cross-presentation by antigen transfer to the cytosol (Imai et al., 2011), recent data support that HSP-70 impairs it (Kato et al., 2012), thus implying that HSP-70 might favor MHC II presentation. Although exposure of DCs to HSP-70 attenuates T cell responses (Stocki et al., 2012) and HSP-70 improves the immunosuppressive functions of Tregs, it also activates effector T cells (Wachstein et al., 2012). However, brain-derived HSP-70 has been involved in the induction of regulatory NK cells that can induce tolerance in experimental autoimmune encephalomyelitis (Galazka et al., 2006, 2007). Therefore, HSP-70 exerts diverse and complex actions in the immune system and further study is required to understand its role in stroke immunity.

ANTIGEN-SPECIFIC T CELLS

Whether the immune response to acute brain injury is non-specific or is directed against specific brain antigens is not yet settled. While tolerogenic effects have been reported with vaccination using neural antigens, several lines of evidence suggest that T cell accumulation at the site of traumatic CNS injury lacks selectivity, as shown after systemic administration of passively transferred T cells recognizing either neural self-antigen or non-self-antigen, since it resulted in accumulation of the T cells in injured optic nerve regardless of the antigen used for immunization (Hirschberg et al., 1998). The latter effects could be more related to non-specific effects of T cells described at early reperfusion following brain ischemia (Kleinschnitz et al., 2010). Nonetheless, evidences for antigen-specific T-cell reactivity have been found in animal models of acute brain injury. Indeed, nerve trauma can trigger the expansion of myelin-reactive T lymphocytes (Olsson et al., 1992) and an abnormal abundance of T cells autoreactive to myelin was reported in peripheral nerve trauma (Olsson et al., 1992), or spinal cord injury (Kil et al., 1999). While in the spinal cord endogenous MBP-reactive lymphocytes activated by traumatic injury can contribute to tissue damage and impair functional recovery (Jones et al., 2002), several lines of evidence support beneficial effects of these cells in the CNS (Graber and Dhib-Jalbut, 2009). Modulation of immune responses by priming T-cells with neural antigens has shown beneficial neuroprotective and anti-inflammatory actions in models of acute brain injury. Notably, autoreactive type-1 and -2 memory T cells pre-primed with myelin oligodendrocyte glycoprotein (MOG), a protein expressed on the surface of oligodendrocytes and myelin sheaths that is exclusive of nervous system, accelerated re-vascularization and healing following post-traumatic brain injury (Hofstetter et al., 2003). Furthermore, passive transfer of MBP-autoimmune T cells protected injured neurons in the CNS from degeneration (Moalem et al., 1999), and a possible contribution of a neurotrophin-related mechanism was proposed (Barouch and Schwartz, 2002). In experimental stroke, systemic inflammation at the time of MCAO in rats induced the development of a deleterious autoimmune response to MBP after 1 month (Becker et al., 2005). Furthermore, in a similar experimental model, impairment of neurological deficits associated with a Th1 response to MBP in the spleen was reported as soon as 48 h after induction of ischemia (Zierath et al., 2010). Further studies are needed to clarify the time-course development of antigen-specific reactions after stroke and their possible negative impact in functional outcome.

In stroke patients, antigen-specific T-cell reactivity (Tarkowski et al., 1991a,b) and *in vivo* expansion of myelin reactive T cells in the CSF (Wang et al., 1992) were observed more than 20 years ago. Increased influx of MOG-specific T cells into the brain was also detected after experimental stroke (Dirnagl et al., 2007). Th1 responses against MBP ranged from 24% in patients with no stroke-associated infection to 60% in patients with pneumonia and more robust Th1 responses to MBP 90 days after human stroke were associated with a decreased likelihood of good functional outcome, even after adjusting for major independent prognostic factors such as baseline stroke severity and age. Responses to another myelin-associated antigen, myelin proteolipid protein (PLP), and to the astrocyte marker GFAP also seemed to be associated to poor outcome, but reactivity to other antigens such as NSE, S-100β, and tetanus toxin were not predictive of outcome (Becker et al., 2011). The diverse prognostic consequences of immune responses to different brain antigens were also seen when analyzing the presence of brain-derived antigens in the lymphoid tissue of stroke patients. Greater reactivity to MBP was correlated with stroke severity on admission, larger infarctions, and worse outcome at follow-up, whereas increased reactivity to neuronal-derived antigens, such as microtubule-associated protein-2 and NMDA receptor subunit NR-2A, was correlated with smaller infarctions and better long-term outcome (Planas et al., 2012). Interestingly, in cervical lymph nodes of multiple sclerosis patients, neuronal antigens were present in pro-inflammatory APCs, whereas the majority of myelin-containing cells were anti-inflammatory (van Zwam et al., 2009). The authors concluded that the presence of myelin and neuronal antigens in functionally distinct APC populations suggests that differential immune responses can be evoked.

It is not settled whether autoimmune responses are the cause or a consequence of severe ischemic damage but the opposing prognostic implications of immune responses to specific brain antigens do suggest a pathogenic role of autoimmune responses against myelin antigens. Fast-conducting myelinated tracts are responsible for long-range connectivity, interhemispheric synchronization, and also have neurotrophic effects (Dan and Poo, 2004; Nave, 2010) and injury to these fibers can therefore impair brain connectivity (Sun et al., 2011; Lawrence et al., 2013), reduce cortical blood flow, and promote cerebral atrophy (Appelman et al., 2008; Chen et al., 2013). Given that myelination is important for neuroplasticity and motor learning (Fields, 2010), greater autoimmune damage to myelin could also compromise recovery after stroke and contribute to cognitive impairment. It is unknown whether antigen-specific responses to molecules widely expressed in the body might also develop after stroke. Patients with antiphospholipid syndrome are at risk of stroke (Sciascia et al., 2014) and this may have additional implications regarding whether existing autoantibodies can impair the functional outcome of stroke, or whether stroke could exacerbate preexisting autoimmune responses.

INDUCTION OF IMMUNOLOGIC TOLERANCE IN STROKE

Seminal studies by the team of J. Hallenbeck, K. Becker and colleagues provided evidences supporting that modulating antigen-specific responses could protect the brain in stroke. They found that oral administration of low doses of bovine MBP to Lewis rats prior to transient (3-h) MCAO reduced infarct volume at days 1 and 4 (Becker et al., 1997) demonstrating induced antigen-specific modulation of the immune response. This strategy reduced delayed-type hypersensitivity to MBP and induced-spleen cell proliferation showing that tolerance to this brain antigen was induced. Similar findings were reproduced using MBP for tolerization through nasal instillation in Lewis rats, which showed reduced infarct volume 24 h after 3-h intraluminal MCAO (Becker et al., 2003). Notably, the latter study showed that the protective effect of MBP tolerization could be transferred by administration of splenocytes from MBP-tolerized donors before induction of MCAO, implying that the protective effect of tolerization can be conferred by splenocyte transplantation. In the same line, nasal vaccination with a MOG peptide prior to transient (2-h) MCAO in C57BL/6 mice reduced infarct volume and was more effective than oral MOG tolerization (Frenkel et al., 2003). Besides tolerization with brain-specific antigens, repetitive nasal administration of small doses of E-selectin was also beneficial in experimental stroke. E-selectin is an adhesion molecule involved in leukocyte trafficking to the tissues across the blood vessels and it is strongly induced in the inflamed endothelium. E-selectin expression in the brain vasculature increases after cerebral ischemia (Huang et al., 2000). In prevention studies, nasal instillation of E-selectin potently inhibited the development of ischemic and hemorrhagic strokes in stroke-prone spontaneously hypertensive rats (SP-SHR; Takeda et al., 2002). Moreover, induction of mucosal tolerance to E-selectin through nasal instillation before induction of permanent MCAO (coagulation) in SP-SHR rats improved the outcome by reducing infarct volume at 48 h (Chen et al., 2003). This study also found that adoptive transfer of splenocytes from E-selectin-tolerized donors was able to reduce infarct volume.

But what is the actual mechanism underlying the protection conferred by antigen-specific tolerization against stroke brain damage? Interleukin-10-producing CD4+ T cells mediated the protective effect of nasal tolerization with MOG (Frenkel et al., 2003, 2005), in agreement with the concept that mucosal administration of proteins preferentially induces IL-10 responses mediated by tolerogenic DCs and Tregs (Weiner et al., 2011). Likewise, oral administration of MOG protected against secondary neurodegeneration in a rat model of acute nerve injury by induction of IL-10 producing myelin-reactive T cells (Monsonego et al., 2003). However, nasal MOG tolerization in stroke induced more IL-10 and less CD11b cells than oral MOG (Frenkel et al., 2003). Interleukin-10 production induces unresponsiveness in innate myeloid cells, which then become less capable of generating IL-17-producing encephalitogenic T cells. Oral MBP tolerization induced TGF-β1 and the immunosuppressive features of this cytokine might underlie the beneficial effects of MBP tolerization in stroke (Becker et al., 1997). Mucosal E-selectin tolerization downregulated MHC class I gene expression (Illoh et al., 2006). This effect could prevent the activation of NK cells or cytotoxic T cells and was associated with reduced numbers of CD8+ cells found after ischemia in the tolerized animals (Chen et al., 2003). Tolerization with E-selectin reprogrammed gene expression to inflammation induced by lipopolysaccharide (LPS) promoting the expression of growth factor genes and genes involved in protection against oxidative stress, and it was suggested that E-selectin tolerization could lead to the expansion of Tregs (Illoh et al., 2006). Again, increased expression of IL-10 was also proposed as a mechanism underlying the protective effects of E-selectin tolerization (Yun et al., 2008). Induction of mucosal tolerance triggers Tregs in an antigen-specific fashion (Weiner et al., 2011). Regulatory T cells attenuate inflammation and prevent autoimmunity through secretion of immunosuppressive cytokines, amongst other effects (Costantino et al., 2008). Then, Tregs can exert a global non-specific suppressive effect locally where they encounter the specific antigen, and this action could mediate, at least in part, the beneficial effects of mucosal tolerization in stroke (Frenkel et al., 2005).

THE EFFECT OF SYSTEMIC INFLAMMATION

Large community studies have found associations between systemic inflammatory conditions, such as osteorarthritis or pelvic inflammatory disease, and cardiovascular disease, including stroke (Chen et al., 2011; Rahman et al., 2013). This could be the result of the profound implication of many components of the immune system in the pathological processes underlying the development of atherosclerosis and in particular in its ischemic complications (Sherer and Shoenfeld, 2006). Acute ischemic brain damage is also exacerbated by systemic inflammation. In an experimental model of cerebral ischemia, systemic inflammation caused sustained disruption of the tight junction protein, claudin-5, and also exacerbated disruption of the basal lamina collagen-IV, and these alterations were associated with an increase in neutrophil-derived MMP-9 (McColl et al., 2008). In the same line, systemic inflammation in IL-10 deficient mice, spontaneously developing colitis when exposed to environmental pathogens, increased mortality after stroke (Pérez-de Puig et al., 2013). Using a murine model of chronic infection leading to a chronic Th1-polarized immune response, Dénes et al. (2010) found upregulation of proinflammatory mediators in the brain and peripheral tissues, as well as an altered Treg response, accelerated platelet aggregation in brain capillaries, increased microvascular injury and MMP activation after experimental ischemia, and a 60% increase in brain damage.

Infections are the most common complication in stroke patients (Kumar et al., 2010; Westendorp et al., 2011). The most frequent infections are respiratory infections and urinary tract infections and the main clinical predictor of infection is the severity of the neurological deficit. Experimental and clinical studies showed that stroke induces a transient immunodepression that increases the susceptibility to systemic infections in the first days after cerebral ischemia. This was first described in a murine model of cerebral ischemia (Prass et al., 2003) where overactivation of the adrenergic system caused apoptotic loss of lymphocytes and a shift from Th1 to Th2 cytokine production. Atrophy of primary and secondary lymphoid organs and increased numbers of Treg cells were also features of the systemic immune changes induced by cerebral ischemia (Prass et al., 2003; Offner et al., 2006). In stroke patients, the best established features of stroke-induced immunodepression are increased levels of stress hormones and anti-inflammatory cytokines like IL-10 (Haeusler et al., 2008; Klehmet et al., 2009; Urra et al., 2009a), decreased numbers of circulating lymphocytes (Haeusler et al., 2008; Vogelgesang et al., 2008; Urra et al., 2009b), and monocyte deactivation with reduced expression of HLA-DR and reduced capacity to produce inflammatory cytokines (Haeusler et al., 2008; Urra et al., 2009a).

Infection triggers inflammation, facilitates the maturation of APCs into potent immunostimulatory cells (Banchereau et al., 2000), and is involved in the development of autoimmune diseases (Getts et al., 2013; Berer and Krishnamoorthy, 2014). Post-stroke infections complicate the clinical course of the patients (Ulm et al., 2012) and could be a source of inflammation favoring autoimmunity. Systemic inflammation and infection in stroke could set an environment in the periphery favorable to promote the development of effector T cells against brain antigens by providing sufficient cytokines and co-stimulatory molecules (Becker, 2012). However, most features of the stroke-induced systemic immune changes modulate antigen presentation and its consequences, presumably favoring tolerogenic immune responses. Therefore, in the absence of infection, immunodepression would be expected to favor tolerance. Catecholamines can inhibit the antigen-presenting capability via β2-adrenoceptors and this effect is at least partly due to impaired CD8+ cell priming by cross-presenting DC (Seiffert et al., 2002; Maestroni and Mazzola, 2003; Hervé et al., 2013). Corticosteroids inhibit the production of inflammatory cytokines in APCs and induce the development of tolerogenic APCs (DeKruyff et al., 1998; de Jong et al., 1999), and glucocorticoid-stimulated monocytes reduce the release of IFN-γ and IL-17 in lymphocytes favoring the generation of Treg (Varga et al., 2014). Interleukin-10 also inhibits autoimmune reactions acting on several immune cells including APCs. Interleukin-10 treated DCs induce anergic T cells that are able to suppress activation and function of T cells in an antigen-specific manner (Steinbrink et al., 2002). In addition, other alterations in the numbers and phenotype of circulating leukocytes, such as lymphocytopenia and reduced HLA-DR expression in monocytes, could further impair the activation of specific T cell responses against brain antigens. For all these reasons, while predisposing patients to systemic infections, immunodepression after stroke could limit detrimental autoimmune responses in the brain. The effect of infection in stroke has been studied in experimental models of brain ischemia. Induction of ischemia in mice intranasally infected with the human influenza A (H1N1) virus increased the number of neutrophils expressing the MMP-9 in the ischemic brain, exacerbated BBB breakdown, and increased the rate of intracerebral hemorrhages after tissue plasminogen activator treatment (Muhammad et al., 2011). Systemic inflammation at the time of experimental stroke has been used experimentally to mimic the clinical situation of infection to increase the likelihood of developing a detrimental autoimmune response to brain antigens (Becker et al., 2011) by favoring Th1 responses to MBP (Becker et al., 2005; Zierath et al., 2010). However, induction of systemic inflammation or infection in experimental animals at the time of cerebral ischemia would possibly mimic better the clinical scenario of infections precipitating a stroke rather than the infections occurring as a complication of stroke, since the latter are usually related to the severity of the lesion and the degree of stroke-induced immunodepression (Chamorro et al., 2007; Dirnagl et al., 2007). Becker et al. (2011) reported that patients who developed an infection after stroke, especially pneumonia, were more likely to show a Th1 response to MBP and GFAP 90 days after stroke. This is very relevant because stronger Th1 responses to MBP were seen associated to poor functional outcome. However, stroke associated infections are especially frequent in patients with severe strokes (Hug et al., 2009; Urra and Chamorro, 2010) and the development of autoimmune responses could be strongly influenced by the severity of the brain lesion. It is also very likely that the timing of the infections is a key factor in modulating the immune response (Emsley and Hopkins, 2008). Infections before stroke can be a source of inflammation and thrombosis, and can precipitate stroke onset (Elkind et al., 2011). A small clinical study showed that patients with previous infection had greater deficits and increased platelet activation and platelet-leukocyte aggregation compared with patients without infection (Zeller et al., 2005). Thus the presence of previous infections, possibly including subclinical infections, could facilitate the occurrence of stroke and impair functional recovery.

PHARMACOLOGIC REGULATION OF AUTOREACTIVE T CELLS AFTER STROKE

Reduction of infarct volume after transient ischemia was achieved by immune regulation of myelin-reactive inflammatory T cells using recombinant T cell receptor ligands (RTL), i.e., partial MHC class II molecules covalently bound to myelin peptides acting as partial agonists that deviate autoreactive T cells to become non-pathogenic (Subramanian et al., 2009; Dziennis et al., 2011), again supporting a negative effect of antigen-specific responses in the lesion caused by stroke. Co-inhibitory molecules, like PD-1, regulate the induction and maintenance of peripheral tolerance (Ceeraz et al., 2013). Accordingly, PD-1-deficient mice showed higher inflammatory responses, infarct volume and neurological deficits after brain ischemia (Ren et al., 2011b). However, mice deficient in PD-1 ligands (PD-L) were protected against ischemic brain damage (Bodhankar et al., 2013b), while it has been reported that PD-1 is necessary for Treg-induced protective effects (Li et al., 2014). Therefore, the role of this pathway in the outcome of brain ischemia seems to be quite complex and is not yet fully characterized.

Regulation of the migration of lymphocyte subsets into the CNS can also control autoimmunity. The egress of lymphocytes from lymph nodes requires lymphocytic S1P1 receptors (Matloubian et al., 2004). The main protective mechanism of fingolimod in multiple sclerosis seems to be mediated by internalization of S1P1 that therefore reduces the responsiveness of T cells to the egress signal S1P and favors CCR7-mediated lymphocyte retention in lymph nodes (Pham et al., 2008). Several experimental studies reported protection after treatment with fingolimod in brain ischemia (Hasegawa et al., 2010; Wei et al., 2011; Kraft et al., 2013), and intracerebral hemorrhage (Rolland et al., 2011), but the mechanisms underlying this protection are not fully understood. While lymphocytopenia could be involved in the effects of fingolimod, one study found that this drug was not protective in experimental cerebral ischemia in spite of reducing lymphocyte influx (Liesz et al., 2011). Other effects of this drug, including BBB protection, decreased microvascular thrombosis (Kraft et al., 2013), and reduced hemorrhagic transformation in thromboembolic stroke (Campos et al., 2013) could account, at least in part, for the reported beneficial effects. Whether fingolimod affects autoimmune responses and autoreactive T cell migration after brain ischemia has not been reported and it is unknown whether fingolimod-induced lymphocytopenia might further increase the risk of infection. Interestingly, the drug appears to be safe for the treatment of intracerebral hemorrhage in humans (Fu et al., 2014). In any case, experimental interventions on the immune system in stroke models should pay particular attention to immunodepression and infection as possible causes of neurological impairment and mortality. However, studies identifying post-stroke infection in experimental animals and its possible neurological consequences are difficult and still infrequent (Braun et al., 2007; Engel and Meisel, 2010; Hetze et al., 2013).

Besides systemic infections, factors such as severe arteriosclerosis or other systemic autoimmune diseases are also likely to promote a proinflammatory environment favoring autoimmunity in ischemic stroke. As vascular risk factors and atherosclerosis are common in stroke patients, clinical and experimental studies assessing this possibility and also the potential of commonly used drugs, such as statins, to modulate the immune reactions to stroke would be relevant. Several beneficial effects of statins may be due to immunomodulatory effects, including impaired maturation of DCs with reduced expression of molecules like MHC class II preventing antigen presentation to T cells (Kwak et al., 2000; Yilmaz et al., 2004) and inducing tolerogenic DCs that increase the numbers of Treg cells (Li et al., 2013c). Vaccination is also an attractive approach to induce protective immunity avoiding the progression of atherosclerosis. In experiments in animals, atherosclerosis was reduced by vaccination with oxidized LDL, bacteria containing certain modified phospholipids, or heat-shock protein 65 (Palinski et al., 1995; Maron et al., 2002; Binder et al., 2003).

FUTURE DIRECTIONS

In this review we described the current evidence suggesting the possibility that stroke can trigger antigen-specific responses. These include the finding of T-cells autoreactive to brain antigens in stroke patients, the presence of brain antigens and autoantibodies in CSF and serum, and APCs carrying brain antigens in the regional lymphoid tissue. Further support to this notion is provided by the beneficial effects of inducing immune tolerance in experimental animal models of stroke. Brain antigens are released after stroke in the presence of inflammatory mediators and danger signals. Soluble molecules can reach the periphery across the leaky BBB or across natural pathways normally allowing fluid efflux, i.e., the drainage of interstitial fluid to the CSF and from there to the blood, and the drainage of CSF through the nasal lymphatics to the cervical lymph nodes. Furthermore, antigens can be internalized locally in the brain by APCs, but whether these cells can migrate to the draining lymph nodes for efficient antigen presentation is currently unknown and deserves further investigation. Since these routes could trigger different immune responses, it is relevant to elucidate their contribution to brain antigen transfer to the lymph nodes. Mechanisms ensuring tolerance to self are tightly regulated. Peripheral tolerance relies on factors including the features of APCs and their interaction with lymphocytes, the cytokine environment, and the presence of danger signals and regulatory or suppressor cells. Although a number of studies have shown specific changes in these factors after stroke, we still lack a complete picture of how these changes are integrated in the organism over time. Furthermore, stroke co-morbidities are often associated with changes in the immune system that could play a crucial role in directing specific immune responses to stroke. Stroke does not consistently trigger autoimmunity, but several lines of evidence support that infection and inflammation could break immune tolerance controls and favor autoreactive responses to brain antigens after stroke. Infection is a frequent complication of stroke that is attributable to stroke-induced immunodepression, characterized by acute lymphopenia and monocyte deactivation. Immunodepression sets a humoral and cellular situation favorable to prevent autoreactivity, but leaves the subjects at risk of infection. In the event of infection, the risk of autoreactivity increases, suggesting a fine balance between the factors regulating tolerance and autoimmunity. Further understanding of these regulatory mechanisms is necessary to elucidate whether antigen-specific reactions could threaten the outcome of stroke patients. Some patients show partial recovery of function and respond to rehabilitation over months after stroke onset. However, certain stroke patients develop complications, as for instance cognitive decline or epilepsy, and it is often difficult to predict such effects. Whether any autoimmune reaction can underlie stroke complications deserves further investigation aiming to prevent or attenuate such adverse events.

ACKNOWLEDGMENTS

Authors receive financial support by the Spanish Ministries of Economy MINECO (SAF2011-30492) and Health (FIS PI12/01437), and the European Community FP7 (ERA-NET program PRI-PIMNEU-2011-1342). Francesc Miró is supported by the "Red Invictus" of the Instituto de Salud Carlos III (RD12/0014/0011). We would like to thank Dr. Vanessa Brait for helpful comments.

REFERENCES

Abbott, N. J. (2004). Evidence for bulk flow of brain interstitial fluid: significance for physiology and pathology. *Neurochem. Int.* 45, 545–552. doi: 10.1016/j.neuint.2003.11.006

Allan, R. S., Waithman, J., Bedoui, S., Jones, C. M., Villadangos, J. A., Zhan, Y., et al. (2006). Migratory dendritic cells transfer antigen to a lymph node-resident dendritic cell population for efficient CTL priming. *Immunity* 25, 153–162. doi: 10.1016/j.immuni.2006.04.017

Appelman, A. P., van der Graaf, Y., Vincken, K. L., Tiehuis, A. M., Witkamp, T. D., Mali, W. P., et al. (2008). Total cerebral blood flow, white matter lesions and brain atrophy: the SMART-MR study. *J. Cereb. Blood Flow Metab.* 28, 633–639. doi: 10.1038/sj.jcbfm.9600563

Arbel-Ornath, M., Hudry, E., Eikermann-Haerter, K., Hou, S., Gregory, J. L., Zhao, L., et al. (2013). Interstitial fluid drainage is impaired in ischemic stroke and Alzheimer's disease mouse models. *Acta Neuropathol.* 126, 353–364. doi: 10.1007/s00401-013-1145-2

Arnold-Schild, D., Hanau, D., Spehner, D., Schmid, C., Rammensee, H. G., de la Salle, H., et al. (1999). Cutting edge: receptor-mediated endocytosis of heat shock proteins by professional antigen-presenting cells. *J. Immunol.* 162, 3757–3760.

Banchereau, J., Briere, F., Caux, C., Davoust, J., Lebecque, S., Liu, Y. J., et al. (2000). Immunobiology of dendritic cells. *Annu. Rev. Immunol.* 18, 767–811. doi: 10.1146/annurev.immunol.18.1.767

Barouch, R., and Schwartz, M. (2002). Autoreactive T cells induce neurotrophin production by immune and neural cells in injured rat optic nerve: implications for protective autoimmunity. *FASEB J.* 16, 1304–1306. doi: 10.1096/fj.01-0467fje

Becker, K. J. (2009). Sensitization and tolerization to brain antigens in stroke. *Neuroscience* 158, 1090–1097. doi: 10.1016/j.neuroscience.2008.07.027

Becker, K. (2012). Autoimmune responses to brain following stroke. *Transl. Stroke Res.* 3, 310–317. doi: 10.1007/s12975-012-0154-0

Becker, K. J., Kalil, A. J., Tanzi, P., Zierath, D. K., Savos, A. V., Gee, J. M., et al. (2011). Autoimmune responses to the brain after stroke are associated with worse outcome. *Stroke* 42, 2763–2769. doi: 10.1161/STROKEAHA.111.619593

Becker, K. J., Kindrick, D. L., Lester, M. P., Shea, C., and Ye, Z. C. (2005). Sensitization to brain antigens after stroke is augmented by lipopolysaccharide. *J. Cereb. Blood Flow Metab.* 25, 1634–1644. doi: 10.1038/sj.jcbfm.9600160

Becker, K., Kindrick, D., McCarron, R., Hallenbeck, J., and Winn, R. (2003). Adoptive transfer of myelin basic protein-tolerized splenocytes to naive animals reduces infarct size: a role for lymphocytes in ischemic brain injury? *Stroke* 34, 1809–1815. doi: 10.1161/01.str.0000078308.77727.ea

Becker, K. J., McCarron, R. M., Ruetzler, C., Laban, O., Sternberg, E., Flanders, K. C., et al. (1997). Immunologic tolerance to myelin basic protein decreases stroke size after transient focal cerebral ischemia. *Proc. Natl. Acad. Sci. U S A* 94, 10873–10878. doi: 10.1073/pnas.94.20.10873

Belz, G. T., Behrens, G. M., Smith, C. M., Miller, J. F., Jones, C., Lejon, K., et al. (2002). The CD8alpha(+) dendritic cell is responsible for inducing peripheral self-tolerance to tissue-associated antigens. *J. Exp. Med.* 196, 1099–1104. doi: 10.1084/jem.20020861

Berer, K., and Krishnamoorthy, G. (2014). Microbial view of central nervous system autoimmunity. *FEBS Lett.* doi: 10.1016/j.febslet.2014.04.007. [Epub ahead of print].

Binder, R. J., Anderson, K. M., Basu, S., and Srivastava, P. K. (2000). Cutting edge: heat shock protein gp96 induces maturation and migration of CD11c+ cells in vivo. *J. Immunol.* 165, 6029–6035. doi: 10.4049/jimmunol.165.11.6029

Binder, C. J., Hörkkö, S., Dewan, A., Chang, M. K., Kieu, E. P., Goodyear, C. S., et al. (2003). Pneumococcal vaccination decreases atherosclerotic lesion formation: molecular mimicry between Streptococcus pneumoniae and oxidized LDL. *Nat. Med.* 9, 736–743. doi: 10.1016/s0214-9168(03)78944-x

Binder, R. J., and Srivastava, P. K. (2005). Peptides chaperoned by heat-shock proteins are a necessary and sufficient source of antigen in the cross-priming of CD8+ T cells. *Nat. Immunol.* 6, 593–599. doi: 10.1038/ni1201

Bodhankar, S., Chen, Y., Vandenbark, A. A., Murphy, S. J., and Offner, H. (2013a). IL-10-producing B-cells limit CNS inflammation and infarct volume in experimental stroke. *Metab. Brain Dis.* 28, 375–386. doi: 10.1007/s11011-013-9413-3

Bodhankar, S., Chen, Y., Vandenbark, A. A., Murphy, S. J., and Offner, H. (2013b). PD-L1 enhances CNS inflammation and infarct volume following experimental stroke in mice in opposition to PD-1. *J. Neuroinflammation* 10:111. doi: 10.1186/1742-2094-10-111

Bokesch, P. M., Izykenova, G. A., Justice, J. B., Easley, K. A., and Dambinova, S. A. (2006). NMDA receptor antibodies predict adverse neurological outcome after cardiac surgery in high-risk patients. *Stroke* 37, 1432–1436. doi: 10.1161/01.str.0000221295.14547.c8

Bornstein, N. M., Aronovich, B., Korczyn, A. D., Shavit, S., Michaelson, D. M., and Chapman, J. (2001). Antibodies to brain antigens following stroke. *Neurology* 56, 529–530. doi: 10.1212/wnl.56.4.529

Braun, J. S., Prass, K., Dirnagl, U., Meisel, A., and Meisel, C. (2007). Protection from brain damage and bacterial infection in murine stroke by the novel caspase-inhibitor Q-VD-OPH. *Exp. Neurol.* 206, 183–191. doi: 10.1016/j.expneurol.2007.03.032

Burster, T., Beck, A., Tolosa, E., Schnorrer, P., Weissert, R., Reich, M., et al. (2005). Differential processing of autoantigens in lysosomes from human monocyte-derived and peripheral blood dendritic cells. *J. Immunol.* 175, 5940–5949. doi: 10.4049/jimmunol.175.9.5940

Caligiuri, G., Nicoletti, A., Poirier, B., and Hansson, G. K. (2002). Protective immunity against atherosclerosis carried by B cells of hypercholesterolemic mice. *J. Clin. Invest.* 109, 745–753. doi: 10.1172/JCI7272

Campisi, J., and Fleshner, M. (2003). Role of extracellular HSP72 in acute stress-induced potentiation of innate immunity in active rats. *J. Appl. Physiol. (1985)* 94, 43–52. doi: 10.1152/japplphysiol.00681.2002

Campos, F., Qin, T., Castillo, J., Seo, J. H., Arai, K., Lo, E. H., et al. (2013). Fingolimod reduces hemorrhagic transformation associated with delayed tissue plasminogen activator treatment in a mouse thromboembolic model. *Stroke* 44, 505–511. doi: 10.1161/STROKEAHA.112.679043

Carare, R. O., Bernardes-Silva, M., Newman, T. A., Page, A. M., Nicoll, J. A., Perry, V. H., et al. (2008). Solutes, but not cells, drain from the brain parenchyma along basement membranes of capillaries and arteries: significance for cerebral amyloid angiopathy and neuroimmunology. *Neuropathol. Appl. Neurobiol.* 34, 131–144. doi: 10.1111/j.1365-2990.2007.00926.x

Carare, R. O., Hawkes, C. A., and Weller, R. O. (2014). Afferent and efferent immunological pathways of the brain. Anatomy, function and failure. *Brain Behav. Immun.* 36, 9–14. doi: 10.1016/j.bbi.2013.10.012

Ceeraz, S., Nowak, E. C., and Noelle, R. J. (2013). B7 family checkpoint regulators in immune regulation and disease. *Trends Immunol.* 34, 556–563. doi: 10.1016/j.it.2013.07.003

Chamorro, Á., Meisel, A., Planas, A. M., Urra, X., van de Beek, D., and Veltkamp, R. (2012). The immunology of acute stroke. *Nat. Rev. Neurol.* 8, 401–410. doi: 10.1038/nrneurol.2012.98

Chamorro, A., Urra, X., and Planas, A. M. (2007). Infection after acute ischemic stroke: a manifestation of brain-induced immunodepression. *Stroke* 38, 1097–1103. doi: 10.1161/01.str.0000258346.68966.9d

Chen, Y., Bodhankar, S., Murphy, S. J., Vandenbark, A. A., Alkayed, N. J., and Offner, H. (2012). Intrastriatal B-cell administration limits infarct size after stroke in B-cell deficient mice. *Metab. Brain Dis.* 27, 487–493. doi: 10.1007/s11011-012-9317-7

Chen, J. J., Rosas, H. D., and Salat, D. H. (2013). The relationship between cortical blood flow and sub-cortical white-matter health across the adult age span. *PLoS One* 8:e56733. doi: 10.1371/journal.pone.0056733

Chen, Y., Ruetzler, C., Pandipati, S., Spatz, M., McCarron, R. M., Becker, K., et al. (2003). Mucosal tolerance to E-selectin provides cell-mediated protection against ischemic brain injury. *Proc. Natl. Acad. Sci. U S A* 100, 15107–15112. doi: 10.1073/pnas.2436538100

Chen, P. C., Tseng, T. C., Hsieh, J. Y., and Lin, H. W. (2011). Association between stroke and patients with pelvic inflammatory disease: a nationwide population-based study in Taiwan. *Stroke* 42, 2074–2076. doi: 10.1161/STROKEAHA.110.612655

Costantino, C. M., Baecher-Allan, C. M., and Hafler, D. A. (2008). Human regulatory T cells and autoimmunity. *Eur. J. Immunol.* 38, 921–924. doi: 10.1002/eji.200738104

Cserr, H. F., Harling-Berg, C. J., and Knopf, P. M. (1992). Drainage of brain extracellular fluid into blood and deep cervical lymph and its immunological significance. *Brain Pathol.* 2, 269–276. doi: 10.1111/j.1750-3639.1992.tb00703.x

Cunningham, L. A., Wetzel, M., and Rosenberg, G. A. (2005). Multiple roles for MMPs and TIMPs in cerebral ischemia. *Glia* 50, 329–339. doi: 10.1002/glia.20169

Czeloth, N., Bernhardt, G., Hofmann, F., Genth, H., and Förster, R. (2005). Sphingosine-1-phosphate mediates migration of mature dendritic cells. *J. Immunol.* 175, 2960–2967. doi: 10.4049/jimmunol.175.5.2960

Dambinova, S. A., Khounteev, G. A., Izykenova, G. A., Zavolokov, I. G., Ilyukhina, A. Y., and Skoromets, A. A. (2003). Blood test detecting autoantibodies to N-methyl-D-aspartate neuroreceptors for evaluation of patients with transient ischemic attack and stroke. *Clin. Chem.* 49, 1752–1762. doi: 10.1373/49.10.1752

Dan, Y., and Poo, M. M. (2004). Spike timing-dependent plasticity of neural circuits. *Neuron* 44, 23–30. doi: 10.1016/j.neuron.2004.09.007

de Jong, E. C., Vieira, P. L., Kalinski, P., and Kapsenberg, M. L. (1999). Corticosteroids inhibit the production of inflammatory mediators in immature monocyte-derived DC and induce the development of tolerogenic DC3. *J. Leukoc. Biol.* 66, 201–204.

DeKruyff, R. H., Fang, Y., and Umetsu, D. T. (1998). Corticosteroids enhance the capacity of macrophages to induce Th2 cytokine synthesis in CD4+ lymphocytes by inhibiting IL-12 production. *J. Immunol.* 160, 2231–2237.

de la Rosa, X., Santalucía, T., Fortin, P. Y., Purroy, J., Calvo, M., Salas-Perdomo, A., et al. (2013). In vivo imaging of induction of heat-shock protein-70 gene expression with fluorescence reflectance imaging and intravital confocal microscopy following brain ischaemia in reporter mice. *Eur. J. Nucl. Med. Mol. Imaging* 40, 426–438. doi: 10.1007/s00259-012-2277-7

Dénes, A., Humphreys, N., Lane, T. E., Grencis, R., and Rothwell, N. (2010). Chronic systemic infection exacerbates ischemic brain damage via a CCL5 (regulated on activation, normal T-cell expressed and secreted)-mediated proinflammatory response in mice. *J. Neurosci.* 30, 10086–10095. doi: 10.1523/JNEUROSCI.1227-10.2010

Denzer, K., Kleijmeer, M. J., Heijnen, H. F., Stoorvogel, W., and Geuze, H. J. (2000). Exosome: from internal vesicle of the multivesicular body to intercellular signaling device. *J. Cell Sci.* 113, 3365–3374.

de Vos, A. F., van Meurs, M., Brok, H. P., Boven, L. A., Hintzen, R. Q., van der Valk, P., et al. (2002). Transfer of central nervous system autoantigens and presentation in secondary lymphoid organs. *J. Immunol.* 169, 5415–5423. doi: 10.4049/jimmunol.169.10.5415

Dirnagl, U., Klehmet, J., Braun, J. S., Harms, H., Meisel, C., Ziemssen, T., et al. (2007). Stroke-induced immunodepression: experimental evidence and clinical relevance. *Stroke* 38, 770–773. doi: 10.1161/01.str.0000251441.89665.bc

Dziennis, S., Mader, S., Akiyoshi, K., Ren, X., Ayala, P., Burrows, G. G., et al. (2011). Therapy with recombinant T-cell receptor ligand reduces infarct size and infiltrating inflammatory cells in brain after middle cerebral artery occlusion in mice. *Metab. Brain Dis.* 26, 123–133. doi: 10.1007/s11011-011-9241-2

Elkind, M. S., Carty, C. L., O'Meara, E. S., Lumley, T., Lefkowitz, D., Kronmal, R. A., et al. (2011). Hospitalization for infection and risk of acute ischemic stroke: the Cardiovascular Health Study. *Stroke* 42, 1851–1856. doi: 10.1161/STROKEAHA.110.608588

Emsley, H. C., and Hopkins, S. J. (2008). Acute ischaemic stroke and infection: recent and emerging concepts. *Lancet Neurol.* 7, 341–353. doi: 10.1016/s1474-4422(08)70061-9

Engel, O., and Meisel, A. (2010). Models of infection before and after stroke: investigating new targets. *Infect. Disord. Drug Targets* 10, 98–104. doi: 10.2174/187152610790963546

Faure-André, G., Vargas, P., Yuseff, M. I., Heuzé, M., Diaz, J., Lankar, D., et al. (2008). Regulation of dendritic cell migration by CD74, the MHC class II-associated invariant chain. *Science* 322, 1705–1710. doi: 10.1126/science.1159894

Felger, J. C., Abe, T., Kaunzner, U. W., Gottfried-Blackmore, A., Gal-Toth, J., McEwen, B. S., et al. (2010). Brain dendritic cells in ischemic stroke: time course, activation state and origin. *Brain Behav. Immun.* 24, 724–737. doi: 10.1016/j.bbi.2009.11.002

Fields, R. D. (2010). Neuroscience. Change in the brain's white matter. *Science* 330, 768–769. doi: 10.1126/science.1199139

Förster, R., Schubel, A., Breitfeld, D., Kremmer, E., Renner-Müller, I., Wolf, E., et al. (1999). CCR7 coordinates the primary immune response by establishing functional microenvironments in secondary lymphoid organs. *Cell* 99, 23–33. doi: 10.1016/s0092-8674(00)80059-8

Frenkel, D., Huang, Z., Maron, R., Koldzic, D. N., Hancock, W. W., Moskowitz, M. A., et al. (2003). Nasal vaccination with myelin oligodendrocyte glycoprotein reduces stroke size by inducing IL-10-producing CD4+ T cells. *J. Immunol.* 171, 6549–6555. doi: 10.4049/jimmunol.171.12.6549

Frenkel, D., Huang, Z., Maron, R., Koldzic, D. N., Moskowitz, M. A., and Weiner, H. L. (2005). Neuroprotection by IL-10-producing MOG CD4+ T cells following ischemic stroke. *J. Neurol. Sci.* 233, 125–132. doi: 10.1016/j.jns.2005.03.022

Fu, Y., Hao, J., Zhang, N., Ren, L., Sun, N., Li, Y. J., et al. (2014). Fingolimod for the Treatment of Intracerebral Hemorrhage: a 2-Arm Proof-of-Concept Study. *JAMA Neurol.* doi: 10.1001/jamaneurol.2014.1065. [Epub ahead of print].

Galazka, G., Jurewicz, A., Orlowski, W., Stasiolek, M., Brosnan, C. F., Raine, C. S., et al. (2007). EAE tolerance induction with Hsp70-peptide complexes depends on H60 and NKG2D activity. *J. Immunol.* 179, 4503–4512. doi: 10.4049/jimmunol.179.7.4503

Galazka, G., Stasiolek, M., Walczak, A., Jurewicz, A., Zylicz, A., Brosnan, C. F., et al. (2006). Brain-derived heat shock protein 70-peptide complexes induce NK cell-dependent tolerance to experimental autoimmune encephalomyelitis. *J. Immunol.* 176, 1588–1599. doi: 10.4049/jimmunol.176.3.1588

Gan, Y., Liu, Q., Wu, W., Yin, J. X., Bai, X. F., Shen, R., et al. (2014). Ischemic neurons recruit natural killer cells that accelerate brain infarction. *Proc. Natl. Acad. Sci. U S A* 111, 2704–2709. doi: 10.1073/pnas.1315943111

Ganguly, D., Haak, S., Sisirak, V., and Reizis, B. (2013). The role of dendritic cells in autoimmunity. *Nat. Rev. Immunol.* 13, 566–577. doi: 10.1038/nri3477

Gee, J. M., Zierath, D., Hadwin, J., Savos, A., Kalil, A., Thullbery, M., et al. (2009). Long term immunologic consequences of experimental stroke and mucosal tolerance. *Exp. Transl. Stroke Med.* 1:3. doi: 10.1186/2040-7378-1-3

Gelderblom, M., Daehn, T., Schattling, B., Ludewig, P., Bernreuther, C., Arunachalam, P., et al. (2013). Plasma levels of neuron specific enolase quantify the extent of neuronal injury in murine models of ischemic stroke and multiple sclerosis. *Neurobiol. Dis.* 59, 177–182. doi: 10.1016/j.nbd.2013.07.017

Gelderblom, M., Leypoldt, F., Steinbach, K., Behrens, D., Choe, C. U., Siler, D. A., et al. (2009). Temporal and spatial dynamics of cerebral immune cell accumulation in stroke. *Stroke* 40, 1849–1857. doi: 10.1161/STROKEAHA.108.534503

Getts, D. R., Chastain, E. M., Terry, R. L., and Miller, S. D. (2013). Virus infection, antiviral immunity and autoimmunity. *Immunol. Rev.* 255, 197–209. doi: 10.1111/imr.12091

Gidday, J. M., Gasche, Y. G., Copin, J. C., Shah, A. R., Perez, R. S., Shapiro, S. D., et al. (2005). Leukocyte-derived matrix metalloproteinase-9 mediates blood-brain barrier breakdown and is proinflammatory after transient focal cerebral ischemia. *Am. J. Physiol. Heart Circ. Physiol.* 289, H558–H568. doi: 10.1152/ajpheart.01275.2004

Gómez-Choco, M., Doucerain, C., Urra, X., Planas, A. M., and Chamorro, A. (2014). Presence of heat shock protein 70 in secondary lymphoid tissue correlates with stroke prognosis. *J. Neuroimmunol.* 270, 67–74. doi: 10.1016/j.jneuroim.2014.03.004

Goodnow, C. C., Sprent, J., Fazekas de St Groth, B., and Vinuesa, C. G. (2005). Cellular and genetic mechanisms of self tolerance and autoimmunity. *Nature* 435, 590–597. doi: 10.1038/nature03724

Graber, J. J., and Dhib-Jalbut, S. (2009). Protective autoimmunity in the nervous system. *Pharmacol. Ther.* 121, 147–159. doi: 10.1016/j.pharmthera.2008.10.001

Haeusler, K. G., Schmidt, W. U., Föhring, F., Meisel, C., Helms, T., Jungehulsing, G. J., et al. (2008). Cellular immunodepression preceding infectious complications after acute ischemic stroke in humans. *Cerebrovasc. Dis.* 25, 50–58. doi: 10.1159/000111499

Hammer, C., Stepniak, B., Schneider, A., Papiol, S., Tantra, M., Begemann, M., et al. (2013). Neuropsychiatric disease relevance of circulating anti-NMDA receptor autoantibodies depends on blood-brain barrier integrity. *Mol. Psychiatry* doi: 10.1038/mp.2013.110. [Epub ahead of print].

Harling-Berg, C., Knopf, P. M., Merriam, J., and Cserr, H. F. (1989). Role of cervical lymph nodes in the systemic humoral immune response to human serum albumin microinfused into rat cerebrospinal fluid. *J. Neuroimmunol.* 25, 185–193. doi: 10.1016/0165-5728(89)90136-7

Harvey, B. P., Gee, R. J., Haberman, A. M., Shlomchik, M. J., and Mamula, M. J. (2007). Antigen presentation and transfer between B cells and macrophages. *Eur. J. Immunol.* 37, 1739–1751. doi: 10.1002/eji.200636452

Hasegawa, Y., Suzuki, H., Sozen, T., Rolland, W., and Zhang, J. H. (2010). Activation of sphingosine 1-phosphate receptor-1 by FTY720 is neuroprotective after ischemic stroke in rats. *Stroke* 41, 368–374. doi: 10.1161/STROKEAHA.109.568899

Hatterer, E., Davoust, N., Didier-Bazes, M., Vuaillat, C., Malcus, C., Belin, M. F., et al. (2006). How to drain without lymphatics? Dendritic cells migrate from the cerebrospinal fluid to the B-cell follicles of cervical lymph nodes. *Blood* 107, 806–812. doi: 10.1182/blood-2005-01-0154

Hawkes, C. A., Hartig, W., Kacza, J., Schliebs, R., Weller, R. O., Nicoll, J. A., et al. (2011). Perivascular drainage of solutes is impaired in the ageing mouse brain and in the presence of cerebral amyloid angiopathy. *Acta Neuropathol.* 121, 431–443. doi: 10.1007/s00401-011-0801-7

Hawkes, C. A., Jayakody, N., Johnston, D. A., Bechmann, I., and Carare, R. O. (2014). Failure of perivascular drainage of β-amyloid in cerebral amyloid angiopathy. *Brain Pathol.* 24, 396–403. doi: 10.1111/bpa.12159

Heath, W. R., and Carbone, F. R. (2001). Cross-presentation in viral immunity and self-tolerance. *Nat. Rev. Immunol.* 1, 126–134. doi: 10.1038/35100512

Herrmann, M., Vos, P., Wunderlich, M. T., de Bruijn, C. H., and Lamers, K. J. (2000). Release of glial tissue-specific proteins after acute stroke: a comparative analysis of serum concentrations of protein S-100B and glial fibrillary acidic protein. *Stroke* 31, 2670–2677. doi: 10.1161/01.str.31.11.2670

Hervé, J., Dubreil, L., Tardif, V., Terme, M., Pogu, S., Anegon, I., et al. (2013). β2-Adrenoreceptor agonist inhibits antigen cross-presentation by dendritic cells. *J. Immunol.* 190, 3163–3171. doi: 10.4049/jimmunol.1201391

Hetze, S., Engel, O., Römer, C., Mueller, S., Dirnagl, U., Meisel, C., et al. (2013). Superiority of preventive antibiotic treatment compared with standard treatment of poststroke pneumonia in experimental stroke: a bed to bench approach. *J. Cereb. Blood Flow Metab.* 33, 846–854. doi: 10.1038/jcbfm.2013.6

Hirschberg, D. L., Moalem, G., He, J., Mor, F., Cohen, I. R., and Schwartz, M. (1998). Accumulation of passively transferred primed T cells independently of their antigen specificity following central nervous system trauma. *J. Neuroimmunol.* 89, 88–96. doi: 10.1016/s0165-5728(98)00118-0

Hofstetter, H. H., Sewell, D. L., Liu, F., Sandor, M., Forsthuber, T., Lehmann, P. V., et al. (2003). Autoreactive T cells promote post-traumatic healing in the central nervous system. *J. Neuroimmunol.* 134, 25–34. doi: 10.1016/s0165-5728(02)00358-2

Hogquist, K. A., Baldwin, T. A., and Jameson, S. C. (2005). Central tolerance: learning self-control in the thymus. *Nat. Rev. Immunol.* 5, 772–782. doi: 10.1038/nri1707

Huang, J., Choudhri, T. F., Winfree, C. J., McTaggart, R. A., Kiss, S., Mocco, J., et al. (2000). Postischemic cerebrovascular E-selectin expression mediates tissue injury in murine stroke. *Stroke* 31, 3047–3053. doi: 10.1161/01.str.31.12.3047

Hug, A., Dalpke, A., Wieczorek, N., Giese, T., Lorenz, A., Auffarth, G., et al. (2009). Infarct volume is a major determiner of post-stroke immune cell function and susceptibility to infection. *Stroke* 40, 3226–3232. doi: 10.1161/strokeaha.109.557967

Hulpke, S., and Tampé, R. (2013). The MHC I loading complex: a multitasking machinery in adaptive immunity. *Trends Biochem. Sci.* 38, 412–420. doi: 10.1016/j.tibs.2013.06.003

Hurn, P. D., Subramanian, S., Parker, S. M., Afentoulis, M. E., Kaler, L. J., Vandenbark, A. A., et al. (2007). T- and B-cell-deficient mice with experimental stroke have reduced lesion size and inflammation. *J. Cereb. Blood Flow Metab.* 27, 1798–1805. doi: 10.1038/sj.jcbfm.9600482

Huseby, E. S., Liggitt, D., Brabb, T., Schnabel, B., Ohlén, C., and Goverman, J. (2001). A pathogenic role for myelin-specific CD8(+) T cells in a model for multiple sclerosis. *J. Exp. Med.* 194, 669–676. doi: 10.1084/jem.194.5.669

Iadecola, C., and Anrather, J. (2011). The immunology of stroke: from mechanisms to translation. *Nat. Med.* 17, 796–808. doi: 10.1038/nm.2399

Illoh, K., Campbell, C., Illoh, O., Diehl, J., Cherry, J., Elkhaloun, A., et al. (2006). Mucosal tolerance to E-selectin and response to systemic inflammation. *J. Cereb. Blood Flow Metab.* 26, 1538–1550. doi: 10.1038/sj.jcbfm.9600308

Imai, T., Kato, Y., Kajiwara, C., Mizukami, S., Ishige, I., Ichiyanagi, T., et al. (2011). Heat shock protein 90 (HSP90) contributes to cytosolic translocation of extracellular antigen for cross-presentation by dendritic cells. *Proc. Natl. Acad. Sci. U S A* 108, 16363–16368. doi: 10.1073/pnas.1108372108

Inaba, K., Pack, M., Inaba, M., Sakuta, H., Isdell, F., and Steinman, R. M. (1997). High levels of a major histocompatibility complex II-self peptide complex on dendritic cells from the T cell areas of lymph nodes. *J. Exp. Med.* 186, 665–672. doi: 10.1084/jem.186.5.665

Janeway, C. A. Jr., and Medzhitov, R. (1999). Lipoproteins take their toll on the host. *Curr. Biol.* 9, R879–R882. doi: 10.1016/s0960-9822(00)80073-1

Jauch, E. C., Lindsell, C., Broderick, J., Fagan, S. C., Tilley, B. C., Levine, S. R., et al. (2006). Association of serial biochemical markers with acute ischemic stroke: the National Institute of Neurological Disorders and Stroke recombinant tissue plasminogen activator Stroke Study. *Stroke* 37, 2508–2513. doi: 10.1161/01.str.0000242290.01174.9e

Joffre, O. P., Segura, E., Savina, A., and Amigorena, S. (2012). Cross-presentation by dendritic cells. *Nat. Rev. Immunol.* 12, 557–569. doi: 10.1038/nri3254

Jones, T. B., Basso, D. M., Sodhi, A., Pan, J. Z., Hart, R. P., MacCallum, R. C., et al. (2002). Pathological CNS autoimmune disease triggered by traumatic spinal cord injury: implications for autoimmune vaccine therapy. *J. Neurosci.* 22, 2690–2700.

Justicia, C., Panés, J., Solé, S., Cervera, A., Deulofeu, R., Chamorro, A., et al. (2003). Neutrophil infiltration increases matrix metalloproteinase-9 in the ischemic brain after occlusion/reperfusion of the middle cerebral artery in rats. *J. Cereb. Blood Flow Metab.* 23, 1430–1440. doi: 10.1097/01.wcb.0000090680.07515.c8

Kato, Y., Kajiwara, C., Ishige, I., Mizukami, S., Yamazaki, C., Eikawa, S., et al. (2012). HSP70 and HSP90 differentially regulate translocation of extracellular antigen to the cytosol for cross-presentation. *Autoimmune Dis.* 2012:745962. doi: 10.1155/2012/745962

Kil, K., Zang, Y. C., Yang, D., Markowski, J., Fuoco, G. S., Vendetti, G. C., et al. (1999). T cell responses to myelin basic protein in patients with spinal cord injury and multiple sclerosis. *J. Neuroimmunol.* 98, 201–207. doi: 10.1016/s0165-5728(99)00057-0

Klehmet, J., Harms, H., Richter, M., Prass, K., Volk, H. D., Dirnagl, U., et al. (2009). Stroke-induced immunodepression and post-stroke infections: lessons from the preventive antibacterial therapy in stroke trial. *Neuroscience* 158, 1184–1193. doi: 10.1016/j.neuroscience.2008.07.044

Kleinschnitz, C., Kraft, P., Dreykluft, A., Hagedorn, I., Göbel, K., Schuhmann, M. K., et al. (2013). Regulatory T cells are strong promoters of acute ischemic stroke in mice by inducing dysfunction of the cerebral microvasculature. *Blood* 121, 679–691. doi: 10.1182/blood-2012-04-426734

Kleinschnitz, C., Schwab, N., Kraft, P., Hagedorn, I., Dreykluft, A., Schwarz, T., et al. (2010). Early detrimental T-cell effects in experimental cerebral ischemia are neither related to adaptive immunity nor thrombus formation. *Blood* 115, 3835–3842. doi: 10.1182/blood-2009-10-249078

Kraft, P., Göb, E., Schuhmann, M. K., Göbel, K., Deppermann, C., Thielmann, I., et al. (2013). FTY720 ameliorates acute ischemic stroke in mice by reducing thrombo-inflammation but not by direct neuroprotection. *Stroke* 44, 3202–3210. doi: 10.1161/STROKEAHA.113.002880

Kumar, S., Selim, M. H., and Caplan, L. R. (2010). Medical complications after stroke. *Lancet Neurol.* 9, 105–118. doi: 10.1016/S1474-4422(09)70266-2

Kwak, B., Mulhaupt, F., Myit, S., and Mach, F. (2000). Statins as a newly recognized type of immunomodulator. *Nat. Med.* 6, 1399–1402. doi: 10.1038/82219

Lawrence, A. J., Patel, B., Morris, R. G., MacKinnon, A. D., Rich, P. M., Barrick, T. R., et al. (2013). Mechanisms of cognitive impairment in cerebral small vessel disease: multimodal MRI results from the St George's cognition and neuroimaging in stroke (SCANS) study. *PLoS One* 8:e61014. doi: 10.1371/journal.pone.0061014

Li, P., Gan, Y., Sun, B. L., Zhang, F., Lu, B., Gao, Y., et al. (2013a). Adoptive regulatory T-cell therapy protects against cerebral ischemia. *Ann. Neurol.* 74, 458–471. doi: 10.1002/ana.23815

Li, X. L., Liu, Y., Cao, L. L., Li, H., Yue, L. T., Wang, S., et al. (2013c). Atorvastatin-modified dendritic cells in vitro ameliorate experimental autoimmune myasthenia gravis by up-regulated Treg cells and shifted Th1/Th17 to Th2 cytokines. *Mol. Cell. Neurosci.* 56, 85–95. doi: 10.1016/j.mcn.2013.03.005

Li, P., Mao, L., Liu, X., Gan, Y., Zheng, J., Thomson, A. W., et al. (2014). Essential role of program death 1-ligand 1 in regulatory T-cell-afforded protection against blood-brain barrier damage after stroke. *Stroke* 45, 857–864. doi: 10.1161/STROKEAHA.113.004100

Li, P., Mao, L., Zhou, G., Leak, R. K., Sun, B. L., Chen, J., et al. (2013b). Adoptive regulatory T-cell therapy preserves systemic immune homeostasis after cerebral ischemia. *Stroke* 44, 3509–3515. doi: 10.1161/STROKEAHA.113.002637

Liesz, A., Sun, L., Zhou, W., Schwarting, S., Mracsko, E., Zorn, M., et al. (2011). FTY720 reduces post-ischemic brain lymphocyte influx but does not improve outcome in permanent murine cerebral ischemia. *PLoS One* 6:e21312. doi: 10.1371/journal.pone.0021312

Liesz, A., Suri-Payer, E., Veltkamp, C., Doerr, H., Sommer, C., Rivest, S., et al. (2009). Regulatory T cells are key cerebroprotective immunomodulators in acute experimental stroke. *Nat. Med.* 15, 192–199. doi: 10.1038/nm.1927

Liesz, A., Zhou, W., Na, S. Y., Hämmerling, G. J., Garbi, N., Karcher, S., et al. (2013). Boosting regulatory T cells limits neuroinflammation in permanent cortical stroke. *J. Neurosci.* 33, 17350–17362. doi: 10.1523/JNEUROSCI.4901-12.2013

Ludewig, P., Sedlacik, J., Gelderblom, M., Bernreuther, C., Korkusuz, Y., Wagener, C., et al. (2013). Carcinoembryonic antigen-related cell adhesion molecule 1 inhibits MMP-9-mediated blood-brain-barrier breakdown in a mouse model for ischemic stroke. *Circ. Res.* 113, 1013–1022. doi: 10.1161/CIRCRESAHA.113.301207

Maestroni, G. J., and Mazzola, P. (2003). Langerhans cells beta 2-adrenoceptors: role in migration, cytokine production, Th priming and contact hypersensitivity. *J. Neuroimmunol.* 144, 91–99. doi: 10.1016/j.jneuroim.2003.08.039

Magnus, T., Wiendl, H., and Kleinschnitz, C. (2012). Immune mechanisms of stroke. *Curr. Opin. Neurol.* 25, 334–340. doi: 10.1097/WCO.0b013e328352ede6

Maron, R., Sukhova, G., Faria, A. M., Hoffmann, E., Mach, F., Libby, P., et al. (2002). Mucosal administration of heat shock protein-65 decreases atherosclerosis and inflammation in aortic arch of low-density lipoprotein receptor-deficient mice. *Circulation* 106, 1708–1715. doi: 10.1161/01.cir.0000029750.99462.30

Matloubian, M., Lo, C. G., Cinamon, G., Lesneski, M. J., Xu, Y., Brinkmann, V., et al. (2004). Lymphocyte egress from thymus and peripheral lymphoid organs is dependent on S1P receptor 1. *Nature* 427, 355–360. doi: 10.1038/nature02284

Mazzini, E., Massimiliano, L., Penna, G., and Rescigno, M. (2014). Oral tolerance can be established via gap junction transfer of fed antigens from CX3CR1$^+$ macrophages to CD103$^+$ dendritic cells. *Immunity* 40, 248–261. doi: 10.1016/j.immuni.2013.12.012

McColl, B. W., Rothwell, N. J., and Allan, S. M. (2008). Systemic inflammation alters the kinetics of cerebrovascular tight junction disruption after experimental stroke in mice. *J. Neurosci.* 28, 9451–9462. doi: 10.1523/JNEUROSCI.2674-08.2008

Millar, D. G., Garza, K. M., Odermatt, B., Elford, A., Ono, N., Li, Z., et al. (2003). Hsp70 promotes antigen presenting cell function and converts T-cell tolerance to autoimmunity in vivo. *Nat. Med.* 9, 1469–1476. doi: 10.1038/nm962

Missler, U., Wiesmann, M., Friedrich, C., and Kaps, M. (1997). S-100 protein and neuron-specific enolase concentrations in blood as indicators of infarction volume and prognosis in acute ischemic stroke. *Stroke* 28, 1956–1960. doi: 10.1161/01.str.28.10.1956

Moalem, G., Leibowitz-Amit, R., Yoles, E., Mor, F., Cohen, I. R., and Schwartz, M. (1999). Autoimmune T cells protect neurons from secondary degeneration after central nervous system axotomy. *Nat. Med.* 5, 49–55. doi: 10.1038/4734

Monsonego, A., Beserman, Z. P., Kipnis, J., Yoles, E., Weiner, H. L., and Schwartz, M. (2003). Beneficial effect of orally administered myelin basic protein in EAE-susceptible Lewis rats in a model of acute CNS degeneration. *J. Autoimmun.* 21, 131–138. doi: 10.1016/s0896-8411(03)00091-x

Muhammad, S., Haasbach, E., Kotchourko, M., Strigli, A., Krenz, A., Ridder, D. A., et al. (2011). Influenza virus infection aggravates stroke outcome. *Stroke* 42, 783–791. doi: 10.1161/STROKEAHA.110.596783

Nagaraja, T. N., Karki, K., Ewing, J. R., Croxen, R. L., and Knight, R. A. (2008). Identification of variations in blood-brain barrier opening after cerebral ischemia by dual contrast-enhanced magnetic resonance imaging and T 1sat measurements. *Stroke* 39, 427–432. doi: 10.1161/STROKEAHA.107.496059

Nave, K. A. (2010). Myelination and support of axonal integrity by glia. *Nature* 468, 244–252. doi: 10.1038/nature09614

Neijssen, J., Herberts, C., Drijfhout, J. W., Reits, E., Janssen, L., and Neefjes, J. (2005). Cross-presentation by intercellular peptide transfer through gap junctions. *Nature* 434, 83–88. doi: 10.1038/nature03290

Noessner, E., Gastpar, R., Milani, V., Brandl, A., Hutzler, P. J., Kuppner, M. C., et al. (2002). Tumor-derived heat shock protein 70 peptide complexes are cross-presented by human dendritic cells. *J. Immunol.* 169, 5424–5432. doi: 10.4049/jimmunol.169.10.5424

Offner, H., Subramanian, S., Parker, S. M., Wang, C., Afentoulis, M. E., Lewis, A., et al. (2006). Splenic atrophy in experimental stroke is accompanied by increased regulatory T cells and circulating macrophages. *J. Immunol.* 176, 6523–6531. doi: 10.4049/jimmunol.176.11.6523

Olsson, T., Diener, P., Ljungdahl, A., Höjeberg, B., van der Meide, P. H., and Kristensson, K. (1992). Facial nerve transection causes expansion of myelin autoreactive T cells in regional lymph nodes and T cell homing to the facial nucleus. *Autoimmunity* 13, 117–126. doi: 10.3109/08916939209001912

Palinski, W., Miller, E., and Witztum, J. L. (1995). Immunization of low density lipoprotein (LDL) receptor-deficient rabbits with homologous malondialdehyde-modified LDL reduces atherogenesis. *Proc. Natl. Acad. Sci. U S A* 92, 821–825. doi: 10.1073/pnas.92.3.821

Pérez-de Puig, I., Miró, F., Salas-Perdomo, A., Bonfill-Teixidor, E., Ferrer-Ferrer, M., Márquez-Kisinousky, L., et al. (2013). IL-10 deficiency exacerbates the brain inflammatory response to permanent ischemia without preventing resolution of the lesion. *J. Cereb. Blood Flow Metab.* 33, 1955–1966. doi: 10.1038/jcbfm.2013.155

Pham, T. H., Okada, T., Matloubian, M., Lo, C. G., and Cyster, J. G. (2008). S1P1 receptor signaling overrides retention mediated by G alpha i-coupled receptors to promote T cell egress. *Immunity* 28, 122–133. doi: 10.1016/j.immuni.2007.11.017

Planas, A. M., Gómez-Choco, M., Urra, X., Gorina, R., Caballero, M., and Chamorro, Á. (2012). Brain-derived antigens in lymphoid tissue of patients with acute stroke. *J. Immunol.* 188, 2156–2163. doi: 10.4049/jimmunol.1102289

Planas, A. M., Soriano, M. A., Estrada, A., Sanz, O., Martin, F., and Ferrer, I. (1997). The heat shock stress response after brain lesions: induction of 72 kDa heat shock protein (cell types involved, axonal transport, transcriptional regulation) and protein synthesis inhibition. *Prog. Neurobiol.* 51, 607–636. doi: 10.1016/s0301-0082(97)00004-x

Prass, K., Meisel, C., Höflich, C., Braun, J., Halle, E., Wolf, T., et al. (2003). Stroke-induced immunodeficiency promotes spontaneous bacterial infections and is mediated by sympathetic activation reversal by poststroke T helper cell type 1-like immunostimulation. *J. Exp. Med.* 198, 725–736. doi: 10.1084/jem.20021098

Prüss, H., Iggena, D., Baldinger, T., Prinz, V., Meisel, A., Endres, M., et al. (2012). Evidence of intrathecal immunoglobulin synthesis in stroke: a cohort study. *Arch. Neurol.* 69, 714–717. doi: 10.1001/archneurol.2011.3252

Rahman, M. M., Kopec, J. A., Cibere, J., Goldsmith, C. H., and Anis, A. H. (2013). The relationship between osteoarthritis and cardiovascular disease in a population health survey: a cross-sectional study. *BMJ Open* 3:e002624. doi: 10.1136/bmjopen-2013-002624

Ransohoff, R. M., Kivisäkk, P., and Kidd, G. (2003). Three or more routes for leukocyte migration into the central nervous system. *Nat. Rev. Immunol.* 3, 569–581. doi: 10.1038/nri1130

Raposo, G., Nijman, H. W., Stoorvogel, W., Liejendekker, R., Harding, C. V., Melief, C. J., et al. (1996). B lymphocytes secrete antigen-presenting vesicles. *J. Exp. Med.* 183, 1161–1172. doi: 10.1084/jem.183.3.1161

Redmond, W. L., and Sherman, L. A. (2005). Peripheral tolerance of CD8 T lymphocytes. *Immunity* 22, 275–284. doi: 10.1016/j.immuni.2005.01.010

Ren, X., Akiyoshi, K., Dziennis, S., Vandenbark, A. A., Herson, P. S., Hurn, P. D., et al. (2011a). Regulatory B cells limit CNS inflammation and neurologic deficits in murine experimental stroke. *J. Neurosci.* 31, 8556–8563. doi: 10.1523/jneurosci.1623-11.2011

Ren, X., Akiyoshi, K., Vandenbark, A. A., Hurn, P. D., and Offner, H. (2011b). Programmed death-1 pathway limits central nervous system inflammation and neurologic deficits in murine experimental stroke. *Stroke* 42, 2578–2583. doi: 10.1161/strokeaha.111.613182

Rescigno, M. (2010). Dendritic cells in tolerance induction for the treatment of autoimmune diseases. *Eur. J. Immunol.* 40, 2119–2123. doi: 10.1002/eji.201040474

Rolland, W. B. 2nd, Manaenko, A., Lekic, T., Hasegawa, Y., Ostrowski, R., Tang, J., et al. (2011). FTY720 is neuroprotective and improves functional outcomes after intracerebral hemorrhage in mice. *Acta Neurochir. Suppl.* 111, 213–217. doi: 10.1007/978-3-7091-0693-8_36

Roström, B., and Link, H. (1981). Oligoclonal immunoglobulin in cerebrospinal fluid in acute cerebrovascular disease. *Neurology* 31, 590–596. doi: 10.1212/wnl.31.5.590

Sakaguchi, S., Sakaguchi, N., Shimizu, J., Yamazaki, S., Sakihama, T., Itoh, M., et al. (2001). Immunologic tolerance maintained by CD25+ CD4+ regulatory T cells: their common role in controlling autoimmunity, tumor immunity and transplantation tolerance. *Immunol. Rev.* 182, 18–32. doi: 10.1034/j.1600-065x.2001.1820102.x

Santambrogio, L., Sato, A. K., Carven, G. J., Belyanskaya, S. L., Strominger, J. L., and Stern, L. J. (1999). Extracellular antigen processing and presentation by immature dendritic cells. *Proc. Natl. Acad. Sci. U S A* 96, 15056–15061. doi: 10.1073/pnas.96.26.15056

Savina, A., Jancic, C., Hugues, S., Guermonprez, P., Vargas, P., Moura, I. C., et al. (2006). NOX2 controls phagosomal pH to regulate antigen processing during crosspresentation by dendritic cells. *Cell* 126, 205–218. doi: 10.1016/j.cell.2006.05.035

Sciascia, S., Sanna, G., Khamashta, M. A., Cuadrado, M. J., Erkan, D., Andreoli, L., et al. (2014). The estimated frequency of antiphospholipid antibodies in young adults with cerebrovascular events: a systematic review. *Ann. Rheum. Dis.* doi: 10.1136/annrheumdis-2014-205663. [Epub ahead of print].

Seiffert, K., Hosoi, J., Torii, H., Ozawa, H., Ding, W., Campton, K., et al. (2002). Catecholamines inhibit the antigen-presenting capability of epidermal Langerhans cells. *J. Immunol.* 168, 6128–6135. doi: 10.4049/jimmunol.168.12.6128

Sherer, Y., and Shoenfeld, Y. (2006). Mechanisms of disease: atherosclerosis in autoimmune diseases. *Nat. Clin. Pract. Rheumatol.* 2, 99–106. doi: 10.1038/ncprheum0092

Singer, B. D., King, L. S., and D'Alessio, F. R. (2014). Regulatory T cells as immunotherapy. *Front. Immunol.* 5:46. doi: 10.3389/fimmu.2014.00046

Spörri, R., and Reis e Sousa, C. (2005). Inflammatory mediators are insufficient for full dendritic cell activation and promote expansion of CD4+ T cell populations lacking helper function. *Nat. Immunol.* 6, 163–170. doi: 10.1038/ni1162

Srivastava, P. (2002). Roles of heat-shock proteins in innate and adaptive immunity. *Nat. Rev. Immunol.* 2, 185–194. doi: 10.1038/nri749

Steinbrink, K., Graulich, E., Kubsch, S., Knop, J., and Enk, A. H. (2002). CD4(+) and CD8(+) anergic T cells induced by interleukin-10-treated human dendritic cells display antigen-specific suppressor activity. *Blood* 99, 2468–2476. doi: 10.1182/blood.v99.7.2468

Steinman, R. M., and Nussenzweig, M. C. (2002). Avoiding horror autotoxicus: the importance of dendritic cells in peripheral T cell tolerance. *Proc. Natl. Acad. Sci. U S A* 99, 351–358. doi: 10.1073/pnas.231606698

Stocki, P., Wang, X. N., and Dickinson, A. M. (2012). Inducible heat shock protein 70 reduces T cell responses and stimulatory capacity of monocyte-derived dendritic cells. *J. Biol. Chem.* 287, 12387–12394. doi: 10.1074/jbc.m111.307579

Strand, T., Alling, C., Karlsson, B., Karlsson, I., and Winblad, B. (1984). Brain and plasma proteins in spinal fluid as markers for brain damage and severity of stroke. *Stroke* 15, 138–144. doi: 10.1161/01.str.15.1.138

Stubbe, T., Ebner, F., Richter, D., Engel, O., Klehmet, J., Royl, G., et al. (2013). Regulatory T cells accumulate and proliferate in the ischemic hemisphere for up to 30 days after MCAO. *J. Cereb. Blood Flow Metab.* 33, 37–47. doi: 10.1038/jcbfm.2012.128

Subramanian, S., Zhang, B., Kosaka, Y., Burrows, G. G., Grafe, M. R., Vandenbark, A. A., et al. (2009). Recombinant T cell receptor ligand treats experimental stroke. *Stroke* 40, 2539–2545. doi: 10.1161/strokeaha.108.543991

Sun, Y. W., Qin, L. D., Zhou, Y., Xu, Q., Qian, L. J., Tao, J., et al. (2011). Abnormal functional connectivity in patients with vascular cognitive impairment, no dementia: a resting-state functional magnetic resonance imaging study. *Behav. Brain Res.* 223, 388–394. doi: 10.1016/j.bbr.2011.05.006

Takeda, H., Spatz, M., Ruetzler, C., McCarron, R., Becker, K., and Hallenbeck, J. (2002). Induction of mucosal tolerance to E-selectin prevents ischemic and hemorrhagic stroke in spontaneously hypertensive genetically stroke-prone rats. *Stroke* 33, 2156–2163. doi: 10.1161/01.str.0000029821.82531.8b

Tarkowski, E., Ekelund, P., and Tarkowski, A. (1991a). Enhancement of antigen-specific T-cell reactivity on the affected side in stroke patients. *J. Neuroimmunol.* 34, 61–67. doi: 10.1016/0165-5728(91)90099-s

Tarkowski, E., Ekelund, P., and Tarkowski, A. (1991b). Increased systemic T-lymphocyte reactivity in patients with established stroke. *J. Clin. Lab. Immunol.* 35, 171–176.

Todryk, S., Melcher, A. A., Hardwick, N., Linardakis, E., Bateman, A., Colombo, M. P., et al. (1999). Heat shock protein 70 induced during tumor cell killing induces Th1 cytokines and targets immature dendritic cell precursors to enhance antigen uptake. *J. Immunol.* 163, 1398–1408.

Tsark, E. C., Wang, W., Teng, Y. C., Arkfeld, D., Dodge, G. R., and Kovats, S. (2002). Differential MHC class II-mediated presentation of rheumatoid arthritis autoantigens by human dendritic cells and macrophages. *J. Immunol.* 169, 6625–6633. doi: 10.4049/jimmunol.169.11.6625

Ulm, L., Harms, H., Ohlraun, S., Reimnitz, P., and Meisel, A. (2012). Impact of infections on long-term outcome after severe middle cerebral artery infarction. *J. Neurol. Sci.* 319, 15–17. doi: 10.1016/j.jns.2012.05.042

Urra, X., Cervera, A., Obach, V., Climent, N., Planas, A. M., and Chamorro, A. (2009a). Monocytes are major players in the prognosis and risk of infection after acute stroke. *Stroke* 40, 1262–1268. doi: 10.1161/strokeaha.108.532085

Urra, X., Cervera, A., Villamor, N., Planas, A. M., and Chamorro, A. (2009b). Harms and benefits of lymphocyte subpopulations in patients with acute stroke. *Neuroscience* 158, 1174–1183. doi: 10.1016/j.neuroscience.2008.06.014

Urra, X., and Chamorro, A. (2010). Stroke-induced immunodepression is a marker of severe brain damage. *Stroke* 41:e110. doi: 10.1161/STROKEAHA.109.566968

Vadasz, Z., Haj, T., Kessel, A., and Toubi, E. (2013). B-regulatory cells in autoimmunity and immune mediated inflammation. *FEBS Lett.* 587, 2074–2078. doi: 10.1016/j.febslet.2013.05.023

van Zwam, M., Huizinga, R., Melief, M. J., Wierenga-Wolf, A. F., van Meurs, M., Voerman, J. S., et al. (2009). Brain antigens in functionally distinct antigen-presenting cell populations in cervical lymph nodes in MS and EAE. *J. Mol. Med. (Berl)* 87, 273–286. doi: 10.1007/s00109-008-0421-4

Varga, G., Ehrchen, J., Brockhausen, A., Weinhage, T., Nippe, N., Belz, M., et al. (2014). Immune suppression via glucocorticoid-stimulated monocytes: a novel mechanism to cope with inflammation. *J. Immunol.* 193, 1090–1099. doi: 10.4049/jimmunol.1300891

Vogelgesang, A., Becker, K. J., and Dressel, A. (2014). Immunological consequences of ischemic stroke. *Acta Neurol. Scand.* 129, 1–12. doi: 10.1111/ane.12165

Vogelgesang, A., and Dressel, A. (2011). Immunological consequences of ischemic stroke: immunosuppression and autoimmunity. *J. Neuroimmunol.* 231, 105–110. doi: 10.1016/j.jneuroim.2010.09.023

Vogelgesang, A., Grunwald, U., Langner, S., Jack, R., Bröker, B. M., Kessler, C., et al. (2008). Analysis of lymphocyte subsets in patients with stroke and their influence on infection after stroke. *Stroke* 39, 237–241. doi: 10.1161/strokeaha.107.493635

Wachstein, J., Tischer, S., Figueiredo, C., Limbourg, A., Falk, C., Immenschuh, S., et al. (2012). HSP70 enhances immunosuppressive function of CD4(+) CD25(+)FoxP3(+) T regulatory cells and cytotoxicity in CD4(+)CD25(-) T cells. *PLoS One* 7:e51747. doi: 10.1371/journal.pone.0051747

Wang, W. Z., Olsson, T., Kostulas, V., Höjeberg, B., Ekre, H. P., and Link, H. (1992). Myelin antigen reactive T cells in cerebrovascular diseases. *Clin. Exp. Immunol.* 88, 157–162. doi: 10.1111/j.1365-2249.1992.tb03056.x

Wei, Y., Yemisci, M., Kim, H. H., Yung, L. M., Shin, H. K., Hwang, S. K., et al. (2011). Fingolimod provides long-term protection in rodent models of cerebral ischemia. *Ann. Neurol.* 69, 119–129. doi: 10.1002/ana.22186

Weiner, H. L., da Cunha, A. P., Quintana, F., and Wu, H. (2011). Oral tolerance. *Immunol. Rev.* 241, 241–259. doi: 10.1111/j.1600-065X.2011.01017.x

Weissman, J. D., Khunteev, G. A., Heath, R., and Dambinova, S. A. (2011). NR2 antibodies: risk assessment of transient ischemic attack (TIA)/stroke in patients with history of isolated and multiple cerebrovascular events. *J. Neurol. Sci.* 300, 97–102. doi: 10.1016/j.jns.2010.09.023

Weller, R. O., Djuanda, E., Yow, H. Y., and Carare, R. O. (2009). Lymphatic drainage of the brain and the pathophysiology of neurological disease. *Acta Neuropathol.* 117, 1–14. doi: 10.1007/s00401-008-0457-0

Weller, R. O., Kida, S., and Zhang, E. T. (1992). Pathways of fluid drainage from the brain–morphological aspects and immunological significance in rat and man. *Brain Pathol.* 2, 277–284. doi: 10.1111/j.1750-3639.1992.tb00704.x

Weller, R. O., Subash, M., Preston, S. D., Mazanti, I., and Carare, R. O. (2008). Perivascular drainage of amyloid-beta peptides from the brain and its failure in cerebral amyloid angiopathy and Alzheimer's disease. *Brain Pathol.* 18, 253–266. doi: 10.1111/j.1750-3639.2008.00133.x

Westendorp, W. F., Nederkoorn, P. J., Vermeij, J. D., Dijkgraaf, M. G., and van de Beek, D. (2011). Post-stroke infection: a systematic review and meta-analysis. *BMC Neurol.* 11:110. doi: 10.1186/1471-2377-11-110

Wilson, N. S., and Villadangos, J. A. (2005). Regulation of antigen presentation and cross-presentation in the dendritic cell network: facts, hypothesis and immunological implications. *Adv. Immunol.* 86, 241–305. doi: 10.1016/s0065-2776(04)86007-3

Yang, Y., and Rosenberg, G. A. (2011). Blood-brain barrier breakdown in acute and chronic cerebrovascular disease. *Stroke* 42, 3323–3328. doi: 10.1161/STROKEAHA.110.608257

Yang, Y., Thompson, J. F., Taheri, S., Salayandia, V. M., McAvoy, T. A., Hill, J. W., et al. (2013). Early inhibition of MMP activity in ischemic rat brain promotes expression of tight junction proteins and angiogenesis during recovery. *J. Cereb. Blood Flow Metab.* 33, 1104–1114. doi: 10.1038/jcbfm.2013.56

Yilmaz, G., Arumugam, T. V., Stokes, K. Y., and Granger, D. N. (2006). Role of T lymphocytes and interferon-gamma in ischemic stroke. *Circulation* 113, 2105–2112. doi: 10.1161/circulationaha.105.593046

Yilmaz, A., Reiss, C., Tantawi, O., Weng, A., Stumpf, C., Raaz, D., et al. (2004). HMG-CoA reductase inhibitors suppress maturation of human dendritic cells: new implications for atherosclerosis. *Atherosclerosis* 172, 85–93. doi: 10.1016/j.atherosclerosis.2003.10.002

Yun, W., Qing-Cheng, L., Lei, Y., and Jia-Yin, M. (2008). Mucosal tolerance to E-selectin provides protection against cerebral ischemia-reperfusion injury in rats. *J. Neuroimmunol.* 205, 73–79. doi: 10.1016/j.jneuroim.2008.09.006

Zeller, J. A., Lenz, A., Eschenfelder, C. C., Zunker, P., and Deuschl, G. (2005). Platelet-leukocyte interaction and platelet activation in acute stroke with and without preceding infection. *Arterioscler. Thromb. Vasc. Biol.* 25, 1519–1523. doi: 10.1161/01.atv.0000167524.69092.16

Zhang, E. T., Richards, H. K., Kida, S., and Weller, R. O. (1992). Directional and compartmentalised drainage of interstitial fluid and cerebrospinal fluid from the rat brain. *Acta Neuropathol.* 83, 233–239. doi: 10.1007/bf00296784

Zierath, D., Thullbery, M., Hadwin, J., Gee, J. M., Savos, A., Kalil, A., et al. (2010). CNS immune responses following experimental stroke. *Neurocrit. Care* 12, 274–284. doi: 10.1007/s12028-009-9270-4

12

Microglia in action: how aging and injury can change the brain's guardians

Athanasios Lourbopoulos[1†], Ali Ertürk[2†] and Farida Hellal[1*†]

[1] Laboratory of Experimental Stroke Research, Institute for Stroke and Dementia Research (ISD), University of Munich Medical School, Munich, Germany
[2] Laboratory of Acute Brain Injury, Institute for Stroke and Dementia Research (ISD), University of Munich Medical School, Munich, Germany

***Correspondence:**
Farida Hellal, Laboratory of Experimental Stroke Research, Institute for Stroke and Dementia Research (ISD), University of Munich Medical School - Campus Großhadern, Feodor-Lynen-Straße 17, 81377 Munich, Germany
e-mail: farida.hellal@med.uni-muenchen.de

[†] These authors have contributed equally to this work.

Neuroinflammation, the inflammatory response in the central nervous system (CNS), is a major determinant of neuronal function and survival during aging and disease progression. Microglia, as the resident tissue-macrophages of the brain, provide constant support to surrounding neurons in healthy brain. Upon any stress signal (such as trauma, ischemia, inflammation) they are one of the first cells to react. Local and/or peripheral signals determine microglia stress response, which can vary within a continuum of states from beneficial to detrimental for neuronal survival, and can be shaped by aging and previous insults. In this review, we discuss the roles of microglia upon an ischemic or traumatic injury, and give our perspective how aging may contribute to microglia behavior in the injured brain. We speculate that a deeper understanding of specific microglia identities will pave the way to develop more potent therapeutics to treat the diseases of aging brain.

Keywords: microglia, stroke, traumatic brain injury, inflammation, aging

INTRODUCTION

Microglia are considered the tissue-resident macrophages that derive from the primitive macrophages produced in the yolk sack. These primitive cells migrate and reach the central nervous system (CNS) at early embryonic stage, prior to development of the bone marrow hematopoietic system (Ginhoux et al., 2010; Schulz et al., 2012; Yona et al., 2013), where they expand and colonize the entire CNS. Depending on the species, microglia account for 5–20% of the total glial cells present in the adult brain (Lawson et al., 1992). Secluded by the blood brain barrier (BBB) and evenly distributed through the brain parenchyma, they form an autonomous population distinct from the peripheral circulating monocytes or macrophages (Ginhoux et al., 2010; Schulz et al., 2012). Microglia play important roles in chronic neurodegeneration as well as in acute lesions in the brain including trauma and stroke, when the BBB is compromised. They express a wide range of receptors allowing them to respond to large number of cytokine signals from other cells circulating in blood and tissue. Therefore, until recently, microglia were mainly seen as the immune-competent cells of the CNS forming the first line of defense against invading pathogens or in case of injury or disease (Nimmerjahn et al., 2005). Recent literature, however, has demonstrated more sophisticated functions of these cells going beyond immune surveillance. Of particular importance, microglia actively participate in plasticity and maintenance of the adult CNS by secreting cytokines and neurotrophic factors including BDNF (Parkhurst et al., 2013) and refining the neuronal circuit by pruning synapses and axonal terminals (Tremblay and Majewska, 2011; Parkhurst et al., 2013; Salter and Beggs, 2014). Hence, in addition to immune surveillance and response, microglia have a number of additional distinct functions compared to immune cells in the blood. Moreover, while monocytes readily replenish from the bone-marrow hematopoietic stem cells, microglia have ~20–30 folds slower self-renewing capacity compared to them under homeostatic conditions (Elmore et al., 2014). Because life span of CNS microglia is longer, they are more prone to accumulating aging-related changes (Gehrmann and Banati, 1995). In addition, it has been proposed that a subtype of monocytes (Ly-6C^{hi}CCR2) could replace microglia by being recruited from the blood circulation and sub-sequentially differentiated into microglia (Mildner et al., 2007; Varvel et al., 2012). However, to which extend these cells could take over different microglia functions is still not yet fully understood.

Hence, the view that microglia act as simple CNS scavengers, cleaning debris and dead cells, is out of date. The microglia are dynamic cells with the capacity of broad spectra of supportive as well as destructive functions in health and disease. The balance between these two opposing roles—undermined by infections, trauma or stroke challenges—are critical for the course of neurodegenerative diseases. Microglia have a high level of plasticity allowing them to change their shape and function in response to environmental cues (Saijo and Glass, 2011). After injury or over time with the aging, their morphology is progressively altered. For example, abnormal microglia morphology and dysfunction have been linked to many neurodegenerative diseases and psychiatric disorders including Alzheimer's disease (AD), Parkinson's disease (PD) and Rett syndrome (Prinz and Priller, 2014). While microglia morphology in general is a good indication of their functions, it is important to assess their cytokine profiles and interactions with the surrounding cells to determine their exact roles in a given situation.

Here we would like to argue that microglia's function and morphology considerably change with the aging. Thus, their response to acute CNS lesions (stroke or trauma) depends on the age of the insult. On the other hand, any acute lesion could confer additional imprints to microglia function, thereby weaken their protective response to future insults and accelerate the aging of the brain.

MICROGLIA IN THE YOUNG HEALTHY BRAIN

While microglia have mainly been studied in the context of disease, recent studies yielded important insights on their significance also in the healthy brain specifically on their contribution to the maintenance of brain's homeostasis (for review, see Schafer et al., 2012, 2013; Wu et al., 2013; Salter and Beggs, 2014). Microglia monitor changes in their environment with their long and motile processes, an activity that is facilitated by their positioning in a grid like fashion within the brain parenchyma. Because of their motility and positioning, they could scan the entire brain tissue every few hours (Davalos et al., 2005; Nimmerjahn et al., 2005). Such microglia dynamics are age-dependent and seem to slow down with the aging (Hefendehl et al., 2014). The homeostatic role of microglia has been linked at least in part to their phagocytic activity to sculpt the developing and young adult brain. Microglia contribute to elimination of sub-numeral Purkinje neurons in the developing cerebellum, a process potentially triggered by free radical release from the microglia (Marín-Teva et al., 2004). However, the molecular mechanisms triggering the engulfment of neurons by microglia are poorly uncovered. One idea is that microglia may recognize the apoptotic targets cells via a "receptor-ligand" interaction as it has been reported during the neurogenesis in the adult hippocampus. The subgranular zone (SGZ) of the dentate gyrus gives rise to numerous new cells. Only a small subset of these cells can reach to the maturity of a neuron and integrate into the hippocampal circuitry while most of them die. During these events, microglia rapidly dispose the dead cells and clear the neurogenic compartment long before migration of the remaining cells to the granular layer (Sierra et al., 2010).

Microglial might also be monitoring neuronal activity via transient contacts with dendritic spines and synapses (Wake et al., 2009; Tremblay et al., 2010). When needed, microglia may prune these dendritic spines and synapses via phagocytic mechanisms (Davalos et al., 2005; Nimmerjahn et al., 2005). For example, physical elimination of the contacted synapse by microglia occurs after an episode of light deprivation in the visual cortex or in the penumbra upon cerebral ischemia (Wake et al., 2009; Tremblay et al., 2010). Proposed microglial phagocytosis of neurons, dendritic spines and axonal shafts depends on the "eat me" and "don't eat me" signals exposed at the neuronal surface (Brown and Neher, 2014). Local flipping of the plasma membrane phospholipids exposing phosphatidylserines to the external layer and synapse tagging with the complement C3 or C1q proteins are part of the signals mediating phagocytosis (Stevens et al., 2007; Berg et al., 2012). Conversely, neurons expressing CD47 and sialylated glycoproteins inhibit this process by binding to the microglial receptors signal regulatory protein 1α (SIRP1α) and sialic acid-binding immunoglobulin-like lectins (SIGLECs), respectively (Brown and Neher, 2014).

MICROGLIA IN AGING BRAIN

Microglia morphology, number and dynamics are altered throughout the aging (Harry, 2013). Studies in young vs. aged retina (Damani et al., 2011) or brain (Hefendehl et al., 2014) have revealed that microglia exhibit age-related soma volume increase, shortening of their processes and loss of homogeneous tissue distribution. In addition, microglia exhibit slower acute and sustained chronic post-injury response, reminiscent of a prolonged inflammatory response (Damani et al., 2011; Hefendehl et al., 2014). Microglia can display swellings, varicosities and retraction of the ramifications, which are indication of unhealthy microglia (Mrak and Griffin, 2005; Miller and Streit, 2007; Norden and Godbout, 2013). Aging *per se* can reduce microglia phagocytic capacities for endogenous proteins such as Abeta peptides (Floden and Combs, 2011; Harry, 2013) and reduce their expression of phagocytosis and/or endocytosis genes (Orre et al., 2014). In addition, *in vitro* data indicate that microglia in the aged brain express more MHC-II molecules and become less sensitive to regulatory signals, such as transforming growth factor beta 1 (TGF beta-1) or colony stimulating factor 1 (CSF1; Rozovsky et al., 1998). During their life span, episodes of systemic inflammation and cytokine stimulation can instruct microglia and increase their reactivity. This mechanism of exposure to multiple noxious stimuli is called priming (Perry and Holmes, 2014). Along with the priming, accumulation of mutations and DNA damage with the aging (Mrak and Griffin, 2005), can lead microglia to gradually acquire resistance to regulation (Norden and Godbout, 2013; Perry and Holmes, 2014).

Upon activation, microglia density is increased several folds (Erturk et al., 2012), which eventually drops back to normal levels during the recovery phase (Streit, 2006). This reduction of microglia numbers in a pathological context is reestablished by apoptosis through activation-induced cell death (AICD), a mechanism triggered by interferon gamma (Takeuchi et al., 2006). Moreover, accumulation of functional and morphological alterations over time also implies that microglia could die independently of AICD, as shown in human brain (Streit, 2004; Streit and Xue, 2009). Potentially these mechanisms could lead to a substantial decrease in the number of microglia, because the proliferation rate is quite low in physiological conditions. While the number of mitotic divisions achieved before death is not known (Saijo and Glass, 2011), telomere shortening along with a significant decrease of telomerase activity—a marker of aging and senescence—in microglia have been reported during normal aging (Flanary et al., 2007). Taken together, this suggests that aged microglia decline in homeostatic functions and become susceptible to deterioration.

Parabiosis experiments have revealed that the source of microglia replenishment depends on the BBB integrity (Wright et al., 2001; Ajami et al., 2007). When the BBB is compromised, Ly-6C^{hi}CCR2^{+} monocytes are recruited from the blood circulation (Mildner et al., 2007). Alternatively, when the BBB is intact, global depletion of microglia by blockage of CSF1 mobilizes a pool of latent progenitors, which, probably originate from the neuroectoderm—a different source than original microglia pool—as they express the specific marker Nestin (Elmore et al., 2014). Whether these substituting cells are really able to recapitulate the very different functions of microglia is unclear. It is possible that reactive microglia during aging could be deriving from the neuroectoderm lineage. Hence, future studies need to characterize different subtypes of microglia in the aging brain and their origins to determine which types support neuronal survival and which are detrimental to neuronal health.

MICROGLIA IN BRAIN LESIONS (STROKE AND TRAUMA)

After a brain lesion, e.g., induced by TBI or ischemic stroke, neuroinflammatory responses are prominent (Liesz et al., 2011). The acute stage begins with the local death of damaged neurons via necrosis and apoptosis (Raghupathi, 2004). It is associated with a rapid inflammatory response involving both resident microglia and infiltrating blood-borne immune cells (neutrophils, monocytes, leukocytes; for a detailed review please refer to Famakin, 2014). This initial neuroinflammation can be both destructive and beneficial depending on the subtype and spatiotemporal distribution of the inflammatory cells and the environmental cues surrounding them (Kreutzberg, 1996; Ramlackhansingh et al., 2011; Aguzzi et al., 2013; Jeong et al., 2013). Neurodegeneration progresses long after acute lesion, perhaps throughout the remaining lifetime, which may result in chronic neurological complications such as dementia (Smith et al., 1997; Pierce et al., 1998; Bramlett and Dietrich, 2002). However, how the initial injury spreads to the rest of the brain and how microglia is involved in this chronic neurodegeneration process are currently unknown (Masel and DeWitt, 2010). Human MRI and PET studies indicate that white matter track pathology after stroke contributes to a secondary degenerative process in the corresponding cortex (Duering et al., 2012) that seems to be associated with microglia/macrophage activation (Radlinska et al., 2009). Could a possible chronic neuroinflammation be a major contributor to long-term degeneration of the brain? In support of this hypothesis, GWAS studies demonstrate that inflammation-related TREM2 (Guerreiro et al., 2013; Jonsson et al., 2013) and CD33 (Hollingworth et al., 2011; Naj et al., 2011) genes are risk factors for AD. In addition, increased microglial response is associated with enhanced pathology and behavioral decline in an experimental model of dementia (Boimel et al., 2010). To our view, detrimental inflammatory response is exacerbated even by aging alone. Additional insults in the brain (e.g., acute injury) might catalyze this inflammatory response and further accelerate aging of the brain (Smith et al., 2013; Jacquin et al., 2014; **Figure 1**).

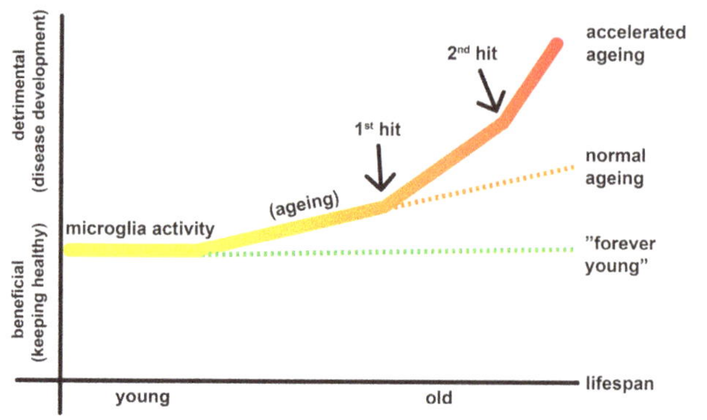

FIGURE 1 | Diagram illustrates putative activities of microglia in aging and lesioned brain. Aging constitutes the continuous factor that transforms some of the microglia to the destructive mode, which may contribute to development of diseases. When there is a lesion, e.g., TBI or stroke (1st hit), some microglia become M1 type, which causes further neurodegeneration while a larger population is still M2 type, which helps healing the lesion environment. In addition, infiltration of the blood-derived immune cells (monocytes/macrophages, lymphocytes) forms the second wing of the inflammatory response and may contribute to neuronal protection and disease development.

Determination of the exact role of microglia in the lesioned CNS is complicated due to the fact that resident microglia cannot easily be distinguished from the blood-borne infiltrating immune cells (e.g., macrophages/monocytes), which come through the leaky BBB. Hence, majority of studies in the context of injuries provided limited information on the specific role of microglia (Hellwig et al., 2013; Perego et al., 2013; Yamasaki et al., 2014). Yet, recent studies demonstrated that indeed microglia and blood-derived immune cells differ in their gene expression signatures, hence, possibly in their functions (Butovsky et al., 2014; Prinz and Priller, 2014). In line with these findings, studies from the traumatic spinal cord injury indicate that blood-derived infiltrating macrophages, but not the resident microglia, are responsible for the secondary axonal dieback (few weeks after the initial insult) (Evans et al., 2014). Similarly, there is supporting data that blood-derived macrophages initiate demyelination in the EAE model, while microglia cleanup the debris and provide trophic support to maintain the tissue homeostasis during the early phases of the disease (Yamasaki et al., 2014). Hence, it is reasonable to consider that the short-lived blood-derived macrophages/monocytes and the long-lived (Elmore et al., 2014) resident microglia are different cell populations with only partially overlapping functions. In the future, accumulation of knowledge on the specificity of each immune cell type (e.g., via the recently generated CCR2-RFP/CX3CR1-GFP transgenic mouse (Saederup et al., 2010)) will be critical to tackle CNS diseases by targeting only the destructive immune cells while preserving the beneficial ones.

Microglia express a repertoire of various receptors such as TREM2, FcγRs, MHC-II, CD200R, RAGE, CX3CR1 (fractalkaline), CXCR3 and 4, purinergic receptors, Toll-like receptors 2 and 4, galectins 1 and 3, scavenger receptors (e.g., CD36), CD47, integrins and SIRPα (Hu et al., 2014). Thereby, they provide both pro-inflammatory and anti-inflammatory response, in a varying range depending on the signals dictated by their environment (Hu et al., 2014, 2015; Peferoen et al., 2015). In the normal brain, it is now understood that microglia activity is repressed by their repeated contacts with normal neurons via inhibitory inputs such as CD200, CX3CL1, CD47, CD22, CD172 or TREM2 (Hellwig et al., 2013). Under acute neuronal injury, inhibitory signals are reduced and danger stimuli (danger-associated molecular patterns, DAMPs) are released (Weinstein et al., 2010). These modifications trigger changes in the microglial response to the environment, collectively resulting in microglia activation, proliferation, migration and response (Patel et al., 2013). The type of microglia response can also vary depending on the mechanisms triggering the lesion (Cherry et al., 2014) (e.g., non-autoimmune, pathogen-associated triggered inflammation vs. adaptive immunity) (Zindler and Zipp, 2010).

Thus, on one hand, microglia can encapsulate dangerous foci and remove the cellular debris via phagocytosis in order to protect the surrounding CNS tissue; on the other hand, they can harm the injured CNS via propagation of inflammation, pro-inflammatory cytokine secretion, antigen-presentation (MHC-II positive) and further immune cell recruitment. Eventually microglia get "deactivated" or cleaned-up by adjacent cells via poorly understood processes that are guided by local and systemic homeostatic signals (Hristova et al., 2010; Saijo and Glass, 2011; Starossom et al., 2012; Patel et al., 2013).

Stroke and TBI initiates a cascade of events (Iadecola and Anrather, 2011) that includes all cellular components of the brain as well as a systemic response from the periphery (Lee et al., 2014). We know that in both ischemic stroke and TBI (Nimmerjahn et al., 2005), microglia respond quickly within the first minutes-hours after the insult (Gelderblom et al., 2009) and the overall neuroinflammatory milieu seems to a peak at around day 5 post-lesion (Turtzo et al., 2014). Interestingly, the initial microglial response in stroke seems to be primarily helping the tissue repair (Hu et al., 2012; **Figure 2**). These microglia secrete and balance anti-inflammatory cytokines and growth factors (IGF1, TGFb1, neurotrophic factors) to promote tissue repair (Wang et al., 2013), indicating that their primary effect after sub-acute ischemia or TBI is to protect the brain and not to kill it (Patel et al., 2013). As mentioned in the review by Hellwig et al. (2013), it is unlikely that the real reason for the presence of numerous inflammatory cells in the vulnerable brain is just to cause harm. In line with this assumption, it has been shown that the enhancement of the microglial population by transplantation of microglia can ameliorate the ischemia-induced injuries via multiple mechanisms, such as upregulation of neurotrophic factors or an active interaction and engulfment of the few neutrophils that might migrate perivascularly after stroke (Neumann et al., 2006, 2008, 2015; Narantuya et al., 2010; Perez-de-Puig et al., 2015). However, microglia dynamically change their phenotypes and they react to the ongoing neuronal death in the peri-infarct regions (Hu et al., 2012) as the lesion extends from core to penumbra over time (Lee et al., 2014; **Figure 2**). Such a change is dictated by the dynamic local ischemic cues (cytokines, chemokines, cells, complement molecules, DAMPs) (Hu et al., 2014). In the lesioned brain, debris are removed via phagocytosis largely by microglia and a lesser extent by infiltrating macrophages (Fu et al., 2014). Removal of debris is beneficial for the tissue and its regeneration (Neumann et al., 2009) but large amounts of debris can overload the microglia and render them dysfunctional over time (Li, 2013). Such a dysfunction can lead to tissue aging as we discuss below.

It is now more evident that neuroinflammation can affect neuronal degeneration and recovery depending on the age of the organism at the time of insult. In other words, we should consider microglia as the brain's guardian of the innate immune compartment that responds to danger and shape a reaction (beneficial or not) (Kigerl et al., 2014) based on their history. Aged microglia are more sensitive to inflammatory stimuli and become resistant to regulation by exposure to multiple noxious stimuli during the life-span of the organism (Norden and Godbout, 2013; Perry and Holmes, 2014). Aging *per se*, can imbalance the repertoire of receptors docked at the membrane and thereby alter the microglial response to environmental cues. Aging decreases some silencing receptors on microglia, e.g., CX3CR1 (Wynne et al., 2010) and CD200 (Lyons et al., 2007), while increases some of the activating ones, thereby priming microglia to become more readily activated upon any trigger (Wong, 2013; Raj et al., 2014). Aged microglia seems to have higher proliferative capacity in response to injury compared to younger adult animals, for example, as observed in facial nerve crush injury (Miller and Streit, 2007) or in mild ischemic injuries (Yan et al., 2014). Moreover, in an aged organism, where a chronic and subtle infection could reside, the intrinsic state of microglia is also *per se* different (increased proinflammatory response) (Püntener et al., 2012) and such microglia may have maladjusted protective response in case of an acute insult. Increased pro-inflammatory or reduced cyto-protective responses related to aging of the organism are indeed a common feature of long-lived resident macrophages reported in various organs including liver (Okaya et al., 2005; Bouchlaka et al., 2013). Conversely, repeated acute lesions can exhaust microglia and reduce their phagocytic function, resulting in chronic, unresolved, sterile inflammation that may propagate over months/years (Li, 2013). The most striking examples for the necessity of a healthy phagocytosis by microglia come from AD (Njie et al., 2012) and multiple sclerosis (Napoli and Neumann, 2010) studies, in which microglial phagocytosis—that is necessary for the clearance of aggregates (e.g., Abeta) or debris—is reduced (Floden and Combs, 2011). In addition to being exhausted by workload, autophagy dysfunction and mitochondrial DNA damage seen in microglia could further contribute to the brain aging and development of neurodegenerative diseases (Nakanishi and Wu, 2009). Eventually, since microglia continuously shape neuronal circuitry and their functions are altered in the post-lesioned brain (Wake et al., 2009), they could also participate in defective circuit remodeling removing not only the degenerating non-functional synapses but also eliminating healthy synapses. Overall, we speculate that multiple acute lesions over the lifespan accelerate aging of the CNS by priming microglia bit-by-bit until they lose their homeostatic and/or repairing capacity (**Figure 2**).

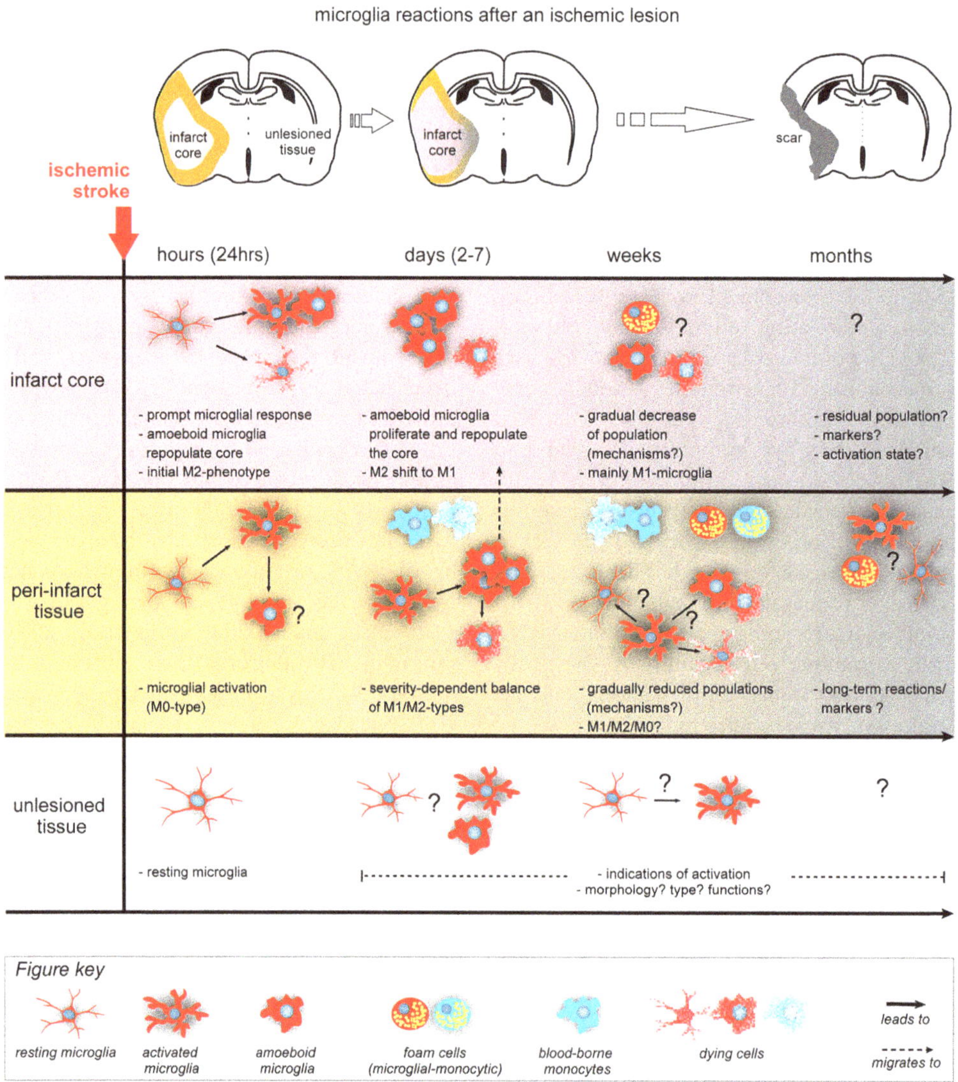

FIGURE 2 | Acute lesions trigger morphological and functional changes from resident microglia. The diagram summarizes the main microglia's temporal (hours to months) and spatial (infarct core, peri-infarct area and unlesioned tissue) kinetics after an ischemic lesion (Ito et al., 2007; Perego et al., 2011, 2013; Hu et al., 2012; Morrison and Filosa, 2013; Patel et al., 2013; Taylor and Sansing, 2013). Infarct core (pink, upper panel) is surrounded by penumbra (orange, middle panel) in the acute phase, a peri-infarct region in the intermediate phases and turns into a scar (gray, with or without cavitation depending on the species) in the chronic phase. During acute phase (first 24 **h**), microglia are the first to respond to the lesion: unless they die immediately by the ischemic processes of the core, they are activated gaining an M2 functional polarization. In the peri-infarct region, microglia are activated but are initially not polarized (M0). In the following **days**, microglia are further activated in the peri-infarct area, proliferate, migrate to the core to repopulate the corresponding cells and some of them die. Depending on the ischemic severity and neuronal damage in the peri-infarct regions, microglia gradually acquire different, region-dependent, polarization states and eventually shift from M2 to M1 microglia as core expands to penumbra and neurons die. At this period, blood-borne monocytes (blue cells) and lymphocytes and neutrophils (not shown here) infiltrate mainly the peri-infarct regions. During the subchronic phase (**weeks**), the core is further cleared from debris (amoeboid microglia turn into foam cells or die) and microglia in the peri-infarct area possibly follow regionally different paths (resting, activation or death), under processes not well studied so far. Foam cells are present (coming from both resident and blood-macrophages), while the numbers of blood-borne cells gradually decline. In the chronic phase (**months**), there are indications of long-term microglial activation and presence of residual foam cells in the peri-infarct tissue, with unknown significance so far. Importantly enough, the **unlesioned tissue** is not well studied so far but probably holds populations of activated microglia that respond or facilitate local degenerative processes. For the simplicity of the figure, we have not included the secreted cytokines produced by the microglia, their changes in their receptors and the contribution of other immune cells. M0: non-polarized microglia, M1: pro-inflammatory or classically activated microglia, M2: anti-inflammatory or alternatively activated microglia (Patel et al., 2013), "?" indicate lack of detailed information.

CONCLUSION

Microglia identity is progressively altered in the aging brain leading to both immunological and homeostasis dysfunctions. In addition to age related decline, microglia accumulate alterations rendering them weaker against protection of the brain after an ischemic or traumatic insult. On the other hand, lesions can prime microglia to age faster, which in return can certainly contribute to escalation of neurodegenerative diseases (**Figure 1**). In fact, resident microglia, which can be imprinted by multiple exposures to insults in the aging brain, should be regarded as "veteran" cells. Therefore, investigating the molecular and cellular mechanisms underlying long-term changes in microglia's identity in response to acute injuries at different times would provide valuable insight for better understanding the aging progression. We believe that novel strategies aiming to reverse the microglia aging could carry high therapeutic potentials for both acute injuries and neurodegenerative diseases.

REFERENCES

Aguzzi, A., Barres, B. A., and Bennett, M. L. (2013). Microglia: scapegoat, saboteur, or something else? *Science* 339, 156–161. doi: 10.1126/science.1227901

Ajami, B., Bennett, J. L., Krieger, C., Tetzlaff, W., and Rossi, F. M. (2007). Local self-renewal can sustain CNS microglia maintenance and function throughout adult life. *Nat. Neurosci.* 10, 1538–1543. doi: 10.1038/nn2014

Berg, A., Zelano, J., Stephan, A., Thams, S., Barres, B. A., Pekny, M., et al. (2012). Reduced removal of synaptic terminals from axotomized spinal motoneurons in the absence of complement C3. *Exp. Neurol.* 237, 8–17. doi: 10.1016/j.expneurol.2012.06.008

Boimel, M., Grigoriadis, N., Lourbopoulos, A., Haber, E., Abramsky, O., and Rosenmann, H. (2010). Efficacy and safety of immunization with phosphorylated tau against neurofibrillary tangles in mice. *Exp. Neurol.* 224, 472–485. doi: 10.1016/j.expneurol.2010.05.010

Bouchlaka, M. N., Sckisel, G. D., Chen, M., Mirsoian, A., Zamora, A. E., Maverakis, E., et al. (2013). Aging predisposes to acute inflammatory induced pathology after tumor immunotherapy. *J. Exp. Med.* 210, 2223–2237. doi: 10.1084/jem.20131219

Bramlett, H. M., and Dietrich, W. D. (2002). Quantitative structural changes in white and gray matter 1 year following traumatic brain injury in rats. *Acta Neuropathol.* 103, 607–614. doi: 10.1007/s00401-001-0510-8

Brown, G. C., and Neher, J. J. (2014). Microglial phagocytosis of live neurons. *Nat. Rev. Neurosci.* 15, 209–216. doi: 10.1038/nrn3710

Butovsky, O., Jedrychowski, M. P., Moore, C. S., Cialic, R., Lanser, A. J., Gabriely, G., et al. (2014). Identification of a unique TGF-β-dependent molecular and functional signature in microglia. *Nat. Neurosci.* 17, 131–143. doi: 10.1038/nn.3599

Cherry, J. D., Olschowka, J. A., and O'Banion, M. K. (2014). Neuroinflammation and M2 microglia: the good, the bad and the inflamed. *J. Neuroinflammation* 11:98. doi: 10.1186/1742-2094-11-98

Damani, M. R., Zhao, L., Fontainhas, A. M., Amaral, J., Fariss, R. N., and Wong, W. T. (2011). Age-related alterations in the dynamic behavior of microglia. *Aging Cell* 10, 263–276. doi: 10.1111/j.1474-9726.2010.00660.x

Davalos, D., Grutzendler, J., Yang, G., Kim, J. V., Zuo, Y., Jung, S., et al. (2005). ATP mediates rapid microglial response to local brain injury in vivo. *Nat. Neurosci.* 8, 752–758. doi: 10.1038/nn1472

Duering, M., Righart, R., Csanadi, E., Jouvent, E., Hervé, D., Chabriat, H., et al. (2012). Incident subcortical infarcts induce focal thinning in connected cortical regions. *Neurology* 79, 2025–2028. doi: 10.1212/WNL.0b013e3182749f39

Elmore, M. R., Najafi, A. R., Koike, M. A., Dagher, N. N., Spangenberg, E. E., Rice, R. A., et al. (2014). Colony-stimulating factor 1 receptor signaling is necessary for microglia viability, unmasking a microglia progenitor cell in the adult brain. *Neuron* 82, 380–397. doi: 10.1016/j.neuron.2014.02.040

Erturk, A., Becker, K., Jahrling, N., Mauch, C. P., Hojer, C. D., Egen, J. G., et al. (2012). Three-dimensional imaging of solvent-cleared organs using 3DISCO. *Nat. Protoc.* 7, 1983–1995. doi: 10.1038/nprot.2012.119

Evans, T. A., Barkauskas, D. S., Myers, J. T., Hare, E. G., You, J. Q., Ransohoff, R. M., et al. (2014). High-resolution intravital imaging reveals that blood-derived macrophages but not resident microglia facilitate secondary axonal dieback in traumatic spinal cord injury. *Exp. Neurol.* 254, 109–120. doi: 10.1016/j.expneurol.2014.01.013

Famakin, B. M. (2014). The immune response to acute focal cerebral ischemia and associated post-stroke immunodepression: a focused review. *Aging Dis.* 5, 307–326. doi: 10.14336/AD.2014.0500307

Flanary, B. E., Sammons, N. W., Nguyen, C., Walker, D., and Streit, W. J. (2007). Evidence that aging and amyloid promote microglial cell senescence. *Rejuvenation Res.* 10, 61–74. doi: 10.1089/rej.2006.9096

Floden, A. M., and Combs, C. K. (2011). Microglia demonstrate age-dependent interaction with amyloid-β fibrils. *J. Alzheimers Dis.* 25, 279–293. doi: 10.3233/JAD-2011-101014

Fu, R., Shen, Q., Xu, P., Luo, J. J., and Tang, Y. (2014). Phagocytosis of microglia in the central nervous system diseases. *Mol. Neurobiol.* 49, 1422–1434. doi: 10.1007/s12035-013-8620-6

Gehrmann, J., and Banati, R. B. (1995). Microglial turnover in the injured CNS: activated microglia undergo delayed DNA fragmentation following peripheral nerve injury. *J. Neuropathol. Exp. Neurol.* 54, 680–688. doi: 10.1097/00005072-199509000-00010

Gelderblom, M., Leypoldt, F., Steinbach, K., Behrens, D., Choe, C. U., Siler, D. A., et al. (2009). Temporal and spatial dynamics of cerebral immune cell accumulation in stroke. *Stroke* 40, 1849–1857. doi: 10.1161/STROKEAHA.108.534503

Ginhoux, F., Greter, M., Leboeuf, M., Nandi, S., See, P., Gokhan, S., et al. (2010). Fate mapping analysis reveals that adult microglia derive from primitive macrophages. *Science* 330, 841–845. doi: 10.1126/science.1194637

Guerreiro, R., Wojtas, A., Bras, J., Carrasquillo, M., Rogaeva, E., Majounie, E., et al. (2013). TREM2 variants in Alzheimer's disease. *N. Engl. J. Med.* 368, 117–127. doi: 10.1056/NEJMoa1211851

Harry, G. J. (2013). Microglia during development and aging. *Pharmacol. Ther.* 139, 313–326. doi: 10.1016/j.pharmthera.2013.04.013

Hefendehl, J. K., Neher, J. J., Suhs, R. B., Kohsaka, S., Skodras, A., and Jucker, M. (2014). Homeostatic and injury-induced microglia behavior in the aging brain. *Aging Cell* 13, 60–69. doi: 10.1111/acel.12149

Hellwig, S., Heinrich, A., and Biber, K. (2013). The brain's best friend: microglial neurotoxicity revisited. *Front. Cell. Neurosci.* 7:71. doi: 10.3389/fncel.2013.00071

Hollingworth, P., Harold, D., Sims, R., Gerrish, A., Lambert, J. C., Carrasquillo, M. M., et al. (2011). Common variants at ABCA7, MS4A6A/MS4A4E, EPHA1, CD33 and CD2AP are associated with Alzheimer's disease. *Nat. Genet.* 43, 429–435. doi: 10.1038/ng.803

Hristova, M., Cuthill, D., Zbarsky, V., Acosta-Saltos, A., Wallace, A., Blight, K., et al. (2010). Activation and deactivation of periventricular white matter phagocytes during postnatal mouse development. *Glia* 58, 11–28. doi: 10.1002/glia.20896

Hu, X., Leak, R. K., Shi, Y., Suenaga, J., Gao, Y., Zheng, P., et al. (2015). Microglial and macrophage polarization-new prospects for brain repair. *Nat. Rev. Neurol.* 11, 56–64. doi: 10.1038/nrneurol.2014.207

Hu, X., Li, P., Guo, Y., Wang, H., Leak, R. K., Chen, S., et al. (2012). Microglia/macrophage polarization dynamics reveal novel mechanism of injury expansion after focal cerebral ischemia. *Stroke* 43, 3063–3070. doi: 10.1161/STROKEAHA.112.659656

Hu, X., Liou, A. K., Leak, R. K., Xu, M., An, C., Suenaga, J., et al. (2014). Neurobiology of microglial action in CNS injuries: receptor-mediated signaling mechanisms and functional roles. *Prog. Neurobiol.* 119–120, 60–84. doi: 10.1016/j.pneurobio.2014.06.002

Iadecola, C., and Anrather, J. (2011). Stroke research at a crossroad: asking the brain for directions. *Nat. Neurosci.* 14, 1363–1368. doi: 10.1038/nn.2953

Ito, U., Nagasao, J., Kawakami, E., and Oyanagi, K. (2007). Fate of disseminated dead neurons in the cortical ischemic penumbra: ultrastructure indicating a novel scavenger mechanism of microglia and astrocytes. *Stroke* 38, 2577–2583. doi: 10.1161/strokeaha.107.484394

Jacquin, A., Binquet, C., Rouaud, O., Graule-Petot, A., Daubail, B., Osseby, G. V., et al. (2014). Post-stroke cognitive impairment: high prevalence and determining factors in a cohort of mild stroke. *J. Alzheimers Dis.* 40, 1029–1038. doi: 10.3233/JAD-131580

Jeong, H. K., Ji, K., Min, K., and Joe, E. H. (2013). Brain inflammation and microglia: facts and misconceptions. *Exp. Neurobiol.* 22, 59–67. doi: 10.5607/en.2013.22.2.59

Jonsson, T., Stefansson, H., Steinberg, S., Jonsdottir, I., Jonsson, P. V., Snaedal, J., et al. (2013). Variant of TREM2 associated with the risk of Alzheimer's disease. *N. Engl. J. Med.* 368, 107–116. doi: 10.1056/NEJMoa1211103

Kigerl, K. A., de Rivero Vaccari, J. P., Dietrich, W. D., Popovich, P. G., and Keane, R. W. (2014). Pattern recognition receptors and central nervous system repair. *Exp. Neurol.* 258, 5–16. doi: 10.1016/j.expneurol.2014.01.001

Kreutzberg, G. W. (1996). Microglia: a sensor for pathological events in the CNS. *Trends Neurosci.* 19, 312–318. doi: 10.1016/0166-2236(96)10049-7

Lawson, L. J., Perry, V. H., and Gordon, S. (1992). Turnover of resident microglia in the normal adult mouse brain. *Neuroscience* 48, 405–415. doi: 10.1016/0306-4522(92)90500-2

Lee, Y., Lee, S. R., Choi, S. S., Yeo, H. G., Chang, K. T., and Lee, H. J. (2014). Therapeutically targeting neuroinflammation and microglia after acute ischemic stroke. *Biomed. Res. Int.* 2014:297241. doi: 10.1155/2014/297241

Li, W. (2013). Phagocyte dysfunction, tissue aging and degeneration. *Ageing Res. Rev.* 12, 1005–1012. doi: 10.1016/j.arr.2013.05.006

Liesz, A., Zhou, W., Mracskó, E., Karcher, S., Bauer, H., Schwarting, S., et al. (2011). Inhibition of lymphocyte trafficking shields the brain against deleterious neuroinflammation after stroke. *Brain* 134, 704–720. doi: 10.1093/brain/awr008

Lyons, A., Downer, E. J., Crotty, S., Nolan, Y. M., Mills, K. H., and Lynch, M. A. (2007). CD200 ligand receptor interaction modulates microglial activation in vivo and in vitro: a role for IL-4. *J. Neurosci.* 27, 8309–8313. doi: 10.1523/jneurosci.1781-07.2007

Marín-Teva, J. L., Dusart, I., Colin, C., Gervais, A., van Rooijen, N., and Mallat, M. (2004). Microglia promote the death of developing Purkinje cells. *Neuron* 41, 535–547. doi: 10.1016/s0896-6273(04)00069-8

Masel, B. E., and DeWitt, D. S. (2010). Traumatic brain injury: a disease process, not an event. *J. Neurotrauma* 27, 1529–1540. doi: 10.1089/neu.2010.1358

Mildner, A., Schmidt, H., Nitsche, M., Merkler, D., Hanisch, U. K., Mack, M., et al. (2007). Microglia in the adult brain arise from Ly-6ChiCCR2+ monocytes only under defined host conditions. *Nat. Neurosci.* 10, 1544–1553. doi: 10.1038/nn2015

Miller, K. R., and Streit, W. J. (2007). The effects of aging, injury and disease on microglial function: a case for cellular senescence. *Neuron Glia Biol.* 3, 245–253. doi: 10.1017/s1740925x08000136

Morrison, H. W., and Filosa, J. A. (2013). A quantitative spatiotemporal analysis of microglia morphology during ischemic stroke and reperfusion. *J. Neuroinflammation* 10:4. doi: 10.1186/1742-2094-10-4

Mrak, R. E., and Griffin, W. S. T. (2005). Glia and their cytokines in progression of neurodegeneration. *Neurobiol. Aging* 26, 349–354. doi: 10.1016/j.neurobiolaging.2004.05.010

Naj, A. C., Jun, G., Beecham, G. W., Wang, L. S., Vardarajan, B. N., Buros, J., et al. (2011). Common variants at MS4A4/MS4A6E, CD2AP, CD33 and EPHA1 are associated with late-onset alzheimer's disease. *Nat. Genet.* 43, 436–441. doi: 10.1038/ng.801

Nakanishi, H., and Wu, Z. (2009). Microglia-aging: roles of microglial lysosome- and mitochondria-derived reactive oxygen species in brain aging. *Behav. Brain Res.* 201, 1–7. doi: 10.1016/j.bbr.2009.02.001

Napoli, I., and Neumann, H. (2010). Protective effects of microglia in multiple sclerosis. *Exp. Neurol.* 225, 24–28. doi: 10.1016/j.expneurol.2009.04.024

Narantuya, D., Nagai, A., Sheikh, A. M., Masuda, J., Kobayashi, S., Yamaguchi, S., et al. (2010). Human microglia transplanted in rat focal ischemia brain induce neuroprotection and behavioral improvement. *PLoS One* 5:e11746. doi: 10.1371/journal.pone.0011746

Neumann, J., Gunzer, M., Gutzeit, H. O., Ullrich, O., Reymann, K. G., and Dinkel, K. (2006). Microglia provide neuroprotection after ischemia. *FASEB J.* 20, 714–716. doi: 10.1096/fj.05-4882fje

Neumann, H., Kotter, M. R., and Franklin, R. J. (2009). Debris clearance by microglia: an essential link between degeneration and regeneration. *Brain* 132, 288–295. doi: 10.1093/brain/awn109

Neumann, J., Riek-Burchardt, M., Herz, J., Doeppner, T. R., Konig, R., Hutten, H., et al. (2015). Very-late-antigen-4 (VLA-4)-mediated brain invasion by neutrophils leads to interactions with microglia, increased ischemic injury and impaired behavior in experimental stroke. *Acta Neuropathol.* 129, 259–277. doi: 10.1007/s00401-014-1355-2

Neumann, J., Sauerzweig, S., Rönicke, R., Gunzer, F., Dinkel, K., Ullrich, O., et al. (2008). Microglia cells protect neurons by direct engulfment of invading neutrophil granulocytes: a new mechanism of CNS immune privilege. *J. Neurosci.* 28, 5965–5975. doi: 10.1523/JNEUROSCI.0060-08.2008

Nimmerjahn, A., Kirchhoff, F., and Helmchen, F. (2005). Resting microglial cells are highly dynamic surveillants of brain parenchyma in vivo. *Science* 308, 1314–1318. doi: 10.1126/science.1110647

Njie, E. G., Boelen, E., Stassen, F. R., Steinbusch, H. W., Borchelt, D. R., and Streit, W. J. (2012). Ex vivo cultures of microglia from young and aged rodent brain reveal age-related changes in microglial function. *Neurobiol. Aging* 33, 195.e1–195.e12. doi: 10.1016/j.neurobiolaging.2010.05.008

Norden, D. M., and Godbout, J. P. (2013). Review: microglia of the aged brain: primed to be activated and resistant to regulation. *Neuropathol. Appl. Neurobiol.* 39, 19–34. doi: 10.1111/j.1365-2990.2012.01306.x

Okaya, T., Blanchard, J., Schuster, R., Kuboki, S., Husted, T., Caldwell, C. C., et al. (2005). Age-dependent responses to hepatic ischemia/reperfusion injury. *Shock* 24, 421–427. doi: 10.1097/01.shk.0000181282.14050.11

Orre, M., Kamphuis, W., Osborn, L. M., Jansen, A. H., Kooijman, L., Bossers, K., et al. (2014). Isolation of glia from Alzheimer's mice reveals inflammation and dysfunction. *Neurobiol. Aging* 35, 2746–2760. doi: 10.1016/j.neurobiolaging.2014.06.004

Parkhurst, C. N., Yang, G., Ninan, I., Savas, J. N., Yates, J. R. 3rd, Lafaille, J. J., et al. (2013). Microglia promote learning-dependent synapse formation through brain-derived neurotrophic factor. *Cell* 155, 1596–1609. doi: 10.1016/j.cell.2013.11.030

Patel, A. R., Ritzel, R., McCullough, L. D., and Liu, F. (2013). Microglia and ischemic stroke: a double-edged sword. *Int. J. Physiol. Pathophysiol. Pharmacol.* 5, 73–90.

Peferoen, L. A., Vogel, D. Y., Ummenthum, K., Breur, M., Heijnen, P. D., Gerritsen, W. H., et al. (2015). Activation status of human microglia is dependent on lesion formation stage and remyelination in multiple sclerosis. *J. Neuropathol. Exp. Neurol.* 74, 48–63. doi: 10.1097/NEN.0000000000000149

Perego, C., Fumagalli, S., and De Simoni, M. G. (2011). Temporal pattern of expression and colocalization of microglia/macrophage phenotype markers following brain ischemic injury in mice. *J. Neuroinflammation* 8:174. doi: 10.1186/1742-2094-8-174

Perego, C., Fumagalli, S., and De Simoni, M. G. (2013). Three-dimensional confocal analysis of microglia/macrophage markers of polarization in experimental brain injury. *J. Vis. Exp.* 79:e50605. doi: 10.3791/50605

Perez-de-Puig, I., Miró-Mur, F., Ferrer-Ferrer, M., Gelpi, E., Pedragosa, J., Justicia, C., et al. (2015). Neutrophil recruitment to the brain in mouse and human ischemic stroke. *Acta Neuropathol.* 129, 239–257. doi: 10.1007/s00401-014-1381-0

Perry, V. H., and Holmes, C. (2014). Microglial priming in neurodegenerative disease. *Nat. Rev. Neurol.* 10, 217–224. doi: 10.1038/nrneurol.2014.38

Pierce, J. E., Smith, D. H., Trojanowski, J. Q., and McIntosh, T. K. (1998). Enduring cognitive, neurobehavioral and histopathological changes persist for up to one year following severe experimental brain injury in rats. *Neuroscience* 87, 359–369. doi: 10.1016/s0306-4522(98)00142-0

Prinz, M., and Priller, J. (2014). Microglia and brain macrophages in the molecular age: from origin to neuropsychiatric disease. *Nat. Rev. Neurosci.* 15, 300–312. doi: 10.1038/nrn3722

Püntener, U., Booth, S. G., Perry, V. H., and Teeling, J. L. (2012). Long-term impact of systemic bacterial infection on the cerebral vasculature and microglia. *J. Neuroinflammation* 9:146. doi: 10.1186/1742-2094-9-146

Radlinska, B. A., Ghinani, S. A., Lyon, P., Jolly, D., Soucy, J. P., Minuk, J., et al. (2009). Multimodal microglia imaging of fiber tracts in acute subcortical stroke. *Ann. Neurol.* 66, 825–832. doi: 10.1002/ana.21796

Raghupathi, R. (2004). Cell death mechanisms following traumatic brain injury. *Brain Pathol.* 14, 215–222. doi: 10.1111/j.1750-3639.2004.tb00056.x

Raj, D. D., Jaarsma, D., Holtman, I. R., Olah, M., Ferreira, F. M., Schaafsma, W., et al. (2014). Priming of microglia in a DNA-repair deficient model of accelerated aging. *Neurobiol. Aging* 35, 2147–2160. doi: 10.1016/j.neurobiolaging.2014.03.025

Ramlackhansingh, A. F., Brooks, D. J., Greenwood, R. J., Bose, S. K., Turkheimer, F. E., Kinnunen, K. M., et al. (2011). Inflammation after trauma: microglial activation and traumatic brain injury. *Ann. Neurol.* 70, 374–383. doi: 10.1002/ana.22455

Rozovsky, I., Finch, C. E., and Morgan, T. E. (1998). Age-related activation of microglia and astrocytes: in vitro studies show persistent phenotypes of aging, increased proliferation and resistance to down-regulation. *Neurobiol. Aging* 19, 97–103. doi: 10.1016/s0197-4580(97)00169-3

Saederup, N., Cardona, A. E., Croft, K., Mizutani, M., Cotleur, A. C., Tsou, C. L., et al. (2010). Selective chemokine receptor usage by central nervous system myeloid cells in CCR2-red fluorescent protein knock-in mice. *PLoS One* 5:e13693. doi: 10.1371/journal.pone.0013693

Saijo, K., and Glass, C. K. (2011). Microglial cell origin and phenotypes in health and disease. *Nat. Rev. Immunol.* 11, 775–787. doi: 10.1038/nri3086

Salter, M. W., and Beggs, S. (2014). Sublime microglia: expanding roles for the guardians of the CNS. *Cell* 158, 15–24. doi: 10.1016/j.cell.2014.06.008

Schafer, D. P., Lehrman, E. K., Kautzman, A. G., Koyama, R., Mardinly, A. R., Yamasaki, R., et al. (2012). Microglia sculpt postnatal neural circuits in an activity and complement-dependent manner. *Neuron* 74, 691–705. doi: 10.1016/j.neuron.2012.03.026

Schafer, D. P., Lehrman, E. K., and Stevens, B. (2013). The "quad-partite" synapse: microglia-synapse interactions in the developing and mature CNS. *Glia* 6, 24–36. doi: 10.1002/glia.22389

Schulz, C., Gomez Perdiguero, E., Chorro, L., Szabo-Rogers, H., Cagnard, N., Kierdorf, K., et al. (2012). A lineage of myeloid cells independent of Myb and hematopoietic stem cells. *Science* 336, 86–90. doi: 10.1126/science.1219179

Sierra, A., Encinas, J. M., Deudero, J. J., Chancey, J. H., Enikolopov, G., Overstreet-Wadiche, L. S., et al. (2010). Microglia shape adult hippocampal neurogenesis through apoptosis-coupled phagocytosis. *Cell Stem Cell* 7, 483–495. doi: 10.1016/j.stem.2010.08.014

Smith, D. H., Chen, X. H., Pierce, J. E., Wolf, J. A., Trojanowski, J. Q., Graham, D. I., et al. (1997). Progressive atrophy and neuron death for one year following brain trauma in the rat. *J. Neurotrauma* 14, 715–727. doi: 10.1089/neu.1997.14.715

Smith, D. H., Johnson, V. E., and Stewart, W. (2013). Chronic neuropathologies of single and repetitive TBI: substrates of dementia? *Nat. Rev. Neurol.* 9, 211–221. doi: 10.1038/nrneurol.2013.29

Starossom, S. C., Mascanfroni, I. D., Imitola, J., Cao, L., Raddassi, K., Hernandez, S. F., et al. (2012). Galectin-1 deactivates classically activated microglia and protects from inflammation-induced neurodegeneration. *Immunity* 37, 249–263. doi: 10.1016/j.immuni.2012.05.023

Stevens, B., Allen, N. J., Vazquez, L. E., Howell, G. R., Christopherson, K. S., Nouri, N., et al. (2007). The classical complement cascade mediates CNS synapse elimination. *Cell* 131, 1164–1178. doi: 10.1016/j.cell.2007.10.036

Streit, W. J. (2004). Microglia and Alzheimer's disease pathogenesis. *J. Neurosci. Res.* 77, 1–8. doi: 10.1002/jnr.20093

Streit, W. J. (2006). Microglial senescence: does the brain's immune system have an expiration date? *Trends Neurosci.* 29, 506–510. doi: 10.1016/j.tins.2006.07.001

Streit, W. J., and Xue, Q. S. (2009). Life and death of microglia. *J. Neuroimmune Pharmacol.* 4, 371–379. doi: 10.1007/s11481-009-9163-5

Takeuchi, H., Wang, J., Kawanokuchi, J., Mitsuma, N., Mizuno, T., and Suzumura, A. (2006). Interferon-gamma induces microglial-activation-induced cell death: a hypothetical mechanism of relapse and remission in multiple sclerosis. *Neurobiol. Dis.* 22, 33–39. doi: 10.1016/j.nbd.2005.09.014

Taylor, R. A., and Sansing, L. H. (2013). Microglial responses after ischemic stroke and intracerebral hemorrhage. *Clin. Dev. Immunol.* 2013:746068. doi: 10.1155/2013/746068

Tremblay, M. E., Lowery, R. L., and Majewska, A. K. (2010). Microglial interactions with synapses are modulated by visual experience. *PLoS Biol.* 8:e1000527. doi: 10.1371/journal.pbio.1000527

Tremblay, M. E., and Majewska, A. K. (2011). A role for microglia in synaptic plasticity? *Commun. Integr. Biol.* 4, 220–222. doi: 10.4161/cib.4.2.14506

Turtzo, L. C., Lescher, J., Janes, L., Dean, D. D., Budde, M. D., and Frank, J. A. (2014). Macrophagic and microglial responses after focal traumatic brain injury in the female rat. *J. Neuroinflammation* 11:82. doi: 10.1186/1742-2094-11-82

Varvel, N. H., Grathwohl, S. A., Baumann, F., Liebig, C., Bosch, A., Brawek, B., et al. (2012). Microglial repopulation model reveals a robust homeostatic process for replacing CNS myeloid cells. *Proc. Natl. Acad. Sci. U S A* 109, 18150–18155. doi: 10.1073/pnas.1210150109

Wake, H., Moorhouse, A. J., Jinno, S., Kohsaka, S., and Nabekura, J. (2009). Resting microglia directly monitor the functional state of synapses in vivo and determine the fate of ischemic terminals. *J. Neurosci.* 29, 3974–3980. doi: 10.1523/JNEUROSCI.4363-08.2009

Wang, J., Yang, Z., Liu, C., Zhao, Y., and Chen, Y. (2013). Activated microglia provide a neuroprotective role by balancing glial cell-line derived neurotrophic factor and tumor necrosis factor-alpha secretion after subacute cerebral ischemia. *Int. J. Mol. Med.* 31, 172–178. doi: 10.3892/ijmm.2012.1179

Weinstein, J. R., Koerner, I. P., and Möller, T. (2010). Microglia in ischemic brain injury. *Future Neurol.* 5, 227–246. doi: 10.2217/fnl.10.1

Wong, W. T. (2013). Microglial aging in the healthy CNS: phenotypes, drivers and rejuvenation. *Front. Cell. Neurosci.* 7:22. doi: 10.3389/fncel.2013.00022

Wright, D. E., Wagers, A. J., Gulati, A. P., Johnson, F. L., and Weissman, I. L. (2001). Physiological migration of hematopoietic stem and progenitor cells. *Science* 294, 1933–1936. doi: 10.1126/science.1064081

Wu, L. J., Stevens, B., Duan, S., and MacVicar, B. A. (2013). Microglia in neuronal circuits. *Neural Plast.* 2013:586426. doi: 10.1155/2013/586426

Wynne, A. M., Henry, C. J., Huang, Y., Cleland, A., and Godbout, J. P. (2010). Protracted downregulation of CX3CR1 on microglia of aged mice after lipopolysaccharide challenge. *Brain Behav. Immun.* 24, 1190–1201. doi: 10.1016/j.bbi.2010.05.011

Yamasaki, R., Lu, H., Butovsky, O., Ohno, N., Rietsch, A. M., Cialic, R., et al. (2014). Differential roles of microglia and monocytes in the inflamed central nervous system. *J. Exp. Med.* 211, 1533–1549. doi: 10.1084/jem.20132477

Yan, B. C., Ohk, T. G., Ahn, J. H., Park, J. H., Chen, B. H., Lee, J. C., et al. (2014). Differences in neuronal damage and gliosis in the hippocampus between young and adult gerbils induced by long duration of transient cerebral ischemia. *J. Neurol. Sci.* 337, 129–136. doi: 10.1016/j.jns.2013.11.034

Yona, S., Kim, K. W., Wolf, Y., Mildner, A., Varol, D., Breker, M., et al. (2013). Fate mapping reveals origins and dynamics of monocytes and tissue macrophages under homeostasis. *Immunity* 38, 79–91. doi: 10.1016/j.immuni.2012.12.001

Zindler, E., and Zipp, F. (2010). Neuronal injury in chronic CNS inflammation. *Best Pract. Res. Clin. Anaesthesiol.* 24, 551–562. doi: 10.1016/j.bpa.2010.11.001

13

Brain immune cell composition and functional outcome after cerebral ischemia: comparison of two mouse strains

Hyun Ah Kim[1], Stephanie C. Whittle[1], Seyoung Lee[1], Hannah X. Chu[1], Shenpeng R. Zhang[1], Zihui Wei[1], Thiruma V. Arumugam[2,3,4], Anthony Vinh[1], Grant R. Drummond[1,5] and Christopher G. Sobey[1,5]*

[1] Department of Pharmacology, Monash University, Clayton, VIC, Australia
[2] Department of Physiology, Yong Loo Lin School of Medicine, National University of Singapore, Singapore, Singapore
[3] School of Pharmacy, Sungkyunkwan University, Suwon, South Korea
[4] School of Biomedical Sciences, The University of Queensland, St Lucia, QLD, Australia
[5] Department of Surgery, Monash Medical Centre, Southern Clinical School, Monash University, Clayton, VIC, Australia

***Correspondence:**
Christopher G. Sobey, Department of Pharmacology, Monash University, Wellington Road, Clayton, VIC 3800, Australia
e-mail: chris.sobey@monash.edu

Inflammatory cells may contribute to secondary brain injury following cerebral ischemia. The C57Bl/6 mouse strain is known to exhibit a T helper 1-prone, pro-inflammatory type response to injury, whereas the FVB strain is relatively T helper 2-prone, or anti-inflammatory, in its immune response. We tested whether stroke outcome is more severe in C57Bl/6 than FVB mice. Male mice of each strain underwent sham surgery or 1 h occlusion of the middle cerebral artery followed by 23 h of reperfusion. Despite no difference in infarct size, C57Bl/6 mice displayed markedly greater functional deficits than FVB mice after stroke, as assessed by neurological scoring and hanging wire test. Total numbers of $CD45^+$ leukocytes tended to be larger in the brains of C57Bl/6 than FVB mice after stroke, but there were marked differences in leukocyte composition between the two mouse strains. The inflammatory response in C57Bl/6 mice primarily involved T and B lymphocytes, whereas neutrophils, monocytes and macrophages were more prominent in FVB mice. Our data are consistent with the concept that functional outcome after stroke is dependent on the immune cell composition which develops following ischemic brain injury.

Keywords: cerebral ischemia-reperfusion, immune cell infiltration, inflammation, middle cerebral artery occlusion, stroke, Th1/Th2 balance

INTRODUCTION

Stroke is the 4th leading cause of death after heart disease, cancer and chronic lower respiratory disease, and over a third of survivors are left with major neurological injury (Go et al., 2013). Approximately 85% of stroke cases are of the ischemic type (Go et al., 2013), in which an embolus or local thrombus causes occlusion of a major cerebral artery and results in disruption of brain blood flow. Whilst thrombolysis by intravenous recombinant tissue plasminogen activator (rt-PA) may be effective in improving outcome by promoting reperfusion, it has a number of limitations, including a short therapeutic window of 3–4.5 h (<10% of stroke patients receive rt-PA) (Gravanis and Tsirka, 2008). For further advances in the clinical treatment of ischemic stroke, the complex mechanisms of cellular injury following cerebral ischemia must be elucidated to provide novel targets for future therapies.

It is now established that the initial insult in ischemic stroke is followed by induction of cytokines and chemokines, which attract numerous inflammatory cell types to the damaged brain region, which ultimately contribute to secondary brain injury (Gelderblom et al., 2009; Chu et al., 2014). Growing evidence indicates the importance of T lymphocytes in cerebral ischemic damage, whereby they become activated and infiltrate the brain within 24 h (Yilmaz et al., 2006; Hurn et al., 2007; Urra et al., 2009a), although the mechanism(s) underlying their actions are not fully clear. Recombination activating gene 1-deficient mice, which lack T and B lymphocytes, have less severe brain injury following cerebral ischemia, and this protection is lost upon reconstitution with T but not B lymphocytes (Yilmaz et al., 2006; Kleinschnitz et al., 2010).

T lymphocytes ($CD3^+$ cells) are mostly comprised of $CD4^+$ T helper (Th) and $CD8^+$ cytotoxic T (Tc) cell subpopulations, both of which are thought to play detrimental roles in ischemic stroke (Yilmaz et al., 2006). There is also evidence that regulatory T lymphocytes (Tregs; $CD4^+CD25^+FoxP3^+$) may modulate the severity of stroke outcome (Liesz et al., 2009), despite exerting acutely detrimental effects by promoting intravascular coagulation during reperfusion (Kleinschnitz et al., 2013). Major distinct Th cell types include Th1 and Th2, and are defined according to the cytokines they release (Abbas et al., 1996). In general terms, Th1 cells promote an inflammatory response through secretion of pro-inflammatory cytokines [e.g., interleukin(IL)-2, IL-12, interferon(IFN)-γ, and tumor necrosis factor(TNF)-α], whereas Th2 cells promote a humoral or allergic response by secretion of anti-inflammatory cytokines (e.g., IL-4, IL-10, and IL-13) (Arumugam et al., 2005; Jin et al., 2010).

Clarification of the importance of Th1 and Th2 immunity in acute stroke is needed to define the complex evolution of cerebral ischemic injury and potentially identify therapeutic strategies to limit stroke injury. Here, we have studied representative mouse strains commonly accepted as Th1-dominant (C57Bl/6) and Th2-dominant (FVB) (Whitehead et al., 2003) to investigate stroke outcome in a prototypical Th1- or Th2-prone immune environment, respectively.

MATERIALS AND METHODS

ANIMALS

This study fully adheres to the Animal Research: Reporting *In Vivo* Experiments (ARRIVE) guidelines (Kilkenny et al., 2010). All animal experiments were conducted in accordance with National Health and Medical Research Council of Australia guidelines for the care and use of animals in research and approved by the Monash University Animal Ethics Committee (Projects SOBSB/2010/10 and SOBSB/2011/112). A total of 201 male mice (C57Bl/6: $n = 89$, 19–33 g; FVB: $n = 112$, 25–39 g) aged 8–15 weeks were studied. The mice had free access to water and food pellets before and after surgery. Thirty-seven mice were excluded from the study because they: (1) died during surgical procedure (C57Bl/6: $n = 12$; FVB: $n = 24$) or (2) were euthanized prior to 24 h as per institutional ethics requirements due to severe functional impairment (C57Bl/6: $n = 1$).

TRANSIENT FOCAL CEREBRAL ISCHEMIA

Focal cerebral ischemia was induced by transient intraluminal filament occlusion of the right middle cerebral artery (MCA) as described previously (Jackman et al., 2009; Brait et al., 2010). Mice were anesthetized with ketamine-xylazine (80 and 10 mg/kg, respectively; intraperitoneal). Rectal temperature was monitored and maintained at 37.5 ± 0.5°C throughout the procedure and until animals regained consciousness using an electronic temperature controller (Testronics, Kinglake, Victoria, Australia) linked to a heat lamp. The right proximal common carotid artery was clamped, and a 6–0 nylon monofilament with silicone-coated tip (Doccol Co., Redlands, CA, USA) was inserted and gently advanced into the distal internal carotid artery, 11–12 mm distal to the carotid bifurcation, occluding the MCA at the junction of the Circle of Willis. Severe (~80%) reduction in regional cerebral blood flow (rCBF) was confirmed using transcranial laser-Doppler flowmetry (Perimed, Järfälla, Sweden) in the area of cerebral cortex supplied by the MCA. The filament was then tied in place and the clamp was removed. After 1 h of cerebral ischemia, the monofilament was retracted to allow reperfusion for 23 h. Reperfusion was confirmed by an immediate increase in rCBF, which reached the pre-ischemic level within 5 min. The wound was then closed and the animal was allowed to recover. Regional CBF was recorded for 30 min after the induction of reperfusion. Sham-operated mice were anesthetized and the right carotid bifurcation was exposed, dissected free from surrounding connective tissue but no filament was inserted. All animals were administered 1 mL of sterile saline via a subcutaneous injection for rehydration after surgery.

NEUROLOGICAL ASSESSMENT

At the end of the experiment (24 h after induction of stroke/sham surgery), neurological assessment was performed using a modified six-point scoring system (Jackman et al., 2009; Brait et al., 2010): 0, normal motor function; 1, flexion of torso and contralateral forelimb when mouse is lifted by the tail; 2, circling when mouse held by the tail on a flat surface; 3, leaning to the one side at rest; 4, no spontaneous motor activity; 5, death within 24 h. A hanging wire test was also performed in which mice were suspended from a wire 30 cm high for up to 180 s, and the average time of 3 trials with 5-min rest periods in between was recorded. Neurological assessment was evaluated by an observer blinded to experimental groups.

CEREBRAL INFARCT AND EDEMA VOLUMES

Mice were killed at 24 h by inhalation of isoflurane, followed by decapitation. The brains were immediately removed and snap frozen with liquid nitrogen. Coronal sections (30 μm) separated by ~420 μm were obtained and stained with thionin (0.1%) to delineate the infarct. Images of the sections were captured with a CCD camera mounted above a light box. Infarct volume was quantified as described previously (Jackman et al., 2009; Kim et al., 2012) using image analysis software (ImageJ, NIH, Bethesda, MD, USA), and corrected for brain edema, estimated using the following formula: corrected infarct volume = [left hemisphere area − (right hemisphere area − right hemisphere infarct area) × (thickness of section + distance between sections)] (Tsuchiya et al., 2003; Xia et al., 2006). Edema-corrected infarct volumes of individual brain sections were then added giving a three-dimensional approximation of the total infarct volume. Total, cortical and subcortical infarct volumes were quantified individually.

GROSS CEREBROVASCULAR ANATOMY

For gross comparison of cerebrovascular anatomy, some naïve animals ($n = 3$ of each strain, without any surgical procedures) were deeply anesthetized by inhalation of isoflurane, the thorax was opened and intracardial perfusion was performed with PBS, followed by 4% paraformaldehyde and finally 4% Evans blue solution in 20% gelatin.

FLOW CYTOMETRY

On each occasion when flow cytometry was utilized, we studied at least one post-stroke mouse together with a time-matched sham-operated control mouse of each strain. Animals were euthanized at 24 h by inhalation of isoflurane, followed by blood removal by cardiac puncture and the whole mouse was then intracardially perfused with phosphate-buffered saline (PBS) and brain, blood, and spleen were collected. Leukocytes were purified from blood using red blood cell lysis buffer (155 mmol/L NH_4Cl, 10 mmol/L $KHCO_3$, and 3 mmol/L EDTA). Spleens were mechanically dissociated and passed through 70 μm nylon cell strainers (BD Falcon, Bedford, MA, USA) to obtain a single-cell suspension. Cells were then lysed with red blood cell lysis buffer and washed with PBS containing 1% bovine serum albumin. The brain was removed from the skull and after removing the cerebellum and olfactory bulb, was separated into left (contralateral) and right (ischemic) hemispheres. Each hemisphere was dissociated mechanically in digestion buffer containing collagenase type XI (125 U/mL), hyaluronidase (60 U/mL), and collagenase type I-S (450 U/mL) in $Ca2^{+}/Mg2^{+}$-supplemented PBS (Sigma, St Louis, MO, USA), and incubated at 37°C for 30 min with gentle agitation. The mixture was then passed through 70 μm nylon cell strainers to obtain a single-cell suspension. After washing with PBS (1200 rpm, 10 min), the cell pellet was resuspended in 3 mL 30% percoll (GE Healthcare, Uppsala, Sweden), underlaid with 70% percoll, and centrifuged for 20 min at 2400 rpm at room temperature without the use of a brake. The cells at the interphase of two density gradients were collected and washed with PBS containing 1% bovine serum albumin (1200 rpm, 10 min) for staining. All cells were incubated with appropriate antibodies listed in **Table 1** at 4°C in darkness for 20 min. After staining, cells were analyzed by LSRII flow cytometer (BD Biosciences, Franklin Lakes, NJ, USA) and FlowJo software (Tree Star Inc., Ashland, OR, USA). Countbright counting beads (Invitrogen, Carlsbad, CA, USA) were included to define the absolute number of cells in the samples.

GATING STRATEGY

Single cells were identified by forward scatter, and dead cells (7-amino actinomycin D^{+}) were excluded. Cells were gated for $CD45^{+high}$ and $CD45^{+med}$ populations as described previously (Chu et al., 2014). $CD45^{+high}$ populations were then divided into lymphoid cells, which include: B cells ($B220^{+}$), T cells ($CD49b^{+}CD90^{-}NK1.1^{-}$), thymocytes ($CD49b^{-}CD90^{+}NK1.1^{-}$), NK cells ($CD49b^{+}CD90^{+}NK1.1^{+}$), and NKT cells ($CD49b^{+}CD90^{-}NK1.1^{+}$); and myeloid cells ($CD11b^{+}$). $CD45^{+med}CD11b^{+}F4/80^{+}$ cells were considered microglia. Two panels of antibodies were used, one of which was employed with each animal. Panel 1 enabled the counting of microglia and myeloid-derived leukocytes (i.e., $CD11b^{+}$ cells), which include: neutrophils ($Ly6G^{+}$), monocytes ($Ly6C^{+}$), macrophages ($F4/80^{+}$), and dendritic cells ($CD11c^{+}$); whereas Panel 2 divided lymphocytes into: B cells ($CD19^{+}$) and T cells ($CD3^{+}$). T cells were then further subdivided into $CD4^{+}$ T cells, $CD8^{+}$ T cells, $CD4^{-}CD8^{-}$ T cells, and $CD4^{+}CD25^{+}$ T cells. Fluorescence-minus-one were included as negative controls to define positive populations for F4/80, CD11c, Ly6C, CD19, CD3, and CD25.

Table 1 | Summary of antibodies used for flow cytometry.

Antigen	Host/Isotype	Supplier
CD8a-APC	Rat IgG2a, kappa	BD Phamingen
CD19-PE	Rat IgG2a, kappa	BioLegend
CD11c-Brilliant Violet 570	ArHam IgG	BioLegend
CD25-PE-Cy7	Rat IgG1, lambda	BioLegend
CD4-FITC	Rat IgG2b, kappa	BioLegend
CD45-APC-Cy7	Rat IgG2b, kappa	BioLegend
CD49b-PE	ArHam IgG	BioLegend
CD90.2-PE	Rat IgG2b, kappa	BioLegend
Ly6C-FITC	Rat IgG2c, kappa	BioLegend
Ly6G-PE-Cy7	Rat IgG2a, kappa	BioLegend
NK1.1-PE	Mouse IgG2a, kappa	BioLegend
CD11b-eFluro450	Rat IgG2b, kappa	eBioscience
CD3-eFluro450	Rat IgG2b, kappa	eBioscience
F4/80-APC	Rat IgG2a, kappa	eBioscience
7-Amino-actinomycin D (7AAD)		Invitrogen

CYTOKINE MEASUREMENT

Single-cell suspensions of brain, blood and spleen were obtained as described for flow cytometry. All cells were resuspended in complete RPMI 1640 media supplemented with heat inactivated fetal bovine serum (10% w/v), streptomycin and penicillin (100 U/mL), L-glutamine (1%) and 2-mercaptoethanol (50 mM). Blood and spleen cells were seeded at 200,000 cells/well in a 96-well plate coated with anti-CD3. All cells in the brain hemisphere were seeded. Blood, spleen, and contralateral brain hemisphere of sham-operated mice was seeded as unstimulated controls. Recombinant mouse IL-2 (20 ng/mL) was added and cells were incubated for 48 h at 37°C in a humidified atmosphere of 5% CO_2 in air. After stimulation, cells were spun down (15,000 rpm, 5 min) and supernatant was collected. Samples were analyzed for 7 key inflammatory cytokines (IL-4, IL-6, IL-10, IL-17A, IFN-γ, and TNF-α) using Cytometric Bead Array Mouse Th1/Th2/Th17 Cytokine kit (BD Biosciences, Franklin Lakes, NJ, USA). Samples and standards were prepared according to manufacturer's protocol. After adding capture beads, cells were analyzed by LSRII flow cytometer (BD Biosciences, Franklin Lakes, NJ, USA) and FCAP Array software (BD Biosciences, Franklin Lakes, NJ, USA).

STATISTICAL ANALYSIS

Values are presented as mean ± standard error. Results of the hanging wire test, infarct volume and flow cytometry, comparing C57Bl/6 and FVB sham- or stroke-operated mice, were analyzed using one-way analysis of variance with Bonferroni *post-hoc* test with selected multiple comparisons or a Student's unpaired *t*-test, as appropriate. The neurological deficit score was expressed as the median result per group and was analyzed using a Kruskal-Wallis test with Dunn's *post-hoc* test. A P value <0.05 was considered statistically significant. Statistical analyses were carried out using GraphPad Prism (GraphPad Software Inc, La Jolla, CA, USA).

RESULTS

CEREBRAL BLOOD FLOW PROFILE AND MORTALITY

CBF was similarly reduced by ~80% in both C57Bl/6 and FVB mice following insertion of the monofilament (**Figure 1A**). No significant differences in CBF profiles were observed between C57Bl/6 and FVB mice. Mortality rates at 24 h after cerebral ischemia were 8.8% (3/34) and 2.9% (1/34) in C57Bl/6 and FVB mice, respectively (**Figure 1B**). Mice of both strains had no significant differences in the cerebrovascular anatomy; in particular, the posterior communicating arteries were present in both strains (Supplementary Figure 1).

NEUROLOGICAL FUNCTION

Mice of both strains typically had no neurological deficit (score of 0) at 24 h after sham surgery (**Figure 1B**). Following cerebral ischemia, both C57Bl/6 and FVB mice had significant

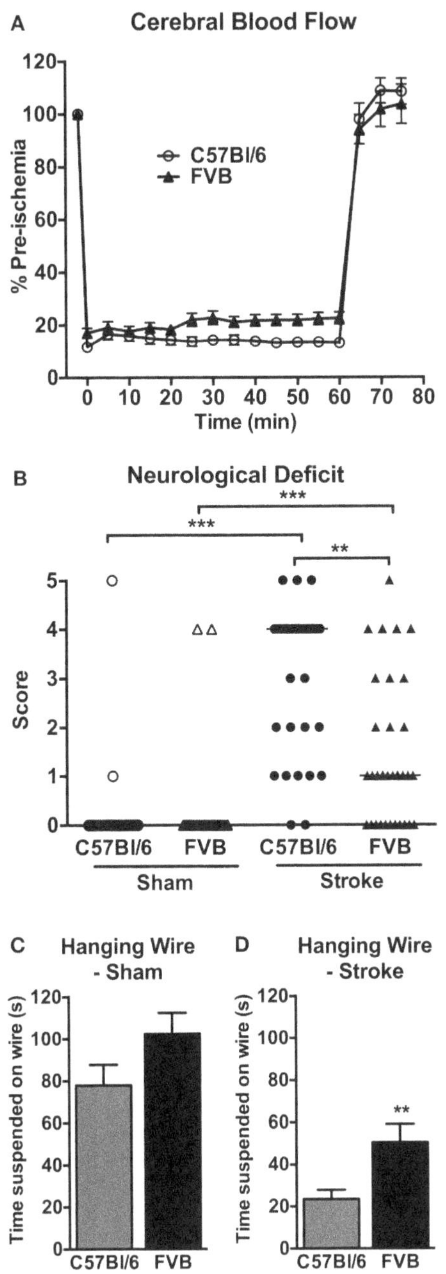

FIGURE 1 | (A) Regional cerebral blood flow during 1 h middle cerebral artery occlusion ($n = 30$–31); (B) neurological deficit ($n = 29$–34; $^{**}P < 0.01$, $^{***}P < 0.001$; Kruskal-Wallis with Dunn's post-tests) and (C,D) hanging wire performance ($n = 28$–33; $^{**}P < 0.01$; Student's unpaired t-test) at 24 h after cerebral ischemia. There was less functional impairment in FVB mice compared to C57Bl/6 mice. Data are mean ± s.e.m. in **(A,C,D)**, and are median scores in **(B)**.

neurological deficit compared to sham-operated mice of the same strain, although C57Bl/6 mice had greater deficit than FVB mice. Similarly, in the hanging wire test sham-operated C57Bl/6 and FVB mice achieved comparable hanging times (**Figure 1C**), whereas FVB mice achieved ~2-fold longer hanging times than C57Bl/6 mice at 24 h following cerebral ischemia (**Figure 1D**).

INFARCT AND EDEMA VOLUMES

Representative coronal sections of C57Bl/6 and FVB brains at 24 h after MCA occlusion are shown in **Figures 2A,B**, respectively. C57Bl/6 and FVB mice had similar total infarct (**Figure 2C**), cortical infarct (**Figure 2E**), subcortical infarct (**Figure 2F**) and edema (**Figure 2D**) volumes.

LEUKOCYTE INFILTRATION IN THE BRAIN

There was a ~4-fold increase in the total number of leukocytes in the ischemic hemisphere of C57Bl/6 mice compared to sham-operated mice ($P < 0.01$, **Figure 3A**). There also tended to be an increase in total leukocytes following ischemia in FVB mice, but there were ~40% fewer leukocytes than in C57Bl/6 mice (**Figure 3A**). Myeloid cells ($CD11b^+$), comprising neutrophils ($Ly6G^+$), dendritic cells ($CD11b^+CD11c^+$), macrophages ($F4/80^+$) and monocytes ($Ly6C^+$), were increased by a ~15-fold in the ischemic hemisphere of FVB mice to levels that were twice those in C57Bl/6 mice ($P < 0.01$, **Figure 3B**). By contrast, lymphoid cells were increased by 2–3-fold following ischemia in C57Bl/6 mice, whereas there was no change in lymphoid cell numbers in the brains of FVB mice following stroke (**Figure 3C**). No significant effect of stroke was observed in the number of microglia ($CD45^{+med}CD11b^+F4/80^+$) in either strain (**Figure 3D**).

Among myeloid cells, neutrophils were most prevalent, with these cells being ~4-fold more numerous in ischemic hemispheres of FVB than in C57Bl6 mice (**Figure 4A**). There was a similar profile of both macrophage and $Ly6C^{low}$ monocyte numbers in the ischemic brain following stroke, with also ~4-fold more of these cells in FVB than C57Bl/6 mice (**Figures 4B,C**). $Ly6C^{high}$ monocytes and total monocytes were present in similar numbers in the ischemic brains of the two strains (**Figures 4D,E**). In contrast, the number of dendritic cells in the ischemic hemisphere was ~3-fold higher in C57Bl/6 than FVB mice (**Figure 4F**).

Among lymphoid cells, there were marked increases in numbers of both B cells and T cells in the post-ischemic brain of C57Bl/6 mice but not FVB mice (**Figures 5A,B**). Further analysis of T cell subpopulations indicated that the increase in C57Bl/6 mice was mostly due to infiltration of $CD4^+CD25^-$ ("T helper") cells and not to $CD8^+$ ("cytotoxic") nor $CD4^+CD25^+$ T cells, which includes Tregs (**Figures 5C–E**).

Overall, despite similar compositions of immune cells in the brains of C57Bl/6 and FVB mice following sham surgery, there were marked differences between strains after stroke with lymphoid:myeloid cells representing ~80:20 in total (**Figure 6**). While a similar ratio persisted in C57Bl/6 mice after ischemia, there was a markedly different leukocyte composition in FVB mice after stroke, with a reversal of the lymphoid:myeloid ratio to ~20:80 (**Figure 6**). There were few differences in blood composition of leukocytes between strains or after stroke (**Figure 7**).

SPLENIC LEUKOCYTE NUMBERS

At 24 h after stroke there was a tendency for a reduction in the total number of splenic leukocytes in both mouse strains (**Figure 8A**). There were fewer splenic myeloid cells in FVB vs. C57Bl/6 mice, due to lower numbers of neutrophils and $Ly6C^{high}$ monocytes (**Figures 8B,D,G**), whereas there were higher

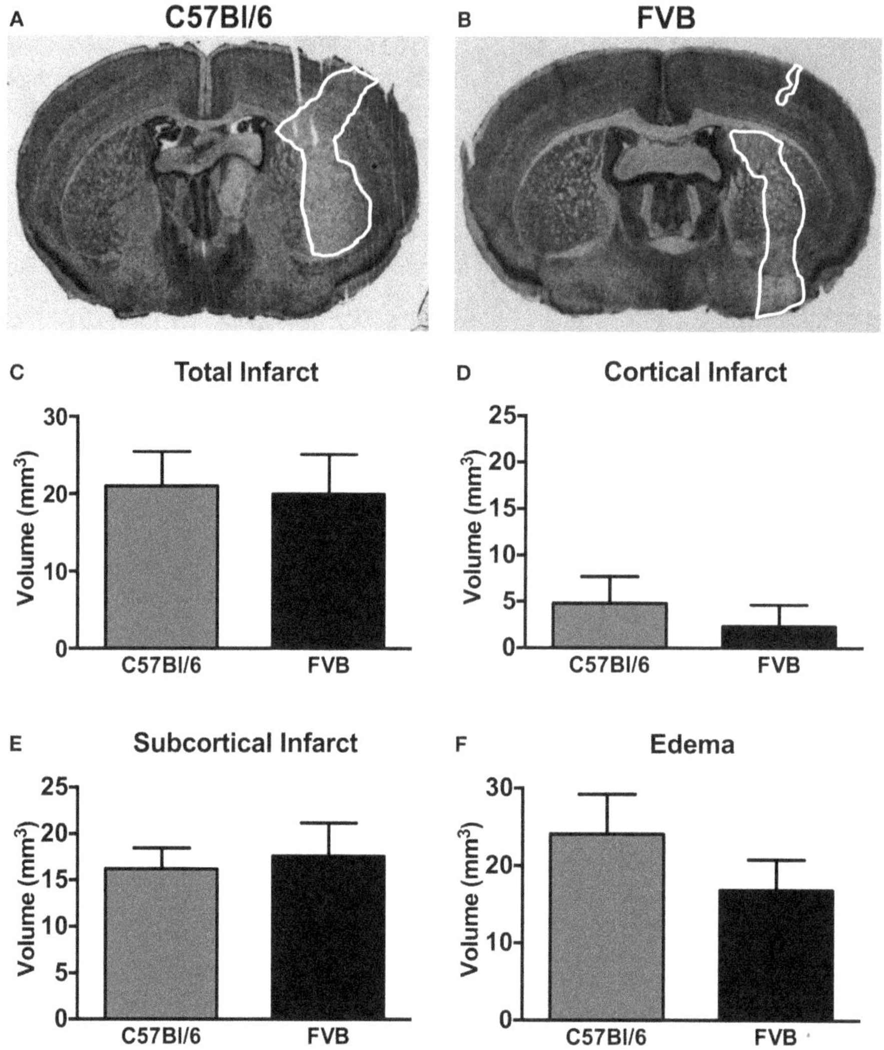

FIGURE 2 | Representative coronal brain sections from a (A) C57Bl/6 mouse and a (B) FVB mouse 24 h after 1 h middle cerebral artery occlusion (infarct areas are outlined in white). Infarct [**(C)**, total; **(D)**, cortical; **(E)**, subcortical] and **(F)** edema volumes are also shown ($n = 11$ per group; Student's unpaired *t*-test). There was no difference in the infarct volume between two strains of mice. Data are mean ± s.e.m.

numbers of $CD4^+$, $CD8^+$, and total T cells in that strain (**Figures 8J–L**). There was no significant reduction in any cell population (**Figures 8C,E,F,H,I**) except for 40–50% fewer T cells in FVB mice (**Figures 8J–L**). Consistent with these data, spleen weight was slightly reduced at 24 h after stroke in both strains, with the difference reaching statistical significance in FVB mice only (Supplementary Figure 2).

CYTOKINE LEVELS

Brain cytokine analysis at 24 h indicated that stroke resulted in substantially higher mean levels of IL-4, IL-6, TNF-α, IFN-γ, IL-10, and IL-17A in both C57Bl/6 and FVB mice (Supplementary Figure 3). There was a tendency for higher levels of IL-4, IL-6, TNF-α, and IFN-γ in the ischemic hemisphere of FVB than of C57Bl/6 (Supplementary Figure 3). There were no clear trends in cytokine levels in blood and spleen were generally similar in sham-operated mice of each strain, and there were no marked effects of stroke after 24 h in either strain (Supplementary Figures 4, 5).

DISCUSSION

There is growing evidence that T lymphocytes may influence the development of ischemic injury and functional deficit following experimental stroke (Iadecola and Anrather, 2011; Brait et al., 2012). For example, mice lacking T cells are reported to have smaller infarcts and improved functional outcome after focal ischemia compared to wild-type mice (Yilmaz et al., 2006; Hurn et al., 2007; Urra et al., 2009a; Kleinschnitz et al., 2013). Furthermore, there may be differential effects of $CD4^+$ T cell subsets on stroke outcome, such as exacerbation by Th1 cells and amelioration by Th2 cells of brain infarct development and functional deficit (Xiong et al., 2011; Gu et al., 2012). There is also clinical evidence that single nucleotide polymorphisms in the genes of Th1 and Th2 cytokines, and molecules that regulate

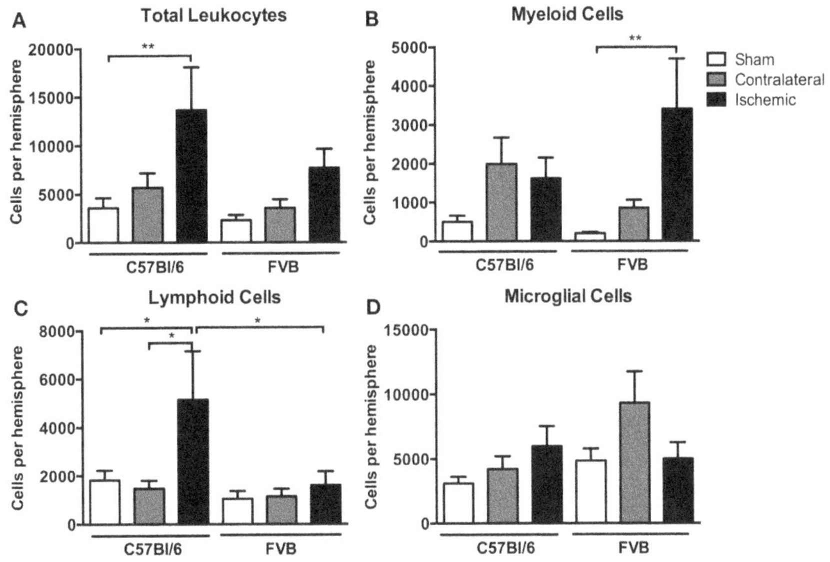

FIGURE 3 | Flow cytometric quantification of (A) total leukocytes and (B–D) leukocyte subsets in the brain at 24 h after 1 h middle cerebral artery occlusion. Data are shown for the contralateral and ischemic hemispheres, and compared with sham control mice of the same strain (n values: total leukocytes $n = 13$–16, subsets $n = 6$–9; $^*P < 0.05$, $^{**}P < 0.01$; One-Way ANOVA with Bonferroni post-tests). There was a greater number of leukocytes, predominantly lymphoid cells, infiltrating the brain of C57Bl/6 mice compared to FVB mice. Data are mean ± s.e.m.

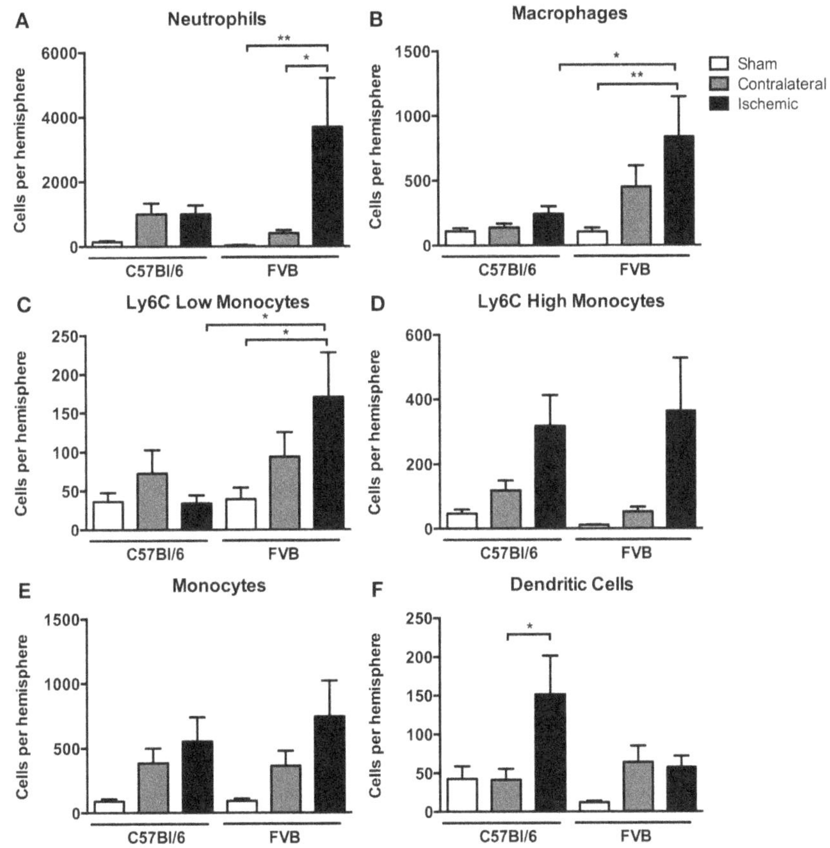

FIGURE 4 | Quantification of myeloid cell subpopulations [(A), neutrophils; (B), macrophages; (C), Ly6C low monocytes; (D), Ly6C high monocytes; (E), monocytes; (F), dendritic cells] in the brain 24 h after 1 h middle cerebral artery occlusion. Data are shown for the contralateral and ischemic hemispheres, and compared with sham control animals of the same strain ($n = 6$–9; $^*P < 0.05$, $^{**}P < 0.01$; One-Way ANOVA with Bonferroni post-tests). Data are mean ± s.e.m.

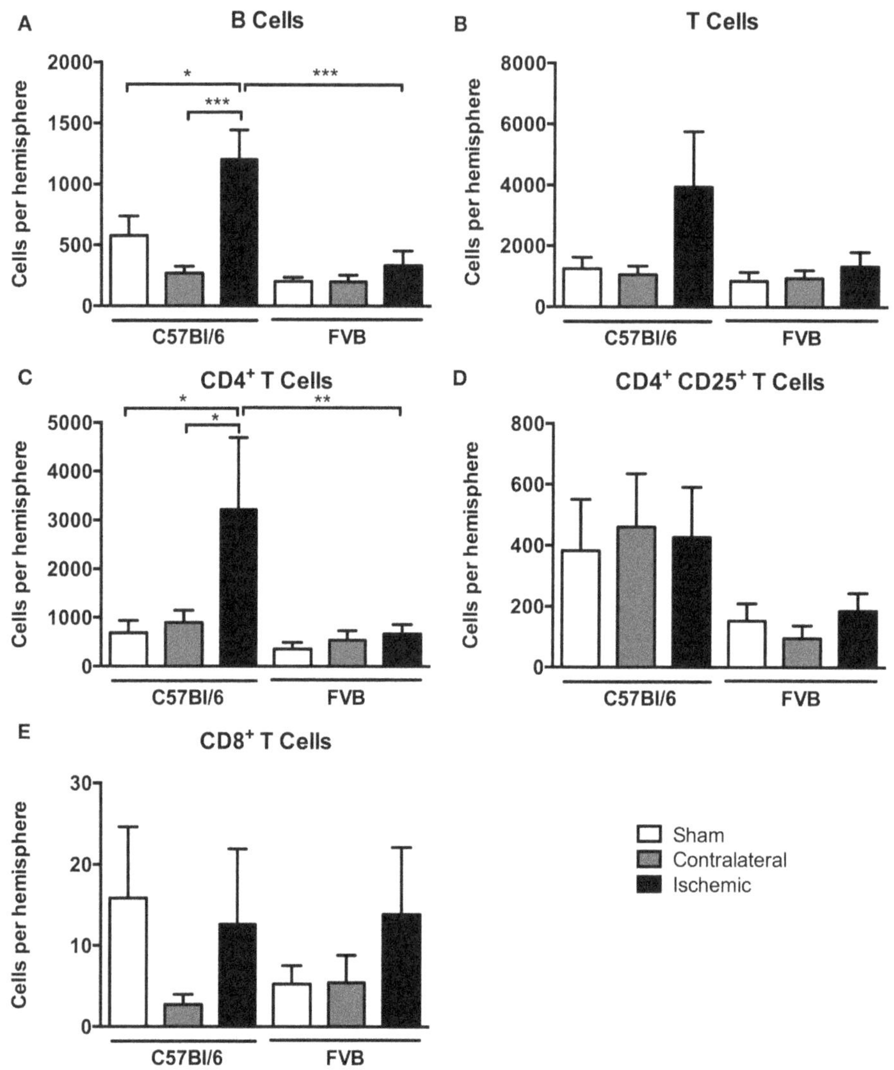

FIGURE 5 | Quantification of lymphocyte subpopulations [(A), B cells; (B), T cells; (C), CD4$^+$ T cells; (D), CD4$^+$ CD25$^+$ T cells; (E), CD8$^+$ T cells] in the brain 24 h after 1 h middle cerebral artery occlusion. Data are shown for the contralateral and ischemic hemispheres, and compared with sham control animals of the same strain ($n = 4$–8; $^*P < 0.05$, $^{**}P < 0.01$, $^{***}P < 0.001$; One-Way ANOVA with Bonferroni post-tests). Data are mean ± s.e.m.

their transcription rate or their functionality, may predispose to immune responses of differing strength and thus contribute to the risk of stroke (Marousi et al., 2008).

Our study has examined representative mouse strains commonly accepted as Th1-dominant (C57Bl/6) and Th2-dominant (FVB) (Whitehead et al., 2003) to investigate stroke outcome at 24 h in prototypical Th1- vs. Th2-prone immune environments, respectively. Our data generally support the concept that Th1-prone immunity in C57Bl/6 results in a more severe functional outcome after stroke compared to Th2-prone FVB mice. For example, spleen levels of IL-4 and IL-10 were 3–4-fold higher in control FVB vs. C57Bl/6 mice. Yet, with no significant differences in cerebrovascular anatomy, degree of ischemic insult caused by MCA occlusion, and ultimately in the developed infarct size between the two mouse strains, there was a markedly different profile of immune cell infiltration in the ischemic hemispheres of C57Bl/6 and FVB mice.

Despite a similar immune cell composition in the brains of sham-operated C57Bl/6 and FVB mice, which comprised myeloid and lymphoid cells in a ~20:80 ratio, after ischemia there was an overall increase in infiltrating cell numbers in both strains whereby this ratio was preserved in C57Bl/6 but was converted to ~80:20 in FVB mice. The magnitude of total leukocyte infiltration into the brain of C57Bl/6 was approximately twice that observed in FVB, and these strain differences occurred in the absence of any notable stroke-related systemic differences such as cell numbers, cell composition or cytokine profile in either blood or spleen. Striking increases were noted to occur particularly in the number of innate immune cells such as neutrophils, macrophages and LyC6^{+low} monocytes infiltrating the ischemic FVB brain, whereas the most prominent increases in C57Bl/6 mice occurred in the numbers of infiltrating T and B lymphocytes and dendritic cells—key cells for adaptive immunity. These responses were associated with some strain differences in the

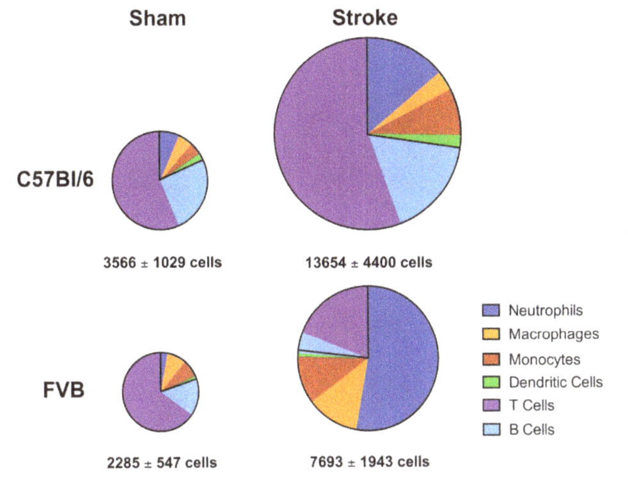

FIGURE 6 | Pie charts summarizing number and composition of immune cells in ischemic hemispheres of C57Bl/6 and FVB mice at 24 h after 1 h middle cerebral artery occlusion. The area of each pie is proportional to the number of leukocytes per hemisphere (also shown as mean ± s.e.m.; total leukocytes $n = 13–16$, myeloid cells $n = 6–9$, lymphocytes $n = 4–8$). There was a greater number of leukocytes, predominantly lymphoid cells, infiltrating the brain of C57Bl/6 mice compared to FVB mice.

mean levels of certain cytokines in the ischemic hemisphere, such as a tendency for larger amounts of both Th1 (IFN-γ, TNF-α) and Th2 (IL-4, IL-6) cytokines to be present in FVB than C57Bl/6 mice. However, it is not possible from the present data to discern whether these differences in brain cytokine levels may have been a cause or effect of the different post-ischemic immune cell profiles.

We found marked differences in neutrophil content of ischemic brains between FVB and C57Bl/6 mice. Clinical and experimental data suggest that neutrophils are the most abundant cell type in the brain after ischemia (Akopov et al., 1996; Gelderblom et al., 2009; Chu et al., 2014) and their accumulation is correlated with the severity of brain infarct and neurological deficit (Akopov et al., 1996). Activated neutrophils have been shown to promote the release of free radicals and cytokines, which further recruit leukocytes to the damaged area (Harris et al., 2005). However, it is controversial whether neutrophils contribute directly to secondary brain damage or have a mild neuroprotective role in cerebral ischemia. Animal studies have shown that increased infarct size is associated with neutrophil elimination (Takizawa et al., 2002) whilst others have shown that neutrophils may not contribute directly to infarct size (Beray-Berthat et al., 2003; Harris et al., 2005; Brait et al., 2011). Our data in FVB mice suggest that neutrophil number is not directly associated with infarct size in that a ~100-fold increase in brain infiltration after ischemia did not result in a bigger infarct size than in C57Bl/6 mice where the increase was markedly less. In previous study of parasite infection, neutrophils were found to play an early role in the induction of the Th2 response that develops in Th2-prone Balb/C mice but not in C57Bl/6 mice (Tacchini-Cottier et al., 2000). Thus, it is possible that the infiltration of neutrophils into the ischemic brains of FVB mice was associated with the induction of a less severe Th2-type immune response.

There were also markedly greater numbers of macrophages and Ly6C^{low} monocytes (the latter are considered to be anti-inflammatory) present in the FVB brains after cerebral ischemia. Macrophages and monocytes produce inflammatory cytokines and upregulate adhesion molecules in endothelial cells, thereby promoting neutrophil accumulation and migration (Chiba and Umegaki, 2013). Analogous to Th cells, macrophages are highly plastic cells and can polarize into two distinct activated macrophage subsets depending on the microenvironment (Kigerl et al., 2009). The classic or M1 activated cells are characterized by their capacity to present antigen, high production of nitric oxide and reactive oxygen species and of pro-inflammatory cytokines. In contrast, alternative or M2 activated cells are involved in scavenging of debris, angiogenesis, tissue remodeling and repair (Kigerl et al., 2009). Macrophages from Th1 strains (e.g., C57Bl/6, B10D2) are known to be more readily activated (e.g., to produce nitric oxide) than macrophages from Th2 strains (e.g., Balb/C, DBA/2) (Mills et al., 2000). Ly6C^{+low} monocytes are known to exhibit M2 characteristics (Geissmann et al., 2010). At the early stages following ischemic stroke, resident microglia and newly recruited macrophages appear to have a M2 phenotype that gradually transforms into an M1 phenotype in peri-infarct regions (Hu et al., 2012). It is possible that the greater number of macrophages and Ly6C^{+low} monocytes in FVB mice at 24 h after stroke represents more numerous M2-like cells contributing to a milder inflammatory environment in that strain. Further insight into the polarity of macrophages in FVB mice is needed.

We observed an increase in dendritic cells in the ischemic brain of C57Bl/6 mice at 24 h. Dendritic cells are involved in antigen presentation during immune cell activation and in the maintenance of peripheral tolerance through modulation of the immune response (Thompson and Thomas, 2002), but their role in outcome after cerebral ischemia is currently unclear.

There was a marked infiltration of lymphoid cells, particularly B and CD4$^+$ T cells (i.e., Th cells), into the ischemic hemisphere of C57Bl/6 mice. T lymphocytes enter the brain by 24 h after ischemic stroke (Gelderblom et al., 2009; Kleinschnitz et al., 2013; Chu et al., 2014), and both CD4$^+$ and CD8$^+$ T cells contribute to post-ischemic injury in mice (Arumugam et al., 2005; Kleinschnitz et al., 2013). It is conceivable that the infiltration of CD4$^+$ cells, which occurred selectively in C57Bl/6 mice following stroke, contributed to a more severe level of brain inflammation than in FVB mice despite a similar infarct volume. Tregs are a subset of CD4$^+$ T cells that are reported to play a protective, immunomodulatory role in the brain over several days after stroke (Liesz et al., 2009), but a detrimental role during more acute conditions (Kleinschnitz et al., 2013). We found no significant changes after stroke in either CD8$^+$ cells or CD4$^+$CD25$^+$ T cells, which will largely consist of Tregs.

Effects of B cells on stroke outcome are poorly understood. B cells can function as antigen-presenting cells to activate cytotoxic CD8$^+$ T cells, but there is also data to suggest that an IL-10-producing subpopulation of regulatory B cells may limit injury in experimental stroke (Ren et al., 2011; Bodhankar

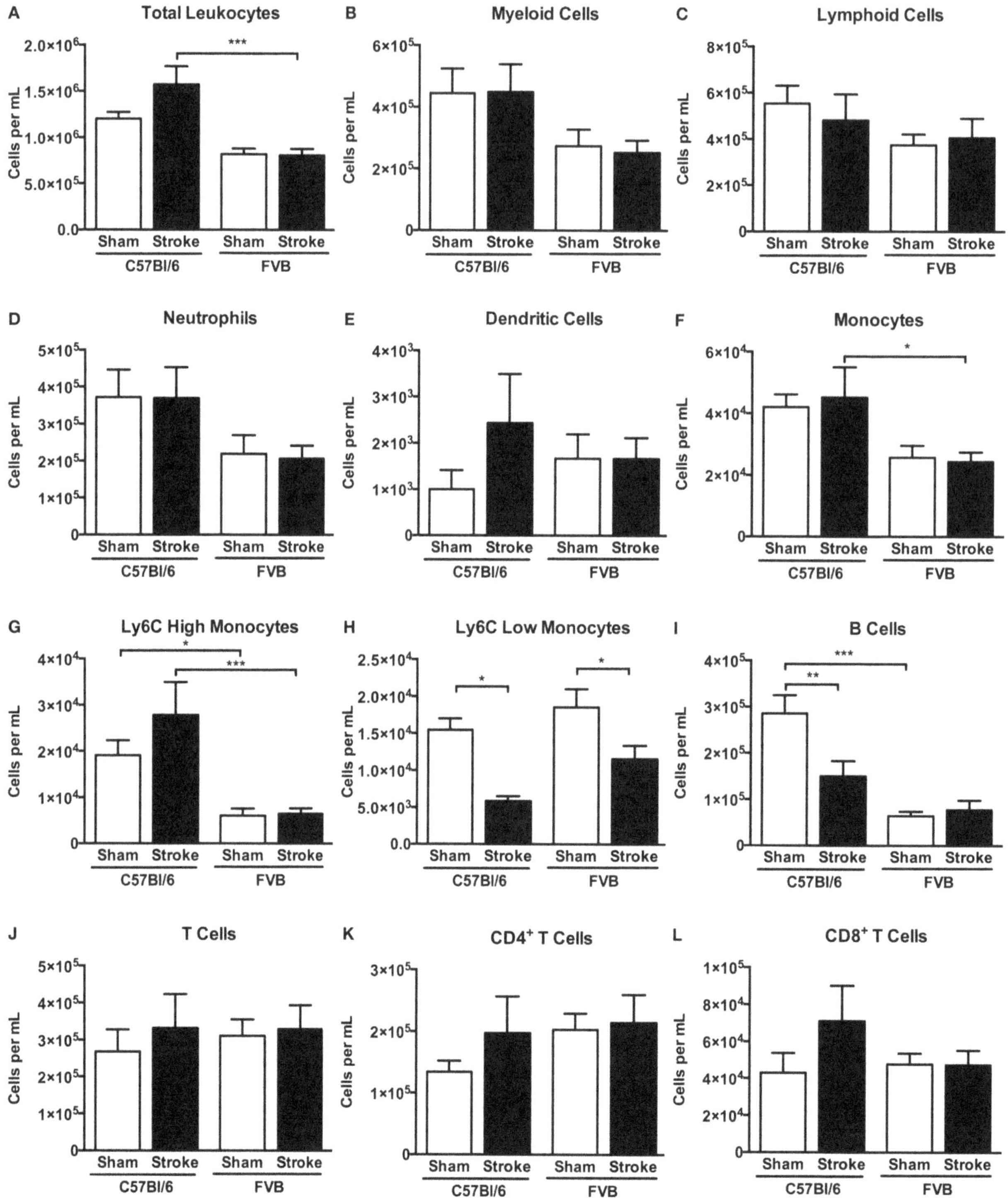

FIGURE 7 | Quantification of (A) total leukocytes and (B–L) leukocyte subsets in blood 24 h after 1 h middle cerebral artery occlusion, compared with sham control animals of the same strain (total leukocytes $n = 16–28$, myeloid cells $n = 9–17$, lymphocytes $n = 7–12$; $^*P < 0.05$, $^{**}P < 0.01$, $^{***}P < 0.001$; One-Way ANOVA with Bonferroni post-tests). Data are mean ± s.e.m.

et al., 2013). In addition, poor outcome in stroke patients is associated with reduced levels of circulating B cells (Urra et al., 2009b). Interestingly, we found that B cell infiltration into the brain following ischemia occurred selectively in C57Bl/6 mice (**Figure 5A**). Furthermore, whereas the number of circulating B cells was ~5-fold higher in control C57Bl/6 vs. FVB mice, stroke selectively reduced the number of B cells in the blood of the former strain (**Figure 7I**). Further study is necessary to clarify

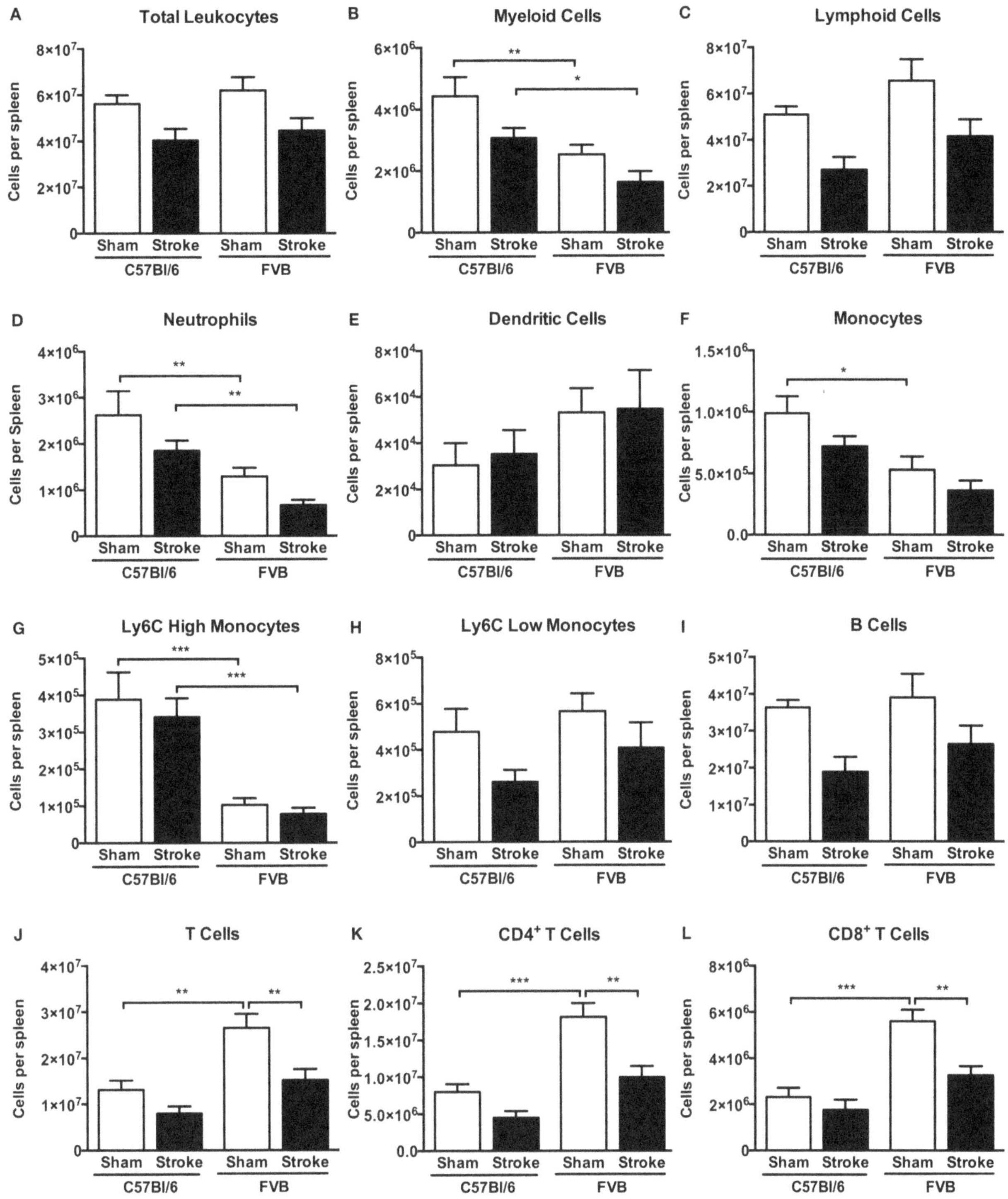

FIGURE 8 | Quantification of (A) total leukocytes and (B–L) leukocyte subsets in spleen 24 h after 1 h middle cerebral artery occlusion, compared with sham control animals of the same strain (total leukocytes $n = 17–29$, myeloid cells $n = 9–17$, lymphocytes $n = 6–12$; $^{*}P < 0.05$, $^{**}P < 0.01$, $^{***}P < 0.001$; One-Way ANOVA with Bonferroni post-tests). Data are mean ± s.e.m.

the importance of these strain differences in B cell number and distribution for stroke outcome.

In summary, we observed a profound difference in post-stroke functional outcome which was associated with a markedly contrasting number and composition of cells infiltrating the injured brain, despite similar systemic immune cell and cytokine profiles between the two mouse strains. The data therefore suggest that the nature of the inflammatory response to brain ischemia can vary considerably, and it may consequently impact the functional outcome independently of the volume of injured tissue. It would appear that the early infiltration into the ischemic brain tissue of certain innate/myeloid cell types, such as neutrophils, macrophages and Ly6C^{+low} monocytes, rather than cells of the adaptive immune system, such as B and T lymphocytes, may assist in achieving a milder level of functional deficit.

We acknowledge that while differences in biological responses between mouse strains that possess varying genetic and immunological profiles may provide a useful tool to gain some mechanistic insight into immune cell-mediated ischemic brain injury, studies of mice of the same genetic background are needed to provide definitive conclusions regarding these complex mechanisms. Moreover, if such findings are relevant for developing effective therapies for stroke patients, it will be interesting to determine whether individuals predisposed to Th2-prone immunity, including conditions such as asthma and allergy, might experience milder brain inflammation and functional deficit after stroke.

ACKNOWLEDGMENT

These studies were supported by Project Grants from the National Health and Medical Research Council of Australia (NHMRC) (ID 1010984 and 1064686). We also acknowledge support from an Australian Research Council Future Fellowship (TVA) and NHMRC Senior Research Fellowships (GRD and CGS).

REFERENCES

Abbas, A. K., Murphy, K. M., and Sher, A. (1996). Functional diversity of helper T lymphocytes. *Nature* 383, 787–793. doi: 10.1038/383787a0

Akopov, S. E., Simonian, N. A., and Grigorian, G. S. (1996). Dynamics of polymorphonuclear leukocyte accumulation in acute cerebral infarction and their correlation with brain tissue damage. *Stroke* 27, 1739–1743. doi: 10.1161/01.STR.27.10.1739

Arumugam, T., Granger, D. N., and Mattson, M. (2005). Stroke and T-cells. *Neuromolecular Med.* 7, 229–242. doi: 10.1385/NMM:7:3:229

Beray-Berthat, V., Palmier, B., Plotkine, M., and Margaill, I. (2003). Neutrophils do not contribute to infarction, oxidative stress, and NO synthase activity in severe brain ischemia. *Exp. Neurol.* 182, 446–454. doi: 10.1016/S0014-4886(03)00106-7

Bodhankar, S., Chen, Y., Vandenbark, A., Murphy, S., and Offner, H. (2013). IL-10-producing B-cells limit CNS inflammation and infarct volume in experimental stroke. *Metab. Brain Dis.* 28, 375–386. doi: 10.1007/s11011-013-9413-3

Brait, V. H., Arumugam, T. V., Drummond, G. R., and Sobey, C. G. (2012). Importance of T lymphocytes in brain injury, immunodeficiency, and recovery after cerebral ischemia. *J. Cereb. Blood Flow Metab.* 32, 598–611. doi: 10.1038/jcbfm.2012.6

Brait, V. H., Rivera, J., Broughton, B. R. S., Lee, S., Drummond, G. R., and Sobey, C. G. (2011). Chemokine-related gene expression in the brain following ischemic stroke: no role for CXCR2 in outcome. *Brain Res.* 1372, 169–179. doi: 10.1016/j.brainres.2010.11.087

Brait, V., Jackman, K., Walduck, A., Selemidis, S., Diep, H., Mast, A., et al. (2010). Mechanisms contributing to cerebral infarct size after stroke: gender, reperfusion, T lymphocytes, and Nox2-derived superoxide. *J. Cereb. Blood Flow Metab.* 30, 1306–1307. doi: 10.1038/jcbfm.2010.14

Chiba, T., and Umegaki, K. (2013). Pivotal Roles of Monocytes/Macrophages in Stroke. *Mediators Inflamm.* 2013, 10. doi: 10.1155/2013/759103

Chu, H. X., Kim, H. A., Lee, S., Moore, J. P., Chan, C. T., Vinh, A., et al. (2014). Immune cell infiltration in malignant middle cerebral artery infarction: comparison with transient cerebral ischemia. *J. Cereb. Blood Flow Metab.* 34, 450–459. doi: 10.1038/jcbfm.2013.217

Geissmann, F., Manz, M., Jung, S., Sieweke, M., Merad, M., and Ley, K. (2010). Development of monocytes, macrophages, and dendritic cells. *Science* 327, 656–661. doi: 10.1126/science.1178331

Gelderblom, M., Leypoldt, F., Steinbach, K., Behrens, D., Choe, C.-U., Siler, D. A., et al. (2009). Temporal and spatial dynamics of cerebral immune cell accumulation in stroke. *Stroke* 40, 1849–1857. doi: 10.1161/STROKEAHA.108.534503

Go, A. S., Mozaffarian, D., Roger, V. L., Benjamin, E. J., Berry, J. D., Blaha, M. J., et al. (2013). Heart disease and stroke statistics—2014 update: a report from the American Heart Association. *Circulation* 129, e28–e292. doi: 10.1161/CIR.0b013e31828124ad

Gravanis, I., and Tsirka, S. (2008). Tissue-type plasminogen activator as a therapeutic target in stroke. *Expert Opin. Ther. Targets* 12, 59–70. doi: 10.1517/14728222.12.2.159

Gu, L., Xiong, X., Zhang, H., Xu, B., Steinberg, G. K., and Zhao, H. (2012). Distinctive effects of T cell subsets in neuronal injury induced by cocultured splenocytes *in vitro* and by *in vivo* stroke in mice. *Stroke* 43, 1941–1946. doi: 10.1161/STROKEAHA.112.656611

Harris, A., Ergul, A., Kozak, A., Machado, L., Johnson, M., and Fagan, S. (2005). Effect of neutrophil depletion on gelatinase expression, edema formation and hemorrhagic transformation after focal ischemic stroke. *BMC Neurosci.* 6:49. doi: 10.1186/1471-2202-6-49

Hu, X., Li, P., Guo, Y., Wang, H., Leak, R. K., Chen, S., et al. (2012). Microglia/macrophage polarization dynamics reveal novel mechanism of injury expansion after focal cerebral ischemia. *Stroke* 43, 3063–3070. doi: 10.1161/STROKEAHA.112.659656

Hurn, P. D., Subramanian, S., Parker, S. M., Afentoulis, M. E., Kaler, L. J., Vandenbark, A. A., et al. (2007). T- and B-cell-deficient mice with experimental stroke have reduced lesion size and inflammation. *J. Cereb. Blood Flow Metab.* 27, 1798–1805. doi: 10.1038/sj.jcbfm.9600482

Iadecola, C., and Anrather, J. (2011). The immunology of stroke: from mechanisms to translation. *Nat. Med.* 17, 796–808. doi: 10.1038/nm.2399

Jackman, K., Miller, A., De Silva, T., Crack, P., Drummond, G., and Sobey, C. (2009). Reduction of cerebral infarct volume by apocynin requires pretreatment and is absent in Nox2-deficient mice. *Br. J. Pharmacol.* 156, 680–688. doi: 10.1111/j.1476-5381.2008.00073.x

Jin, R., Yang, G., and Li, G. (2010). Inflammatory mechanisms in ischemic stroke: role of inflammatory cells. *J. Leukoc. Biol.* 87, 779–789. doi: 10.1189/jlb.1109766

Kigerl, K. A., Gensel, J. C., Ankeny, D. P., Alexander, J. K., Donnelly, D. J., and Popovich, P. G. (2009). Identification of two distinct macrophage subsets with divergent effects causing either neurotoxicity or regeneration in the injured mouse spinal cord. *J. Neurosci.* 29, 13435–13444. doi: 10.1523/JNEUROSCI.3257-09.2009

Kilkenny, C., Browne, W., Cuthill, I. C., Emerson, M., and Altman, D. G. (2010). Animal research: reporting *in vivo* experiments: the ARRIVE guidelines. *J. Gene. Med.* 12, 561–563. doi: 10.1002/jgm.1473

Kim, H. A., Brait, V. H., Lee, S., De Silva, T. M., Diep, H., Eisenhardt, A., et al. (2012). Brain infarct volume after permanent focal ischemia is not dependent on Nox2 expression. *Brain Res.* 1483, 105–111. doi: 10.1016/j.brainres.2012.09.023

Kleinschnitz, C., Kraft, P., Dreykluft, A., Hagedorn, I., Göbel, K., Schuhmann, M. K., et al. (2013). Regulatory T cells are strong promoters of acute ischemic stroke in mice by inducing dysfunction of the cerebral microvasculature. *Blood* 121, 679–691. doi: 10.1182/blood-2012-04-426734

Kleinschnitz, C., Schwab, N., Kraft, P., Hagedorn, I., Dreykluft, A., Schwarz, T., et al. (2010). Early detrimental T-cell effects in experimental cerebral ischemia are neither related to adaptive immunity nor thrombus formation. *Blood* 115, 3835–3842. doi: 10.1182/blood-2009-10-249078

Liesz, A., Suri-Payer, E., Veltkamp, C., Doerr, H., Sommer, C., Rivest, S., et al. (2009). Regulatory T cells are key cerebroprotective immunomodulators in acute experimental stroke. *Nat. Med.* 15, 192–199. doi: 10.1038/nm.1927

Marousi, S., Ellul, J., and Karakantza, M. (2008). Genetic polymorphisms of Type-1 and Type-2 inflammatory cytokines in ischaemic stroke. *Vasc. Dis. Prev.* 5, 89–103. doi: 10.2174/156727008784223981

Mills, C. D., Kincaid, K., Alt, J. M., Heilman, M. J., and Hill, A. M. (2000). M-1/M-2 macrophages and the Th1/Th2 paradigm. *J. Immunol.* 164, 6166–6173. doi: 10.4049/jimmunol.164.12.6166

Ren, X., Akiyoshi, K., Dziennis, S., Vandenbark, A., Herson, P., Hurn, P., et al. (2011). Regulatory B cells limit CNS inflammation and neurologic deficits in murine experimental stroke. *J. Neurosci.* 8, 8556–8563. doi: 10.1523/JNEUROSCI.1623-11.2011

Tacchini-Cottier, F., Zweifel, C., Belkaid, Y., Mukankundiye, C., Vasei, M., Launois, P., et al. (2000). An immunomodulatory function for neutrophils during the induction of a $CD4^+$ Th2 response in BALB/c mice infected with *Leishmania major*. *J. Immunol.* 165, 2628–2636. doi: 10.4049/jimmunol.165.5.2628

Takizawa, S., Aratani, Y., Fukuyama, N., Maeda, N., Hirabayashi, H., Koyama, H., et al. (2002). Deficiency of myeloperoxidase increases infarct volume and nitrotyrosine formation in mouse brain. *J. Cereb. Blood Flow Metab.* 22, 50–54. doi: 10.1097/00004647-200201000-00006

Thompson, A. G., and Thomas, R. (2002). Induction of immune tolerance by dendritic cells: implications for preventative and therapeutic immunotherapy of autoimmune disease. *Immunol. Cell Biol.* 80, 509–519. doi: 10.1046/j.1440-1711.2002.01114.x

Tsuchiya, D., Hong, S., Kayama, T., Panter, S. S., and Weinstein, P. R. (2003). Effect of suture size and carotid clip application upon blood flow and infarct volume after permanent and temporary middle cerebral artery occlusion in mice. *Brain Res.* 970, 131–139. doi: 10.1016/S0006-8993(03)02300-X

Urra, X., Cervera, A., Villamor, N., Planas, A. M., and Chamorro, A. (2009a). Harms and benefits of lymphocyte subpopulations in patients with acute stroke. *Neuroscience* 158, 1174–1183. doi: 10.1016/j.neuroscience.2008.06.014

Urra, X., Villamor, N., Amaro, S., Gomez-Choco, M., Obach, V., Oleaga, L., et al. (2009b). Monocyte subtypes predict clinical course and prognosis in human stroke. *J. Cereb. Blood Flow Metab.* 29, 994–1002. doi: 10.1038/jcbfm.2009.25

Whitehead, G. S., Walker, J. K. L., Berman, K. G., Foster, W. M., and Schwartz, D. A. (2003). Allergen-induced airway disease is mouse strain dependent. *Am. J. Physiol. Lung Cell. Mol. Physiol.* 285, L32–L42. doi: 10.1152/ajplung.00390.2002

Xia, C.-F., Smith, R. S., Shen, B., Yang, Z.-R., Borlongan, C. V., Chao, L., et al. (2006). Postischemic brain injury is exacerbated in mice lacking the kinin B2 receptor. *Hypertension* 47, 752–761. doi: 10.1161/01.HYP.0000214867.35632.0e

Xiong, X., Barreto, G. E., Xu, L., Ouyang, Y. B., Xie, X., and Giffard, R. G. (2011). Increased brain injury and worsened neurological outcome in interleukin-4 knockout mice after transient focal cerebral ischemia. *Stroke* 42, 2026–2032. doi: 10.1161/STROKEAHA.110.593772

Yilmaz, G., Arumugam, T. V., Stokes, K. Y., and Granger, D. N. (2006). Role of T lymphocytes and interferon-γ in ischemic stroke. *Circulation* 113, 2105–2112. doi: 10.1161/CIRCULATIONAHA.105.593046

14

Role of the kallikrein–kinin system in traumatic brain injury

Christiane Albert-Weissenberger[1]*, Stine Mencl[1], Sarah Hopp[1], Christoph Kleinschnitz[1†] and Anna-Leena Sirén[2†]

[1] *Department of Neurology, University Hospital of Würzburg, Würzburg, Germany*
[2] *Department of Neurosurgery, University Hospital of Würzburg, Würzburg, Germany*

***Correspondence:**
*Christiane Albert-Weissenberger, Department of Neurology, University Hospital of Würzburg, Josef-Schneider-Str. 11, 97080 Würzburg, Germany
e-mail: Albert_c2@ukw.de*

† These authors have contributed equally to this work.

Traumatic brain injury (TBI) is a major cause of mortality and morbidity worldwide. Despite improvements in acute intensive care, there are currently no specific therapies to ameliorate the effects of TBI. Successful therapeutic strategies for TBI should target multiple pathophysiologic mechanisms that occur at different stages of brain injury. The kallikrein–kinin system is a promising therapeutic target for TBI as it mediates key pathologic events of traumatic brain damage, such as edema formation, inflammation, and thrombosis. Selective and specific kinin receptor antagonists and inhibitors of plasma kallikrein and coagulation factor XII have been developed, and have already shown therapeutic efficacy in animal models of stroke and TBI. However, conflicting preclinical evaluation, as well as limited and inconclusive data from clinical trials in TBI, suggests that caution should be taken before transferring observations made in animals to humans. This review summarizes current evidence on the pathologic significance of the kallikrein–kinin system during TBI in animal models and, where available, the experimental findings are compared with human data.

Keywords: traumatic brain injury, kallikrein–kinin system, bradykinin, factor XII, kinin receptor

INTRODUCTION

Traumatic brain injury (TBI) accounts for one-third of all injury-related deaths. An estimated 1.74 million TBIs occur annually in the United States (Faul et al., 2010; Ma et al., 2014). About 43% of people discharged with TBI after acute hospitalization, develop TBI-related long-term disability. Moreover, individuals with a history of TBI are more likely to receive welfare or disability payments and to develop neurologic disorders that are disabling in their own right (Ma et al., 2014)— for example, Alzheimer's disease (Fleminger et al., 2003). The incidence of TBI is particularly high in younger age groups, with motor vehicle accidents being the leading cause (Asemota et al., 2013). The direct costs of TBI have been estimated at \$13.1 billion per year (in 2013) in the United States (Ma et al., 2014); additionally, \$64.7 billion per year are lost through missed work and lost productivity, and total medical costs range from \$63.4 to \$79.1 billion per year (Ma et al., 2014). The significant economic impact of TBI is at variance with the lack of therapies available to ameliorate the effects of TBI.

To better understand the pathobiology of TBI and to evaluate potential therapeutic approaches, various animal models have been developed to mimic certain components of clinical TBI. Closed-head weight-drop models—with a weight that falls onto the exposed skull—probably mimic most closely clinical TBI cases. Depending on the experimental settings, the impact of the weight results in largely focal or diffuse brain injury. In controlled cortical impact models an impact onto the dura, inflicted by a pneumatic pistol, predominantly results in focal brain injury. For fluid percussion models it is inconsistently reported to what extend the brain injury is diffuse or focal. Here, tissue damage is induced by a fluid pulse onto the intact dura through a craniotomy. A solely focal brain injury can be achieved by cold lesion models, which commonly utilize a cold rod that is exposed to the dura or skull (for a comprehensive review, see Albert-Weissenberger and Sirén, 2010). Despite promising results from these experimental TBI models, more than 30 phase III trials of TBI in humans have failed to generate favorable results in terms of developing potential therapeutic strategies (Doppenberg et al., 2004; Maas et al., 2010). In part, these failures likely reflect the heterogeneity of TBI (e.g., severity and location of the injury—focal vs. diffuse injury). Therefore, future therapeutic approaches are more likely to succeed if they target diverse pathophysiologic mechanisms. As the kallikrein–kinin system links edema formation, inflammation, and thrombosis (Costa-Neto et al., 2008; Langhauser et al., 2012), it seems to be a promising target.

In this review, current available evidence on the pathologic significance of the kallikrein–kinin system during TBI is summarized. Findings from experimental models are compared with human data, where available.

THE KALLIKREIN–KININ SYSTEM

Kinins play key roles in regulating vascular permeability and inflammatory processes following tissue injury (Leeb-Lundberg et al., 2005). They are released either by the tissue or the plasma. In the tissue, kallikrein is activated by proteases and it releases a kinin called kallidin from the inactive precursors, the kininogens. Plasma kallikrein is released from prekallikrein by activated factor XII (FXII) and reciprocally activates FXII (Revak et al., 1978). Subsequently, plasma kallikrein releases bradykinin from

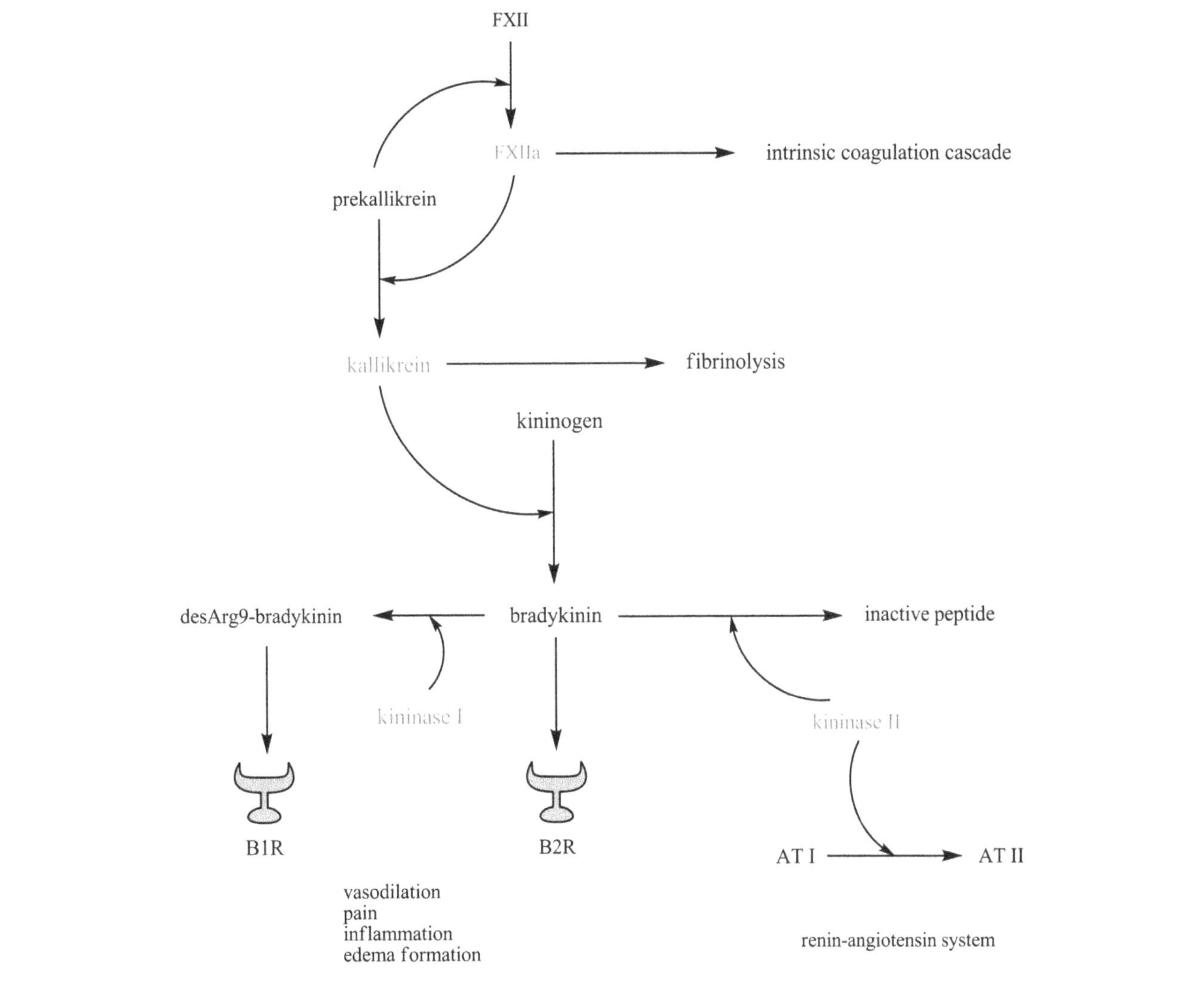

FIGURE 1 | The plasma kallikrein–kinin system is linked to thrombosis, fibrinolysis, and the renin–angiotensin system. Abbreviations: AT, angiotensin; B1R, kinin receptor B1; B2R, kinin receptor B2; FXII, factor XII; FXIIa, activated factor XII.

the kininogens. Kallidin and bradykinin mediate their effects via kinin receptor B2. Both kallidin and bradykinin are converted by the action of kininase I-type carboxypeptidases into des-Arg9-bradykinin and des-Arg10-kallidin, respectively, which specifically bind to kinin receptor B1 (**Figure 1**).

Interestingly, the plasma kallikrein–kinin system is linked to thrombosis, fibrinolysis, and the renin–angiotensin system: FXII has an essential role in thrombosis (Renné et al., 2012), and mice selectively depleted of plasma kallikrein or FXII are protected from pathogenic thrombus formation without increased risk of bleeding (Revenko et al., 2011). Plasma kallikrein (and, to a lesser extent, activated FXII) converts plasminogen to plasmin, linking the kallikrein–kinin system to fibrinolysis (Colman, 1969). In addition, bradykinin is mainly inactivated by kininase II (also known as angiotensin converting enzyme (ACE)), an enzyme that also degrades angiotensin I into angiotensin II (Bernstein et al., 2011; **Figure 1**).

ROLE OF THE KININ RECEPTORS IN TRAUMATIC BRAIN INJURY

All essential components of the kallikrein–kinin system are present in the rodent and human brain (Kariya et al., 1985; Kizuki et al., 1994; Ongali et al., 2003; Trabold et al., 2010). Moreover, it has been reported that their expression is induced after brain injury but the expression pattern varies depending on the brain injury model used (Ongali et al., 2006; Raslan et al., 2010; Trabold et al., 2010; Albert-Weissenberger et al., 2012). In a controlled cortical impact model, bradykinin concentrations in the brain were significantly increased at 2 h post-injury, and then subsequently declined (Trabold et al., 2010). Kinin receptor B1 transcripts peaked at 6 h post-injury and remained elevated until day 2, whereas kinin receptor B2 was constitutively expressed at lower levels (Trabold et al., 2010). In a cold lesion model, a strong but transient mRNA expression of kinin receptor B1 was observed in the first 12 h after injury, whereas the enhanced mRNA expression of kinin receptor B2 was more sustained, lasting up to 48 h (Raslan et al., 2010). In our hand, a closed-head weight-drop trauma in mice resulting in a mixed brain injury pattern (focal and diffuse brain injury) caused a slight increase of kinin receptor mRNA levels one week after injury induction (Albert-Weissenberger et al., 2012).

Kinins mediate their physiologic effects via kinin receptors B1 and B2. Support for a pathologic role of kinin receptors in TBI was obtained through the use of genetically engineered mice that lack either kinin receptor B1 or kinin receptor B2. After controlled cortical impact, kinin receptor B2-deficient mice, but not kinin receptor B1-deficient mice, had less brain edema, smaller lesion volumes, and a better functional outcome as compared with wild-type mice (Trabold et al., 2010). Another study also reported that the kinin receptor B2 mediates detrimental effects after TBI in mice (Hellal et al., 2003). On the contrary, findings from our group point out that kinin receptor B1 plays an important role in the pathophysiology of TBI (Raslan et al., 2010). Kinin receptor B1-deficient mice subjected to cold lesion displayed smaller lesion volumes, less blood–brain barrier disruption, and less inflammation in the injured brain area, whereas kinin receptor B2-deficient mice were fully susceptible to brain trauma. Supporting these results, application of the kinin receptor B1-inhibitor R-715 reduced lesion size even in a therapeutic setting (administered 1 h after injury induction), whereas application of the kinin receptor B2-inhibitor Hoe140 (Icatibant) had no significant effect on lesion volume in wild-type mice (Raslan et al., 2010). Importantly, application of the kinin receptor B2-inhibitor Hoe140 in kinin receptor B1-deficient mice had no additive benefit on the reduction in brain lesion size. However, Hoe140 treatment has been shown to result in a moderate reduction in brain lesion size after cold lesion in rats and mice (by 19% and 14%, respectively) (Görlach et al., 2001). We recently reported that kinin receptor B1 deficiency in mice is associated with diminished functional deficits and a reduction in axonal injury, astrogliosis, and neuronal apoptosis after a weight-drop-induced brain trauma (Albert-Weissenberger et al., 2012). Inhibition of kinin receptor B1 in wild-type mice by the specific kinin receptor B1-blocker R-715, starting from 1 h after trauma, confirmed these results. By contrast, deficiency of kinin receptor B2 was ineffective in this trauma model (Albert-Weissenberger et al., 2012).

Kinin receptor inhibitors, other than the kinin receptor B1-inhibitor R-715 and the kinin receptor B2-inhibitor Hoe140, have also been tested in experimental and clinical settings of TBI. Treatment with the kinin receptor B2-antagonist LF 18-1505T resulted in reduced brain edema and improved neurologic outcome in a closed-head trauma model in rats (Ivashkova et al., 2006). In rats subjected to closed-head trauma, a continuous infusion of the nonpeptide kinin receptor B2-inhibitor LF 16-0687 (Anatibant), from 1 h to 24 h after injury, resulted in diminished brain edema formation on day 1 and less neurologic deficits on day 1, day 3, and day 7 (Pruneau et al., 1999). Administered as a single dose 1 h after trauma, LF 16-0687 was able to reduce brain swelling and to improve the recovery of neurologic function following closed-head trauma in rats (Kaplanski et al., 2002). Similar results were obtained after controlled cortical impact or cold lesion (Schulz et al., 2000; Stover et al., 2000; Zweckberger and Plesnila, 2009). It was suggested that stabilization of the blood–brain barrier and mitigation of inflammatory processes are the underlying mechanisms. However, it remains questionable whether LF 16-0687 is effective within a clinically relevant time window (Plesnila et al., 2001). LF 16-0687 was investigated in a phase I clinical study (Marmarou et al., 2005) in patients with severe TBI. In this trial, patients with TBI and Glasgow Coma Scale <8 received LF 16-0687 as a single subcutaneous injection within 8–12 h after TBI, and Marmarou et al. concluded that LF 16-0687 provides a potential therapeutic approach to treating cerebral edema following brain damage, as the compound was well tolerated. A phase II trial using LF 16-0687 in TBI patients with a Glasgow Coma Scale score of ≤ 12 was unable to recruit a sufficient number of patients (Shakur et al., 2009). Moreover, results from this trial were disappointing in that there was a non-significant trend towards worse outcomes in the LF 16-0687 treatment group.

Bradycor (Deltibant, CP-0127), a peptide compound kinin receptor B2-antagonist, was tested in a pilot, single-blinded clinical pilot study in 20 patients with focal head injury. Results indicated that CP-0127 treatment diminished the pathologic rise of intracranial pressure (Narotam et al., 1998). A phase II trial in severely brain injured patients reported a slight trend towards a better outcome in the CP-0127 treatment group (Marmarou et al., 1999). However, a Cochrane analysis concluded that those clinical trials do not provide reliable evidence that kinin receptor B2-antagonists are effective in improving outcome after TBI (Ker and Blackhall, 2008). Reports on the clinical use of kinin receptor B1-inhibitors in patients with TBI are not yet available.

ROLE OF THE KALLIKREINS AND FACTOR XII IN TRAUMATIC BRAIN INJURY

In 1978, it was reported that patients with severe trauma have increased protease activity in the cerebrospinal fluid, the activity of which could be inhibited by aprotinin treatment. In rabbits subjected to cold injury, aprotinin treatment resulted in reduced brain edema formation (Unterberg et al., 1986). Aprotinin is known to inhibit several serine proteases, including plasma kallikrein, and a reduced protease activity has been associated with a lower mortality rate (Auer et al., 1979).

There are promising results from recent studies suggesting a therapeutic potential for the serine protease inhibitor C1-inhibitor. C1-inhibitor is an endogenous regulator with various physiologic functions (Singer and Jones, 2011), including the inhibition of activated FXII and plasma kallikrein. Application of C1-inhibitor has proven to be beneficial in ischemic stroke (Heydenreich et al., 2012). Similarly, in mice subjected to controlled cortical impact, C1-inhibitor treatment at 10 min (Longhi et al., 2008) or 1 h (Longhi et al., 2009) after injury resulted in less pronounced functional deficits and smaller brain lesions compared with control mice.

ROLE OF THE KININASE II IN TRAUMATIC BRAIN INJURY

Indirect support for a pathologic role of kinins in TBI was obtained through inhibition of kininase II, an enzyme that hydrolyzes proteins such as bradykinin, substance P, and angiotensin I. Inhibition of kininase II results in downregulation of angiotensin II production. Moreover, it has been reported that kininase II inhibition potentiates the physiologic effects of kinins and all kinin-related peptides are subject to less hydrolyzation. Using the kininase II inhibitor Captopril, Harford-Wright et al. (2010) showed, in a diffuse TBI model, that inhibition of kininase II results in increased "dark cell changes" and in exacerbated motor function deficits. However, they did not consider the effects of kininase II inhibition on the kallikrein–kinin system; instead, the authors conclude that kininase II inhibitors worsen outcome following TBI, presumably because they impair the degradation of substance P—as shown by the increase in substance P immunoreactivity. However, the fact that bradykinin potentiates the release of substance P should also be noted (for a review, see Geppetti, 1993). Interestingly, a kininase II polymorphism in humans influences the neuropsychologic subacute performance of patients with moderate or severe TBI (Ariza et al., 2006).

PERSPECTIVE

There is accumulating evidence that the kallikrein–kinin system is critically involved in various brain diseases (e.g., stroke, multiple sclerosis, Alzheimer's disease, epilepsy, depression) and its modulation might be a promising strategy to combat these diseases. The reported effects of specific components of the kallikrein–kinin system, however, are often inconsistent.

The paucity of therapies for brain trauma has resulted in a pressing clinical demand for new treatment options. The findings summarized in this review indicate that modulation of the components of the kallikrein–kinin system, which links edema formation, inflammation, and thrombosis, might be a promising strategy to combat TBI. Another tempting approach might be inhibition of the starting point of the kallikrein–kinin system, e.g., by the C1-inhibitor.

AUTHOR CONTRIBUTIONS

Christiane Albert-Weissenberger wrote the manuscript. Stine Mencl corrected the manuscript and checked the references. Sarah Hopp corrected the manuscript and build the figure. Christoph Kleinschnitz revised the manuscript for important intellectual content and approved the final version of the manuscript. Anna-Leena Sirén revised the manuscript critically for important intellectual content and approved the final version of the manuscript.

ACKNOWLEDGMENTS

Part of the work referenced in this review article was supported by the Else Kröner-Fresenius Foundation, the Interdisciplinary Center for Clinical Research (IZKF) Würzburg (Project A226), the Deutsche Forschungsgemeinschaft (SFB 688) and CSL Behring GmbH, Marburg, Germany.

REFERENCES

Albert-Weissenberger, C., and Sirén, A. L. (2010). Experimental traumatic brain injury. *Exp. Transl. Stroke Med.* 2:16. doi: 10.1186/2040-7378-2-16

Albert-Weissenberger, C., Stetter, C., Meuth, S. G., Göbel, K., Bader, M., Sirén, A. L., et al. (2012). Blocking of bradykinin receptor B1 protects from focal closed head injury in mice by reducing axonal damage and astroglia activation. *J. Cereb. Blood Flow Metab.* 32, 1747–1756. doi: 10.1038/jcbfm.2012.62

Ariza, M., Matarin, M. D., Junqué, C., Mataró, M., Clemente, I., Moral, P., et al. (2006). Influence of Angiotensin-converting enzyme polymorphism on neuropsychological subacute performance in moderate and severe traumatic brain injury. *J. Neuropsychiatry Clin. Neurosci.* 18, 39–44. doi: 10.1176/appi.neuropsych.18.1.39

Asemota, A. O., George, B. P., Bowman, S. M., Haider, A. H., and Schneider, E. B. (2013). Causes and trends in traumatic brain injury for United States adolescents. *J. Neurotrauma* 30, 67–75. doi: 10.1089/neu.2012.2605

Auer, L. M., Marth, E., Heppner, F., and Holasek, A. (1979). Proteolytic enzyme activity in patienst with severe head injury and the effect of a proteinase inhibitor. *Acta Neurochir. (Wien)* 49, 207–217. doi: 10.1007/bf01808960

Bernstein, K. E., Shen, X. Z., Gonzalez-Villalobos, R. A., Billet, S., Okwan-Duodu, D., Ong, F. S., et al. (2011). Different in vivo functions of the two catalytic domains of angiotensin-converting enzyme (ACE). *Curr. Opin. Pharmacol.* 11, 105–111. doi: 10.1016/j.coph.2010.11.001

Colman, R. W. (1969). Activation of plasminogen by human plasma kallikrein. *Biochem. Biophys. Res. Commun.* 35, 273–279. doi: 10.1016/0006-291x(69)90278-2

Costa-Neto, C. M., Dillenburg-Pilla, P., Heinrich, T. A., Parreiras-e-Silva, L. T., Pereira, M. G., Reis, R. I., et al. (2008). Participation of kallikrein-kinin system in different pathologies. *Int. Immunopharmacol.* 8, 135–142. doi: 10.1016/j.intimp.2007.08.003

Doppenberg, E. M., Choi, S. C., and Bullock, R. (2004). Clinical trials in traumatic brain injury: lessons for the future. *J. Neurosurg. Anesthesiol.* 16, 87–94. doi: 10.1097/00008506-200401000-00019

Faul, M., Xu, L., Wald, M. M., and Coronado, V. G. (2010). *Traumatic Brain Injury in the United States: Emergency Department Visits, Hospitalizations and Deaths, 2002–2006.* Atlanta: U.S. Department of Health and Human Services, Centers for Disease Control and Prevention, National Center for Injury Prevention and Control.

Fleminger, S., Oliver, D. L., Lovestone, S., Rabe-Hesketh, S., and Giora, A. (2003). Head injury as a risk factor for Alzheimer's disease: the evidence 10 years on; a partial replication. *J. Neurol. Neurosurg. Psychiatry* 74, 857–862. doi: 10.1136/jnnp.74.7.857

Geppetti, P. (1993). Sensory neuropeptide release by bradykinin: mechanisms and pathophysiological implications. *Regul. Pept.* 47, 1–23. doi: 10.1016/0167-0115(93)90268-d

Görlach, C., Hortobágyi, T., Hortobágyi, S., Benyó, Z., Relton, J., Whalley, E. T., et al. (2001). Bradykinin B2, but not B1, receptor antagonism has a neuroprotective effect after brain injury. *J. Neurotrauma* 18, 833–838. doi: 10.1089/089771501316919193

Harford-Wright, E., Thornton, E., and Vink, R. (2010). Angiotensin-converting enzyme (ACE) inhibitors exacerbate histological damage and motor deficits after experimental traumatic brain injury. *Neurosci. Lett.* 481, 26–29. doi: 10.1016/j.neulet.2010.06.044

Hellal, F., Pruneau, D., Palmier, B., Faye, P., Croci, N., Plotkine, M., et al. (2003). Detrimental role of bradykinin B2 receptor in a murine model of diffuse brain injury. *J. Neurotrauma* 20, 841–851. doi: 10.1089/089771503322385773

Heydenreich, N., Nolte, M. W., Göb, E., Langhauser, F., Hofmeister, M., Kraft, P., et al. (2012). C1-inhibitor protects from brain ischemia-reperfusion injury by combined antiinflammatory and antithrombotic mechanisms. *Stroke* 43, 2457–2467. doi: 10.1161/strokeaha.112.660340

Ivashkova, Y., Svetnitsky, A., Mayzler, O., Pruneau, D., Benifla, M., Fuxman, Y., et al. (2006). Bradykinin B2 receptor antagonism with LF 18-1505T reduces brain edema and improves neurological outcome after closed head trauma in rats. *J. Trauma* 61, 879–885. doi: 10.1097/01.ta.0000234722.98537.01

Kaplanski, J., Pruneau, D., Asa, I., Artru, A. A., Azez, A., Ivashkova, Y., et al. (2002). LF 16–0687 Ms, a bradykinin B2 receptor antagonist, reduces brain edema and improves long-term neurological function recovery after closed head trauma in rats. *J. Neurotrauma* 19, 953–964. doi: 10.1089/089771502320317104

Kariya, K., Yamauchi, A., and Sasaki, T. (1985). Regional distribution and characterization of kinin in the CNS of the rat. *J. Neurochem.* 44, 1892–1897. doi: 10.1111/j.1471-4159.1985.tb07185.x

Ker, K., and Blackhall, K. (2008). Beta-2 receptor antagonists for acute traumatic brain injury. *Cochrane Database Syst. Rev.* 23:CD006686. doi: 10.1002/14651858.cd006686.pub2

Kizuki, K., Suzuki, T., Sugaya, K., Noguchi, T., and Kudo, M. (1994). Tissue kallikrein in rat and mouse neurons. *Braz. J. Med. Biol. Res.* 27, 1891–1896.

Langhauser, F., Göb, E., Kraft, P., Geis, C., Schmitt, J., Brede, M., et al. (2012). Kininogen deficiency protects from ischemic neurodegeneration in mice by reducing thrombosis, blood-brain barrier damage and inflammation. *Blood* 120, 4082–4092. doi: 10.1182/blood-2012-06-440057

Leeb-Lundberg, L. M., Marceau, F., Müller-Esterl, W., Pettibone, D. J., and Zuraw, B. L. (2005). International union of pharmacology. XLV. Classification of the kinin receptor family: from molecular mechanisms to pathophysiological consequences. *Pharmacol. Rev.* 57, 27–77. doi: 10.1124/pr.57.1.2

Longhi, L., Perego, C., Ortolano, F., Zanier, E. R., Bianchi, P., Stocchetti, N., et al. (2009). C1-inhibitor attenuates neurobehavioral deficits and reduces contusion volume after controlled cortical impact brain injury in mice. *Crit. Care Med.* 37, 659–665. doi: 10.1097/ccm.0b013e318195998a

Longhi, L., Perego, C., Zanier, E. R., Ortolano, F., Bianchi, P., Stocchetti, N., et al. (2008). Neuroprotective effect of C1-inhibitor following traumatic brain injury in mice. *Acta Neurochir. Suppl.* 102, 381–384. doi: 10.1007/978-3-211-85578-2_73

Ma, V. Y., Chan, L., and Carruthers, K. J. (2014). Incidence, prevalence, costs and impact on disability of common conditions requiring rehabilitation in the United States: stroke, spinal cord injury, traumatic brain injury, multiple sclerosis, osteoarthritis, rheumatoid arthritis, limb loss and back pain. *Arch. Phys. Med. Rehabil.* 95, 986.e1–995.e1. doi: 10.1016/j.apmr.2013.10.032

Maas, A. I., Roozenbeek, B., and Manley, G. T. (2010). Clinical trials in traumatic brain injury: past experience and current developments. *Neurotherapeutics* 7, 115–126. doi: 10.1016/j.nurt.2009.10.022

Marmarou, A., Guy, M., Murphey, L., Roy, F., Layani, L., Combal, J. P., et al. (2005). A single dose, three-arm, placebo-controlled, phase I study of the bradykinin B2 receptor antagonist Anatibant (LF16–0687Ms) in patients with severe traumatic brain injury. *J. Neurotrauma* 22, 1444–1455. doi: 10.1089/neu.2005.22.1444

Marmarou, A., Nichols, J., Burgess, J., Newell, D., Troha, J., Burnham, D., et al. (1999). Effects of the bradykinin antagonist Bradycor (deltibant, CP-1027) in severe traumatic brain injury: results of a multi-center, randomized, placebo-controlled trial. American Brain Injury Consortium Study Group. *J. Neurotrauma* 16, 431–444. doi: 10.1089/neu.1999.16.431

Narotam, P. K., Rodell, T. C., Nadvi, S. S., Bhoola, K. D., Troha, J. M., Parbhoosingh, R., et al. (1998). Traumatic brain contusions: a clinical role for the kinin antagonist CP-0127. *Acta Neurochir. (Wien)* 140, 793–802; discussion 802–803. doi: 10.1007/s007010050181

Ongali, B., Campos, M. M., Bregola, G., Rodi, D., Regoli, D., Thibault, G., et al. (2003). Autoradiographic analysis of rat brain kinin B1 and B2 receptors: normal distribution and alterations induced by epilepsy. *J. Comp. Neurol.* 461, 506–519. doi: 10.1002/cne.10706

Ongali, B., Hellal, F., Rodi, D., Plotkine, M., Marchand-Verrecchia, C., Pruneau, D., et al. (2006). Autoradiographic analysis of mouse brain kinin B1 and B2 receptors after closed head trauma and ability of Anatibant mesylate to cross the blood-brain barrier. *J. Neurotrauma* 23, 696–707. doi: 10.1089/neu.2006.23.696

Plesnila, N., Schulz, J., Stoffel, M., Eriskat, J., Pruneau, D., and Baethmann, A. (2001). Role of bradykinin B2 receptors in the formation of vasogenic brain edema in rats. *J. Neurotrauma* 18, 1049–1058. doi: 10.1089/08977150152693746

Pruneau, D., Chorny, I., Benkovitz, V., Artru, A., Roitblat, L., and Shapira, Y. (1999). Effect of LF 16–0687MS, a new nonpeptide bradykinin B2 receptor antagonist, in a rat model of closed head trauma. *J. Neurotrauma* 16, 1057–1065. doi: 10.1089/neu.1999.16.1057

Raslan, F., Schwarz, T., Meuth, S. G., Austinat, M., Bader, M., Renné, T., et al. (2010). Inhibition of bradykinin receptor B1 protects mice from focal brain injury by reducing blood-brain barrier leakage and inflammation. *J. Cereb. Blood Flow Metab.* 30, 1477–1486. doi: 10.1038/jcbfm.2010.28

Renné, T., Schmaier, A. H., Nickel, K. F., Blombäck, M., and Maas, C. (2012). In vivo roles of factor XII. *Blood* 120, 4296–4303. doi: 10.1182/blood-2012-07-292094

Revak, S. D., Cochrane, C. G., Bouma, B. N., and Griffin, J. H. (1978). Surface and fluid phase activities of two forms of activated Hageman factor produced during contact activation of plasma. *J. Exp. Med.* 147, 719–729. doi: 10.1084/jem.147.3.719

Revenko, A. S., Gao, D., Crosby, J. R., Bhattacharjee, G., Zhao, C., May, C., et al. (2011). Selective depletion of plasma prekallikrein or coagulation factor XII inhibits thrombosis in mice without increased risk of bleeding. *Blood* 118, 5302–5311. doi: 10.1182/blood-2011-05-355248

Schulz, J., Plesnila, N., Eriskat, J., Stoffel, M., Pruneau, D., and Baethmann, A. (2000). LF16–0687 a novel non-peptide bradykinin B2 receptor antagonist reduces vasogenic brain edema from a focal lesion in rats. *Acta Neurochir. Suppl.* 76, 137–139. doi: 10.1007/978-3-7091-6346-7_28

Shakur, H., Andrews, P., Asser, T., Balica, L., Boeriu, C., Quintero, J. D., et al. (2009). The BRAIN TRIAL: a randomised, placebo controlled trial of a Bradykinin B2 receptor antagonist (Anatibant) in patients with traumatic brain injury. *Trials* 10:109. doi: 10.1186/1745-6215-10-109

Singer, M., and Jones, A. M. (2011). Bench-to-bedside review: the role of C1-esterase inhibitor in sepsis and other critical illnesses. *Crit. Care* 15:203. doi: 10.1186/cc9304

Stover, J. F., Dohse, N. K., and Unterberg, A. W. (2000). Bradykinin 2 receptor antagonist LF 16–0687Ms reduces posttraumatic brain edema. *Acta Neurochir. Suppl.* 76, 171–175. doi: 10.1007/978-3-7091-6346-7_34

Trabold, R., Erös, C., Zweckberger, K., Relton, J., Beck, H., Nussberger, J., et al. (2010). The role of bradykinin B(1) and B(2) receptors for secondary brain damage after traumatic brain injury in mice. *J. Cereb. Blood Flow Metab.* 30, 130–139. doi: 10.1038/jcbfm.2009.196

Unterberg, A., Dautermann, C., Baethmann, A., and Müller-Esterl, W. (1986). The kallikrein-kinin system as mediator in vasogenic brain edema. Part 3: Inhibition of the kallikrein-kinin system in traumatic brain swelling. *J. Neurosurg.* 64, 269–276. doi: 10.3171/jns.1986.64.2.0269

Zweckberger, K., and Plesnila, N. (2009). Anatibant, a selective non-peptide bradykinin B2 receptor antagonist, reduces intracranial hypertension and histopathological damage after experimental traumatic brain injury. *Neurosci. Lett.* 454, 115–117. doi: 10.1016/j.neulet.2009.02.014

15

Post-ischemic inflammation regulates neural damage and protection

Takashi Shichita[1,2], Minako Ito[1] and Akihiko Yoshimura[1] *

[1] *Department of Microbiology and Immunology, School of Medicine, Keio University, Tokyo, Japan*
[2] *Precursory Research for Embryonic Science and Technology, Japan Science and Technology Agency, Tokyo, Japan*

***Correspondence:**
Akihiko Yoshimura, Department of Microbiology and Immunology, School of Medicine, Keio University, 35 Shinanomachi, Shinjuku-ku, Tokyo 160-8582, Japan
e-mail: yoshimura@a6.keio.jp

Post-ischemic inflammation is important in ischemic stroke pathology. However, details of the inflammation process, its resolution after stroke and its effect on pathology and neural damage have not been clarified. Brain swelling, which is often fatal in ischemic stroke patients, occurs at an early stage of stroke due to endothelial cell injury and severe inflammation by infiltrated mononuclear cells including macrophages, neutrophils, and lymphocytes. At early stage of inflammation, macrophages are activated by molecules released from necrotic cells [danger-associated molecular patterns (DAMPs)], and inflammatory cytokines and mediators that increase ischemic brain damage by disruption of the blood–brain barrier are released. After post-ischemic inflammation, macrophages function as scavengers of necrotic cell and brain tissue debris. Such macrophages are also involved in tissue repair and neural cell regeneration by producing tropic factors. The mechanisms of inflammation resolution and conversion of inflammation to neuroprotection are largely unknown. In this review, we summarize information accumulated recently about DAMP-induced inflammation and the neuroprotective effects of inflammatory cells, and discuss next generation strategies to treat ischemic stroke.

Keywords: damage-associated molecular patterns (DAMPs), inflammation, cytokines, inflammasome, resolution of inflammation

INTRODUCTION

Inflammation is implicated in almost all of central nervous system (CNS) diseases (Lo, 2010; Moskowitz et al., 2010; Iadecola and Anrather, 2011). Neurodegeneration, infection, trauma, and ischemia stimulate immune responses in the brain, although to varying degrees. The process in neuronal injury involves various intracellular mechanisms (abnormal metabolism and degeneration of protein, dysfunction of organelles, etc.), which cause the activation of microglia and the infiltration of circulating immune cells (Lo, 2010). Inflammation may not be always main process in the pathology of CNS diseases; nonetheless, the distinct characteristics of ischemic stroke are large amount of necrotic neuronal death and extreme infiltration of immune cells (Moskowitz et al., 2010; Iadecola and Anrather, 2011).

Severe inflammation causes cerebral swelling, which is often fatal in ischemic stroke patients. Broad necrotic lesion generates abundant inflammatory mediators and damage-associated molecular patterns (DAMPs), which enhance the chemotaxis of circulating immune cells and make them more efficient participants to promote inflammation (Moskowitz et al., 2010; Iadecola and Anrather, 2011). Cerebral inflammation exaggerates vascular dysfunction and induces further neuronal cell death (Dirnagl et al., 1999). Thus, post-ischemic inflammation is an essential process in the pathophysiology of ischemic stroke and is closely related to the prognosis after stroke (Dirnagl et al., 1999; Lo, 2010; Moskowitz et al., 2010; Iadecola and Anrather, 2011). In addition, inflammation is generally considered useful for the clearance of the large amount of debris caused by brain cell necrotic death (Moskowitz et al., 2010; Iadecola and Anrather, 2011). Inflammation, resolution of inflammation, and repair of neural damage are sequential pivotal events after stroke. To clarify the detailed mechanisms of each step of cerebral inflammation is indispensable to develop next generation therapies for ischemic stroke. The molecular basis of these steps is now being clarified by the recent accumulating evidences. We summarize these findings and discuss the principles of post-ischemic inflammation from beginning to end.

INFLAMMATORY DAMPs

Brain ischemia induces various large metabolic changes in brain cells. Hypoxic stress, nutrients stress, and ER stress will cause cell death and trigger post-ischemic inflammation. Although receptors for pathogens such as Toll-like receptors (TLRs) are thought to be involved in early step of inflammation, brain is a sterile organ. Thus, endogenous molecules, i.e., DAMPs derived from injured brain cells, must trigger the inflammatory response in immune cells (**Table 1**). These DAMPs induce the activation of TLRs and other pattern recognition receptors [receptor for advanced glycation end products (RAGE) and c-type lectin receptors], which promote inflammatory mediator expression and tissue injury (**Figure 1**; Tang et al., 2007; Yanai et al., 2009; Suzuki et al., 2013). Recent scientific advances have suggested the existence of various types of DAMPs in ischemic brain.

NUCLEIC ACIDS AND NUCLEOTIDES

Various intracellular components are released into the extracellular space by necrotic brain cell death. Among these,

Table 1 | List of inflammatory DAMPs.

		DAMPs	Receptor	Reference
Signal 1	Nucleic acid	Mitochondrial DNA	TLR9	Zhang et al. (2010), Sun et al. (2013), Maeda and Fadeel (2014), Walko et al. (2014), Wenceslau et al. (2014)
		Self RNA, DNA	TLR7,9	Hyakkoku et al. (2010), Kawai and Akira (2010), Brea et al. (2011), Stevens et al. (2011), Leung et al. (2012)
	Lipid	Carboxyalkylpyrroles	TLR2	West et al. (2010)
		Oxidized phospholipids	CD36	Cho et al. (2005), Gao et al. (2006), Abe et al. (2010), Haider et al. (2011), Miller et al. (2011), Ho et al. (2012), Matt et al. (2013)
	Protein	HMGB1	TLR2,4, RAGE	Qiu et al. (2008), Zhang et al. (2011)
		Peroxiredoxin	TLR2,4	Shichita et al. (2012), Kuang et al. (2014)
		S100A8, A9	TLR4	Tsai et al. (2014)
		Mrp8, 14	TLR4	Loser et al. (2010)
		CIRP	TLR2,4	Qiang et al. (2013)
Signal 2	Nucleotide	ATP	P2X, P2Y	Martinon et al. (2002), Abulafia et al. (2009), Ceruti et al. (2009), Denes et al. (2013), Fann et al. (2013), Yang et al. (2014),
	Lipid	Phospholipids	?	Clemens et al. (1996), Bonventre et al. (1997), Muralikrishna Adibhatla and Hatcher (2006), Shanta et al. (2012), Iyer et al. (2013), Zhong et al. (2013)
	Protein	ASC specks	?	Baroja-Mazo et al. (2014), Franklin et al. (2014)

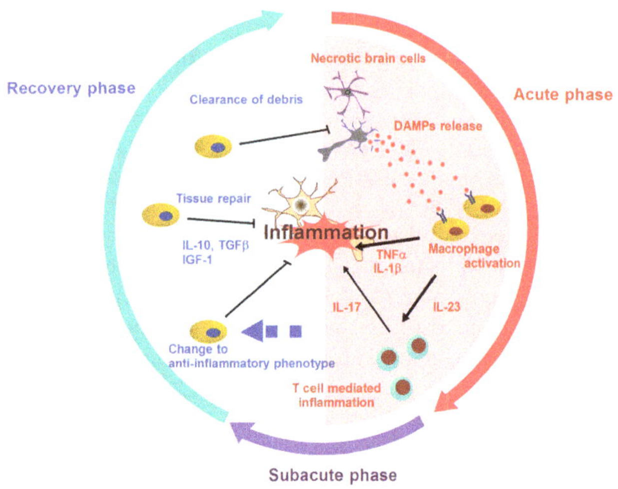

FIGURE 1 | Mechanisms of post-ischemic inflammation. DAMPs are released into extracellular compartment and activate infiltrating immune cells by two ways: Signal 1 (via the activation of pattern recognition receptor) and Signal 2 (via the activation of inflammasome). Various inflammatory cytokines promote neuronal injury, and induce further inflammation mediated by T cells in subacute phase. After days and week after stroke onset, the resolution of post-ischemic inflammation is brought by the clearance of debris including DAMPs or inflammatory mediators, and the production of anti-inflammatory molecules or neurotrophic factors. In this recover phase, inflammatory immune cells turn into neuroprotective cells.

nucleic acids and nucleotides are major DAMPs that have recently received much attention. Mitochondrial DNA released by cellular injury can be detected as DAMPs by immune cells, because mitochondria are considered to have a symbiotic origin that carries numerous characteristics resembling bacteria. Mitochondrial DNA is a sensor molecule of innate immunity by activating TLR9 and can be detected in cerebrospinal fluid after traumatic brain injury (Zhang et al., 2010; Walko et al., 2014). Vascular permeability is also increased by circulating mitochondrial DNA after injury (Sun et al., 2013; Wenceslau et al., 2014). Recently accumulated data indicates that mitochondrial DAMPs could be an important candidate for the trigger of post-ischemic inflammation, even if there is not yet any direct evidence (Maeda and Fadeel, 2014).

Self RNA and DNA (in complex with LL37 peptide) activate immune cells via TLR7 or TLR9 (Kawai and Akira, 2010). TLR7 is associated with the deterioration in ischemic stroke patients; in contrast, ischemic brain damage was not reduced in TLR9-deficient mice (Hyakkoku et al., 2010; Brea et al., 2011). Several reports demonstrate the implications of TLR7 and TLR9 in ischemic preconditioning. In these articles, the pretreatment using a TLR7 or TLR9 agonist reveals significant neuroprotection after cerebral ischemia by activating interferon regulatory factor 3/7- (IRF3/7)-induced type I interferon (IFN) signaling pathway (Stevens et al., 2011; Leung et al., 2012). Although the interaction between self nucleic acids and TLRs in the ischemic brain remains controversial, ischemic preconditioning via the TLR7 or TLR9 signaling pathway may represent a therapeutic strategy.

Purines (ATP and UTP) released from injured brain cells and their receptors, P2X and P2Y, function as alerting signals in CNS (Ceruti et al., 2009). Importantly, ATP also activates inflammasomes, which are large multimolecular complexes that control the activity of the proteolytic enzyme caspase-1 that cleaves pro-IL-1β to an active 17 kDa form (Martinon et al., 2002). The activation of the NLRP1 or NALP3 inflammasome has been recently reported to promote post-ischemic inflammation and neuronal death (Abulafia et al., 2009; Fann et al., 2013; Yang et al., 2014). Because IL-1β produced from both infiltrating immune cells and brain cells is important (Denes et al., 2013), it should be clarified how the inflammasome is activated in ischemic brain or hematopoietic cells. Inhibition of the inflammasome activation pathway may be a possible therapeutic strategy for ischemic stroke.

LIPIDS

Various types of lipids are also important regulators of innate immunity. For example, oxidized low density lipoprotein (oxLDL) is a popular inflammatory mediator, which activates TLRs through binding with its receptor, CD36 (Stewart et al., 2010). Although the function of oxLDL in ischemic brain remains unclear, recent research has indicated that end products of lipid oxidation may be implicated in cerebral post-ischemic inflammation (Uchida, 2013). Carboxyalkylpyrroles, which are generated in inflammatory tissue, activate TLR2 and promote angiogenesis in ischemic organs (West et al., 2010). Oxidized phospholipids are also generated during cerebral inflammation and are considered to be DAMPs (Gao et al., 2006; Haider et al., 2011; Ho et al., 2012). Oxidized phospholipids are CD36 ligands that promote inflammation via TLR2 activation in ischemic brain (Cho et al., 2005; Abe et al., 2010). The recognition and endocytosis of oxidized lipids by pattern recognition receptors could regulate post-ischemic inflammation (Miller et al., 2011; Matt et al., 2013).

Phospholipids could also be inflammasome activators. Phospholipid metabolism is drastically altered by cerebral ischemia (Shanta et al., 2012). There are several reports showing the activation of phospholipase A2 (PLA2) in ischemic brain, which results in hydrolysis of membrane phospholipids (Clemens et al., 1996; Bonventre et al., 1997; Muralikrishna Adibhatla and Hatcher, 2006). Phospholipid hydrolysis and mitochondrial dysfunction induced by cerebral ischemia generate reactive oxygen species (ROS). Two recent studies have identified both ROS-dependent and ROS-independent pathways for inflammasome activation. The former is demonstrated by a charged phospholipid liposome that consecutively induces ROS-dependent calcium influx and NLRP3 inflammasome activation (Zhong et al., 2013). In the latter case, mitochondrial cardiolipin has been reported to directly bind to and activate the NLRP3 inflammasome (Iyer et al., 2013). Thus, the metabolism and modification of lipids during cerebral ischemia may be closely associated with the post-ischemic inflammation start signal.

PROTEINS

High mobility group box 1 (HMGB1) and peroxiredoxin (Prx) family proteins are two major DAMPs in ischemic brain. There is a difference in the functional phase of these two proteins (Shichita et al., 2012). HMGB1, which is included in the nucleus of brain cells, is released extracellularly at the hyperacute phase (several hours after the stroke onset; Qiu et al., 2008). On the other hand, Prx family proteins function at the acute and subacute phases (12–72 h after the onset), especially in the penumbral area (Shichita et al., 2012). This is because Prx family protein expression is induced by an intracellular increase in ROS, which results from ischemic change. HMGB1 directly breaks down the blood–brain barrier and increases vascular permeability (Zhang et al., 2011). However, Prx directly induces the activation of infiltrating immune cells via TLR signaling. Ligustilide has been reported as a therapeutic candidate that suppresses cerebral post-ischemic inflammation by inhibiting the Prx/TLR4 signaling pathway (Kuang et al., 2014).

S100A8, S100A9, Mrp8, Mrp14, and cold-inducible RNA binding protein (CIRP) have also been reported to be protein DAMPs, although their relevance in post-ischemic inflammation has not yet been clarified (Loser et al., 2010; Qiang et al., 2013; Tsai et al., 2014). Inflammatory responses by these protein DAMPs occur through the activation of TLR2, TLR4, and RAGE. TLR2 and TLR4 signaling pathways are essential for sterile inflammation, including ischemic stroke (Chen et al., 2007). TLR2-blocking antibody is neuroprotective against ischemic brain injury (Ziegler et al., 2011). Similarly, resatorvid, which inhibits the TLR4 signaling pathway, attenuates ischemic brain injury and also suppresses Nox4-induced oxidative stress and neuronal apoptosis (Suzuki et al., 2012). It is also possible that DAMP-mediated TLR activation requires other adaptor molecules (Chun and Seong, 2010). CD14, a TLR4 co-receptor, may be implicated in post-ischemic inflammation (Reed-Geaghan et al., 2009). Heat shock protein gp96 is another candidate molecule that functions as an adaptor for both TLR2 and TLR4 (Yang et al., 2007).

It is not known whether protein DAMPs can activate inflammasomes. Recently, aggregated ASC (apoptosis-associated speck-like protein containing a caspase recruitment domain) has been reported to be released into the extracellular space after cell death and it activates inflammasomes in the surrounding immune cells (Baroja-Mazo et al., 2014; Franklin et al., 2014). Inflammasome activation, which occurs through ASC polymerization, results in caspase-1 activation and pyroptotic cell death. Extracellularly released ASC is internalized by surrounding macrophages and induces lysosomal damage and inflammasome activation. These mechanisms of inflammasome activation remain to be elucidated in ischemic brain injury.

OTHER INFLAMMATORY DAMPs

Basic research may neglect the influence of aging and life habits by using healthy young rodents. These are important factors for the generation of DAMPs. Aging and continuous high serum glucose levels increase lipid peroxidation and AGEs in body systems (Basta et al., 2004; Cai et al., 2014). AGEs are proteins that are modified by sugar, through the Amadori and Maillard reaction. AGEs are found in chronic lesions; for example, the amyloid deposits that are surrounded by macrophages in patients with dialysis-related amyloidosis (Miyata et al., 1993). Thus, AGEs usually take a long time (more than a month) to generate; however, AGEs can be generated in a short period of time during inflammation (Weil, 2012). Glyoxal and glyceraldehyde induce AGE formation within 1 week (Takeuchi et al., 2001). In addition, the pivotal role of the RAGE in post-ischemic inflammation has been demonstrated (Muhammad et al., 2008). AGEs can be a potential DAMP, especially in aged human ischemic stroke patients.

INFLAMMATION SUPPRESSION AND RESOLUTION

Activated immune cells and brain cells are the major players after various DAMPs trigger post-ischemic inflammation. These cells produce inflammatory cytokines, chemokines, and other cytotoxic mediators, and this leads to prolonged inflammation and progressive brain edema during several days after the stroke onset (**Figure 1**). However, post-ischemic inflammation rarely lasts for a long period of time, and the most intense inflammatory phase takes place within 7 days after stroke onset (Dirnagl et al., 1999; Iadecola and Anrather, 2011). In this phase, the number of infiltrating immune cells decreases remarkably, and remaining immune cells in ischemic brain produce anti-inflammatory or neurotrophic factors (Shichita et al., 2009; Smirkin et al., 2010). For example, the detailed mechanisms about the infiltration and the change to anti-inflammatory phenotype of neutrophils have been recently clarified (Cuartero et al., 2013; Gorina et al., 2014). The period of cerebral post-ischemic inflammation always ends, and thus, the mechanisms of its resolution must exist in ischemic brain.

Three major points on the resolution of inflammation have been discussed in a recent publication (Buckley et al., 2012). These points are the production of anti-inflammatory mediators, the depletion of inflammatory mediators, and the induction of anti-inflammatory immune cells. After post-ischemic inflammation, infiltrating macrophages turn into anti-inflammatory macrophages, which produce neurotropic factors and clear necrotic debris. Inflammatory DAMPs will also be implicated in the induction of anti-inflammatory macrophages, although its mechanism still remains to be clarified. We introduce recent advantages of the relationship between post-ischemic inflammation and its resolution.

ANTI-INFLAMMATORY MEDIATOR PRODUCTION

Many molecules have been reported to be neuroprotective factors. However, most of these molecules failed to improve neurological deficits in ischemic stroke patients, even if they are effective in animal stroke models. It has been suggested that neuroprotection alone is not sufficient to improve the prognosis of human ischemic stroke. Anti-inflammatory mechanisms in the entire brain and how these mechanisms are triggered needs to be determined. Because most brain cells are dead in the ischemic region several days after the stroke onset, infiltrating immune cells and reactive glial cells could be major players in the tissue repair. In practice, accelerating their effect is a potential next generation therapeutic strategy, and direct *in vivo* reprogramming of reactive glial cells into functional neurons after cerebral injury by retroviral transduction of the NeuroD1 gene was recently reported (Guo et al., 2014).

IL-10 and TGF-β are major anti-inflammatory molecules in various organ injuries. Both are produced by infiltrating immune cells and reactive glial cells after ischemic brain injury. Viral overexpression of IL-10 in ischemic brain is neuroprotective (Ooboshi et al., 2006). One recent report demonstrated the anti-inflammatory effect of TGF-β by inhibiting excessive neuroinflammation during the subacute phase of brain ischemia (Cekanaviciute et al., 2014). Although the anti-inflammatory effects of IL-10 and TGF-β have been pivotal, it remains to be clarified whether these effects last up to 1 week after the stroke onset (Pál et al., 2012). If the mechanisms for stimulating TGF-β and IL-10 expression can be controlled, this may become a strong therapeutic method.

DEPLETION OF INFLAMMATORY MEDIATORS AND CELLS

Infiltrating immune cells and reactive glial cells produce various inflammatory mediators. TNF-α and IL-1β directly induce neuronal cell death. IL-23 and IL-1β activate T cell-mediated innate immunity and promote secondary ischemic damage during the subacute phase of ischemic brain injury (Shichita et al., 2009; Konoeda et al., 2010). The existence of these inflammatory mediators, including DAMPs, prolongs post-ischemic inflammation and will be a threat to neuronal survival and repair. However, inflammatory mediator degradation mechanisms remain mostly unknown. Inflammatory molecules may be degraded by some enzymes or consumed by receptor-mediated endocytosis. It is expected that nucleotides and lipids are rapidly metabolized in the ischemic brain, and transfer by the blood stream or cerebrospinal fluid (CSF) will help to scavenge inflammatory mediator. Further research should clarify the detailed mechanisms to scavenge inflammatory molecules produced in the ischemic brain, and antibody therapy will be a pivotal therapeutic method targeting this potential mechanism. TNF-α and IL-23 neutralizing antibody have been used clinically for rheumatoid arthritis and psoriasis patients, respectively. Natalizumab is the neutralizing antibody for integrin-α4, which is necessary for T cell infiltration into the inflammatory tissue, and has already been used for multiple sclerosis (Yednock et al., 1992). T cell depletion from ischemic brain has received attention as a potential next generation therapy for ischemic stroke (Meisel and Meisel, 2011; Wei et al., 2011). Thus, antibody therapies may be used to help treat ischemic stroke patients in the near future.

Activation of inflammasomes in immune cells induces the production of IL-1β in its mature form, and finally results in the rapid cell death of the same cells, which is called pyroptosis. Pyroptosis may be a possible mechanism for the clearance of inflammatory immune cells. This is supported by the fact that dying cells detected using the TdT-mediated dUTP nick end labeling (TUNEL) staining method include macrophages and glial cells in the ischemic brain (Mabuchi et al., 2000).

INDUCTION OF IMMUNE CELL REPAIR

The repair process for damaged brain tissues and regeneration of neural cells takes place during resolution of inflammation. It is difficult to separate this process from the anti-inflammatory mechanism, because they may overlap each other. We will further discuss neuroprotective factors and repairing the damage to immune cells.

NEUROPROTECTIVE FACTORS

Various growth factors are also produced by immune cells and glial cells (Gudi et al., 2011). Among these, IGF-1 and FGF-2 are produced by infiltrating macrophages and microglia during the recovery phase of ischemic brain injury (which occurs

1 week after the stroke onset). IGF-1 and FGF-2 improve the neurological outcome by saving neuron and glial cells from cell death (Ness et al., 2004; Ikeda et al., 2005; Zhu et al., 2008; Hill et al., 2012; Lalancette-Hébert et al., 2012). IGF-1 also enhances repair after ischemic stroke by promoting neural regeneration, remyelination, and synaptogenesis (Lecker et al., 2007; Zhu et al., 2008, 2009; Kooijman et al., 2009). Further investigation should clarify the mechanisms of IGF-1 and FGF-2 induction in the ischemic brain. Recently, transfer of mesenchymal stem cells (MSCs) has been explored as a next generation therapy for ischemic stroke (Kalladka and Muir, 2014). MSCs produce various growth factors and promote neuronal survival and neurogenesis (Calió et al., 2014). By improving the transfer method, cell therapy may become a pivotal therapeutic strategy (Guo et al., 2013).

The neuroprotective effect of prostaglandin E2 (PGE2) and its receptor signaling pathway has received recent attention. PGE2 has an effect via four distinct G protein-coupled EP receptors (E-prostanoid: EP1, EP2, EP3, and EP4). The activation of EP2 signaling has a neuroprotective effect in ischemic brain injury, which was shown in the significant increase in infarct volume in mice lacking the EP2 receptor (McCullough et al., 2004). Similarly, signaling via the EP4 receptor, which is expressed in both neurons and ischemic endothelial cells, has neuroprotective effects against ischemic brain injury (Liang et al., 2011). The administration of an EP4 agonist reduces infarct volume and neurological deficits. In a neonatal hypoxic-ischemic encephalopathy model, the inhibition of EP1 receptor signaling or the activation of EP2, EP3, and EP4 receptor signaling reveals attenuation of the ischemic injury (Taniguchi et al., 2011). PGE2 and EP receptor signaling pathways have various functions, which are dependent on distinct pathology of cerebral diseases (Furuyashiki and Narumiya, 2011). Targeting specific EP receptors in ischemic brain may become a novel therapeutic method.

Similar to PGE2, some lipids have been reported to have anti-inflammatory effects and promote neuroregeneration (Serhan, 2014). Cerebral ischemia increases PLA2 activity, which results in the hydrolysis of phospholipids in the cellular membrane (Shanta et al., 2012). Although the PLA2 effect itself is cytotoxic because it disrupts the cellular membrane, PLA2 also generates docosahexaenoic acid (DHA) derivatives and lysophospholipids through phospholipid hydrolysis (Bonventre et al., 1997). Resolvin and Neuroprotectin have been investigated for their anti-inflammatory function in ischemic stroke (Marcheselli et al., 2003; Bazan, 2009). Lysophospholipids also increase in ischemic brain and promote neurite outgrowth (Ikeno et al., 2005; Spohr et al., 2011; Shanta et al., 2012). Regulating the effect of these lipids is expected for the resolution of post-ischemic inflammation.

NEUROPROTECTIVE CELLS

Inflammatory DAMPs activate glial cells and infiltrating immune cells to promote post-ischemic inflammation. Paradoxically, this mechanism results in the infiltrating macrophage cell death and also induces anti-inflammatory and tissue-repairing immune cells.

Immune cell activation also induces anti-inflammatory cells. These cells have been called M2 macrophages, in contrast to the inflammatory M1 macrophages. Many researches have described the M2 macrophage markers; these markers include: arginase-1 (Arg1), chitinase3l3 (Ym), and Relmα (Fizz1). These markers are intracellular enzymes that are implicated in collagen synthesis and cell division; therefore, M2 enzymes are considered to promote tissue repair. Arg1 is the only marker that was reported to function as a neuroprotective enzyme (Estévez et al., 2006). However, these M2 markers may not be a good indicator for recovery after ischemic stroke. M2 markers are rapidly expressed in macrophages by TLR activation or other pattern recognition receptors, which also induce inflammatory cytokine expression (Hu et al., 2012). M2 markers appear in ischemic brain mostly during the same phase as the inflammatory mediators, the M1 markers, are expressed. In addition, the transfer of M2 marker positive-macrophages has not been reported to be sufficiently neuroprotective (Desestret et al., 2013).

During post-ischemic inflammation, some populations of macrophages and microglia become neuroprotective (Lalancette-Hébert et al., 2007). Galectin-1 has been suggested to be an inducer of anti-inflammatory macrophage/microglial cells (Starossom et al., 2012; Quintá et al., 2014). Galectin-1 is produced by astrocytes and has a neuroprotective effect against ischemic brain damage (Qu et al., 2011). Thus, the resolution of post-ischemic inflammation can be enhanced by the induction of a specific macrophage/microglial cell population. However, it is not clear whether the M2 markers truly reflect the neuroprotective function of macrophages and microglial cells. Suppressing inflammation alone is not enough to protect the brain from ischemic injury. IGF-1 and FGF-2 production seems to be a good index of repairing function (Lalancette-Hébert et al., 2012).

Further study is required to clarify whether sufficient clearance of inflammatory mediators (including DAMPs) begins neuronal regeneration after ischemic stroke. A recent study has suggested that there is a relationship between TLR activation and neuronal repair (Bohacek et al., 2012). It is possible that DAMPs triggers the secondary signals, which lead to resolution of post-ischemic inflammation, even if the primary signals via pattern recognition receptors promote ischemic damage. What is this mechanism? The role of immune cells, other than macrophages and microglia in part of the repair process, is not fully understood. This understanding may be critical for the establishment of next generation therapies for ischemic stroke.

CONCLUSION

Immunity and various physiological mechanisms are implicated in the triggering, persistence, and resolution of post-ischemic inflammation. Recent accumulating evidences clarify the complexity of these mechanisms to understand the entire mechanisms. They will show promising potential targets to develop therapies for ischemic stroke.

REFERENCES

Abe, T., Shimamura, M., Jackman, K., Kurinami, H., Anrather, J., Zhou, P., et al. (2010). Key role of CD36 in Toll-like receptor 2 signaling in cerebral ischemia. *Stroke* 41, 898–904. doi: 10.1161/STROKEAHA.109.572552

Abulafia, D. P., de Rivero Vaccari, J. P., Lozano, J. D., Lotocki, G., Keane, R. W., and Dietrich, W. D. (2009). Inhibition of the inflammasome complex reduces the inflammatory response after thromboembolic stroke in mice. *J. Cereb. Blood Flow Metab.* 29, 534–544. doi: 10.1038/jcbfm.2008.143

Baroja-Mazo, A., Martín-Sánchez, F., Gomez, A., Martínez, C. M., Amores-Iniesta, J., Compan, V., et al. (2014). The NLRP3 inflammasome is released as a particulate danger signal that amplifies the inflammatory response. *Nat. Immunol.* 15, 738–748. doi: 10.1038/ni.2919

Basta, G., Schmidt, A. M., and De Caterina, R. (2004). Advanced glycation end products and vascular inflammation: implications for accelerated atherosclerosis in diabetes. *Cardiovasc. Res.* 63, 582–592. doi: 10.1016/j.cardiores.2004.05.001

Bazan, N. G. (2009). Neuroprotectin D1-mediated anti-inflammatory and survival signaling in stroke, retinal degenerations, and Alzheimer's disease. *J. Lipid Res.* 50, S400–S405. doi: 10.1194/jlr.R800068-JLR200

Bohacek, I., Cordeau, P., Lalancette-Hébert, M., Gorup, D., Weng, Y. C., Gajovic, S., et al. (2012). Toll-like receptor 2 deficiency leads to delayed exacerbation of ischemic injury. *J. Neuroinflammation* 9, 191. doi: 10.1186/1742-2094-9-191

Bonventre, J. V., Huang, Z., Taheri, M. R., O'Leary, E., Li, E., Moskowitz, M. A., et al. (1997). Reduced fertility and postischaemic brain injury in mice deficient in cytosolic phospholipase A2. *Nature* 390, 622–625. doi: 10.1038/37635

Brea, D., Sobrino, T., Rodríguez-Yáñez, M., Ramos-Cabrer, P., Agulla, J., Rodríguez-González, R., et al. (2011). Toll-like receptors 7 and 8 expression is associated with poor outcome and greater inflammatory response in acute ischemic stroke. *Clin. Imunol.* 139, 193–198. doi: 10.1016/j.clim.2011.02.001

Buckley, C. D., Gilroy, D. W., Serhan, C. N., Stockinger, B., and Tak, P. P. (2012). The resolution of inflammation. *Nat. Rev. Immunol.* 13, 59–66. doi: 10.1038/nri3362

Cai, W., Uribarri, J., Zhu, L., Chen, X., Swamy, S., Zhao, Z., et al. (2014). Oral glycotoxins are a modifiable cause of dementia and the metabolic syndrome in mice and humans. *Proc. Natl. Acad. Sci. U.S.A.* 111, 4940–4945. doi: 10.1073/pnas.1316013111

Calió, M. L., Marinho, D. S., Ko, G. M., Ribeiro, R. R., Carbonel, A. F., Oyama, L. M., et al. (2014). Transplantation of bone marrow mesenchymal stem cells decreases oxidative stress, apoptosis, and hippocampal damage in brain of a spontaneous stroke model. *Free Radic. Biol. Med.* 70, 141–154. doi: 10.1016/j.freeradbiomed.2014.01.024

Cekanaviciute, E., Fathali, N., Doyle, K. P., Williams, A. M., Han, J., and Buckwalter, M. S. (2014). Astrocytic transforming growth factor-beta signaling reduces subacute neuroinflammation after stroke in mice. *Glia* 62, 1227–1240. doi: 10.1002/glia.22675

Ceruti, S., Villa, G., Genovese, T., Mazzon, E., Longhi, R., Rosa, P., et al. (2009). The P2Y-like receptor GPR17 as a sensor of damage and a new potential target in spinal cord injury. *Brain* 132(Pt 8), 2206–2218. doi: 10.1093/brain/awp147

Chen, C. J., Kono, H., Golenbock, D., Reed, G., Akira, S., and Rock, K. L. (2007). Identification of a key pathway required for the sterile inflammatory response triggered by dying cells. *Nat. Med.* 13, 851–856. doi: 10.1038/nm1603

Cho, S., Park, E. M., Febbraio, M., Anrather, J., Park, L., Racchumi, G., et al. (2005). The class B scavenger receptor CD36 mediates free radical production and tissue injury in cerebral ischemia. *J. Neurosci.* 25, 2504–2512. doi: 10.1523/JNEUROSCI.0035-05.2005

Chun, K. H., and Seong, S. Y. (2010). CD14 but not MD2 transmit signals from DAMP. *Int. Immunopharmaol.* 10, 98–106. doi: 10.1016/j.intimp.2009.10.002

Clemens, J. A., Stephenson, D. T., Smalstig, E. B., Roberts, E. F., Johnstone, E. M., Sharp, J. D., et al. (1996). Reactive glia express cytosolic phospholipase A2 after transient global forebrain ischemia in the rat. *Stroke* 27, 527–535. doi: 10.1161/01.STR.27.3.527

Cuartero, M. I., Ballesteros, I., Moraga, A., Nombela, F., Vivancos, J., Hamilton, J. A., et al. (2013). N2 neutrophils, novel players in brain inflammation after stroke: modulation by the PPARg agonist rosiglitazone. *Stroke* 44, 3498–3508. doi: 10.1161/STROKEAHA.113.002470

Denes, A., Wilkinson, F., Bigger, B., Chu, M., Rothwell, N. J., and Allan, S. M. (2013). Central and haematopoietic interleukin-1 both contribute to ischaemic brain injury. *Dis. Model. Mech.* 6, 1043–1048. doi: 10.1242/dmm.011601

Desestret, V., Riou, A., Chauveau, F., Cho, T. H., Devillard, E., Marinescu, M., et al. (2013). *In vitro* and *in vivo* models of cerebral ischemia show discrepancy in therapeutics effects of M2 macrophages. *PLoS ONE.* 8:e67063. doi: 10.1371/journal.pone.0067063

Dirnagl, U., Iadecola, C., and Moskowitz, M. A. (1999). Pathobiology of ischaemic stroke: an integrated view. *Trends Neurosci.* 22, 391–397. doi: 10.1016/S0166-2236(99)01401-0

Estévez, A. G., Sahawneh, M. A., Lange, P. S., Bae, N., Egea, M., and Ratan, R. R. (2006). Arginase 1 regulation of nitric oxide production is key to survival of trophic factor-deprived motor neurons. *J. Neurosci.* 26, 8512–8516. doi: 10.1523/JNEUROSCI.0728-06.2006

Fann, D. Y., Lee, S. Y., Manzanero, S., Tang, S. C., Gelderblom, M., Chunduri, P., et al. (2013). Intravenous immunoglobulin suppresses NLRP1 and NLRP3 inflammasome-mediated neuronal death in ischemic stroke. *Cell Death Dis.* 4, e790. doi: 10.1038/cddis.2013.326

Franklin, B. S., Bossaller, L., De Nardo, D., Ratter, J. M., Stutz, A., Engels, G., et al. (2014). The adaptor ASC has extracellular and 'prionoid' activities that propagate inflammation. *Nat. Immunol.* 15, 727–737. doi: 10.1038/ni.2913

Furuyashiki, T., and Narumiya, S. (2011). Stress responses: the contribution of prostaglandin E_2 and its receptors. *Nat. Rev. Endocrinol.* 7, 163–175. doi: 10.1038/nrendo.2010.194

Gao, S., Zhang, R., Greenberg, M. E., Sun, M., Chen, X., Levison, B. S., et al. (2006). Phospholipid hydroxyalkenals, a subset of recently discovered endogenous CD36 ligands, spontaneously generate novel furan-containing phospholipids lacking CD36 binding activity *in vivo*. *J. Biol. Chem.* 281, 31298–31308. doi: 10.1074/jbc.M604039200

Gorina, R., Lyck, R., Vestweber, D., and Engelhardt, B. (2014). β2 integrin-mediated crawling on endothelial ICAM-1 and ICAM-2 is a prerequisite for transcellular neutrophil diapedesis across the inflamed blood–brain barrier. *J. Immunol.* 192, 324–337. doi: 10.4049/jimmunol.1300858

Gudi, V., Škuljec, J., Yildiz, Ö., Frichert, K., Skripuletz, T., Moharregh-Khiabani, D., et al. (2011). Spatial and temporal profiles of growth factor expression during CNS demyelination reveal the dynamics of repair priming. *PLoS ONE* 6:e22623. doi: 10.1371/journal.pone.0022623

Guo, L., Ge, J., Wang, S., Zhou, Y., Wang, X., and Wu, Y. (2013). A novel method for efficient delivery of stem cells to the ischemic brain. *Stem Cell Res. Ther.* 4, 116. doi: 10.1186/scrt327

Guo, Z., Zhang, L., Wu, Z., Chen, Y., Wang, F., and Chen, G. (2014). In Vivo direct reprogramming of reactive glial cells into functional neurons after brain injury and in an Alzheimer's disease model. *Cell Stem Cell* 14, 188–202. doi: 10.1016/j.stem.2013.12.001

Haider, L., Fischer, M. T., Frishcer, J. M., Bauer, J., Höftberger, R., Botond, G., et al. (2011). Oxidative damage in multiple sclerosis lesions. *Brain* 134(Pt 7), 1914–1924. doi: 10.1093/brain/awr128

Hill, J. J., Jin, K., Mao, X. O., Xie, L., and Greenberg, D. A. (2012). Intracerebral chondroitinase ABC and heparan sulfate proteoglycan glypican improve outcome from chronic stroke in rats. *Proc. Natl. Acad. Sci. U.S.A.* 109, 9155–9160. doi: 10.1073/pnas.1205697109

Ho, P. P., Kanter, J. L., Johnson, A. M., Srinagesh, H. K., Chang, E. J., Purdy, T. M., et al. (2012). Identification of naturally occurring fatty acids of the myelin sheath that resolve neuroinflammation. *Sci. Transl. Med.* 4, 137ra73. doi: 10.1126/scitranslmed.3003831

Hu, X., Li, P., Guo, Y., Wang, H., Leak, R. K., Chen, S., et al. (2012). Microglia/macrophage polarization dynamics reveal novel mechanism of injury expansion after focal cerebral ischemia. *Stroke* 43, 3063–3070. doi: 10.1161/STROKEAHA.112.659656

Hyakkoku, K., Hamanaka, J., Tsuruma, K., Shimazawa, M., Tanaka, H., Uematsu, S., et al. (2010). Toll-like receptor 4 (TLR4), but not TLR3 or TLR9, knock-out mice have neuroprotective effects against focal cerebral ischemia. *Neuroscience* 171, 258–267. doi: 10.1016/j.neuroscience.2010.08.054

Iadecola, C., and Anrather, J. (2011). The immunology of stroke: from mechanisms to translation. *Nat. Med.* 17, 796–808. doi: 10.1038/nm.2399

Ikeda, N., Nonoguchi, N., Zhao, M. Z., Watanabe, T., Kajimoto, Y., Furutama, D., et al. (2005). Bone marrow stromal cells that enhanced fibroblast growth factor-2 secretion by herpes simplex virus vector improve neurological outcome after transient focal cerebral ischemia in rats. *Stroke* 36, 2725–2730. doi: 10.1161/01.STR.0000190006.88896.d3

Ikeno, Y., Konno, N., Cheon, S. H., Bolchi, A., Ottonello, S., Kitamoto, K., et al. (2005). Secretory phospholipases A2 induce neurite outgrowth in PC12 cells through lysophosphatidylcholine generation and activation of G2A receptor. *J. Biol. Chem.* 280, 28044–28052. doi: 10.1074/jbc.M503343200

Iyer, S. S., He, Q., Janczy, J. R., Elliott, E. I., Zhong, Z., Olivier, A. K., et al. (2013). Mitochondrial cardiolipin is required for Nlrp3 inflammasome activation. *Immunity* 39, 311–323. doi: 10.1016/j.immuni.2013.08.001

Kalladka, D., and Muir, K. W. (2014). Brain repair: cell therapy in stroke. *Stem Cells Cloning* 7, 31–44.

Kawai, T., and Akira, S. (2010). The role of pattern-recognition receptors in innate immunity: update on Toll-like receptors. *Nat. Immunol.* 11, 373–384. doi: 10.1038/ni.1863

Konoeda, F., Shichita, T., Yoshida, H., Sugiyama, Y., Muto, G., Hasegawa, E., et al. (2010). Therapeutic effect of IL-12/23 and their signaling pathway blockade on brain ischemia model. *Biochem. Biophys. Res. Commun.* 402, 500–506. doi: 10.1016/j.bbrc.2010.10.058

Kooijman, R., Sarre, S., Michotte, Y., and De Keyser, J. (2009). Insulin-like growth factor I: a potential neuroprotective compound for the treatment of acute ischemic stroke? *Stroke* 40, e83–e88. doi: 10.1161/STROKEAHA.108.528356

Kuang, X., Wang, L. F., Yu, L., Li, Y. J., Wang, Y. N., He, Q., et al. (2014). Ligustilide ameliorates neuroinflammation and brain injury in focal cerebral ischemia/reperfusion rats: involvement of inhibition of TLR4/peroxiredoxin 6 signaling. *Free Radic. Biol. Med.* 71, 165–175. doi: 10.1016/j.freeradbiomed.2014.03.028

Lalancette-Hébert, M., Gowing, G., Simard, A., Weng, Y. C., and Kriz, J. (2007). Selective ablation of proliferating microglial cells exacerbates ischemic injury in the brain. *J. Neurosci.* 27, 2596–2605. doi: 10.1523/JNEUROSCI.5360-06.2007

Lalancette-Hébert, M., Swarup, V., Beaulieu, J. M., Bohacek, I., Abdelhamid, E., Weng, Y. C., et al. (2012). Galectin-3 is required for resident microglia activation and proliferation in response to ischemic injury. *J. Neurosci.* 32, 10383–10395. doi: 10.1523/JNEUROSCI.1498-12.2012

Lecker, R. R., Soldner, F., Velasco, I., Gavin, D. K., Androutsellis-Theotokis, A., and McKay, R. D. (2007). Long-lasting regeneration after ischemia in the cerebral cortex. *Stroke* 38, 153–161. doi: 10.1161/01.STR.0000252156.65953.a9

Leung, P. Y., Stevens, S. L., Packard, A. E., Lessov, N. S., Yang, T., Conrad, V. K., et al. (2012). Toll-like receptor 7 preconditioning induces robust neuroprotection against stroke by a novel type I interferon-mediated mechanism. *Stroke* 43, 1383–1389. doi: 10.1161/STROKEAHA.111.641522

Liang, X., Lin, L., Woodling, N. S., Wang, Q., Anacker, C., Pan, T., et al. (2011). Signaling via the prostaglandin E2 receptor EP4 exerts neuronal and vascular protection in a mouse model of cerebral ischemia. *J. Clin. Invest.* 121, 4362–4371. doi: 10.1172/JCI46279

Lo, E. H. (2010). Degeneration and repair in central nervous system disease. *Nat. Med.* 16, 1205–1209. doi: 10.1038/nm.2226

Loser, K., Vogl, T., Voskort, M., Leuken, A., Kupas, V., Nacken, W., et al. (2010). The Toll-like receptor 4 ligands Mrp8 and Mrp14 are crucial in the development of autoreactive $CD8^+$ T cells. *Nat. Med.* 16, 713–717. doi: 10.1038/nm.2150

Mabuchi, T., Kitagawa, K., Ohtsuki, T., Kuwabara, K., Yagita, Y., Yanagihara, T., et al. (2000). Contribution of microglia/macrophages to expansion of infarction and response of oligodendrocytes after focal cerebral ischemia in rats. *Stroke* 31, 1735–1743. doi: 10.1161/01.STR.31.7.1735

Maeda, A., and Fadeel, B. (2014). Mitochondria released by cells undergoing TNF-α-induced necroptosis act as danger signals. *Cell Death Dis.* 5, e1312. doi: 10.1038/cddis.2014.277

Marcheselli, V. L., Hong, S., Lukiw, W. J., Tian, X. H., Gronert, K., Musto, A., et al. (2003). Novel docosanoids inhibit brain ischemia-reperfusion-mediated leukocyte infiltration and pro-inflammatory gene expression. *J. Biol. Chem.* 278, 43807–43817. doi: 10.1074/jbc.M305841200

Martinon, F., Burns, K., and Tschopp, J. (2002). The inflammasome: a molecular platform triggering activation of inflammatory caspases and processing of proIL-β. *Mol. Cell* 10, 417–426. doi: 10.1016/S1097-2765(02)00599-3

Matt, U., Sharif, O., Martins, R., Furtner, T., Langeberg, L., Gawish, R., et al. (2013). WAVE1 mediates suppression of phagocytosis by phospholipid-derived DAMPs. *J. Clin. Invest.* 123, 3014–3024. doi: 10.1172/JCI60681

McCullough, L., Wu, L., Haughey, N., Liang, X., Hand, T., Wang, Q., et al. (2004). Neuroprotective function of the PGE_2 EP2 receptor in cerebral ischemia. *J. Neurosci.* 24, 257–268. doi: 10.1523/JNEUROSCI.4485-03.2004

Meisel, C., and Meisel, A. (2011). Suppressing immunosuppression after stroke. *N. Engl. J. Med.* 365, 2134–2136. doi: 10.1056/NEJMcibr1112454

Miller, Y. I., Choi, S. H., Wiesner, P., Fang, L., Harkewicz, R., Hartvigsen, K., et al. (2011). Oxidation-specific epitopes are danger-associated molecular patterns recognized by pattern recognition receptors of innate immunity. *Circ. Res.* 108, 235–248. doi: 10.1161/CIRCRESAHA.110.223875

Miyata, T., Oda, O., Inagi, R., Iida, Y., Araki, N., Yamada, N., et al. (1993). beta 2-Microglobulin modified with advanced glycation end products is a major component of hemodialysis-associated amyloidosis. *J. Clin. Invest.* 92, 1243–1252. doi: 10.1172/JCI116696

Moskowitz, M. A., Lo, E. H., and Iadecola, C. (2010). The science of stroke: mechanisms in search of treatments. *Neuron* 67, 181–198. doi: 10.1016/j.neuron.2010.07.002

Muhammad, S., Barakat, W., Stoyanov, S., Murikinati, S., Yang, H., Tracey, K. J., et al. (2008). The HMGB1 receptor RAGE mediates ischemic brain damage. *J. Neurosci.* 28, 12023–12031. doi: 10.1523/JNEUROSCI.2435-08.2008

Muralikrishna Adibhatla, R., and Hatcher, J. F. (2006). Phospholipase A2, reactive oxygen species, and lipid peroxidation in cerebral ischemia. *Free Radic. Biol. Med.* 40, 376–387. doi: 10.1016/j.freeradbiomed.2005.08.044

Ness, J. K., Scaduto, R. C. Jr., and Wood, T. L. (2004). IGF-I prevents glutamate-mediated bax translocation and cytochrome C release in $O4^+$ oligodendrocyte progenitors. *Glia* 46, 183–194. doi: 10.1002/glia.10360

Ooboshi, H., Ibayashi, S., Shichita, T., Kumai, Y., Takada, J., Ago, T., et al. (2006). Postischemic gene transfer of interleukin-10 protects against both focal and global brain ischemia. *Circulation* 111, 913–919. doi: 10.1161/01.CIR.0000155622.68580.DC

Pál, G., Vincze, C., Renner, É., Wappler, E. A., Nagy, Z., Lovas, G., et al. (2012). Time course, distribution and cell types of induction of transforming growth factor betas following middle cerebral artery occlusion in the rat brain. *PLoS ONE* 7:e46731. doi: 10.1371/journal.pone.0046731

Qiang, X., Yang, W. L., Wu, R., Zhou, M., Jacob, A., Dong, W., et al. (2013). Cold-inducible RNA-binding protein (CIRP) triggers inflammatory responses in hemorrhagic shock and sepsis. *Nat. Med.* 19, 1489–1495. doi: 10.1038/nm.3368

Qiu, J., Nishimura, M., Wang, Y., Sims, J. R., Qiu, S., Savitz, S. I., et al. (2008). Early release of HMGB-1 from neurons after the onset of brain ischemia. *J. Cereb. Blood Flow Metab.* 28, 927–938. doi: 10.1038/sj.jcbfm.9600582

Qu, W. S., Wang, Y. H., Ma, J. F., Tian, D. S., Zhang, Q., Pan, D. J., et al. (2011). Galectin-1 attenuates astrogliosis-associated injuries and improves recovery of rats following focal cerebral ischemia. *J. Neurochem.* 116, 217–226. doi: 10.1111/j.1471-4159.2010.07095.x

Quintá, H. R., Pasquini, J. M., Rabinovich, G. A., and Pasquini, L. A. (2014). Glycan-dependent binding of galectin-1 to neuropilin-1 promotes axonal regeneration after spinal cord injury. *Cell Death. Differ.* 21, 941–955. doi: 10.1038/cdd.2014.14

Reed-Geaghan, E. G., Savage, J. C., Hise, A. G., and Landreth, G. E. (2009). CD14 and toll-like receptors 2 and 4 are required for fibrillar Aβ-stimulated microglial activation. *J. Neurosci.* 29, 11982–11992. doi: 10.1523/JNEUROSCI.3158-09.2009

Serhan, C. N. (2014). Pro-resolving lipid mediators are leads for resolution physiology. *Nature* 510, 92–101. doi: 10.1038/nature13479

Shanta, S. R., Choi, C. S., Lee, J. H., Shin, C. Y., Kim, Y. J., Kim, K. H., et al. (2012). Global changes in phospholipids identified by MALDI MS in rats with focal cerebral ischemia. *J. Lipid Res.* 53, 1823–1831. doi: 10.1194/jlr.M022558

Shichita, T., Hasegawa, E., Kimura, A., Morita, R., Sakaguchi, R., Takada, I., et al. (2012). Peroxiredoxin family proteins are key initiators of post-ischemic inflammation in the brain. *Nat. Med.* 18, 911–917. doi: 10.1038/nm.2749

Shichita, T., Sugiyama, Y., Ooboshi, H., Sugimori, H., Nakagawa, R., Takada, I., et al. (2009). Pivotal role of cerebral interleukin-17-producing γδT cells in the delayed phase of ischemic brain injury. *Nat. Med.* 215, 946–950. doi: 10.1038/nm.1999

Smirkin, A., Matsumoto, H., Takahashi, H., Inoue, A., Tagawa, M., Ohue, S., et al. (2010). $Iba1^+/NG2^+$ macrophage-like cells expressing a variety of neuroprotective factors ameliorate ischemic damage of the brain. *J. Cereb. Blood Flow Metab.* 30, 603–615. doi: 10.1038/jcbfm.2009.233

Spohr, T. C., Dezonne, R. S., Rehen, S. K., and Gomes, F. C. (2011). Astrocytes treated by lysophosphatidic acid induce axonal outgrowth of cortical progenitors through extracellular matrix protein and epidermal growth factor signaling pathway. *J. Neurochem.* 119, 113–123. doi: 10.1111/j.1471-4159.2011.07421.x

Starossom, S. C., Mascanfroni, I. D., Imitola, J., Cao, L., Raddassi, K., Hernandez, S. F., et al. (2012). Galectin-1 deactivates classically activated microglia and protects from inflammation-induced neurodegeneration. *Immunity* 37, 249–263. doi: 10.1016/j.immuni.2012.05.023

Stevens, S. L., Leung, P. Y., Vartanian, K. B., Gopalan, B., Yang, T., Simon, R. P., et al. (2011). Multiple preconditioning paradigms converge on interferon regulatory factor-dependent signaling to promote tolerance to ischemic brain injury. *J. Neurosci.* 31, 8456–8463. doi: 10.1523/JNEUROSCI.0821-11.2011

Stewart, C. R., Stuart, L. M., Wilkinson, K., van Gils, J. M., Deng, J., Halle, A., et al. (2010). CD36 ligands promote sterile inflammation through assembly of a Toll-like receptor 4 and 6 heterodimer. *Nat. Immunol.* 11, 155–161. doi: 10.1038/ni.1836

Sun, S., Sursal, T., Adibnia, Y., Zhao, C., Zheng, Y., Li, H., et al. (2013). Mitochondrial DAMPs increase endothelial permeability through neutrophil dependent and independent pathways. *PLoS ONE* 8:e59989. doi: 10.1371/journal.pone.0059989

Suzuki, Y., Hattori, K., Hamanaka, J., Murase, T., Egashira, Y., Mishiro, K., et al. (2012). Pharmacological inhibition of TLR4-NOX4 signal protects against neuronal death in transient focal ischemia. *Sci. Rep.* 2, 896. doi: 10.1038/srep00896

Suzuki, Y., Nakano, Y., Mishiro, K., Takagi, T., Tsuruma, K., Nakamura, M., et al. (2013). Involvement of Mincle and Syk in the changes to innate immunity after ischemic stroke. *Sci. Rep.* 3, 3177. doi: 10.1038/srep03177

Takeuchi, M., Yanase, Y., Matsuura, N., Yamagishi Si, S., Kameda, Y., Bucala, R., et al. (2001). Immunological detection of a novel advanced glycation end-product. *Mol. Med.* 7, 783–791.

Tang, S. C., Arumugam, T. V., Xu, X., Cheng, A., Mughal, M. R., Jo, D. G., et al. (2007). Pivotal role for neuronal Toll-like receptors in ischemic brain injury and functional deficits. *Proc. Natl. Acad. Sci. U.S.A.* 104, 13798–13803. doi: 10.1073/pnas.0702553104

Taniguchi, H., Anacker, C., Suarez-Mier, G. B., Wang, Q., and Andreasson, K. (2011). Function of prostaglandin E2 EP receptors in the acute outcome of rodent hypoxic ischemic encephalopathy. *Neurosci. Lett.* 504, 185–190. doi: 10.1016/j.neulet.2011.09.005

Tsai, S. Y., Segovia, J. A., Chang, T. H., Morris, I. R., Berton, M. T., Tessier, P. A., et al. (2014). DAMP molecule S100A9 acts as a molecular pattern to enhance inflammation during influenza A virus infection: role of DDX21-TRIF-TLR4-MyD88 pathway. *PLoS Pathog.* 10:e1003848. doi: 10.1371/journal.ppat.1003848

Uchida, K. (2013). Redox-derived damage-associated molecular patterns: ligand function of lipid peroxidation adducts. *Redox Biol.* 1, 94–96. doi: 10.1016/j.redox.2012.12.005

Walko, T. D. 3rd, Bola, R. A., Hong, J. D., Au, A. K., Bell, M. J., Kochanek, P. M., et al. (2014). Cerebrospinal fluid mitochondrial DNA: a novel DAMP in pediatric traumatic brain injury. *Shock* 41, 499–503. doi: 10.1097/SHK.0000000000000160

Wei, Y., Yemisci, M., Kim, H. H., Yung, L. M., Shin, H. K., Hwang, S. K., et al. (2011). Fingolimod provides long-term protection in rodent models of cerebral ischemia. *Ann. Neurol.* 69, 119–129. doi: 10.1002/ana.22186

Weil, Z. M. (2012). Ischemia-induced hyperglycemia: consequences, neuroendocrine regulation, and a role for RAGE. *Horm. Behav.* 62, 280–285. doi: 10.1016/j.yhbeh.2012.04.001

Wenceslau, C. F., McCarthy, C. G., Szasz, T., Spitler, K., Goulopoulou, S., Webb, R. C., et al. (2014). Mitochondrial damage-associated molecular patterns and vascular function. *Eur. Heart J.* 35, 1172–1177. doi: 10.1093/eurheartj/ehu047

West, X. Z., Malinin, N. L., Merkulova, A. A., Tischenko, M., Kerr, B. A., Borden, E. C., et al. (2010). Oxidative stress induces angiogenesis by activating TLR2 with novel endogenous ligands. *Nature* 467, 972–976. doi: 10.1038/nature09421

Yanai, H., Ban, T., Wang, Z., Choi, M. K., Kawamura, T., Negishi, H., et al. (2009). HMGB proteins function as universal sentinels for nucleic-acid-mediated innate immune responses. *Nature* 462, 99–103. doi: 10.1038/nature08512

Yang, F., Wang, Z., Wei, X., Han, H., Meng, X., Zhang, Y., et al. (2014). NLRP3 deficiency ameliorates neurovascular damage in experimental ischemic stroke. *J. Cereb. Blood Flow Metab.* 34, 660–667. doi: 10.1038/jcbfm.2013.242

Yang, Y., Liu, B., Dai, J., Srivastava, P. K., Zammit, D. J., Lefrançois, L., et al. (2007). Heat shock protein gp96 is a master chaperone for Toll-like receptors and is important in the innate function of macrophages. *Immunity* 26, 215–226. doi: 10.1016/j.immuni.2006.12.005

Yednock, T. A., Cannon, C., Fritz, L. C., Sanchez-Madrid, F., Steinman, L., and Karin, N. (1992). Prevention of experimental autoimmune encephalomyelitis by antibodies against α4β1 integrin. *Nature* 356, 63–66. doi: 10.1038/356063a0

Zhang, J., Takahashi, H. K., Liu, K., Wake, H., Liu, R., Maruo, T., et al. (2011). Anti-high mobility group box-1 monoclonal antibody protects the blood–brain barrier from ischemia-induced disruption in rats. *Stroke* 42, 1420–1428. doi: 10.1161/STROKEAHA.110.598334

Zhang, Q., Raoof, M., Chen, Y., Sumi, Y., Sursal, T., Junger, W., et al. (2010). Circulating mitochondrial DAMPs cause inflammatory responses to injury. *Nature* 464, 104–107. doi: 10.1038/nature08780

Zhong, Z., Zhai, Y., Liang, S., Mori, Y., Han, R., Sutterwala, F. S., et al. (2013). TRPM2 links oxidative stress to NLRP3 inflammasome activation. *Nat. Commun.* 4, 1611. doi: 10.1038/ncomms2608

Zhu, W., Fan, Y., Frenzel, T., Gasmi, M., Bartus, R. T., Young, W. L., et al. (2008). Insulin growth factor-1 gene transfer enhances neurovascular remodeling and improves long-term stroke outcome in mice. *Stroke* 39, 1254–1261. doi: 10.1161/STROKEAHA.107.500801

Zhu, W., Fan, Y., Hao, Q., Shen, F., Hashimoto, T., Yang, G. Y., et al. (2009). Postischemic IGF-1 gene transfer promotes neurovascular regeneration after experimental stroke. *J. Cereb. Blood Flow Metab.* 29, 1528–1537. doi: 10.1038/jcbfm.2009.75

Ziegler, G., Freyer, D., Harhausen, D., Khojasteh, U., Nietfeld, W., and Trendelenburg, G. (2011). Blocking TLR2 in vivo protects against accumulation of inflammatory cells and neuronal injury in experimental stroke. *J. Cereb. Blood Flow Metab.* 31, 757–766. doi: 10.1038/jcbfm.2010.161

16

$\gamma\delta$ T cells as early sensors of tissue damage and mediators of secondary neurodegeneration

Mathias Gelderblom *, Priyadharshini Arunachalam and Tim Magnus *

Department of Neurology, University Medical Center Hamburg-Eppendorf, Hamburg, Germany

Correspondence:
Mathias Gelderblom and Tim Magnus, Department of Neurology, University Medical Center Hamburg-Eppendorf, Martinistraße 52, 20246 Hamburg, Germany
e-mail: m.gelderblom@uke.de; t.magnus@uke.de

Spontaneous or medically induced reperfusion occurs in up to 70% of patients within 24 h after cerebral ischemia. Reperfusion of ischemic brain tissue can augment the inflammatory response that causes additional injury. Recently, T cells have been shown to be an essential part of the post-ischemic tissue damage, and especially IL-17 secreting T cells have been implicated in the pathogenesis of a variety of inflammatory reactions in the brain. After stroke, it seems that the innate $\gamma\delta$ T cells are the main IL-17 producing cells and that the $\gamma\delta$ T cell activation constitutes an early and mainly damaging immune response in stroke. Effector mechanism of $\gamma\delta$ T cell derived IL-17 in the ischemic brain include the induction of metalloproteinases, proinflammatory cytokines and neutrophil attracting chemokines, leading to a further amplification of the detrimental inflammatory response. In this review, we will give an overview on the concepts of $\gamma\delta$ T cells and IL-17 in stroke pathophysiology and on their potential importance for human disease conditions.

Keywords: $\gamma\delta$ T cell, stroke, inflammation, IL-17, lymphocyte, brain, ischemia, neutrophils

INTRODUCTION

Ischemic stroke is the primary reason for sustained disability and the third leading cause of death in the western world. In 85% of these patients, occlusion of an artery in the brain is the cause of stroke. Early restoration of blood flow (reperfusion) remains the treatment of choice for limiting brain injury following stroke. The reperfusion, which enhances the oxygen and glucose content in the tissue also increases an inflammatory response (Iadecola and Anrather, 2011). The idea that inflammation causes further brain injury is supported by a large number of reports that describe a reduction in infarct size and brain edema in animal models of stroke that receive blocking antibodies against specific cell adhesion molecules that mediate leukocyte recruitment (Yilmaz and Granger, 2008), anti-inflammatory treatment (Sharkey and Butcher, 1994), and immune deficient animals (Yilmaz et al., 2006; Hurn et al., 2007; Kleinschnitz et al., 2010; Gelderblom et al., 2012).

$\alpha\beta$ T CELLS AND REGULATORY T CELLS IN STROKE

Compared to resident microglia, infiltrating macrophages and neutrophils, lymphocytes and NK cells infiltrate the ischemic hemisphere in small numbers. Nevertheless, T cells have a great impact on stroke outcome. The initial observation by Yilmaz et al. that lymphocyte deficient rag1$^{-/-}$ mice are protected from stroke (Yilmaz et al., 2006) could be extended to mice with severe combined immunodeficiency lacking T cells and B cells (Hurn et al., 2007) and to CD4^{+} and CD8^{+} T cell-deficient animals (Yilmaz et al., 2006). Direct detrimental mechanisms elicited by $\alpha\beta$ T cell in stroke pathophysiology include CD8^{+} T cell derived perforin mediated cytotoxicity (Liesz et al., 2011) and IL-21 secreted by CD4^{+} T cells (Clarkson et al., 2014).

The classical activation of $\alpha\beta$ T cells requires several coincident signals: (1) engagement of the antigen receptor; (2) co-stimulatory receptors; (3) cytokine receptors such IL-2 receptor; a process requiring at least 3–5 d (Jensen et al., 2008). Multiple studies using antigen specific mucosal tolerization protocols against myelin antigens suggest the involvement of adaptive mechanism in stroke pathophysiology. Already in 1997 the group from Hallenbeck demonstrated that rodents tolerized with myelin peptides are protected from ischemic stroke (Becker et al., 1997). Mechanistically the protective effects could be attributed to IL-10 producing T cells (Frenkel et al., 2005) and transforming growth factor-β1 (Becker et al., 2003).

These classical concepts of T cell activation are challenged by the observation that detrimental T cell dependent effects following cerebral ischemia can be observed already 24 h post stroke, in an antigen independent fashion (Kleinschnitz et al., 2010). Similarly controversial is the role of regulatory T_{regs} and B cells in stroke. Liesz and colleagues showed that endogenous T_{regs} are protective in later stages following stroke when the lesions were small (Liesz et al., 2009) and that their beneficial functions depend on IL-10 (Liesz et al., 2013). However, a lot of the observed effects of T_{regs} cannot be attributed to concepts of adaptive immunity. For example, an early direct inhibitory effect of T_{regs} on the MMP9 production from neutrophils was a recently suggested mechanism (Li et al., 2013). In this model, transfer of regulatory T_{regs} conferred protective effects on the outcome already on day one after stroke even before T_{regs} infiltrated the

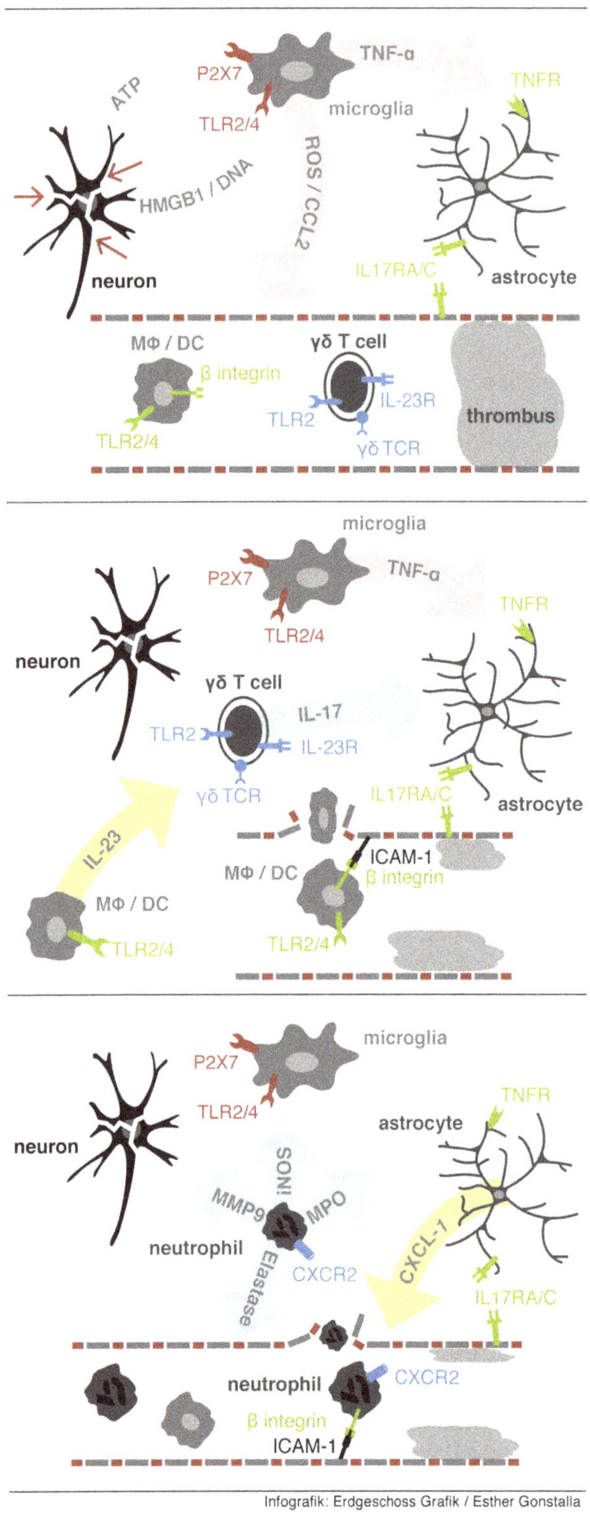

FIGURE 1 | Sequential events leading to neutrophil infiltration. First, release from DAMPs from injured cells activates resident microglia via PPRs to release proinflammatory factors including TNF-α. Second, IL-23 activates γδ T cells to rapidly secrete IL-17 in the ischemic tissue. Third, neutrophil infiltration is initiated via IL-17 and TNF-α synergistically induced expression of CXCL-1 in astrocytes.

ischemic brain. Protective effects could be attributed to program death-1 ligand 1 (PD-L1) dependent inhibition on MMP9 production in neutrophils in the peripheral circulation which then led to a consecutive protection of the blood brain barrier (Li et al., 2014). Further studies even challenged the overall concept of T_{regs} as endogenous protective immune cell population in stroke (Ren et al., 2011) and a recent study suggests that T_{regs} have an early detrimental role, by inducing dysfunction of the cerebral microcirculation (Kleinschnitz et al., 2013). While the data on T cell effects in particular T_{regs} in stroke is still controversial, it is clear that most of the important immunological effects are not following classical concepts of adaptive immunity, suggesting an innate like behavior of lymphocytes. In this line, atypical T cells such as γδ T cell and NK cells are likely to participate in the early orchestration of the inflammatory reaction. For NK cells it has been shown that neuronal cell death is mediated by IFN-γ- and Perforin-dependent pathways as early as 3 h post reperfusion (Gan et al., 2014). A lot more data exist on γδ T cell, which we will focus on in the following section.

BIOLOGY OF γδ T CELLS SUBPOPULATIONS

Like αβ T cells, γδ T cells develop in the thymus using the recombinase activated gene product (RAG) for the somatic rearrangement of V (variable), D (Diversity and J (joining) gene segments of the γ and δ chains of their T cell receptor (TcR) (reviewed in Raulet, 1989). Compared to αβ TcR, the sets of TcR detected on γδ T cells are limited. Many γδ subsets, primarily the ones populating certain tissues such as the epidermis, dermis, intestine, lungs and uterus are displaying an even higher limitation of their TcR diversity. These tissue-specific γδ T cell subsets show a biased use of certain TcR V gene segments. Since some of them express "invariant" TcRs with identical (canonical) junctional sequences, they are also named canonical γδ T cells. As reviewed by Vantourout and Hayday, the limited TcR diversity implies that these cells recognize either pathogen encoded antigens, that are likely to be encountered in specific tissues such as the epidermis, or self-encoded molecules that reflect a dysregulated state of that tissue (Vantourout and Hayday, 2013). Since these γδ T cell subsets can be rapidly activated without the requirement of prior clonal expansion they are also called "innate like" T cells. In contrast to canonical γδ T cells so-called non-canonical γδ T cells, which are characterized by an expression of more diverse γδ TcRs, are homing into secondary lymphoid tissues. Here they make up a minor fraction of rodent and human T cells after birth (in mice 1–4% of all T cells). In the context of immune responses non-canonical γδ T cells are capable to participate distant from their original site of residence, by trafficking to the site of inflammation in solid organs (reviewed by Korn and Petermann, 2012). Similar to αβ T cells, γδ T cells can be divided by their cytokine profile. Mouse γδ T cells which are developing from fetal liver progenitors undergo functional pre-programming, which leads to a subpopulation of IL-17 producing Scart-2^+ and $CCR6^+$ γδ T cells on one side and IFN-γ producing $NK.1.1^+$ and $CD27^+$ γδ T cells on the other side. Both subpopulations have an innate like phenotype, since they can be rapidly activated without prior clonal expansion (Vantourout and Hayday, 2013). γδ T cells fulfill important sentinel functions in the immune system. The ability of γδ T cells to recognize molecules that are rapidly displayed after stress without requiring extensive clonal expansion permits γδ T cells to participate in early stages of immune responses. In such scenarios γδ T cells act in parallel with cells of the innate immune system as sensors of dysregulation. γδ T cells may respond to classical signals of the adaptive immune system or to cytokine signals and either Toll-like receptor (TLR) or dectin stimuli in the absence of TcR ligation. Activation of the γδ TcR can occur through major histocompatibility complex (MHC)-related and unrelated TcR ligands, which are including foreign- and self-antigens. This allows γδ T cells to respond to infection and sterile tissue dysregulation such as ischemia. Beside TcR dependent mechanisms γδ T cell activation can be mediated through engagement of the activating natural killer receptors (NKRs) such as NK group 2 member D (NKD2D), by patter recognition receptors including TLRs (reviewed by Bonneville et al., 2010) and through cytokines such as IL-1β and/or IL-23 (Sutton et al., 2009). The constitutive expression of IL-23 and IL-1β receptors by γδ T cells assures this rapid responsiveness. Within hours upon activation and without prior expansion systemic γδ T cells can express high levels of effector cytokines, such as IFN-γ, IL-17, TNF-α and granzymes. In addition, γδ T cells are capable of producing numerous chemokines and regulatory factors including IL-13 and insulin-like-growth factor 1 (IGF-1), allowing them to interact with other immune cells, such as B cells and αβ T cells in the afferent phase of the immune response. Regarding the cellular interplay between γδ T cells and innate immune cells neutrophils play a central role. Once activated, γδ T cells can stimulate the release of potent chemoattractants for neutrophils. In this respect, γδ T cells were recently shown to be the primary sources of the neutrophil-attracting IL-17 in mouse models of infection (Shibata et al., 2007), hypersensitivity (Simonian et al., 2009) and autoimmunity (Roark et al., 2007). Often the activation of the innate immune system results in a feed back loop that increasingly stimulates γδ T cells.

γδ T CELLS AS SENSORS OF TISSUE DAMAGE IN STROKE

Stroke resembles classical features of a "sterile inflammation", which is characterized by a inflammation in response to tissue disruption without the involvement of pathogenic microorganisms (See **Figure 1**; Chen and Nuñez, 2010). Sterile inflammation shares similar mechanisms with inflammation during infection. Receptors essential for sensing microorganisms are collectively called pattern recognition receptors (PPRs). PRRs sense conserved structural moieties that are found in microorganisms and are often called pathogen-associated molecular patterns (PAMPs) (for review see Chen and Nuñez, 2010). Following ligand recognition these receptors activate downstream signaling pathways, such as the nuclear factor-κb (NF-κb), mitogen-activated protein kinase (MAPK) and type I interferon pathways, which result in the upregulation of pro-inflammatory cytokines and chemokines that are important in inflammatory responses. In non-infectious conditions immune cells can be activated via recognition of endogenous material by PPRs. These endogenous molecules have been named danger-associated molecular patterns (DAMPs). Under physiological conditions these DAMPs are localized intracellularly. Under conditions of apoptotic cells death, cells are cleared immunologically silent without significant release of DAMPs into the extracellular environment. In contrast, necrosis following ischemia leads to loss of cell integrity and release of the cell content into the extracellular space. DAMPs derived from necrotic cells include the chromatin-associated protein high-mobility group box 1 (HMGB1), heat shock proteins (HSPs), mitochondrial peptides and purine metabolites, such as adenosine triphosphate (ATP) and uric acid (reviewed by Chen and Nuñez, 2010 and Shen et al., 2013). Consecutively, activated receptors and signaling pathways include TLR2/4/9, CD24, CD44, NLRP3, formyl peptide receptor 1, RAGE and IL-1 receptor. In the context of stroke DAMPs are massively released into the extracellular compartment. In stroke several pathways have been described, including TLR2/4, CD38, P2X7 and RAGE, which are associated with an worsened outcome (Liu et al., 2007; Tang et al., 2008; Choe et al., 2011; Arbeloa et al., 2012). As we discussed above γδ T cells can be activated directly by DAMPs via TLR1/2 and dectin receptors and cytokines, such as IL-1β and IL-23 (Martin et al., 2009; Sutton et al., 2012). Following stroke, there is clear evidence that IL-23 activates IL-17 production in γδ T cells (Shichita et al., 2009). Even though it is likely that further signals via TcR and TLR/dectin receptors are necessary to fully activate γδ T cells, the actual experimental data is outstanding.

EFFECTOR MECHANISMS OF γδ T CELLS IN STROKE

Several papers have shown a significant contribution of γδ T cells and IL-17 in stroke and other conditions of central nervous system inflammation (Kebir et al., 2007; Shichita et al., 2009; Caccamo et al., 2011; Gelderblom et al., 2012). In ischemia reperfusion injury of the brain we and others have observed a pathogenic role of γδ T cells, which can be detected in ischemic brain tissue as early as 6 h post ischemia (Shichita et al., 2009; Gelderblom et al., 2012). Effector mechanisms of γδ T cells in stroke primarily depend on their IL-17 production. In stroke, synergistic stimulation of astrocytes by IL-17 and TNF-α induces a massive induction of neutrophil attracting chemokines including CXCL-1 (Gelderblom et al., 2012), resulting in a subsequent neutrophil infiltration, which is leading to an increased tissue damage. Activated macrophages and microglia are secreting high amounts of TNF-α in the ischemic tissue. In the presence of the TNF-α rich milieu the additional IL-17 signal leads to the rapid increase of CXCL-1 via a stabilizing effect on the CXCL-1 RNA in astrocytes. Blocking either signal, IL-17 or the CXCL-1/CXCR2-axis, results in a robust reduction in infarct size and a significant improved neurological outcome. Even if an anti-IL-17 antibody is administered 6 h after stroke, neutrophil invasion can be blocked (Gelderblom et al., 2012). Neutrophil independent effects of IL-17 secreted by γδ T cells in stroke include the induction of MMP3 and MMP9 which are associated with blood brain barrier breakdown (Shichita et al., 2009; Gelderblom et al., 2012). Other potential effector functions of γδ T are engagement of death inducing receptors such as CD95 or TNF-related apoptosis-inducing ligand receptors (TRAILR), and the release of cytotoxic effector molecules, such as perforin and granzymes (See **Figure 1**). Molecular signals directing γδ T cell into the ischemic brain is another unresolved issue. γδ T cell subpopulations can be divided by Scart-2 and CCR6 vs. NK.1.1 and CD27 expression into IL-17 vs. IFN-γ producing T cells, respectively. The functional relevance of the CCR6 expression on IL-17 producing γδ T cells is supported by experimental data, showing that the migration of γδ T cells into the inflamed liver depends on the CCL20/CCR6 axis (Hammerich et al., 2014). Nevertheless, in stroke it is so far unclear which chemokines/chemokine receptors are essential for the entry of γδ T cells into the ischemic brain and which γδ T cell subpopulations are migrating into the ischemic brain.

ROLE OF γδ T CELLS IN HUMAN STROKE PATHOPHYSIOLOGY

Most of the data on inflammation in stroke is derived from studies in rodent models. These models have several drawback, including differences between the immune system of rodents and humans. Further, the vast majority of stroke patients are older that 65 and are characterized by co-morbidities, which are not reflected in rodent models (Heuschmann et al., 2010). Despite these discrepancies, results from post-mortem and imaging studies in human stroke demonstrate that a rapid activation of the resident and systemic immune system are hallmarks of human stroke pathophysiology (Mena et al., 2004; Price et al., 2004; Thiel and Heiss, 2011). Similar to experimental stroke, neutrophils are recruited into the ischemic brain within 24 h after symptom onset (Chuaqui and Tapia, 1993; Price et al., 2004) and microglia undergo rapid activation in the infarct core but also remote areas such as fiber tracts or relay nuclei (Thiel and Heiss, 2011). These findings let to several clinical trials targeting neutrophils in human stroke. Studies employing inhibitors of the neutrophil—endothelial cell interaction including CD18 and ICAM-1 were conducted, none of them showing favorable results on the clinical outcome parameters (del Zoppo, 2010). Nevertheless, the immunological understanding of the post ischemic inflammatory response was limited when these human trials were designed. Regarding our current understanding of the stroke induced inflammation IL-17 seems to be promising target. Infiltration by γδ T cells and secretion of IL-17 have been demonstrated in ischemic pathological human brain tissue (Li et al., 2005; Gelderblom et al., 2012). Similarly, IL-17 induced downstream pathways can be found. The IL-17 presence in the ischemic brain is early and short-lived and has most likely only pro-inflammatory effects. Therefore a short anti-IL-17 intervention could be beneficial without producing side effects, for example enhancing the systemic immune suppression. Recent data from human clinical trials with humanized neutralizing IL-17A antibodies in patients with autoimmune disease showed that treatment is well tolerized and effective (Hueber et al., 2010).

SUMMARY

Inflammation can enhance ischemic damage and lymphocytes seem to be important component of this process. Interestingly, the classical concepts of adaptive immune responses do not explain all observed effects. Several innate like features of lymphocytes dominate the early pro-inflammatory events. Particularly atypical T cells such as γδ T cells could explain some of these discrepancies and targeted treatment against their signature cytokine IL-17 might be a promising treatment option.

REFERENCES

Arbeloa, J., Pérez-Samartín, A., Gottlieb, M., and Matute, C. (2012). P2X7 receptor blockade prevents ATP excitotoxicity in neurons and reduces brain damage after ischemia. *Neurobiol. Dis.* 45, 954–961. doi: 10.1016/j.nbd.2011.12.014

Becker, K., Kindrick, D., McCarron, R., Hallenbeck, J., and Winn, R. (2003). Adoptive transfer of myelin basic protein-tolerized splenocytes to naive animals reduces infarct size: a role for lymphocytes in ischemic brain injury? *Stroke* 34, 1809–1815. doi: 10.1161/01.str.0000078308.77727.ea

Becker, K. J., McCarron, R. M., Ruetzler, C., Laban, O., Sternberg, E., Flanders, K. C., et al. (1997). Immunologic tolerance to myelin basic protein decreases stroke size after transient focal cerebral ischemia. *Proc. Natl. Acad. Sci. U S A* 94, 10873–10878. doi: 10.1073/pnas.94.20.10873

Bonneville, M., O'Brien, R. L., and Born, W. K. (2010). Gammadelta T cell effector functions: a blend of innate programming and acquired plasticity. *Nat. Rev. Immunol.* 10, 467–478. doi: 10.1038/nri2781

Caccamo, N., La Mendola, C., Orlando, V., Meraviglia, S., Todaro, M., Stassi, G., et al. (2011). Differentiation, phenotype and function of interleukin-17-producing human Vγ9Vδ2 T cells. *Blood* 118, 129–138. doi: 10.1182/blood-2011-01-331298

Chen, G. Y., and Nuñez, G. (2010). Sterile inflammation: sensing and reacting to damage. *Nat. Rev. Immunol.* 10, 826–837. doi: 10.1038/nri2873

Choe, C.-U., Lardong, K., Gelderblom, M., Ludewig, P., Leypoldt, F., Koch-Nolte, F., et al. (2011). CD38 exacerbates focal cytokine production, postischemic inflammation and brain injury after focal cerebral ischemia. *PLoS One* 6:e19046. doi: 10.1371/journal.pone.0019046

Chuaqui, R., and Tapia, J. (1993). Histologic assessment of the age of recent brain infarcts in man. *J. Neuropathol. Exp. Neurol.* 52, 481–489. doi: 10.1097/00005072-199309000-00006

Clarkson, B. D. S., Ling, C., Shi, Y., Harris, M. G., Rayasam, A., Sun, D., et al. (2014). T cell-derived interleukin (IL)-21 promotes brain injury following stroke in mice. *J. Exp. Med.* 211, 595–604. doi: 10.1084/jem.20131377

del Zoppo, G. J. (2010). Acute anti-inflammatory approaches to ischemic stroke. *Ann. N Y Acad. Sci.* 1207, 143–148. doi: 10.1111/j.1749-6632.2010.05761.x

Frenkel, D., Huang, Z., Maron, R., Koldzic, D. N., Moskowitz, M. A., and Weiner, H. L. (2005). Neuroprotection by IL-10-producing MOG CD4+ T cells following ischemic stroke. *J. Neurol. Sci.* 233, 125–132. doi: 10.1016/j.jns.2005.03.022

Gan, Y., Liu, Q., Wu, W., Yin, J. X., Bai, X. F., Shen, R., et al. (2014). Ischemic neurons recruit natural killer cells that accelerate brain infarction. *Proc. Natl. Acad. Sci. U S A* 111, 2704–2709. doi: 10.1073/pnas.1315943111

Gelderblom, M., Weymar, A., Bernreuther, C., Velden, J., Arunachalam, P., Steinbach, K., et al. (2012). Neutralization of the IL-17 axis diminishes neutrophil invasion and protects from ischemic stroke. *Blood* 120, 3793–3802. doi: 10.1182/blood-2012-02-412726

Hammerich, L., Bangen, J. M., Govaere, O., Zimmermann, H. W., Gassler, N., Huss, S., et al. (2014). Chemokine receptor CCR6-dependent accumulation of γδ T cells in injured liver restricts hepatic inflammation and fibrosis. *Hepatology* 59, 630–642. doi: 10.1002/hep.26697

Heuschmann, P., Busse, O., Wagner, M., Endres, M., Villringer, A., Röther, J., et al. (2010). Schlaganfallhäufigkeit und Versorgung von Schlaganfallpatienten in Deutschland. *Akt. Neurol.* 37, 333–340. doi: 10.1055/s-0030-1248611

Hueber, W., Patel, D. D., Dryja, T., Wright, A. M., Koroleva, I., Bruin, G., et al. (2010). Effects of AIN457, a fully human antibody to Interleukin-17A, on Psoriasis, Rheumatoid Arthritis and Uveitis. *Sci. Transl. Med.* 2:52ra72. doi: 10.1126/scitranslmed.3001107

Hurn, P. D., Subramanian, S., Parker, S. M., Afentoulis, M. E., Kaler, L. J., Vandenbark, A. A., et al. (2007). T- and B-cell-deficient mice with experimental stroke have reduced lesion size and inflammation. *J. Cereb. Blood Flow Metab.* 27, 1798–1805. doi: 10.1038/sj.jcbfm.9600482

Iadecola, C., and Anrather, J. (2011). The immunology of stroke: from mechanisms to translation. *Nat. Med.* 17, 796–808. doi: 10.1038/nm.2399

Jensen, K. D. C., Su, X., Shin, S., Li, L., Youssef, S., Yamasaki, S., et al. (2008). Thymic selection determines γδ T cell effector fate: antigen-naive cells make interleukin-17 and antigen-experienced cells make interferon γ. *Immunity* 29, 90–100. doi: 10.1016/j.immuni.2008.04.022

Kebir, H., Kreymborg, K., Ifergan, I., Dodelet-Devillers, A., Cayrol, R., Bernard, M., et al. (2007). Human TH17 lymphocytes promote blood-brain barrier disruption and central nervous system inflammation. *Nat. Med.* 13, 1173–1175. doi: 10.1038/nm1651

Kleinschnitz, C., Kraft, P., Dreykluft, A., Hagedorn, I., Göbel, K., Schuhmann, M. K., et al. (2013). Regulatory T cells are strong promoters of acute ischemic stroke in mice by inducing dysfunction of the cerebral microvasculature. *Blood* 121, 679–691. doi: 10.1182/blood-2012-04-426734

Kleinschnitz, C., Schwab, N., Kraft, P., Hagedorn, I., Dreykluft, A., Schwarz, T., et al. (2010). Early detrimental T-cell effects in experimental cerebral ischemia are neither related to adaptive immunity nor thrombus formation. *Blood* 115, 3835–3842. doi: 10.1182/blood-2009-10-249078

Korn, T., and Petermann, F. (2012). Development and function of interleukin 17-producing γδ T cells. *Ann. N Y Acad. Sci.* 1247, 34–45. doi: 10.1111/j.1749-6632.2011.06355.x

Li, P., Gan, Y., Sun, B.-L., Zhang, F., Lu, B., Gao, Y., et al. (2013). Adoptive regulatory T-cell therapy protects against cerebral ischemia. *Ann. Neurol.* 74, 458–471. doi: 10.1002/ana.23815

Li, P., Mao, L., Liu, X., Gan, Y., Zheng, J., Thomson, A. W., et al. (2014). Essential role of program death 1-Ligand 1 in regulatory T-cell-afforded protection against blood-brain barrier damage after stroke. *Stroke* 45, 857–864. doi: 10.1161/STROKEAHA.113.004100

Li, G.-Z., Zhong, D., Yang, L.-M., Sun, B., Zhongy, Z.-H., Yin, Y.-H., et al. (2005). Expression of interleukin-17 in ischemic brain tissue. *Scand. J. Immunol.* 62, 481–486. doi: 10.1111/j.1365-3083.2005.01683.x

Liesz, A., Suri-Payer, E., Veltkamp, C., Doerr, H., Sommer, C., Rivest, S., et al. (2009). Regulatory T cells are key cerebroprotective immunomodulators in acute experimental stroke. *Nat. Med.* 15, 192–199. doi: 10.1038/nm.1927

Liesz, A., Zhou, W., Mracskó, E., Karcher, S., Bauer, H., Schwarting, S., et al. (2011). Inhibition of lymphocyte trafficking shields the brain against deleterious neuroinflammation after stroke. *Brain* 134, 704–720. doi: 10.1093/brain/awr008

Liesz, A., Zhou, W., Na, S. Y., Hämmerling, G. J., Garbi, N., Karcher, S., et al. (2013). Boosting regulatory T cells limits neuroinflammation in permanent cortical stroke. *J. Neurosci.* 33, 17350–17362. doi: 10.1523/JNEUROSCI.4901-12.2013

Liu, K., Mori, S., Takahashi, H. K., Tomono, Y., Wake, H., Kanke, T., et al. (2007). Anti-high mobility group box 1 monoclonal antibody ameliorates brain infarction induced by transient ischemia in rats. *FASEB J.* 21, 3904–3916. doi: 10.1096/fj.07-8770com

Martin, B., Hirota, K., Cua, D. J., Stockinger, B., and Veldhoen, M. (2009). Interleukin-17-producing gammadelta T cells selectively expand in response to pathogen products and environmental signals. *Immunity* 31, 321–330. doi: 10.1016/j.immuni.2009.06.020

Mena, H., Cadavid, D., and Rushing, E. J. (2004). Human cerebral infarct: a proposed histopathologic classification based on 137 cases. *Acta Neuropathol.* 108, 524–530. doi: 10.1007/s00401-004-0918-z

Price, C. J. S., Menon, D. K., Peters, A. M., Ballinger, J. R., Barber, R. W., Balan, K. K., et al. (2004). Cerebral neutrophil recruitment, histology and outcome in acute ischemic stroke: an imaging-based study. *Stroke* 35, 1659–1664. doi: 10.1161/01.str.0000130592.71028.92

Raulet, D. H. (1989). The structure, function, and molecular genetics of the gamma/delta T cell receptor. *Annu. Rev. Immunol.* 7, 175–207. doi: 10.1146/annurev.immunol.7.1.175

Ren, X., Akiyoshi, K., Vandenbark, A. A., Hurn, P. D., and Offner, H. (2011). CD4+FoxP3+ regulatory T-cells in cerebral ischemic stroke. *Metab. Brain Dis.* 26, 87–90. doi: 10.1007/s11011-010-9226-6

Roark, C. L., French, J. D., Taylor, M. A., Bendele, A. M., Born, W. K., and O'Brien, R. L. (2007). Exacerbation of collagen-induced arthritis by oligoclonal, IL-17-producing γδ T cells. *J. Immunol.* 179, 5576–5583. doi: 10.4049/jimmunol.179.8.5576

Sharkey, J., and Butcher, S. P. (1994). Immunophilins mediate the neuroprotective effects of Fk506 in focal cerebral-ischemia. *Nature* 371, 336–339. doi: 10.1038/371336a0

Shen, H., Kreisel, D., and Goldstein, D. R. (2013). Processes of Sterile Inflammation. *J. Immunol.* 191, 2857–2863. doi: 10.4049/jimmunol.1301539

Shibata, K., Yamada, H., Hara, H., Kishihara, K., and Yoshikai, Y. (2007). Resident Vdelta1+ gammadelta T cells control early infiltration of neutrophils after Escherichia coli infection via IL-17 production. *J. Immunol.* 178, 4466–4472. doi: 10.4049/jimmunol.178.7.4466

Shichita, T., Sugiyama, Y., Ooboshi, H., Sugimori, H., Nakagawa, R., Takada, I., et al. (2009). Pivotal role of cerebral interleukin-17-producing gammadeltaT cells in the delayed phase of ischemic brain injury. *Nat. Med.* 15, 946–950. doi: 10.1038/nm.1999

Simonian, P. L., Roark, C. L., Wehrmann, F., Lanham, A. M., Born, W. K., O'Brien, R. L., et al. (2009). IL-17A-Expressing T Cells are essential for bacterial clearance in a Murine Model of Hypersensitivity Pneumonitis. *J. Immunol.* 182, 6540–6549. doi: 10.4049/jimmunol.0900013

Sutton, C. E., Lalor, S. J., Sweeney, C. M., Brereton, C. F., Lavelle, E. C., and Mills, K. H. G. (2009). Interleukin-1 and IL-23 induce innate IL-17 production from gammadelta T cells, amplifying Th17 responses and autoimmunity. *Immunity* 31, 331–341. doi: 10.1016/j.immuni.2009.08.001

Sutton, C. E., Mielke, L. A., and Mills, K. H. G. (2012). IL-17-producing γδ T cells and innate lymphoid cells. *Eur. J. Immunol.* 42, 2221–2231. doi: 10.1002/eji.201242569

Tang, S.-C., Lathia, J. D., Selvaraj, P. K., Jo, D.-G., Mughal, M. R., Cheng, A., et al. (2008). Toll-like receptor-4 mediates neuronal apoptosis induced by amyloid beta-peptide and the membrane lipid peroxidation product 4-hydroxynonenal. *Exp. Neurol.* 213, 114–121. doi: 10.1016/j.expneurol.2008.05.014

Thiel, A., and Heiss, W.-D. (2011). Imaging of microglia activation in stroke. *Stroke* 42, 507–512. doi: 10.1161/STROKEAHA.110.598821

Vantourout, P., and Hayday, A. (2013). Six-of-the-best: unique contributions of. *Nat. Rev. Immunol.* 13, 88–100. doi: 10.1038/nri3384

Yilmaz, G., Arumugam, T. V., Stokes, K. Y., and Granger, D. N. (2006). Role of T lymphocytes and interferon-gamma in ischemic stroke. *Circulation* 113, 2105–2112. doi: 10.1161/circulationaha.105.593046

Yilmaz, G., and Granger, D. N. (2008). Cell adhesion molecules and ischemic stroke. *Neurol. Res.* 30, 783–793. doi: 10.1179/174313208X341085

17

Fingolimod for the treatment of neurological diseases—state of play and future perspectives

Robert Brunkhorst[1], Rajkumar Vutukuri[2] and Waltraud Pfeilschifter[1]*

[1] *Cerebrovascular Research Group, Department of Neurology, Frankfurt University Hospital, Frankfurt am Main, Germany*
[2] *Institute of General Pharmacology and Toxicology, pharmazentrum frankfurt, Goethe University Frankfurt, Frankfurt am Main, Germany*

***Correspondence:**
Waltraud Pfeilschifter, Cerebrovascular Research Group, Department of Neurology, Frankfurt University Hospital, Theodor-Stern-Kai 7, 60590 Frankfurt am Main, Germany
e-mail: Waltraud.Pfeilschifter@kgu.de

Sphingolipids are a fascinating class of signaling molecules derived from the membrane lipid sphingomyelin. They show abundant expression in the brain. Complex sphingolipids such as glycosphingolipids (gangliosides and cerebrosides) regulate vesicular transport and lysosomal degradation and their dysregulation can lead to storage diseases with a neurological phenotype. More recently, simple sphingolipids such ceramide, sphingosine and sphingosine 1-phosphate (S1P) were discovered to signal in response to many extracellular stimuli. Forming an intricate signaling network, the balance of these readily interchangeable mediators is decisive for cell fate under stressful conditions. The immunomodulator fingolimod is the prodrug of an S1P receptor agonist. Following receptor activation, the drug leads to downregulation of the $S1P_1$ receptor inducing functional antagonism. As the first drug to modulate the sphingolipid signaling pathway, it was marketed in 2010 for the treatment of multiple sclerosis (MS). At that time, immunomodulation was widely accepted as the key mechanism of fingolimod's efficacy in MS. But given the excellent passage of this lipophilic compound into the brain and its massive brain accumulation as well as the abundant expression of S1P receptors on brain cells, it is conceivable that fingolimod also affects brain cells directly. Indeed, a seminal study showed that the protective effect of fingolimod in experimental autoimmune encephalitis (EAE), a murine MS model, is lost in mice lacking the $S1P_1$ receptor on astrocytes, arguing for a specific role of astrocytic S1P signaling in MS. In this review, we discuss the role of sphingolipid mediators and their metabolizing enzymes in neurologic diseases and putative therapeutic strategies arising thereof.

Keywords: sphingosine 1-phosphate, ceramides, sphingosine kinase, sphingosine 1-phosphate receptors, multiple sclerosis, stroke, epilepsy, dementia

THE SPHINGOLIPID SIGNALING PATHWAY

Sphingolipids have first been described by the German physician Ludwig Thudichum, then living in London (Great Britain) in the end of the 19th century in his book "A treatise on the chemical constitution of the brain". The more complex cerebrosides) are required for cell functions such as cell recognition, vesicular transport and lysosomal degradation and their dysregulation can lead to storage diseases with a neurological phenotype (Sandhoff and Christomanou, 1979), for example Tay-Sachs disease, Sandhoff disease or Niemann-Pick disease. The physiological relevance of sphingomyelin and its derivatives as signaling molecules gradually came into focus during the last decades, spurred by the discovery of sphingosine as an inhibitor of protein kinase C (Hannun et al., 1986; Wilson et al., 1986, reviewed by Kolesnick, 1991). Numerous reviews focus on the intricate regulation of the sphingolipid pathway (Huwiler et al., 2000; Hannun and Obeid, 2008; Huwiler and Pfeilschifter, 2008) with ceramides and sphingosine 1-phosphate (S1P) functioning as key signaling molecules (**Figure 1**). The pathway forms a rheostat and the substrates are readily interconvertible. Ceramide, which is derived either from the membrane lipid sphingomyelin by sphingomyelinases or synthesized de novo can be induced by many cell stressors. It acts on defined intracellular targets (reviewed by Huwiler et al., 2000; Ruvolo, 2003) and in general has proinflammatory and proapototic effects. It is degraded to sphingosine, which can be phosphorylated to S1P by sphingosine

Abbreviations: AD, Alzheimer's disease; BBB, blood-brain barrier; BDNF, brain-derived neurotrophic factor; CNS, central nervous system; EAE, experimental autoimmune encephalitis; ERK1/2, extracellular signal-regulated kinase; GBM, multiform glioblastoma; Gd, gadolinium; HDAC, histone deacetylase; HIF, hypoxia-inducible factor; HP, hypoxic preconditioning; HRE, hypoxia-responsive element; IFNγ, interferon γ; IL-1β, Interleukin-1β; LPP3, lysophospholipid phosphatase 3; LPS, lipopolysaccharide; LTP, long-term potentiation; MRI, magnetic resonance imaging; MS, multiple sclerosis; PKB/Akt, protein kinase B/Akt kinase; RRMS, relapsing-remitting MS; NMDA, N-methyl-D-aspartate; S1P, sphingosine 1-phosphate; $S1P_{1-5}$, S1P receptor types 1 to 5; S1PL, sphingosine 1-phosphate lyase; SphK1, sphingosine kinase 1; SphK2, sphingosine kinase 2; SPP, sphingosine 1-phosphate phosphatase; TNFα, tumor necrosis factor α; t-PA, tissue-type plasminogen activator; TrkB, tropomyosin receptor kinase B; VEGFα, vascular endothelial growth factor α.

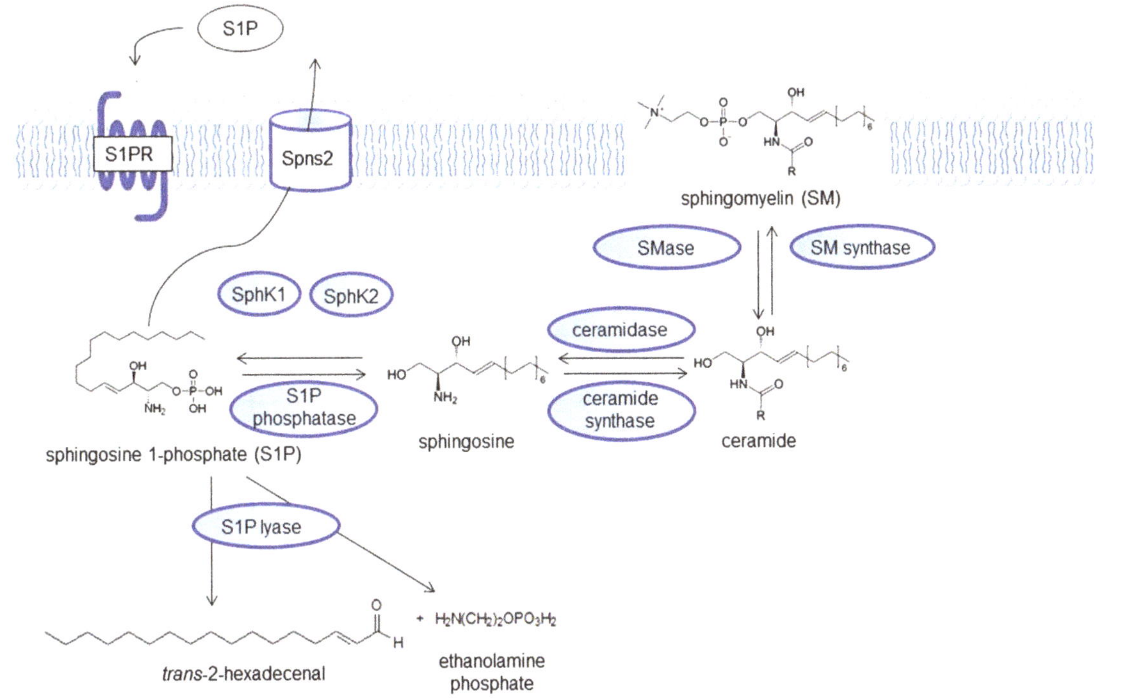

FIGURE 1 | The sphingolipid signaling pathway. Sphingolipid signaling molecules are derived from the membrane lipid sphingomyelin and intricately regulated forming a "rheostat" that can be imbalanced in disease states.

kinase (SphK), an enzyme that exists in two isoforms with different subcellular distribution, SphK1 and SphK2. S1P is an antiinflammtory, proproliferative and antiapoptotic signaling molecule. It was first assumed to act as an intracellular second messenger, because its cellular levels increased upon growth factor stimulation of SphK. However, it took years to identify the first intracellular targets of S1P, whereas it was soon discovered that S1P can signal from the extracellular side through a family of G protein-coupled receptors (GPCRs), formerly known as Endothelial Differentiation Genes (EDG; Kluk and Hla, 2002). Previously, they had been orphan receptors without known ligands. In 2002, they were renamed by the IUPHAR into $S1P_{1-5}$ (Chun et al., 2002). Kawahara et al. (2009) identified Spinster 2 (Spns2) as a specific outward transporter for S1P (**Figure 2**).

Mouse models with genetic deletions of S1P receptors and the use of pharmacological tools have been helpful to shed light on the role of S1P in lymphocyte homeostasis, in the development of the cardiovascular and the central nervous system (CNS), and maintenance of endothelial barriers (reviewed by Brinkmann, 2007). $S1P_{1-3}$ show a practically ubiquitous expression, whereas $S1P_4$ expression is mainly detectable on leukocytes but not relevantly in the brain, and $S1P_5$ shows a high expression in oligodendrocytes, the main myelinating cells of the brain. The receptors couple to different G proteins (Gαi, Gαq, Gα12/13). From the point-of-view of drug development, the differential receptor expression patterns in different organs, a modulation of receptor expression in disease states, as well as the differential coupling to G proteins, may afford a sufficient degree of specificity to make S1P receptors drugable targets (**Figure 2**).

Currently, many of the pathophysiologically relevant processes seem to be regulated by the $S1P_1$ receptor. Studies of S1P receptor knockout mice showed embryonic lethality for $S1P_1$-deficient mice with defects in vasculogenesis and neural tube formation, supporting the important role of this receptor in developmental processes, but not for mice deficient for one of the other four S1P receptors. The $S1P_1$ receptor has also been shown to be the relevant receptor to mediate the decisive effect of the vascular S1P gradient on the number of circulating immune cells. S1P concentrations are close to the micromolar range in the bloodstream and concentrations in interstitial fluids are around three orders of magnitude lower. Most prominent are the effects on T lymphocytes: antigen-induced activation of T cells leads to an up-regulation of $S1P_1$ and therefore increases the responsiveness to S1P. $S1P_1$ regulates T cell trafficking at multiple stages of T cell development as well as their responses, e.g., thymocyte egress into the periphery, egress of mature T cells out of lymph nodes during systemic trafficking and retention of T cells in non-lymphoid tissues. B cells do not require $S1P_1$ to leave the bone marrow but, like T cells, they need the receptor to exit secondary lymphoid organs (Matloubian et al., 2004; Ledgerwood et al., 2008; Skon et al., 2013). The egress of other immune cells such as eosinophils (Sugita et al., 2010) and natural killer cells (Walzer et al., 2007) also depends on S1P receptors. In dendritic cells, the functional S1P antagonist fingolimod increased the production of the anti-inflammatory

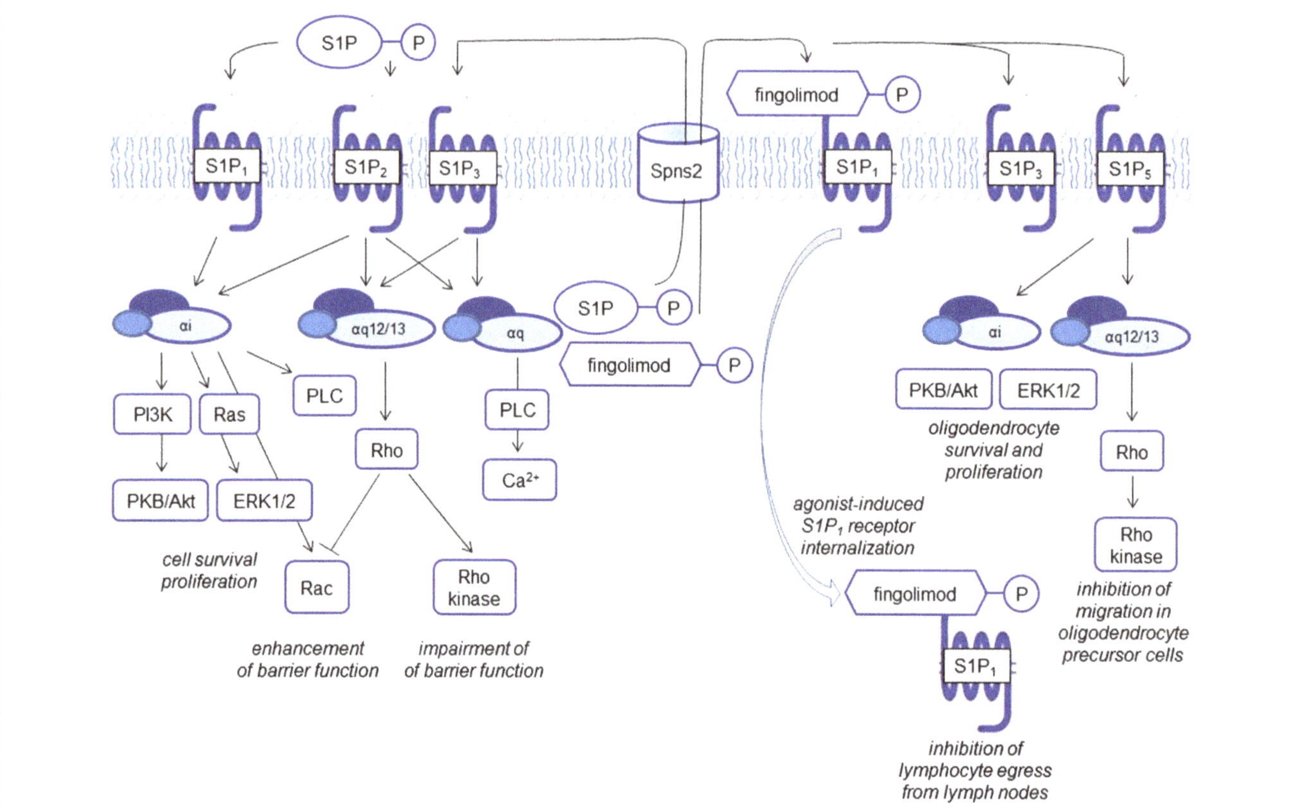

FIGURE 2 | Biological functions of S1P receptor signaling. S1P signals via five G protein-coupled receptors, termed $S1P_{1-5}$. Each of the receptors couples to several G proteins eliciting different downstream events. FTY720 phosphate activates all S1P receptors except $S1P_2$. S1P and FTY720 phosphate are generated by intracellular phosphorylation of sphingosine and FTY270, respectively and transported outwards to elicit signaling via S1P receptors. Characteristically, FTY720 phosphate leads to agonist-induced receptor internalization of the $S1P_1$ receptor.

cytokine IL-10 and reduced IL-12 secretion (Durafourt et al., 2011).

The vascular S1P gradient also seems to serve as a "tonic" regulator of endothelial barrier integrity. The intricate regulation of barrier function via cytoskeletal rearrangement with opposing functions of the S1P receptors $S1P_1$, $S1P_2$ and $S1P_3$ signaling via small GTPases of the Rho family and the functional consequences in several disease models have been reviewed by Xiong and Hla (2014; **Figure 2**).

Besides the S1P receptors, also the SphKs catalyzing S1P formation, SphK1 with cytoplasmic localization and SphK2, the predominant SphK isoform in the brain, with primarily nuclear localization (Igarashi et al., 2003) as well as the S1P degrading enzymes S1P lyase (S1PL; Le Stunff et al., 2002), S1P phosphatases (SPP1 and SPP2), and the lysophospholipid phosphatase 3 (LPP3; Brindley and Pilquil, 2009) have been found to be altered in several neurological diseases and also represent putative targets for drug development (**Figure 1**).

DISCOVERY AND DEVELOPMENT OF FINGOLIMOD/FTY720

The substance fingolimod (also known as FTY720) has made a very long and interesting journey from traditional asian medicine to a drug tested in large scale international multicenter randomized-controlled placebo-or standard of care-controlled trials proving its efficacy in the treatment of multiple sclerosis (MS) (reviewed by Im, 2003). It evolved from derivatization of ISP-1 that has been isolated from the fungus Isaria sinclairii. This fungus contributes to the fascinating phenomenon of "vegetable wasps and plant worms", also termed "vegetative wesps" or "winter-insect and summer-plant" according to its Chinese characters, caused by the fungus infecting the living insect host, feeding on it during winter time and growing out of the host insect's cadaver in summer (Fujita et al., 1994). ISP-1 showed 10-100fold greater immunosuppressant activity than ciclosporin A in experimental models (Fujita et al., 1994) and was modified for less gastric toxicity to fingolimod (Kiuchi et al., 2000). In contrast to all known immunosuppressants known at that time, fingolimod acts via a sequestration of circulating mature lymphocytes to the lymph nodes (Chiba et al., 1998) without major alterations of their immune functions such as cytokine secretion (Yanagawa et al., 1998), and thus seemed to promise the prevention of allograft rejection without a severe general immunosuppression (reviewed by Brinkmann et al., 2000). Inspired by the structural similarity of FTY720 to sphingosine (**Figure 3**) and the fact that S1P receptors had been identified on lymphocytes, Brinkmann et al. (2002) discovered that fingolimod was phosphorylated by

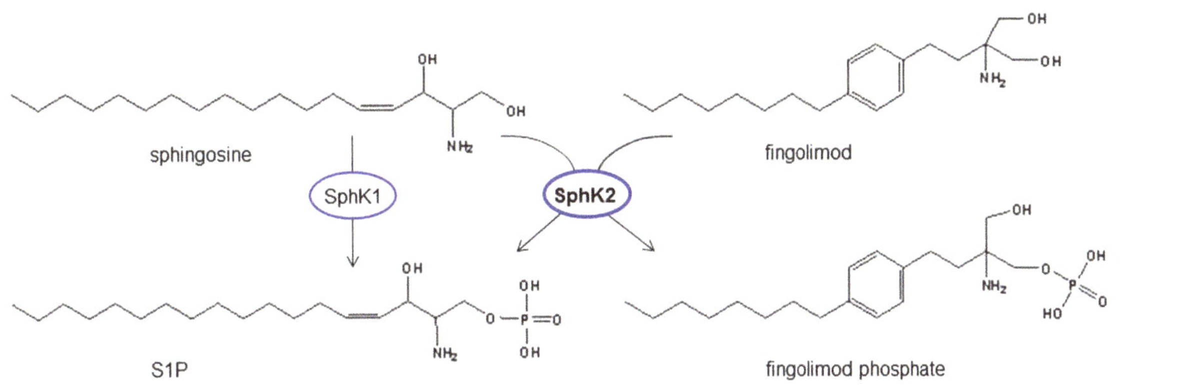

FIGURE 3 | Phosphorylation of fingolimod generates a structural analog to S1P. Fingolimod shows high analogy to sphingosine and is phosphorylated by spingosine kinases, mainly SphK2, which is the predominant SphK isoform in the brain. Fingolimod is a prodrug of fingolimod phosphate that can signal via S1P receptors and activate intracellular targets of S1P.

SphKs to fingolimod phosphate and targeted S1P receptors and thereby could prevent experimental autoimmune encephalitis (EAE), the rodent disease model for MS, in rats. Mandala et al. (2002) provided evidence for lymphocyte sequestration in the lymph nodes secondary to S1P receptor activation. Matloubian et al. (2004) established the $S1P_1$ receptor to be essential for sensing of the S1P gradient by lymphocytes leading to recirculation and regulation of lymphocyte egress from both thymus and peripheral lymphoid organs. The inhibition of lymphocyte recirculation by fingolimod argues for a functional antagonism of fingolimod phosphate at the $S1P_1$ receptor. Indeed, Gräler and Goetzl (2004) described a downregulation of S1P receptors upon treatment with fingolimod and Pham et al. (2008) showed *in vivo* that treatment with fingolimod reduced membrane expression of $S1P_1$ on lymphocytes. This proposed functional antagonism of fingolimod at $S1P_1$ is in line with the observation that mutant mice that express an internalization-defective $S1P_1$ have delayed lymphopenia kinetics in response to fingolimod (Thangada et al., 2010) and that a lymphocytic knock-down of $S1P_1$ also inhibits their egress from thymus (Allende et al., 2004).

Fingolimod was advanced into large scale randomized controlled trials to prevent allograft rejection in patients with renal transplantations but finally its further development was abandoned because high doses (2.5 mg/d and 5 mg/d) did not provide sufficient immunosuppression to allow reduction of co-immunosuppressants and was not superior to standard care. There was an increased incidence of macular edema and transient decreases in heart rate (reviewed by Mansoor and Melendez, 2008). Since 10–100–fold lower doses than those required in animal models of organ graft survival had been highly efficient in EAE (Brinkmann et al., 2010), the focus of clinical development shifted from transplant medicine to MS as an autoimmune disease.

Fingolimod might also have receptor-independent effects on inflammation, especially by binding to intracellular targets of S1P (Hait et al., 2014) or interacting with metabolism and signaling of other lipids. Fingolimod can inhibit both S1P generating as well as degrading enzymes such as SphK1 (Lim et al., 2011), S1PL (Bandhuvula et al., 2005), the ceramide synthases (Lahiri et al., 2009) and the acid sphingomyelinase (ASM; Dawson and Qin, 2011; **Figure 4**).

Ceramides could also play a role in MS pathophysiology (Qin et al., 2010; Schiffmann et al., 2012) and evidence for an interaction of fingolimod with ceramides has been shown (van Doorn et al., 2012). Fingolimod also appears to inhibit the cannabinoid receptor CB1 (Paugh et al., 2006), which has been shown to have some proinflammatory properties in EAE (Zhang et al., 2009). Additionally, fingolimod can inhibit phospholipase A_2 (PLA_2) activity in mast cells and therefore prostaglandin and thromboxane secretion (Payne et al., 2007). This could contribute to the therapeutic effect of fingolimod in MS, as PLA_2 has been shown to be highly expressed in EAE plaques (Kalyvas and David, 2004) and arachidonic acid is increased in cerebrospinal fluid of MS patients (Dore-Duffy et al., 1991).

CLINICAL EFFICACY OF FINGOLIMOD IN RELAPSING-REMITTING MULTIPLE SCLEROSIS

MS is an autoimmune disease of the CNS. The primary mechanism is the aberrant formation of autoreactive immune cells directed against CNS antigens. Upon passing the blood-brain barrier (BBB), they meet their antigen and incite inflammatory demyelination leading to subacute neurological symptoms that can remit and, given the chronicity of the disease, relapse. In the early inflammatory phase of the disease, immunomodulation with beta-interferons or glatiramer acetate have been shown to slow disease progression. In later stages of the disease, neurodegenerative processes also play a role.

Fingolimod was approved by the regulatory authorities worldwide as the first oral agent to treat relapsing-remitting multiple sclerosis (RRMS) after the successful completion of two phase III studies in 2010 showed its efficacy. FREEDOMS (Kappos et al., 2010) was a placebo controlled trial and TRANSFORMS (Cohen et al., 2010) even showed the superiority of fingolimod over treatment with intramuscular interferon beta-1a, the standard of care for RRMS. FREEDOMS showed a relative reduction of the

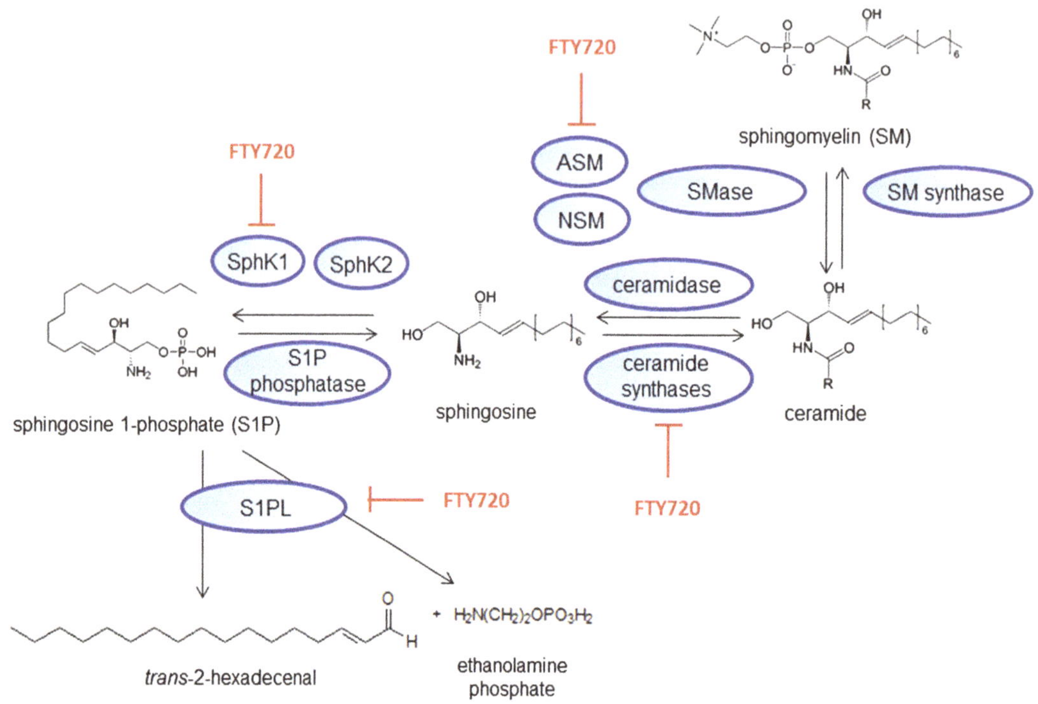

FIGURE 4 | Fingolimod interacts with sphingolipid metabolizing enzymes. Inhibitory effects on SphK1 (Lim et al., 2011), S1PL (Bandhuvula et al., 2005), ceramide synthases (Lahiri et al., 2009) and the acid sphingomyelinase (ASM; Dawson and Qin, 2011) have been shown. NSM—neutral sphingomyelinases.

relapse rate by 54–60% and a corresponding effect on disability progression (Kappos et al., 2006). TRANSFORMS showed similar relapse rates, although no significant effect on disability. FREEDOMS II, another Phase III placebo controlled trial (Calabresi et al., 2014) initiated by Novartis recently, could reproduce the positive effect of fingolimod on relapse rate. In clinical practice, due to its presumed superiority over interferon beta, fingolimod is one of the first line therapeutic choices for highly active RRMS.

Besides the positive effect on clinical outcome, previous clinical trials (Kappos et al., 2006; Comi et al., 2010) as well as the following phase III studies FREEDOMS, TRANSFORMS and FREEDOMS II have shown effects of fingolimod on magnetic resonance imaging (MRI) outcomes: Gadolinium (Gd) enhanced lesions, the morphological correlates of clinical as well as subclinical relapses, were reduced in the fingolimod treatment group compared to the patients receiving interferon beta-1a or placebo. Gd enhancement indicates BBB leakage, which is one of the initial steps in the pathophysiological cascade resulting in a MS plaque. Furthermore, BBB failure is a hallmark of almost every inflammatory reaction in the CNS. Another secondary endpoint of some of the studies cited above was brain atrophy—which was also reduced in fingolimod treated patients. The reduction of Gd-positive lesions demonstrates a direct or indirect anti-neuroinflammatory effect of fingolimod in patients, whereas the relatively crude parameter brain atrophy might be attributable to a direct neuroprotective mechanism or secondary to a reduced accumulation of MS plaques and secondary neurodegeneration.

As expected from the preceding animal studies, peripheral lymphocyte counts of fingolimod-treated patients are significantly reduced as compared to patients receiving placebo and interferon beta-1a (Cohen et al., 2010; Kappos et al., 2010). In contrast to other cytotoxic immunosuppressive drugs resulting in lymphopenia, the effect of fingolimod on the peripheral circulation of subsets of lymphocytes is reversible (Boulton et al., 2012). In line with the available experimental data, other studies showed that fingolimod selectively inhibits the egress of CCR7-positive naive and central memory T lymphocytes from the lymph node of treated patients (Pham et al., 2008). Effector memory cells represent the largest T cell population in the blood of patients receiving fingolimod and are important to maintain immune competence (Masopust et al., 2001). Furthermore, these cells did not lose the capacity to produce interferon-γ (IFNγ; Mehling et al., 2008). On the other hand, the CD4+TH17 subset of lymphocytes, which are trapped by fingolimod is believed to have a more pro-inflammatory role in the pathophysiology of MS (Lock et al., 2002; Tzartos et al., 2008). TH17 cells produce proinflammatory IL-17 and IL-22, transmigrate efficiently across the BBB, disrupt tight junctions, highly express neurotoxic substances, and promote CNS inflammation through additional CD4+ T cell and neutrophil recruitment (Kebir et al., 2007). In fingolimod-treated patients, the remaining CD8+ T cells are less responsive to the chemokine CCL2 (Johnson et al., 2010) and, therefore, probably less likely recruited to sites of antigen-induced inflammation (Carr et al., 1994). Fingolimod also strongly reduces certain sets of B cell counts in the blood of MS patients (Kowarik et al., 2011).

The remaining lymphocyte populations appear to be sufficient to protect patients against most infections (Francis et al., 2014). However, there is some evidence for more viral infections, e.g., severe herpes/varizella virus reactivation (Cohen et al., 2010), pointing towards a compromised T cell function. The broad range of immune regulatory functions of fingolimod seen in patient blood samples and those of experimental animals goes far beyond lymphocyte trafficking and has recently been reviewed by Garris et al. (2014).

In summary, the clinical data on the efficacy of fingolimod in RRMS is robust and has been shown in several independent phase III trials. Additional drugs that modulate S1P signaling are in the pipeline, some of them in advanced clinical trials (reviewed by Bigaud et al., 2014). The dose of 0.5 mg/d approved for MS treatment, which is decisively lower than doses used in animal models to treat EAE, also leads to peripheral lymphopenia and other immune cell mediated effects in patients. But the MRI findings that fingolimod has unequivocal effects on BBB disruption and brain atrophy suggests additional direct effects of fingolimod in brain cells.

FINGOLIMOD IN EXPERIMENTAL MODELS OF MULTIPLE SCLEROSIS

Fingolimod was first shown to be effective in EAE in the rat by Brinkmann et al. (2002) at a dose of 0.3 mg/kg/d. Later studies confirmed these results in different models of MS and different species (Webb et al., 2004; Kataoka et al., 2005). The suppression of EAE in mice and rats by fingolimod correlated with reduced numbers of lymphocytes in the blood and the CNS (Brinkmann et al., 2002; Kataoka et al., 2005).

Besides a prophylactic effect, which is comparable to relapse prevention in patients, a therapeutic effect could also be shown (Kataoka et al., 2005). Even a very late-initiated treatment is able to reverse paralysis (Balatoni et al., 2007), downregulates inflammatory genes such as matrix metalloproteinases and reduces BBB leakiness (Foster et al., 2009). This effect is only one of the mechanisms which appears to be independent of the "classical" role of fingolimod in lymphocyte trafficking. In EAE several additional effects on the immune system have been shown: Fingolimod changes CD8+ effector T cell function and inhibits their cytotoxic function by inhibition of cytosolic PLA_2 and the reduction of IFNγ and Granzyme B expression. Interestingly, this effect appears to be independent of S1P receptor modulation as fingolimod phosphate did not elicit these effects (Ntranos et al., 2014). In some EAE-studies, the effect of fingolimod on CNS physiology was analyzed. The observed clinical benefit was accompanied by improvement of electrophysiological abnormalities (Balatoni et al., 2007), demyelination (Papadopoulos et al., 2010) and synaptic dysfunction (Rossi et al., 2012).

At least some of these outcome parameters might be due to an additional effect of fingolimod directly within the CNS. Fingolimod readily penetrates into the CNS and accumulates in the brain and in the spinal cord (Foster et al., 2007). S1P receptors are expressed in cells of the CNS. Interstingly, short-term fingolimod administration can fail to suppress EAE, albeit producing a rapid and substantial reduction of lymphocyte counts (Foster et al., 2007). Moreover, neurological deficits reappear before lymphocyte numbers normalize if treatment with fingolimod is stopped (Webb et al., 2004). CYM-5442, an $S1P_1$-selective fingolimod analog that leads to significant levels of the drug in CNS but not in plasma, also improves the disease course in EAE. There was no persisting lymphopenia in these mice but a cyclical recovery from lymphopenia. Nevertheless, $S1P_1$ expression on neurons and astrocytes was reduced, and levels of cytokines in the CNS were suppressed (Gonzalez-Cabrera et al., 2012).

Furthermore, in alternative MS models, which are based on lymphocyte-independent demyelination, an effect of fingolimod could be observed: Fingolimod enhances remyelination following demyelination of organotypic cerebellar slices (Miron et al., 2010) and in the cuprizone model (Kim et al., 2011), although there is some controversy about the latter model (Hu et al., 2011). Another animal model for MS is the delayed-type hypersensitivity model (DTH) in Lewis rats. Again, an effect of fingolimod could be shown independently of lymphocyte infiltration and BBB leakage (Anthony et al., 2014).

So what could be the cellular target of fingolimod within the CNS? There is accumulating evidence for a specific role of astrocytes, a cell type which is supposed to play an important role in MS pathophysiology (Brosnan and Raine, 2013). Strong evidence points to an anti-inflammatory effect of fingolimod on astrocytes *in vitro* (Wu et al., 2013). A particularly illuminating study of Choi et al. (2010) made use of a conditional, cell-specific knock down of the $S1P_1$ receptor on all cells of the CNS (nestin-cre), neurons (synapsin-cre) and astrocytes (GFAP-cre). They found that $S1P_1$-deficiency on astrocytes led to an attenuation of EAE and that the protective effect of fingolimod in EAE was lost in mice with astrocytic but not with neuronal $S1P_1$ deletion (Choi et al., 2010). Finally, therapeutic administration of fingolimod to EAE mice has specific effects on astrocyte activation and nitric oxide production (Colombo et al., 2014).

Oligodendrocytes also express S1P receptors, especially the $S1P_5$ receptor, which shows a relatively restricted expression pattern. Interestingly, genetically modified mice with $S1P_5$ deficiency do not show defects in myelination (Brinkmann, 2007). At least *in vitro* and in slice cultures direct effects of fingolimod on myelination could be shown (Miron et al., 2008, 2010). A possible role for microglia in the therapeutic effect of fingolimod can be derived from studies of so called microvesicles. They were shown to be significantly reduced in EAE mice treated with fingolimod and are increased in cerebrospinal fluid of MS patients (Verderio et al., 2012). Furthermore, fingolimod treatment leads to a reduced microglial production of pro-inflammatory cytokines such as tumor necrosis factor α (TNFα), interleukin 1β (IL-1β), and interleukin 6 (IL-6; Noda et al., 2013).

An analysis of fingolimod's effects in EAE clearly points towards several contributing mechanisms. Beyond the effect on lymphocyte trafficking, a direct immunmodulatory effect as well as direct effects of fingolimod in the CNS seem to be involved. As new, more receptor-specific agents will enter the scene in the future, it is possible that we will realize that fingolimod as a rather "dirty" drug acting on multiple targets may even prove to be superior to receptor-specific agents.

STROKE

Stroke is an acute brain attack caused by the sudden thromboembolic occlusion of a brain vessel with the consequence of cerebral ischemia, the more frequent cause of stroke, or by a rupture of a brain artery causing a hemorrhage into the brain parenchyma. These different stroke entities show the same clinical presentation consisting of a focal neurological deficit such as hemiparesis or aphasia of sudden onset.

CEREBRAL ISCHEMIA

The embolic blockade of a brain vessel leads to hypoperfusion of the dependent vascular territory in the brain with an almost immediate loss of brain function. However, we know from experimental studies (Astrup et al., 1981) and clinical imaging (Thijs et al., 2002) that the affected brain tissue remains viable for a few hours with the infarct gradually expanding from the core to the periphery of the hypoperfused territory. This is the pathophysiologic correlate of a therapeutic time window for vessel recanalization with thrombolytics or catheter-based interventions. The only approved stroke therapy to date is thrombolysis with recombinant human tissue-type plasminogen activator (t-PA), which is safe and effective within 4.5 h after symptom onset (Lees et al., 2010). The pathophysiological cascades taking place in the ischemic brain are well characterized and can be roughly summarized by the three interleaving phenomena of excitotoxicity, inflammation and apoptosis (Dirnagl et al., 1999).

In recent years, experimental stroke research has produced strong evidence that cellular immunity and especially T cells play a decisive role in the fate of brain tissue following cerebral ischemia. Different experimental strategies aiming at a reduction of lymphocyte counts such as the use of genetic models (Hurn et al., 2007; Kleinschnitz et al., 2010); splenectomy prior to stroke (Ajmo et al., 2009), immunosuppressive drugs (Sharkey et al., 1996) or the induction of lymphocytic tolerance (Becker et al., 1997) have shown therapeutic efficacy in experimental stroke models. Therefore, to test the potent immunomodulator fingolimod with its specific lymphocyte-directed immunomodulation in experimental stroke models was a straightforward approach.

Meanwhile, over 10 experimental studies have shown therapeutic efficacy of fingolimod in stroke models in mice and rats (Czech et al., 2009; Shichita et al., 2009; Hasegawa et al., 2010; Pfeilschifter et al., 2011a,b; Wei et al., 2011; Kraft et al., 2013) with doses from 0.25 to 1 mg/kg applied systemically, leading to a robust lymphocytopenia in rodents (Czech et al., 2009). Reproducible therapeutic effects on lesion size and functional outcome were accompanied by a reduction in pro-apoptotic processes in the infarcted brain areas such as reduced nuclear translocation of apoptosis inducing factor (AIF; Czech et al., 2009), less caspase-3 cleavage and TUNEL positive neurons (Hasegawa et al., 2010), and an activation of pro-survival pathways such as extracellular signal-regulated kinase (ERK1/2), protein kinase B/Akt kinase (PKB/Akt) and Bcl-2 upregulation (Hasegawa et al., 2010; Wei et al., 2011). Cell culture experiments did not show relevant neuroprotection by fingolimod in neuronal cells subjected to "ischemia in the dish" stimuli such as glutamate, H_2O_2 or hypoxia (Wei et al., 2011; Kraft et al., 2013) but a reduced inflammatory activation of microvascular brain endothelial cells (Wei et al., 2011). Most topical, Kraft et al. (2013) found a reduction of microvascular thromboses in the periinfarct area after fingolimod treatment, a phenomenon that has been observed also previously by the group secondary to several T cell-directed therapies (Kleinschnitz et al., 2013). Since these findings argue for a role of lymphocytes to boost microvascular thrombus formation in cerebral ischemia, they coined the term thromboinflammation. Of note, there was also one study that reported no therapeutic effect on lesion size and outcome in two different stroke models despite efficient systemic lymphocyte depletion, and decreased cerebral lymphocyte infiltration (Liesz et al., 2011). Similar findings were reported in a recent study on traumatic brain injury (TBI) by Mencl et al. (2014), who assessed the effect of FTY720 in two different experimental models of TBI mimicking focal and diffuse brain injury. FTY720 applied directly prior to the induction of the brain lesion did not reduce lesion size or improve functional neurological outcome neither early or 1 week after the induction of the brain lesion, even though it led to a reduced infiltration of neutrophils and macrophages and/or a reduced microglial activation. TBI, however, is a clearly different entity of brain injury than ischemic stroke. The role of circulating immune cells in lesion development after TBI is less unequivocal and there is most probably not as much microvascular endothelial activation as in ischemic stroke.

Concerning the signaling pathway mediating the protective effect of fingolimod, Hasegawa et al. (2010) demonstrated that this therapeutic effect could also be elicited by the $S1P_1$-selective agonist SEW2871 and abrogated by the $S1P_1/S1P_3$-selective competitive antagonist VPC23019, argueing for an $S1P_1$-mediated effect. This assumption was supported by findings of Pfeilschifter et al. (2011b) showing that the neuroprotective effect of fingolimod is lost in SphK2 deficient mice, which cannot efficiently phosphorylate and thus activate fingolimod, arguing against a direct effect of non-phosphorylated fingolimod. Hasegawa et al. (2013) examined the expression of the SphK and the $S1P_1$ receptor in the ischemic area with a focus on neurons 6 h and 24 h after stroke by immunohistochemistry, and found a significantly decreased expression of $S1P_1$, $SphK_1$, and $SphK_2$ starting at 6 h and significant at 24 h after MCAO. Labeling of $S1P_1$ and both SphKs was reduced in the infarct cortex but remained present in the periinfarct cortex, allowing fingolimod to be phosphorylated and act via inside-out signaling on the $S1P_1$ receptor.

In analogy to the findings of Choi et al. (2010) in the EAE model, it could be possible that the protective effect of fingolimod only partially depends on the peripheral immunomodulation and also relies on direct effects in the CNS. To weigh the effect of lymphocyte depletion against other putative mechanisms, Kraft et al. (2013) applied fingolimod to recombination activating gene-1 (Rag1)-deficient mice that are devoid of T and B lymphocytes. While these mice *per se* developed smaller infarcts than wild type mice, they were not further protected by fingolimod, showing that the neuroprotective effects of fingolimod largely depends on immunomodulation.

Stroke-associated infections, especially pneumonia, are the most important factor of mortality in the acute phase. They are promoted by a stroke-associated immunodepression

(Meisel et al., 2005) and will have to be considered prior to any clinical application of fingolimod in the context of stroke. In an experimental stroke model, Pfeilschifter et al. (2011b) did not find an increase of bacterial colonalization in the lungs of fingolimod-treated animals in comparison to control animals 24 h after stroke. Beyond the acute phase, the fate of stroke survivors is mainly determined by the success of rehabilitative stroke care aiming at functional recovery. Brunkhorst et al. (2013) showed that fingolimod applied from day 3 to day 7 (1 mg/kg b.i.d.) after a photothrombotic lesion directed to the motor cortex of mice relevantly ameliorated functional impairment over an observation period of 31 days, reduced astroglial scarring and increased the size of post-synaptic densities. In this model, fingolimod increased the expression of the trophic factor vascular endothelial growth factor α (VEGFα) but not of brain-derived neurotrophic factor (BDNF), which has been shown to increase secondary to fingolimod treatment in other models of neurodegenerative diseases.

Another event of importance in the context of stroke, but also intensive care medicine and transplant surgery, which has been shown to be regulated by S1P and fingolimod is preconditioning. Following the principle of "what does not kill you makes you stronger", preconditioning is a process that uses a sublethal noxious stimulus to induce or increase tolerance towards a second noxious stimulus. In stroke research, well established preconditioning stimuli include hypoxic preconditioning (HP), transient ischemia, inhalational anesthetics such as isoflurane or inflammatory agents such as bacterial lipopolysaccharide (LPS). HP is based on a hypoxia-induced stabilization of hypoxia-inducible factor (HIF) that is continuously degraded by an oxygen-sensing degradative pathway under normoxic conditions. Stabilized by hypoxia, HIF, which exists in three isoforms, binds to hypoxia-responsive elements (HRE) of hypoxia-regulated genes to promote their transcription. Besides hypoxia and ischemia, also non-hypoxic stimuli such as isoflurane (Sun et al., 2013) or LPS (He et al., 2014) can stabilize HIF. SphK2, but not SphK1 has been shown to be upregulated by HP and isoflurane in the brain (Wacker et al., 2009; Yung et al., 2012) in a HIF-dependent manner (Wacker et al., 2012) and pharmacological inhibition (Wacker et al., 2009) and genetic deletion of SphK2 (Wacker et al., 2012; Yung et al., 2012) were shown to abrogate the protective effects of preconditioning in experimental stroke. There are conflicting findings whether genetic deletion of SphK2, the predominant SphK isoform in the brain (Blondeau et al., 2007) *per se* exacerbates ischemic damage in stroke or not (Pfeilschifter et al., 2011b; Yung et al., 2012). In other cell systems, HIF-mediated upregulation has also been shown for SphK1 (Ader et al., 2008; Schwalm et al., 2008) and both isoforms contain HREs in their respective promotor regions. Wacker et al. (2009, 2012) showed that fingolimod given 48 h prior to stroke also reduced lesion size and had a strong synergistic effect in conjuction with HP. Therefore, they concluded that fingolimod is a preconditioning agent. While the protective effect after a remote pretreatment 48 h prior to the insult could be explained by the long-lasting lymphocyte depletion after a single dose of FTY720 (Chiba et al., 1998) and the accumulation of fingolimod in the brain (Foster et al., 2007), the finding that coadministration of R59949, which inhibits HIF accumulation was able to abolish the protective effect of remote fingolimod pretreatment (Wacker et al., 2012) clearly suggests that HIF-mediated gene regulation is downstream of fingolimod. The finding of Yung et al. (2012) that HIF-1α stabilization following isoflurane preconditioning is lost in SphK2-deficient mice also supports a regulation of HIF-mediated signaling by S1P. In synthesis, these findings suggest that in the context of preconditioning and stroke, the signaling between SphK2 and its products fingolimod phosphate or S1P is bidirectional with an induction of SphK2 following preconditioning stimuli and a lost efficacy of HIF-stabilizing factors in SphK2-deficient mice on the one hand and a HIF-dependency of the preconditioning effect of fingolimod on the other hand. The preconditioning effect of HP, the HIF stabilizer cobalt chloride, and of fingolimod was abolished by pretreatment with the $S1P_1$-specific antagonist W146, supporting an auto- and paracrine propagation of preconditioning by the $S1P_1$ receptor. Functionally, SphK2 deficiency not only abrogates the neuroprotection by HP but also BBB preserving effects of HP by an alteration in the expression of adhesion molecules in homogenated cortical brain tissue from SphK2-deficient mice analyzed 48 h after the hypoxic stimulus in comparison to WT mice (Wacker et al., 2012).

THROMBOLYSIS WITH TISSUE PLASMINOGEN ACTIVATOR (t-PA)

The vascular S1P gradient with high concentrations in the bloodstream and low concentrations in the interstitial fluids is generally viewed as a tonic barrier preserving mechanism for endothelial barriers (reviewed by Xiong and Hla, 2014). Several reports of the efficacy of S1P or fingolimod in experimental states of vascular leakage such as acute lung injury (Peng et al., 2004) or anaphylaxis (Camerer et al., 2009) have sparked interest on a putative therapeutic effect of fingolimod on BBB disruption after stroke that contributes to potentially fatal brain edema. So far, the data from experimental stroke models on this question are not unequivocal. Cerebral ischemia induces BBB disruption and the thrombolytic t-PA has been shown to aggravate this process (Latour et al., 2004) which accelerates with time from symptom onset, representing the underlying cause of an increased bleeding risk associated with late t-PA treatment, the main obstacle to a more widespread use of this stroke therapy. In a model of moderate size thromboembolic stroke, a faithful model for recanalization by t-PA treatment, fingolimod reduced infarct growth and BBB disruption secondary to late application of t-PA (Campos et al., 2013). By contrast, in a model of large hemispheric strokes and t-PA treatment, fingolimod did not show a beneficial effect (Cai et al., 2013). These contradictory findings can in part be reconciled by the possibility that this massive infarction might have led to an overly rapid loss of SphK and S1P receptors in the infarct and periinfarct region explaining a non-response to fingolimod treatment. Concerning possible future clinical trials of fingolimod in stroke, this would argue against the inclusion of patients with severe stroke symptoms and massive infarctions on brain imaging.

INTRACEREBRAL HEMORRHAGE

Intracerebral hemorrhage (ICH) is often denoted as "the most untreatable cause of stroke" because there is no causal treatment and it is charged with a high mortality. Noteworthy, Asian populations display higher rates of ICH, with ICH representing over 30% of all first ever strokes in China in a meta-analysis of population-based studies (Tsai et al., 2013). Fingolimod has shown therapeutic efficacy in experimental models of ICH (Rolland et al., 2011, 2013; Lu et al., 2014) with a reduced infiltration of CD3+ lymphocytes and reduced endothelial ICAM-1 expression. Rolland et al. (2013) conducted a 10 week follow-up of their experimental animals after ICH induction and a single injection or a 3-day course of 1 mg/kg FTY720 and auspiciously found an improved outcome in neurocognitive scores and brain atrophy with a stronger effect in the animals treated for 3 days. These findings support the observations of a proregenerative effect of FTY720 by Brunkhorst et al. (2013). Lu et al. (2014) described a reduction of apoptotic cell death both in the center and at the edge of the hematoma but no alteration of in the numbers of CD68+ monocytes/macrophages and resident microglia and also reported positive long-term results concerning neurological function and brain atrophy after 2 weeks.

Recently, a first clinical trial was conducted in China, which recruited 23 patients with deep primary ICH. They were randomized to a treatment with placebo or 0.5 mg/d FTY720 (Gilenya®) orally for 3 consecutive days (Fu et al., 2014). This very small clinical trial did not detect differences in adverse events such as increased susceptibility to infections. The group reported an improvement of magnetic resonance imaging-based measurements of perihematomal edema volume, but the patient number seems too small to draw valid conclusions about efficacy yet.

NEURODEGENERATIVE DISEASES

ALZHEIMER'S DISEASE

Alzheimer's disease (AD) is the most common age-related neurodegenerative disorder and shows a rising prevalence along with global trends towards increasing life spans. AD leads to a cognitive decline that is attributable to neuronal loss predominantly affecting higher cortical functions (visuospatial orientation, memory, planning and execution of activities, language and arithmetics) whereas cognitive working tempo and drive seem unaltered. Patients are often able to maintain an unremarkable "façade" even in later stages of the disease when brain atrophy, predominantly of the hippocampus and the temporal lobe can be seen in clinical brain imaging. Currently, there is no causal treatment of this devastating disease. While the disease-triggering mechanisms are yet unknown, the neuropathological hallmarks of AD consist of the deposition of amyloid-β (Aβ) plaques and the formation of neurofibrillary tangles consisting of hyperphosphorylated tau protein (Braak and Braak, 1991, 1995). Following an ascending course from the entorhinal region to the neocortex, these changes are accompanied by a loss of cortical synapses, which correlates with cognitive decline (DeKosky and Scheff, 1990). Inflammatory processes such as activation of microglia and astrocytes as well as production of inflammatory cytokines occur within and around amyloid plaques (Lukiw and Bazan, 2006). Recently, autopsy studies on brains of AD patients but also data from experimental disease models of AD have provided evidence that alterations of the sphingolipid linked to the pathological mechanisms of AD and that S1P receptor modulation by fingolimod represents a promising therapeutic approach reducing both the production (Takasugi et al., 2013) and the neurotoxicity (Asle-Rousta et al., 2013; Doi et al., 2013; Hemmati et al., 2013; Fukumoto et al., 2014) of Aβ peptide. Aβ is produced from Aβ precursor protein (APP) in the amyloidogenic pathway through sequential cleavage by two aspartate proteases, β- and γ-secretases (Zheng and Koo, 2011). Several studies have implicated cholesterol and sphingolipid-rich membrane microdomains, termed lipid rafts, in the amyloidogenic processing of APP, and the activities of the secretases are influenced by the composition of these lipid rafts (Kalvodova et al., 2005; Osenkowski et al., 2008; Holmes et al., 2012).

There is ample evidence that the sphingolipid metabolism is altered in AD brains, leading to an accumulation of proapoptotic and proinflammatory ceramides (Han et al., 2001). The expression of the ceramide-generating acid and neutral sphingomyelinases (NSM) has been shown to be upregulated in brains of patients suffering from AD (Filippov et al., 2012) and elevated ceramide levels are linked to an inhibition of glycolysis (Arboleda et al., 2007) and the induction of nitric oxide synthase and oxidative stress (Cutler et al., 2004). Cutler et al. showed elevations of cholesterol levels and ceramide species (especially C18 and C24) that gradually increased in correlation to disease severity in brain samples from AD patients and over time in a murine model of AD. The accumulation of ceramide species or cholesterol in cultured hippocampal neurons could be reversed by anti-oxidative treatment with α-tocopherol. Mechanistically, this may be attributed to an activation of the neutral sphingomyelinase by Aβ, as Jana and Pahan (2010) had shown previously that Aβ induces neutral sphingomyelinase in an NADPH-dependent pathway leading to ceramide accumulation that has a propapototic effect on cultured neurons. Elevated ceramide levels stabilize the Aβ-cleaving enzyme BACE-1 (Puglielli et al., 2003) whereas a reduction of ceramide levels in turn leads to a reduced secretion of APP and Aβ in human neuroblastoma cells (Tamboli et al., 2005), indicating a vicious cycle involving Aβ production, cellular stress and ceramide accumulation. The clinical significance of increased ceramide levels in the pathophysiology of AD is supported by studies on patient serum and CSF samples that indentified ceramide species as potential biomarkers of AD (Mielke et al., 2014) and HIV-associated dementia (Bandaru et al., 2007).

Less is known about the role of S1P, the functional opponent of ceramide, in the development of AD. An analysis of post-mortem brain tissues of 9 individuals with a clinical and histopathological diagnosis of AD and 6 age-matched control individuals by He et al. (2010) revealed a pattern of elevated ASM and acid ceramidase (AC) expression in AD, along with a reduction in sphingomyelin and elevation of ceramide. Sphingosine levels were higher in the AD brains, but levels of the downstream lipid mediator S1P were reduced. This finding was corroborated by a very recent study of Couttas et al. (2014) reporting on sphingosine/S1P levels and SphK activity in post-mortem brain samples from 34 individuals. Not all of the patients had received a clinical diagnosis of AD and the cohort was composed of carriers of the protective apolipoprotein (APO) ε2 genotype as well as the risk-bearing APO ε4 genotype. In this cohort, the S1P to sphingosine ratio was higher in hippocampal regions of Apo ε2 carriers and S1P levels declined in a regiospecific manner most strongly in brain regions with the most advanced histopathological changes. The activity of SphK1 and SphK2, which generate S1P from sphingosine, also decreased with higher histopathological disease scores. Besides a loss of SphK activity, lower S1P levels in AD patients could also be explained by increased activities of the S1P degrading enzymes S1PL and S1PP. Indeed, S1PP1 has been shown to be markedly up-regulated in AD brains using microarray technology (Katsel et al., 2007).

Seemingly in contrast to these findings, Takasugi et al. (2011) described that the activity of β-site APP cleaving enzyme-1 (BACE1), the major β secretase and rate-limiting enzyme for amyloid-β peptide (Aβ) production, is positively modulated by S1P in mouse neurons. They found that β-cleavage of APP was inhibited by genetic knockdown of the S1P-generating SphKs in cultured neuronal cells, an effect that was more pronounced when SphK2 was targeted, or by pharmacological inhibition with the SphK-selective inhibitor SKII. Congruently, increasing S1P levels via inhibition of S1PL or the S1PP1 enhanced Aβ secretion. Modifications of extracellular levels of the poorly permeating lipid mediator S1P failed to modulate BACE1 activity and BACE1 was specifically pulled down to matrices carrying S1P. Therefore Takasugi et al. (2011) concluded that the S1P-BACE1 interaction was of a direct intracellular nature and not mediated via membrane-bound S1P receptors. Translating these findings into a mouse model of AD, they found a protective effect of the SphK inhibitor SKII against Aβ secretion. Since SphK2 is the predominant isoform of the two S1P synthesizing enzymes in the brain (Blondeau et al., 2007) they analyzed SphK2 expression levels and activity in brain specimens from AD patients in comparison to non-demented individuals. While the overall SphK2 protein levels were decreased in the brains of individuals suffering from dementia, which was explained by progressive neuronal loss and the predominantly neuronal expression of SphK2 in the brain (Blondeau et al., 2007) the relative *in vitro* activitiy of SphK2 normalized to SphK2 protein levels was significantly increased in AD brains (Takasugi et al., 2011). Due to the normalization of total SphK2 protein levels, these findings do not necessarily stand in contrast to the above-mentioned observations of Couttas et al. (2014) who found a decreased SphK activity of both isoenzymes in post-mortem brain specimens from individuals with histopathological features of AD.

A very recent report from Karaca et al. (2014) on the influence of S1P levels in models of S1PL deficiency on APP metabolism sustained detrimental effects of elevated intracellular S1P levels concerning Aβ accumulation. This group found that inhibition of SphK2 reduced the accumulation of amyloidogenic C-terminal fragments of APP whereas genetic deletion of S1PL or downregulation by siRNA, which both were effective in raising intracellular S1P levels, increased their accumulation. This effect could be mimicked by extracellular addition of the easily cell-permeating sphingosine but not by extracellular addition of the polar mediator S1P. Karaca et al. found that the processing of APP C-terminal fragments to Aβ1-40 and Aβ1-42 was reduced due to an impaired γ-secretase activity in S1PL-deficient cells and APP C-terminal fragments accumulated in the lysosomal compartments, along with a deregulated expression of other lysosomal proteins and an impairment of the final stage of autophagy. Interestingly, these pathophysiological processes could be alleviated by a mobilization of intracellular calcium from the endoplasmic reticulum, a process that has been shown to be impaired in a model for the lysosomal storage disease Nieman Pick type C (Lloyd-Evans et al., 2008).

Concerning a putative therapeutic effect of fingolimod on AD progression in experimental models of established disease, there are several reports presenting promising evidence. In a model of intrahippocampal injection of Aβ1-42 in rats, a 2 week course of fingolimod treatment (1 mg/kg daily i.p.) ameliorated spatial learning and memory in the Morris water maze test at the end of the 2 week course and reduced neuronal damage and caspase-3 activation in the hippocampus (Asle-Rousta et al., 2013). Of note, fingolimod did not enhance learning and memory in control animals who received saline injections into the hippocampus. Fingolimod showed equal efficacy as the NMDA receptor antagonist memantine, an approved drug to treat AD symptoms in the same disease model (Hemmati et al., 2013) and both were able to partly reverse changes of the gene expression pattern induced by Aβ injection. So far, the mechanism underlying these therapeutic effects is not yet clear. It is possible that the systemic immunomodulation dampens the inflammatory reaction to Aβ deposition. Specifically, fingolimod may interfere with the migration of phagocytes in the brain since it has been shown to reduce Aβ-triggered whole blood cell migration along an Aβ gradient in a Boyden chamber assay in a dose-dependent manner (Kaneider et al., 2004).

Takasugi et al. (2013) analyzed the effects of fingolimod and the $S1P_1$-specific receptor agonist KRP203 on Aβ production in cultured neuronal cells and brain Aβ levels in a murine AD model (Takasugi et al., 2013). In cell culture, they found a dose-dependent reduction of Aβ production by both compounds. Contrary to S1P, fingolimod and KRP203 affected the activity of γ- but not β-secretases. Phosphorylation of both compounds by SphK2 was a prerequisite for their activity as demonstrated by pharmacological inhibition and genetic knockdown of this enzyme. The effects of fingolimod and KRP203 seem to be receptor-independent since Aβ production was not affected by the $S1P_1$ agonist SEW2871 or the $S1P_1$ antagonist W123, and neither W123 nor the Gαi protein inhibitor suramin altered the inhibition of Aβ production by fingolimod. These findings point towards intracellular effects of fingolimod requiring prior phosphorylation by SphK2, and this hypothesis was further corroborated by the finding that extracellular addition of the polar fingolimod phosphate, which poorly permeates cell membranes, also did not effect Aβ production. Takasugi et al. translated these findings into an animal model of transgenic mice overexpressing human APP and could show opposite effects of a short-course treatment with fingolimod (0.5 mg/kg for 6 days) on the production of Aβ1-40 (decreased) and Aβ1-42 (increased), thus showing that fingolimod affects Aβ levels also *in vivo* (Takasugi et al., 2013).

Furthermore, direct effects of fingolimod on brain cells have been shown, such as a dose-dependent induction of BDNF production in cultured neurons on mRNA and protein levels that inhibited Aβ-induced neurotoxicity in a dose-dependent fashion (Doi et al., 2013). The trophic effects of BDNF were shown to be mediated via the tropomyosin receptor kinase B (TrkB) involving the main downstream pathway ERK1/2 phosphorylation. BDNF was also induced by fingolimod in a murine AD as shown by a BDNF ELISA from mouse brain homogenates (Fukumoto et al., 2014). The translational relevance of these findings is further sustained by the fact that BDNF expression levels are lower in patients with AD.

ANIMAL MODELS OF LEARNING AND MEMORY

There is increasing evidence that S1P signaling also plays a physiological role in learning processes. S1P has been shown to increase glutamate release from presynaptic terminals in the CA3 pyramidal neurons of the hippocampus in an $S1P_3$ receptor-dependent manner (Kanno et al., 2010). S1P induced the translocation of $S1P_3$ receptors to presynaptic mossy fiber terminals in the CA3 region and long term potentiation depending on the mossy fiber—CA3 pyramidal neuron interaction was inhibited by a SphK inhibitor, an effect that could be reversed by addition of S1P. Again, the positive effect of S1P on long-term potentiation (LTP) could be inhibited by $S1P_3$ receptor antagonism. SphK1 is highly expressed in mossy fibers of the hippocampus and LTP was significantly impaired in SphK1 knockout mice, showing that SphK1 is required for hippocampal S1P generation. Congruently, mice with genetic deletion of SphK1 showed an impairment of spatial learning and memomory in the Morris water maze. Interestingly, somewhat opposing findings have recently been described by Hait et al. (2014), see below.

Topical work of the last few years has established a role for coagulation factors such as thrombin, plasmin and activated protein C (aPC) and protease-activated receptors (PAR) in hippocampal learning processes (Maggio et al., 2008; Mannaioni et al., 2008; Yuan et al., 2009). Interestingly, Maggio et al. (2014) characterized aPC as a metaplastic molecule that enhances LTP upon delivery of a subthreshold stimulation. They propose a model in which upon binding to the endothelial protein C receptor, which is also expressed on astrocytes, aPC activates PAR1, which triggers the SphK-dependent production of S1P. In turn, S1P binds to the $S1P_1$ receptor and stimulates intracellular Ca^{2+} stores, ultimately leading to enhanced LTP.

Very recently, Hait et al. (2014) showed that fingolimod affects learning and memory function by epigenetic regulation of gene expression. After SphK2 dependent phosphorylation, fingolimod phosphate binds to class 1 histone deacetylases (HDAC), some of the few defined targets of intracellular S1P signaling (Hait et al., 2009). Primary hippocampal neurons as well as a neuroblastoma cell line showed a robust, predominantly nuclear expression and activity of SphK2, showing abundant fingolimod phosphorylation within hours of fingolimod treatment. Most of the fingolimod phosphate remained intracellularly, and interfering with SphK2 expression crucially regulated fingolimod phosphate levels. Interestingly, treatment with fingolimod reduced nuclear S1P levels, probably by competition for phosphorylation by SphK2. As shown for S1P in non-neuronal systems (Hait et al., 2009), fingolimod treatment led to histone acetylation, and the negative modulation of this effect by SphK down-regulation in a cell membrane-free system of highly purified nuclei as well as the inefficacy of extracellularly-added S1P or fingolimod phosphate showed that this is a purely intracellular inhibitory effect of phosphorylated fingolimod on HDAC activity while the activity of histone acetyltransferases, which have opposing effects, is not influenced by S1P or fingolimod phosphate.

To test the physiological relevance of these observations and following reports on the role of epigenetic regulation, especially histone acetylation in memory and learning processes (Fischer et al., 2010), Hait et al. (2014) chose an experimental model of contextual fear extinction to evaluate the effects of FTY720 on learning and memory *in vivo*. To exclude well-established complex effects of the immune system on cognitive functions (Kipnis et al., 2004; Brynskikh et al., 2008), T and B cell deficient severe combined immunodeficiency (SCID) mice were used. The contextual fear extinction test evaluates freezing as an expression of acquired fear secondary to an adversive stimulus, and fear extinction upon re-exposure to the same environment without this stimulus and hence is a model for how the individual reduces fear-related reactions to a no longer dangerous stimulus, a mechanism that is impaired in anxiety disorders. Here, fingolimod, which accumulated in the hippocampus, did not change fear acquisition and fear extinction, but alleviated delayed extinction deficits in comparison to saline-treated SCID mice. By contrast, performance in paradigms of tone-dependent fear conditioning that is acquired independently of the hippocampus, exploratory behavior, basal anxiety-like behavior and spatial learning were not influenced by fingolimod treatment in SCID mice. The amelioration of contextual fear extinction in the foot-shock model was accompanied by increased histone acetylation in the hippocampus and alterations in gene expression of genes linked to synaptic plasticity and learning. In electrophysiological recordings from hippocampal slices, Hait et al. (2014) could show that like other HDAC inhibitors, fingolimod increased LTP as a marker of synaptic plasticity. To confirm the role of SphK2 in hippocampal learning processes and especially SphK2 dependent phosphorylation of fingolimod, they used SphK2 deficient mice, which spontaneously showed impaired visuospatial memory in the Morris water maze and decreased contextual fear extinction. Consistent with the hypothesis that nuclear phosphorylation of fingolimod by SphK2 is a prerequisite of HDAC inhibition, fingolimod failed to rescue fear extinction in this model.

HUNTINGTON DISEASE

Huntington disease (HD) is an inherited neurodegenerative brain disease with autosomal-dominant inheritance. It is characterized by mutations of the huntingtin gene with extended CAG trinucleotide repeats encoding a dysfunctional mutant huntingtin protein (mHtt). mHtt forms aggregates that are cytotoxic and interfere with many physiological cell functions, such as the expression of neurotrophins, e.g., BDNF (Zuccato et al., 2001). mHtt accumulation has also been shown to influence lipid metabolism (Maglione et al., 2010) and intraventricular infusion of ganglioside GM1 induced phosphorylation and detoxification of mutant huntingtin (Di Pardo et al., 2012). Clinically, this disease which predominantly affects the striatum and the cortex manifests as a hyperkinetic movement disorder with unvoluntary dance-like movements accompanied by a cognitive and psychosocial decline. Symptoms usually begin around the age of 40 and characteristically show an "anticipation" (earlier onset and heavier symptoms from generation to generation) that is linked to an increasing extension of the CAG repeats. Di Pardo et al. (2014) assessed a potential therapeutic effect of fingolimod in transgenic mice expressing exon 1 of the human HD gene carrying a CAG repeat (line R6/2). These mice develop a progressive neurological phenotype with motor symptoms resembling those seen in HD (Carter et al., 1999). Daily fingolimod injections over several weeks, starting in the subtle phase of HD symptoms, significantly ameliorated motor signs of HD and prevented weight loss usually associated with this disease but had no effect on motor tests in WT mice. This was accompanied by activation of the prosurvival pathways of PKB/Akt and ERK1/2 in the striatum. Fingolimod-treated R6/2 mice showed a reduction of brain atrophy and a dramatic reduction of mHtt aggregates in comparison to untreated mice. Fingolimod was able to partially prevent the reduction in corpus callosum thickness that is observed in R6/2 mice compared to WT mice, a hint towards brain-specific and disease-modifying properties of this drug, which were also supported by increases in DARPP-32, a specific marker of medium spiny neurons and myelin-associated glycoprotein (MAG), a marker of myelin and white matter integrity in R6/2 mice after fingolimod treatment. DiPardo et al. also found a significant increase of cortical BDNF mRNA levels both in R6/2 and WT mice treated with FTY720 and the treatment improved cortical neuronal activity. Interestingly, FTY720-treated mice showed a less pronounced loss of GM1 gangliosides in the striatum, so one putative protective mechanism of FTY720 is preventing the disturbance of the lipid balance.

RETT DISEASE

Rett disease is a rare congenital neurodegenerative disease with postnatal onset, usually at the age of 6–18 months, linked to a mutation in the MeCP2 gene located on the x chromosome. Typical for this disease is a relatively normal appearance of infants at birth followed by a developmental regression with severe motor and cognitive deficits. So far, there is no causal treatment. Experiments with MeCP2 -deficient mice have shown an improvement of symptoms by the administration of a small molecule agonist to the neurotrophin receptor TrkB that is activated by BDNF (Schmid et al., 2012). The fact that BDNF levels in MeCP2 mice did not increase in the first weeks after birth as in WT mice (Kolbeck et al., 1999; Chang et al., 2006) as well as a more severe phenotype of MeCP2 null mice crossed with BDNF-deficient mice or an ameliorated phenotype if MeCP2 null mice were crossed with mice overexpressing BDNF (Chang et al., 2006) pointed towards an influence of BDNF on the course of Rett disease. Furthermore, mice lacking MeCP2 and BDNF in neurons show behavioral similarities (Rauskolb et al., 2010). This makes MeCP2-deficient mice a useful tool to study functional consequences of therapies that raise BDNF levels in the brain. Due to its excellent brain permeability, its confirmed neuroprotective properties in models of cerebral ischemia and the fact that it activates ERK1/2 in neurons–a pathway that is activated by BDNF via the TrkB receptor–prompted Deogracias et al. (2012) to investigate the effects of fingolimod on BDNF levels and disease severity in MeCP2 knockout mice. They found that fingolimod phosphate increased BDNF mRNA and protein in a time- and dose-dependent manner in cultured neuronal cells that were shown to express the S1P receptors $S1P_{1-3}$. The phosphorylation of ERK1/2 and PKB/Akt that occurred in parallel could be shown to be $S1P_1$ dependent by use of specific agonists and antagonists whereas it was not further clarified whether BDNF induction was an S1P receptor-mediated or direct intracellular effect. In organotypic cortical cultures, Deogracias et al. (2012) showed that addition of fingolimod phosphate increases network activity and by addition of a monoclonal BDNF-blocking antibody could prove that BDNF is in part responsible for this increased activity. This neutralizing BDNF antibody also reversed the antiapoptotic effect of fingolimod phosphate protecting neurons from NMDA-induced death. *In vivo*, treatment of healthy animals with fingolimod led to increased ERK1/2 phosphorylation and BDNF levels in cortical neurons. In the Rett disease model of MeCP2-deficient mice, a 4 week course of fingolimod treatment at a rather low dose (0.5 mg/kg every 4d) lead to increased levels of BDNF in affected brain structures and even to an amelioration of motor impairment and survival. This was the first description of a fingolimod-elicited production of the neurotrophin BDNF which could be attributed primarily to neurons by immunohistochemistry and cell culture experiments while a relevant contribution of astrocytes could be excluded (Deogracias et al., 2012).

EPILEPSY

Epilepsy is a chronic neurological disorder characterized by repetitive seizures, either of genetic (caused by mutations of genes encoding for excitatory or inhibitory signal tranducers in neurons or glial cells) or structural (caused by a brain lesion such as cerebral infarcts or brain tumors) origin. While epilepsies are well controllable by anticonvulsant medication in the majority of cases, series of recurrent seizures or non-terminating status epilepticus represent a serious threat for patients with epilepsy. The processes happening in the propagation from single seizures to prolonged epileptic activity have been characterized in experimental models and emcompass cell death, axonal and dendritic plasticity, neurogenesis and neuroinflammation (Lukasiuk et al., 2006). Especially neuroinflammatory processes such as glial cell activation and increases in inflammatory cytokines such as IL-1β and TNFα have recently gained interest (Ravizza et al., 2011; Vezzani and Friedman, 2011) and the blockade of IL-1β (Maroso et al., 2011) or TNFα (Rao et al., 2008) were shown to effectively decrease seizure activity. Gao et al. (2012) reported a significant decrease in the incidence and duration of spontaneous recurrent seizures by fingolimod treatment in rats that were subjected to an experimental model of lithium/pilocarpine-induced status epilepticus. Rats were treated with fingolimod 1 mg/kg daily starting 24 h after the induced status epilepticus and showed a reduced activation of microglia and astrocytes in the hippocampus in comparison to vehicle-treated mice as well as reduced hippocampal expression of the proinflammatory cytokines IL-1β and TNFα. Concerning a putative effect on neurons, there was abundant staining for the neuronal marker NeuN in immunohistochemical stainings of the hippocampus of healthy rats that was lost to a great degree 4 days after status epilepticus and partially rescued by FTY720 treatment. The loss of NeuN-positive Neurons in the hippocampus was accompanied by mossy fiber sprouting which was also reduced by treatment with FTY720.

Concerning putative non-immunomodulatory effects of FTY720 in epilepsy, it should be noted that mice with a genetic deletion of the $S1P_2$ receptor develop spontaneous, sporadic, and occasionally lethal seizures between 3 and 7 weeks of age (MacLennan et al., 2001). At a cellular level, loss of the $S1P_2$ receptor leads to a large increase in the excitability of neocortical pyramidal neurons, demonstrating that $S1P_2$ plays an essential and functionally important role in the control of neuronal excitability.

BRAIN TUMORS

Primary brain tumors most commonly originate from glial cells. Among them, high grade gliomas such as the glioblastoma multiforme (GBM) are the most malignant forms with aggressive growth and invasion of the surrounding brain tissue. Due to their infiltrating nature, they cannot be completely excised and the majority will recur locally (Giese et al., 2004). Life expectancy of patients diagnosed with GBM operated and treated with radiotherapy ranges around 12 months and can be extended by chemotherapy with the DNA alkylating chemotherapeutic temozolomid (TMZ), the current standard of care (Hart et al., 2013). There is increasing evidence that dysregulations of S1P metabolizing enzymes with increased levels of S1P are correlated with malignant properties of GBM. Van Brocklyn et al. (2005) showed that high expression levels of the SphK isoform SphK1 in human astrocytomas correlates with a 3fold shorter median survival of patients whereas in glioblastoma cell lines, RNA interference to knock down SphK2 even had a greater effect on tumor cell proliferation than knock down of SphK1 (Van Brocklyn et al., 2005). Exogenously added S1P has been found to stimulate motility and invasiveness of human GBM cells (Van Brocklyn et al., 2003). GBM cell lines express the S1P receptors $S1P_1$, $S1P_2$ and $S1P_3$. From cellular the lower affinity S1P receptor ligands dihydro-sphingosine and sphingosylphosphorylcholine in the high nanomolar to low micromolar range, Van Brocklyn et al. (2002) concluded that the proproliferative effects of S1P on astrocytic tumor cell lines are mediated by the S1P1 receptor involving PI3K and ERK1/2 activation rather than by intracellular effects of S1P. This is supported by (partial) abolishments of S1P effects by the Gi protein inhibitor pertussis toxin or the phosphatidylinositol 3-kinase (PI3K) inhibitors wortmannin and LY294002 and the ERK1/2 kinase inhibiting MEK inhibitor U0126.

A thorough analysis of Young and Van Brocklyn (2009) on the contribution of the single S1P receptors to glioma cell proliferation, migration and invasiveness by means of differential overexpression or RNAi knockdown of the receptors on glioma cell lines established that $S1P_1$, $S1P_2$ and $S1P_3$ all contribute positively to S1P-stimulated glioma cell proliferation, with $S1P_1$ being the major contributor. Stimulation of glioma cell proliferation by these receptors correlated with activation of ERK1/2. Activation of $S1P_5$ inhibited glioma cell proliferation and ERK1/2 activation. $S1P_1$ and $S1P_3$ enhance glioma cell migration and invasion. $S1P_2$ inhibited migration through Rho activation, Rho kinase signaling and stress fiber formation, but enhanced invasiveness of glioma cells by stimulating cell adhesion. Thus, while $S1P_2$ decreases glioma cell motility, it may enhance tumor cell invasion (Van Brocklyn et al., 2003; Lepley et al., 2005).

This may be in part mediated through induction of proteins that modulate glioma cell interaction with the extracellular matrix. $S1P_2$ potently enhances expression of CCN1/Cyr61, a matricellular protein which stimulates cellular adhesion, migration, angiogenesis and invasion. A neutralizing antibody to CCN1 blocked $S1P_2$-stimulated glioma invasion (Van Brocklyn et al., 2003). Expression of CCN1 has been shown to correlate with tumor progression and poor patient prognosis in glioma patients (Xie et al., 2004a) and to enhance tumorigenicity of glioma cells (Xie et al., 2004b). Besides that, uPA and its receptor uPAR, have been established as critical mediators of tumor cell invasiveness (Andreasen et al., 1997). In a subsequent study, Young et al. (2009) found that both CCN1 and uPA are upregulated in a GBM cell line upon treatment with S1P (100 nM). The expression of both proteins was induced through different individual S1P receptor subtypes that were overexpressed in a GBM cell line that normally expresses very low levels of S1P receptors. $S1P_1$ and $S1P_2$ receptors contribute to CCN1 induction while all three receptors, with $S1P_1$ being the most potent, contribute to induce expression of members of the uPA system. Neutralizing antibodies directed against uPA or CCN1 significantly decreased both basal and S1P-stimulated GBM cell invasiveness. uPA activity and glioma invasion were potently blocked by SphK inhibition. Thus, the SphK/S1P/S1P receptor subtypes have a profound and coordinated effect on expression of several genes which are known to be involved in GBM invasiveness (Young et al., 2009).

Growth factors, including EGF, are known to stimulate SphK1 in several cell types and their overexpression in tumor cells is often associated with worse prognosis (Salomon et al., 1995). Especially the EGF receptor (EGFR) is often overexpressed and mutated in gliomas (Frederick et al., 2000). Estrada-Bernal et al. (2011) showed that treatment of glioma cell lines with EGF led to increases in SphK1 expression and activity. Expression of the constitutively active EGFRvIII mutant in glioma cells mimicked this effect. In addition, siRNA to SphK1 partially inhibited EGFRvIII-induced growth and survival of glioma cells as well as ERK1/2 activation. Interestingly, this effect could be overridden by treatment with high concentrations (10 μM) of S1P but not by lower concentrations. Since 10 μM S1P have been shown to activate the intracellular S1P target TRAF2, while lower concentrations of S1P (10 nM) are sufficient to activate the membrane-bound receptors, this hints to receptor-independent intracellular effects (Alvarez et al., 2010). Pharmacological blockade of the EGFR by gefetinib had a rather modest inhibitory effect on glioma cell proliferation whereas pharmacological inhibition of SphK1 strongly blocked proliferation and induced apoptosis of a GBM-derived neurosphere cell line (Estrada-Bernal et al., 2011). These data showed that EGF/EGFR and EGFRvIII signaling induces SphK1 in glioblastoma cells and that SphK1 is necessary to maintain survival of glioblastoma cells.

A putative therapeutic effect of fingolimod in the context of glioma research was evaluated as early as 2001 (Sonoda et al., 2001), spurred by the finding that higher concentrations of fingolimod in the micromolar range were shown to induce apoptosis in mature T lymphocytes (Enosawa et al., 1996). Sonoda et al. found that fingolimod at rather high concentrations (ED50 between 1–10 μg/ml) induced apoptosis in the human glioma cell line T89G. FTY720 led to tyrosine dephosphorylation of the focal adhesion kinase (FAK) and inhibited the protective FAK/PI3K pathway leading to an activation of caspase 6. Conversely, the inhibition of protein tyrosine phosphatases by orthovanadate prevented FAK dephosphorylation and inhibited fingolimod-induced cell death. An antitumor effect of fingolimod has been described in many tumor cell types (reviewed by Pitman et al., 2012; Zhang et al., 2013). In most cases, these antitumor effects are caused by unphosphorylated fingolimod, not fingolimod phosphate in cell culture systems and seem to involve direct intracellular effects of fingolimod such as an activation of phosphatase 2A (PP2A), the tumor suppressor PTEN, an inhibition of the PI3K/AKT/mTOR pathway or even an inhibition of SphKs. Estrada-Bernal et al. (2012) reproduced the propapoptotic effect of fingolimod on glioma cells in the pathophysiologically more relevant model of brain tumor stem cells (BTSCs) derived from human GBM tissue. These cells develop neurosphere-like aggregates in cell culture and develop into faithful histological models of human gliomas when injected into the brains of mice. Four different BTSC lines underwent apoptosis at FTY720 concentrations of 1 μg/ml and higher whereas toxicity to non-malignant primary astrocytes began at 10 μg/ml and was thus one order of magnitude higher. Fingolimod led to a rapid dephosphorylation of ERK1/2, upregulation of the BH3-only protein Bim, and cleavage of caspases 9 and 7 or caspase 3. Fingolimod also reduced BTSC invasiveness and, most importantly, had a synergistic effect in addition to TMZ, the current standard chemotherapeutic agent to treat malignant gliomas, allowing a reduction of the fingolimod dose required for BTSC toxicity. By contrast, fingolimod phosphate was much less effective at inducing apoptosis of BTSC. Generally, in animal models of many cancers, exceedingly high FTY720 doses of 5–10 mg/kg are required for satisfying effectiveness, as compared to 0.5–1 mg/kg that were found to be effective in models of cerebral ischemia (Czech et al., 2009; Hasegawa et al., 2010; Wei et al., 2011; Kraft et al., 2013) or neurodegeneration (Deogracias et al., 2012; Takasugi et al., 2013) and even lower doses required in EAE (Brinkmann et al., 2002). This was also described in the experimental glioma model of Estrada-Bernal et al. (2012), who injected glioma BTSCs into nude mice that were treated with either fingolimod (10 mg/kg), TMZ (5 mg/kg) or a combination of both drugs. This experiment confirmed the efficacy of fingolimod as an experimental glioma therapy that significantly prolonged survival and reduced tumor growth even though it was somewhat less effective than TMZ. The combination of both drugs showed the greatest efficacy. Even if due to yet undefined reasons, the *in vivo* effect of fingolimod was somewhat weaker than the stunning *in vitro* effects, fingolimod seems to be a promising (adjuvant) drug to treat gliomas, whose progression is yet barely controlled by the current standard therapies.

SUMMARY AND FUTURE PERSPECTIVES

According to experimental data, the sphingolipid signaling pathway seems to be of central relevance in the pathophysiology of many diverse neurological diseases. The versatile sphingosine analog fingolimod, prodrug of the S1P-modulating fingolimod phosphate, provides scientifically proven reduction of relapse rate and amelioration of disease progression in MS. But data from experimental animal models suggest that fingolimod has additional therapeutic applications in store. Many of the diseases reviewed here follow a fatal course and treatment options yet are scarce and their efficacy often short-lived. Given the growing body of experience with fingolimod accumulated by clinical neurologists and the favorable safety profile in the indication of MS, there is hope for a translation of some of these experimental findings into the clinics.

ACKNOWLEDGMENTS

Rajkumar Vutukuri is a stipendiary of the International Research Training Group "Dr. Hans Kröner Graduiertenkolleg" funded by the Else Kröner Fresenius-Stiftung. The publication of this manuscript was supported by a publication grant from NEUROWIND e.V.

REFERENCES

Ader, I., Brizuela, L., Bouquerel, P., Malavaud, B., and Cuvillier, O. (2008). Sphingosine kinase 1: a new modulator of hypoxia inducible factor 1alpha during hypoxia in human cancer cells. *Cancer Res.* 68, 8635–8642. doi: 10.1158/0008-5472.CAN-08-0917

Ajmo, C. T., Collier, L. A., Leonardo, C. C., Hall, A. A., Green, S. M., Womble, T. A., et al. (2009). Blockade of adrenoreceptors inhibits the splenic response to stroke. *Exp. Neurol.* 218, 47–55. doi: 10.1016/j.expneurol.2009.03.044

Allende, M. L., Dreier, J. L., Mandala, S., and Proia, R. L. (2004). Expression of the sphingosine 1-phosphate receptor, S1P1, on T-cells controls thymic emigration. *J. Biol. Chem.* 279, 15396–15401. doi: 10.1074/jbc.m314291200

Alvarez, S. E., Harikumar, K. B., Hait, N. C., Allegood, J., Strub, G. M., Kim, E. Y., et al. (2010). Sphingosine-1-phosphate is a missing cofactor for the E3 ubiquitin ligase TRAF2. *Nature* 465, 1084–1088. doi: 10.1038/nature09128

Andreasen, P. A., Kjøller, L., Christensen, L., and Duffy, M. J. (1997). The urokinase-type plasminogen activator system in cancer metastasis: a review. *Int. J. Cancer* 72, 1–22. doi: 10.1002/(sici)1097-0215(19970703)72:1<1::aid-ijc1>3.0.co;2-z

Anthony, D. C., Sibson, N. R., Losey, P., Meier, D. P., and Leppert, D. (2014). Investigation of immune and CNS-mediated effects of fingolimod in the focal delayed-type hypersensitivity multiple sclerosis model. *Neuropharmacology* 79, 534–541. doi: 10.1016/j.neuropharm.2013.12.022

Arboleda, G., Huang, T.-J., Waters, C., Verkhratsky, A., Fernyhough, P., and Gibson, R. M. (2007). Insulin-like growth factor-1-dependent maintenance of neuronal metabolism through the phosphatidylinositol 3-kinase-Akt pathway is inhibited by C2-ceramide in CAD cells. *Eur. J. Neurosci.* 25, 3030–3038. doi: 10.1111/j.1460-9568.2007.05557.x

Asle-Rousta, M., Kolahdooz, Z., Oryan, S., Ahmadiani, A., and Dargahi, L. (2013). FTY720 (fingolimod) attenuates beta-amyloid peptide (Aβ42)-induced impairment of spatial learning and memory in rats. *J. Mol. Neurosci.* 50, 524–532. doi: 10.1007/s12031-013-9979-6

Astrup, J., Siesjö, B. K., and Symon, L. (1981). Thresholds in cerebral ischemia—the ischemic penumbra. *Stroke* 12, 723–725. doi: 10.1161/01.str.12.6.723

Balatoni, B., Storch, M. K., Swoboda, E.-M., Schönborn, V., Koziel, A., Lambrou, G. N., et al. (2007). FTY720 sustains and restores neuronal function in the DA rat model of MOG-induced experimental autoimmune encephalomyelitis. *Brain Res. Bull.* 74, 307–316. doi: 10.1016/j.brainresbull.2007.06.023

Bandaru, V. V. R., McArthur, J. C., Sacktor, N., Cutler, R. G., Knapp, E. L., Mattson, M. P., et al. (2007). Associative and predictive biomarkers of dementia in HIV-1-infected patients. *Neurology* 68, 1481–1487. doi: 10.1212/01.wnl.0000260610.79853.47

Bandhuvula, P., Tam, Y. Y., Oskouian, B., and Saba, J. D. (2005). The immune modulator FTY720 inhibits sphingosine-1-phosphate lyase activity. *J. Biol. Chem.* 280, 33697–33700. doi: 10.1074/jbc.c500294200

Becker, K. J., McCarron, R. M., Ruetzler, C., Laban, O., Sternberg, E., Flanders, K. C., et al. (1997). Immunologic tolerance to myelin basic protein decreases stroke size after transient focal cerebral ischemia. *Proc. Natl. Acad. Sci. U S A* 94, 10873–10878. doi: 10.1073/pnas.94.20.10873

Bigaud, M., Guerini, D., Billich, A., Bassilana, F., and Brinkmann, V. (2014). Second generation S1P pathway modulators: research strategies and clinical developments. *Biochim. Biophys. Acta* 1841, 745–758. doi: 10.1016/j.bbalip.2013.11.001

Blondeau, N., Lai, Y., Tyndall, S., Popolo, M., Topalkara, K., Pru, J. K., et al. (2007). Distribution of sphingosine kinase activity and mRNA in rodent brain. *J. Neurochem.* 103, 509–517. doi: 10.1111/j.1471-4159.2007.04755.x

Boulton, C., Meiser, K., David, O. J., and Schmouder, R. (2012). Pharmacodynamic effects of steady-state fingolimod on antibody response in healthy volunteers: a 4-week, randomized, placebo-controlled, parallel-group, multiple-dose study. *J. Clin. Pharmacol.* 52, 1879–1890. doi: 10.1177/0091270011427908

Braak, H., and Braak, E. (1991). Demonstration of amyloid deposits and neurofibrillary changes in whole brain sections. *Brain Pathol.* 1, 213–216. doi: 10.1111/j.1750-3639.1991.tb00661.x

Braak, H., and Braak, E. (1995). Staging of Alzheimer's disease-related neurofibrillary changes. *Neurobiol. Aging* 16, 271–278. doi: 10.1016/0197-4580(95)00021-6

Brindley, D. N., and Pilquil, C. (2009). Lipid phosphate phosphatases and signaling. *J. Lipid Res.* 50(Suppl), S225–S230. doi: 10.1194/jlr.R800055-JLR200

Brinkmann, V. (2007). Sphingosine 1-phosphate receptors in health and disease: mechanistic insights from gene deletion studies and reverse pharmacology. *Pharmacol. Ther.* 115, 84–105. doi: 10.1016/j.pharmthera.2007.04.006

Brinkmann, V., Billich, A., Baumruker, T., Heining, P., Schmouder, R., Francis, G., et al. (2010). Fingolimod (FTY720): discovery and development of an oral drug to treat multiple sclerosis. *Nat. Rev. Drug Discov.* 9, 883–897. doi: 10.1038/nrd3248

Brinkmann, V., Davis, M. D., Heise, C. E., Albert, R., Cottens, S., Hof, R., et al. (2002). The immune modulator FTY720 targets sphingosine 1-phosphate receptors. *J. Biol. Chem.* 277, 21453–21457. doi: 10.1074/jbc.c200176200

Brinkmann, V., Pinschewer, D., Chiba, K., and Feng, L. (2000). FTY720: a novel transplantation drug that modulates lymphocyte traffic rather than activation. *Trends Pharmacol. Sci.* 21, 49–52. doi: 10.1016/s0165-6147(99)01419-4

Brosnan, C. F., and Raine, C. S. (2013). The astrocyte in multiple sclerosis revisited. *Glia* 61, 453–465. doi: 10.1002/glia.22443

Brunkhorst, R., Kanaan, N., Koch, A., Ferreirós, N., Mirceska, A., Zeiner, P., et al. (2013). FTY720 treatment in the convalescence period improves functional recovery and reduces reactive astrogliosis in photothrombotic stroke. *PLoS One* 8:e70124. doi: 10.1371/journal.pone.0070124

Brynskikh, A., Warren, T., Zhu, J., and Kipnis, J. (2008). Adaptive immunity affects learning behavior in mice. *Brain Behav. Immun.* 22, 861–869. doi: 10.1016/j.bbi.2007.12.008

Cai, A., Schlunk, F., Bohmann, F., Kashefiolasl, S., Brunkhorst, R., Foerch, C., et al. (2013). Coadministration of FTY720 and rt-PA in an experimental model of large hemispheric stroke-no influence on functional outcome and blood-brain barrier disruption. *Exp. Transl. Stroke Med.* 5:11. doi: 10.1186/2040-7378-5-11

Calabresi, P. A., Radue, E.-W., Goodin, D., Jeffery, D., Rammohan, K. W., Reder, A. T., et al. (2014). Safety and efficacy of fingolimod in patients with relapsing-remitting multiple sclerosis (FREEDOMS II): a double-blind, randomised, placebo-controlled, phase 3 trial. *Lancet Neurol.* 13, 545–556. doi: 10.1016/s1474-4422(14)70049-3

Camerer, E., Regard, J. B., Cornelissen, I., Srinivasan, Y., Duong, D. N., Palmer, D., et al. (2009). Sphingosine-1-phosphate in the plasma compartment regulates basal and inflammation-induced vascular leak in mice. *J. Clin. Invest.* 119, 1871–1879. doi: 10.1172/jci38575

Campos, F., Qin, T., Castillo, J., Seo, J. H., Arai, K., Lo, E. H., et al. (2013). Fingolimod reduces hemorrhagic transformation associated with delayed tissue plasminogen activator treatment in a mouse thromboembolic model. *Stroke* 44, 505–511. doi: 10.1161/STROKEAHA.112.679043

Carr, M. W., Roth, S. J., Luther, E., Rose, S. S., and Springer, T. A. (1994). Monocyte chemoattractant protein 1 acts as a T-lymphocyte chemoattractant. *Proc. Natl. Acad. Sci. U S A* 91, 3652–3656. doi: 10.1073/pnas.91.9.3652

Carter, R. J., Lione, L. A., Humby, T., Mangiarini, L., Mahal, A., Bates, G. P., et al. (1999). Characterization of progressive motor deficits in mice transgenic for the human Huntington's disease mutation. *J. Neurosci.* 19, 3248–3257.

Chang, Y.-C., Tzeng, S.-F., Yu, L., Huang, A.-M., Lee, H.-T., Huang, C.-C., et al. (2006). Early-life fluoxetine exposure reduced functional deficits after hypoxic-ischemia brain injury in rat pups. *Neurobiol. Dis.* 24, 101–113. doi: 10.1016/j.nbd.2006.06.001

Chiba, K., Yanagawa, Y., Masubuchi, Y., Kataoka, H., Kawaguchi, T., Ohtsuki, M., et al. (1998). FTY720, a novel immunosuppressant, induces sequestration of circulating mature lymphocytes by acceleration of lymphocyte homing in rats. I. FTY720 selectively decreases the number of circulating mature lymphocytes by acceleration of lymphocyte homing. *J. Immunol.* 160, 5037–5044. doi: 10.1046/j.1365-2567.1998.00639.x

Choi, J. W., Gardell, S. E., Herr, D. R., Rivera, R., Lee, C. W., Noguchi, K., et al. (2010). FTY720 (fingolimod) efficacy in an animal model of multiple sclerosis requires astrocyte sphingosine 1-phosphate receptor 1 (S1P1) modulation. *Proc. Natl. Acad. Sci. U S A* 108, 751–756. doi: 10.1073/pnas.1014154108

Chun, J., Goetzl, E. J., Hla, T., Igarashi, Y., Lynch, K. R., Moolenaar, W., et al. (2002). International Union of Pharmacology. XXXIV. Lysophospholipid receptor nomenclature. *Pharmacol. Rev.* 54, 265–269. doi: 10.1124/pr.54.2.265

Cohen, J. A., Barkhof, F., Comi, G., Hartung, H.-P., Khatri, B. O., Montalban, X., et al. (2010). Oral fingolimod or intramuscular interferon for relapsing multiple sclerosis. *N. Engl. J. Med.* 362, 402–415. doi: 10.1056/NEJMoa0907839

Colombo, E., Dario, M. D., Capitolo, E., Chaabane, L., Newcombe, J., Martino, G., et al. (2014). Fingolimod may support neuroprotection via blockade of astrocyte nitric oxide. *Ann. Neurol.* doi: 10.1002/ana.24217. [Epub ahead of print].

Comi, G., O'Connor, P., Montalban, X., Antel, J., Radue, E.-W., Karlsson, G., et al. (2010). Phase II study of oral fingolimod (FTY720) in multiple sclerosis: 3-year results. *Mult. Scler.* 16, 197–207. doi: 10.1177/1352458509357065

Couttas, T. A., Kain, N., Daniels, B., Lim, X. Y., Shepherd, C., Kril, J., et al. (2014). Loss of the neuroprotective factor Sphingosine 1-phosphate early in Alzheimer's disease pathogenesis. *Acta Neuropathol. Commun.* 2:9. doi: 10.1186/2051-5960-2-9

Cutler, R. G., Kelly, J., Storie, K., Pedersen, W. A., Tammara, A., Hatanpaa, K., et al. (2004). Involvement of oxidative stress-induced abnormalities in ceramide and cholesterol metabolism in brain aging and Alzheimer's disease. *Proc. Natl. Acad. Sci. U S A* 101, 2070–2075. doi: 10.1073/pnas.0305799101

Czech, B., Pfeilschifter, W., Mazaheri-Omrani, N., Strobel, M. A., Kahles, T., Neumann-Haefelin, T., et al. (2009). The immunomodulatory sphingosine 1-phosphate analog FTY720 reduces lesion size and improves neurological outcome in a mouse model of cerebral ischemia. *Biochem. Biophys. Res. Commun.* 389, 251–256. doi: 10.1016/j.bbrc.2009.08.142

Dawson, G., and Qin, J. (2011). Gilenya (FTY720) inhibits acid sphingomyelinase by a mechanism similar to tricyclic antidepressants. *Biochem. Biophys. Res. Commun.* 404, 321–323. doi: 10.1016/j.bbrc.2010.11.115

DeKosky, S. T., and Scheff, S. W. (1990). Synapse loss in frontal cortex biopsies in Alzheimer's disease: correlation with cognitive severity. *Ann. Neurol.* 27, 457–464. doi: 10.1002/ana.410270502

Deogracias, R., Yazdani, M., Dekkers, M. P. J., Guy, J., Ionescu, M. C. S., Vogt, K. E., et al. (2012). Fingolimod, a sphingosine-1 phosphate receptor modulator, increases BDNF levels and improves symptoms of a mouse model of Rett syndrome. *Proc. Natl. Acad. Sci. U S A* 109, 14230–14235. doi: 10.1073/pnas.1206093109

Di Pardo, A., Amico, E., Favellato, M., Castrataro, R., Fucile, S., Squitieri, F., et al. (2014). FTY720 (fingolimod) is a neuroprotective and disease-modifying agent in cellular and mouse models of Huntington disease. *Hum. Mol. Genet.* 23, 2251–2265. doi: 10.1093/hmg/ddt615

Di Pardo, A., Maglione, V., Alpaugh, M., Horkey, M., Atwal, R. S., Sassone, J., et al. (2012). Ganglioside GM1 induces phosphorylation of mutant huntingtin and restores normal motor behavior in Huntington disease mice. *Proc. Natl. Acad. Sci. U S A* 109, 3528–3533. doi: 10.1073/pnas.1114502109

Dirnagl, U., Iadecola, C., and Moskowitz, M. A. (1999). Pathobiology of ischaemic stroke: an integrated view. *Trends Neurosci.* 22, 391–397. doi: 10.1016/s0166-2236(99)01401-0

Doi, Y., Takeuchi, H., Horiuchi, H., Hanyu, T., Kawanokuchi, J., Jin, S., et al. (2013). Fingolimod phosphate attenuates oligomeric amyloid β-induced neurotoxicity via increased brain-derived neurotrophic factor expression in neurons. *PLoS One* 8:e61988. doi: 10.1371/journal.pone.0061988

Dore-Duffy, P., Ho, S. Y., and Donovan, C. (1991). Cerebrospinal fluid eicosanoid levels: endogenous PGD2 and LTC4 synthesis by antigen-presenting cells that migrate to the central nervous system. *Neurology* 41, 322–324. doi: 10.1212/wnl.41.2_part_1.322

Durafourt, B. A., Lambert, C., Johnson, T. A., Blain, M., Bar-Or, A., and Antel, J. P. (2011). Differential responses of human microglia and blood-derived myeloid cells to FTY720. *J. Neuroimmunol.* 230, 10–16. doi: 10.1016/j.jneuroim.2010.08.006

Enosawa, S., Suzuki, S., Kakefuda, T., Li, X. K., and Amemiya, H. (1996). Induction of selective cell death targeting on mature T-lymphocytes in rats by a novel immunosuppressant, FTY720. *Immunopharmacology* 34, 171–179. doi: 10.1016/0162-3109(96)00132-4

Estrada-Bernal, A., Lawler, S. E., Nowicki, M. O., Ray Chaudhury, A., and Van Brocklyn, J. R. (2011). The role of sphingosine kinase-1 in EGFRvIII-regulated growth and survival of glioblastoma cells. *J. Neurooncol.* 102, 353–366. doi: 10.1007/s11060-010-0345-z

Estrada-Bernal, A., Palanichamy, K., Ray Chaudhury, A., and Van Brocklyn, J. R. (2012). Induction of brain tumor stem cell apoptosis by FTY720: a potential therapeutic agent for glioblastoma. *Neuro. Oncol.* 14, 405–415. doi: 10.1093/neuonc/nos005

Filippov, V., Song, M. A., Zhang, K., Vinters, H. V., Tung, S., Kirsch, W. M., et al. (2012). Increased ceramide in brains with Alzheimer's and other neurodegenerative diseases. *J. Alzheimers Dis.* 29, 537–547. doi: 10.3233/JAD-2011-111202

Fischer, A., Sananbenesi, F., Mungenast, A., and Tsai, L.-H. (2010). Targeting the correct HDAC(s) to treat cognitive disorders. *Trends Pharmacol. Sci.* 31, 605–617. doi: 10.1016/j.tips.2010.09.003

Foster, C. A., Howard, L. M., Schweitzer, A., Persohn, E., Hiestand, P. C., Balatoni, B., et al. (2007). Brain penetration of the oral immunomodulatory drug FTY720 and its phosphorylation in the central nervous system during experimental autoimmune encephalomyelitis: consequences for mode of action in multiple sclerosis. *J. Pharmacol. Exp. Ther.* 323, 469–475. doi: 10.1124/jpet.107.127183

Foster, C. A., Mechtcheriakova, D., Storch, M. K., Balatoni, B., Howard, L. M., Bornancin, F., et al. (2009). FTY720 rescue therapy in the dark agouti rat model of experimental autoimmune encephalomyelitis: expression of central nervous system genes and reversal of blood-brain-barrier damage. *Brain Pathol.* 19, 254–266. doi: 10.1111/j.1750-3639.2008.00182.x

Francis, G., Kappos, L., O'Connor, P., Collins, W., Tang, D., Mercier, F., et al. (2014). Temporal profile of lymphocyte counts and relationship with infections with fingolimod therapy. *Mult. Scler.* 20, 471–480. doi: 10.1177/1352458513500551

Frederick, L., Wang, X. Y., Eley, G., and James, C. D. (2000). Diversity and frequency of epidermal growth factor receptor mutations in human glioblastomas. *Cancer Res.* 60, 1383–1387.

Fu, Y., Hao, J., Zhang, N., Ren, L., Sun, N., Li, Y.-J., et al. (2014). Fingolimod for the treatment of intracerebral hemorrhage: a 2-arm proof-of-concept study. *JAMA Neurol.* doi: 10.1001/jamaneurol.2014.1065. [Epub ahead of print].

Fujita, T., Inoue, K., Yamamoto, S., Ikumoto, T., Sasaki, S., Toyama, R., et al. (1994). Fungal metabolites. Part 11. A potent immunosuppressive activity found in Isaria sinclairii metabolite. *J. Antibiot. (Tokyo)* 47, 208–215. doi: 10.7164/antibiotics.47.208

Fukumoto, K., Mizoguchi, H., Takeuchi, H., Horiuchi, H., Kawanokuchi, J., Jin, S., et al. (2014). Fingolimod increases brain-derived neurotrophic factor levels and ameliorates amyloid β-induced memory impairment. *Behav. Brain Res.* 268, 88–93. doi: 10.1016/j.bbr.2014.03.046

Gao, F., Liu, Y., Li, X., Wang, Y., Wei, D., and Jiang, W. (2012). Fingolimod (FTY720) inhibits neuroinflammation and attenuates spontaneous convulsions in lithium-pilocarpine induced status epilepticus in rat model. *Pharmacol. Biochem. Behav.* 103, 187–196. doi: 10.1016/j.pbb.2012.08.025

Garris, C. S., Blaho, V. A., Hla, T., and Han, M. H. (2014). Sphingosine-1-phosphate receptor 1 signalling in T cells: trafficking and beyond. *Immunology* 142, 347–353. doi: 10.1111/imm.12272

Giese, A., Kucinski, T., Knopp, U., Goldbrunner, R., Hamel, W., Mehdorn, H. M., et al. (2004). Pattern of recurrence following local chemotherapy with biodegradable carmustine (BCNU) implants in patients with glioblastoma. *J. Neurooncol.* 66, 351–360. doi: 10.1023/b:neon.0000014539.90077.db

Gonzalez-Cabrera, P. J., Cahalan, S. M., Nguyen, N., Sarkisyan, G., Leaf, N. B., Cameron, M. D., et al. (2012). S1P(1) receptor modulation with cyclical recovery from lymphopenia ameliorates mouse model of multiple sclerosis. *Mol. Pharmacol.* 81, 166–174. doi: 10.1124/mol.111.076109

Gräler, M. H., and Goetzl, E. J. (2004). The immunosuppressant FTY720 down-regulates sphingosine 1-phosphate G-protein-coupled receptors. *FASEB J.* 18, 551–553.

Hait, N. C., Allegood, J., Maceyka, M., Strub, G. M., Harikumar, K. B., Singh, S. K., et al. (2009). Regulation of histone acetylation in the nucleus by sphingosine-1-phosphate. *Science* 325, 1254–1257. doi: 10.1126/science.1176709

Hait, N. C., Wise, L. E., Allegood, J. C., O'Brien, M., Avni, D., Reeves, T. M., et al. (2014). Active, phosphorylated fingolimod inhibits histone deacetylases and facilitates fear extinction memory. *Nat. Neurosci.* 17, 971–980. doi: 10.1038/nn.3728

Han, X., Holtzman, D. M., and McKeel, D. W. (2001). Plasmalogen deficiency in early Alzheimer's disease subjects and in animal models: molecular characterization using electrospray ionization mass spectrometry. *J. Neurochem.* 77, 1168–1180. doi: 10.1046/j.1471-4159.2001.00332.x

Hannun, Y. A., Loomis, C. R., Merrill, A. H., and Bell, R. M. (1986). Sphingosine inhibition of protein kinase C activity and of phorbol dibutyrate binding in vitro and in human platelets. *J. Biol. Chem.* 261, 12604–12609.

Hannun, Y. A., and Obeid, L. M. (2008). Principles of bioactive lipid signalling: lessons from sphingolipids. *Nat. Rev. Mol. Cell Biol.* 9, 139–150. doi: 10.1038/nrm2329

Hart, M. G., Garside, R., Rogers, G., Stein, K., and Grant, R. (2013). Temozolomide for high grade glioma. *Cochrane Database Syst. Rev.* 4:CD007415. doi: 10.1002/14651858.CD007415

Hasegawa, Y., Suzuki, H., Altay, O., Rolland, W., and Zhang, J. H. (2013). Role of the sphingosine metabolism pathway on neurons against experimental cerebral ischemia in rats. *Transl. Stroke Res.* 4, 524–532. doi: 10.1007/s12975-013-0260-7

Hasegawa, Y., Suzuki, H., Sozen, T., Rolland, W., and Zhang, J. H. (2010). Activation of sphingosine 1-phosphate receptor-1 by FTY720 is neuroprotective after ischemic stroke in rats. *Stroke* 41, 368–374. doi: 10.1161/STROKEAHA.109.568899

He, K., Chen, X., Han, C., Xu, L., Zhang, J., Zhang, M., et al. (2014). Lipopolysaccharide-induced cross-tolerance against renal ischemia-reperfusion injury is mediated by hypoxia-inducible factor-2α-regulated nitric oxide production. *Kidney Int.* 85, 276–288. doi: 10.1038/ki.2013.342

He, X., Huang, Y., Li, B., Gong, C.-X., and Schuchman, E. H. (2010). Deregulation of sphingolipid metabolism in Alzheimer's disease. *Neurobiol. Aging* 31, 398–408. doi: 10.1016/j.neurobiolaging.2008.05.010

Hemmati, F., Dargahi, L., Nasoohi, S., Omidbakhsh, R., Mohamed, Z., Chik, Z., et al. (2013). Neurorestorative effect of FTY720 in a rat model of Alzheimer's disease: comparison with memantine. *Behav. Brain Res.* 252, 415–421. doi: 10.1016/j.bbr.2013.06.016

Holmes, O., Paturi, S., Ye, W., Wolfe, M. S., and Selkoe, D. J. (2012). Effects of membrane lipids on the activity and processivity of purified γ-secretase. *Biochemistry* 51, 3565–3575. doi: 10.1021/bi300303g

Hu, Y., Lee, X., Ji, B., Guckian, K., Apicco, D., Pepinsky, R. B., et al. (2011). Sphingosine 1-phosphate receptor modulator fingolimod (FTY720) does not promote remyelination in vivo. *Mol. Cell. Neurosci.* 48, 72–81. doi: 10.1016/j.mcn.2011.06.007

Hurn, P. D., Subramanian, S., Parker, S. M., Afentoulis, M. E., Kaler, L. J., Vandenbark, A. A., et al. (2007). T- and B-cell-deficient mice with experimental stroke have reduced lesion size and inflammation. *J. Cereb. Blood Flow Metab.* 27, 1798–1805. doi: 10.1038/sj.jcbfm.9600482

Huwiler, A., Kolter, T., Pfeilschifter, J., and Sandhoff, K. (2000). Physiology and pathophysiology of sphingolipid metabolism and signaling. *Biochim. Biophys. Acta* 1485, 63–99. doi: 10.1016/s1388-1981(00)00042-1

Huwiler, A., and Pfeilschifter, J. (2008). New players on the center stage: sphingosine 1-phosphate and its receptors as drug targets. *Biochem. Pharmacol.* 75, 1893–1900. doi: 10.1016/j.bcp.2007.12.018

Igarashi, N., Okada, T., Hayashi, S., Fujita, T., Jahangeer, S., and Nakamura, S. (2003). Sphingosine kinase 2 is a nuclear protein and inhibits DNA synthesis. *J. Biol. Chem.* 278, 46832–46839. doi: 10.1074/jbc.m306577200

Im, D. S. (2003). Linking Chinese medicine and G-protein-coupled receptors. *Trends Pharmacol. Sci.* 24, 2–4. doi: 10.1016/s0165-6147(02)00012-3

Jana, A., and Pahan, K. (2010). Fibrillar amyloid-beta-activated human astroglia kill primary human neurons via neutral sphingomyelinase: implications for

Alzheimer's disease. *J. Neurosci.* 30, 12676–12689. doi: 10.1523/JNEUROSCI.1243-10.2010

Johnson, T. A., Lapierre, Y., Bar-Or, A., and Antel, J. P. (2010). Distinct properties of circulating CD8+ T cells in FTY720-treated patients with multiple sclerosis. *Arch. Neurol.* 67, 1449–1455. doi: 10.1001/archneurol.2010.312

Kalvodova, L., Kahya, N., Schwille, P., Ehehalt, R., Verkade, P., Drechsel, D., et al. (2005). Lipids as modulators of proteolytic activity of BACE: involvement of cholesterol, glycosphingolipids and anionic phospholipids in vitro. *J. Biol. Chem.* 280, 36815–36823. doi: 10.1074/jbc.m504484200

Kalyvas, A., and David, S. (2004). Cytosolic phospholipase A2 plays a key role in the pathogenesis of multiple sclerosis-like disease. *Neuron* 41, 323–335. doi: 10.1016/s0896-6273(04)00003-0

Kaneider, N. C., Lindner, J., Feistritzer, C., Sturn, D. H., Mosheimer, B. A., Djanani, A. M., et al. (2004). The immune modulator FTY720 targets sphingosine-kinase-dependent migration of human monocytes in response to amyloid beta-protein and its precursor. *FASEB J.* 18, 1309–1311.

Kanno, T., Nishizaki, T., Proia, R. L., Kajimoto, T., Jahangeer, S., Okada, T., et al. (2010). Regulation of synaptic strength by sphingosine 1-phosphate in the hippocampus. *Neuroscience* 171, 973–980. doi: 10.1016/j.neuroscience.2010.10.021

Kappos, L., Antel, J., Comi, G., Montalban, X., O'Connor, P., Polman, C. H., et al. (2006). Oral fingolimod (FTY720) for relapsing multiple sclerosis. *N. Engl. J. Med.* 355, 1124–1140. doi: 10.1056/NEJMoa052643

Kappos, L., Radue, E.-W., O'Connor, P., Polman, C., Hohlfeld, R., Calabresi, P., et al. (2010). A placebo-controlled trial of oral fingolimod in relapsing multiple sclerosis. *N. Engl. J. Med.* 362, 387–401. doi: 10.1056/NEJMoa0909494

Karaca, I., Tamboli, I. Y., Glebov, K., Richter, J., Fell, L. H., Grimm, M. O., et al. (2014). Deficiency of Sphingosine-1-phosphate Lyase Impairs Lysosomal Metabolism of the Amyloid Precursor Protein. *J. Biol. Chem.* 289, 16761–16772. doi: 10.1074/jbc.M113.535500

Kataoka, H., Sugahara, K., Shimano, K., Teshima, K., Koyama, M., Fukunari, A., et al. (2005). FTY720, sphingosine 1-phosphate receptor modulator, ameliorates experimental autoimmune encephalomyelitis by inhibition of T cell infiltration. *Cell. Mol. Immunol.* 2, 439–448.

Katsel, P., Li, C., and Haroutunian, V. (2007). Gene expression alterations in the sphingolipid metabolism pathways during progression of dementia and Alzheimer's disease: a shift toward ceramide accumulation at the earliest recognizable stages of Alzheimer's disease? *Neurochem. Res.* 32, 845–856. doi: 10.1007/s11064-007-9297-x

Kawahara, A., Nishi, T., Hisano, Y., Fukui, H., Yamaguchi, A., and Mochizuki, N. (2009). The sphingolipid transporter spns2 functions in migration of zebrafish myocardial precursors. *Science* 323, 524–527. doi: 10.1126/science.1167449

Kebir, H., Kreymborg, K., Ifergan, I., Dodelet-Devillers, A., Cayrol, R., Bernard, M., et al. (2007). Human TH17 lymphocytes promote blood-brain barrier disruption and central nervous system inflammation. *Nat. Med.* 13, 1173–1175. doi: 10.1038/nm1651

Kim, H. J., Miron, V. E., Dukala, D., Proia, R. L., Ludwin, S. K., Traka, M., et al. (2011). Neurobiological effects of sphingosine 1-phosphate receptor modulation in the cuprizone model. *FASEB J.* 25, 1509–1518. doi: 10.1096/fj.10-173203

Kipnis, J., Cohen, H., Cardon, M., Ziv, Y., and Schwartz, M. (2004). T cell deficiency leads to cognitive dysfunction: implications for therapeutic vaccination for schizophrenia and other psychiatric conditions. *Proc. Natl. Acad. Sci. U S A* 101, 8180–8185. doi: 10.1073/pnas.0402268101

Kiuchi, M., Adachi, K., Kohara, T., Minoguchi, M., Hanano, T., Aoki, Y., et al. (2000). Synthesis and immunosuppressive activity of 2-substituted 2-aminopropane-1,3-diols and 2-aminoethanols. *J. Med. Chem.* 43, 2946–2961. doi: 10.1021/jm000173z

Kleinschnitz, C., Kraft, P., Dreykluft, A., Hagedorn, I., Göbel, K., Schuhmann, M. K., et al. (2013). Regulatory T cells are strong promoters of acute ischemic stroke in mice by inducing dysfunction of the cerebral microvasculature. *Blood* 121, 679–691. doi: 10.1182/blood-2012-04-426734

Kleinschnitz, C., Schwab, N., Kraft, P., Hagedorn, I., Dreykluft, A., Schwarz, T., et al. (2010). Early detrimental T-cell effects in experimental cerebral ischemia are neither related to adaptive immunity nor thrombus formation. *Blood* 115, 3835–3842. doi: 10.1182/blood-2009-10-249078

Kluk, M. J., and Hla, T. (2002). Signaling of sphingosine-1-phosphate via the S1P/EDG-family of G-protein-coupled receptors. *Biochim. Biophys. Acta* 1582, 72–80. doi: 10.1016/s1388-1981(02)00139-7

Kolbeck, R., Bartke, I., Eberle, W., and Barde, Y. A. (1999). Brain-derived neurotrophic factor levels in the nervous system of wild-type and neurotrophin gene mutant mice. *J. Neurochem.* 72, 1930–1938. doi: 10.1046/j.1471-4159.1999.0721930.x

Kolesnick, R. N. (1991). Sphingomyelin and derivatives as cellular signals. *Prog. Lipid Res.* 30, 1–38. doi: 10.1016/0163-7827(91)90005-p

Kowarik, M. C., Pellkofer, H. L., Cepok, S., Korn, T., Kümpfel, T., Buck, D., et al. (2011). Differential effects of fingolimod (FTY720) on immune cells in the CSF and blood of patients with MS. *Neurology* 76, 1214–1221. doi: 10.1212/WNL.0b013e3182143564

Kraft, P., Göb, E., Schuhmann, M. K., Göbel, K., Deppermann, C., Thielmann, I., et al. (2013). FTY720 ameliorates acute ischemic stroke in mice by reducing thrombo-inflammation but not by direct neuroprotection. *Stroke* 44, 3202–3210. doi: 10.1161/STROKEAHA.113.002880

Lahiri, S., Park, H., Laviad, E. L., Lu, X., Bittman, R., and Futerman, A. H. (2009). Ceramide synthesis is modulated by the sphingosine analog FTY720 via a mixture of uncompetitive and noncompetitive inhibition in an Acyl-CoA chain length-dependent manner. *J. Biol. Chem.* 284, 16090–16098. doi: 10.1074/jbc.M807438200

Latour, L. L., Kang, D.-W., Ezzeddine, M. A., Chalela, J. A., and Warach, S. (2004). Early blood-brain barrier disruption in human focal brain ischemia. *Ann. Neurol.* 56, 468–477. doi: 10.1002/ana.20199

Ledgerwood, L. G., Lal, G., Zhang, N., Garin, A., Esses, S. J., Ginhoux, F., et al. (2008). The sphingosine 1-phosphate receptor 1 causes tissue retention by inhibiting the entry of peripheral tissue T lymphocytes into afferent lymphatics. *Nat. Immunol.* 9, 42–53. doi: 10.1038/ni1534

Lees, K. R., Bluhmki, E., von Kummer, R., Brott, T. G., Toni, D., Grotta, J. C., et al. (2010). Time to treatment with intravenous alteplase and outcome in stroke: an updated pooled analysis of ECASS, ATLANTIS, NINDS and EPITHET trials. *Lancet* 375, 1695–1703. doi: 10.1016/S0140-6736(10)60491-6

Lepley, D., Paik, J.-H., Hla, T., and Ferrer, F. (2005). The G protein-coupled receptor S1P2 regulates Rho/Rho kinase pathway to inhibit tumor cell migration. *Cancer Res.* 65, 3788–3795. doi: 10.1158/0008-5472.can-04-2311

Le Stunff, H., Peterson, C., Liu, H., Milstien, S., and Spiegel, S. (2002). Sphingosine-1-phosphate and lipid phosphohydrolases. *Biochim. Biophys. Acta* 1582, 8–17. doi: 10.1016/s1388-1981(02)00132-4

Liesz, A., Sun, L., Zhou, W., Schwarting, S., Mracsko, E., Zorn, M., et al. (2011). FTY720 reduces post-ischemic brain lymphocyte influx but does not improve outcome in permanent murine cerebral ischemia. *PLoS One* 6:e21312. doi: 10.1371/journal.pone.0021312

Lim, K. G., Tonelli, F., Li, Z., Lu, X., Bittman, R., Pyne, S., et al. (2011). FTY720 analogues as sphingosine kinase 1 inhibitors: enzyme inhibition kinetics, allosterism, proteasomal degradation, and actin rearrangement in MCF-7 breast cancer cells. *J. Biol. Chem.* 286, 18633–18640. doi: 10.1074/jbc.M111.220756

Lloyd-Evans, E., Morgan, A. J., He, X., Smith, D. A., Elliot-Smith, E., Sillence, D. J., et al. (2008). Niemann-Pick disease type C1 is a sphingosine storage disease that causes deregulation of lysosomal calcium. *Nat. Med.* 14, 1247–1255. doi: 10.1038/nm.1876

Lock, C., Hermans, G., Pedotti, R., Brendolan, A., Schadt, E., Garren, H., et al. (2002). Gene-microarray analysis of multiple sclerosis lesions yields new targets validated in autoimmune encephalomyelitis. *Nat. Med.* 8, 500–508. doi: 10.1038/nm0502-500

Lu, L., Barfejani, A. H., Qin, T., Dong, Q., Ayata, C., and Waeber, C. (2014). Fingolimod exerts neuroprotective effects in a mouse model of intracerebral hemorrhage. *Brain Res.* 1555, 89–96. doi: 10.1016/j.brainres.2014.01.048

Lukasiuk, K., Dabrowski, M., Adach, A., and Pitkänen, A. (2006). Epileptogenesis-related genes revisited. *Prog. Brain Res.* 158, 223–241. doi: 10.1016/s0079-6123(06)58011-2

Lukiw, W. J., and Bazan, N. G. (2006). Survival signalling in Alzheimer's disease. *Biochem. Soc. Trans.* 34, 1277–1282. doi: 10.1042/bst0341277

MacLennan, A. J., Carney, P. R., Zhu, W. J., Chaves, A. H., Garcia, J., Grimes, J. R., et al. (2001). An essential role for the H218/AGR16/Edg-5/LP(B2) sphingosine 1-phosphate receptor in neuronal excitability. *Eur. J. Neurosci.* 14, 203–209. doi: 10.1046/j.0953-816x.2001.01634.x

Maggio, N., Itsekson, Z., Ikenberg, B., Strehl, A., Vlachos, A., Blatt, I., et al. (2014). The anticoagulant activated protein C (aPC) promotes metaplasticity in the hippocampus through an EPCR-PAR1–S1P1 receptors dependent mechanism. *Hippocampus* 24, 1030–1038. doi: 10.1002/hipo.22288

Maggio, N., Shavit, E., Chapman, J., and Segal, M. (2008). Thrombin induces long-term potentiation of reactivity to afferent stimulation and facilitates epileptic seizures in rat hippocampal slices: toward understanding the functional consequences of cerebrovascular insults. *J. Neurosci.* 28, 732–736. doi: 10.1523/JNEUROSCI.3665-07.2008

Maglione, V., Marchi, P., Di Pardo, A., Lingrell, S., Horkey, M., Tidmarsh, E., et al. (2010). Impaired ganglioside metabolism in Huntington's disease and neuroprotective role of GM1. *J. Neurosci.* 30, 4072–4080. doi: 10.1523/JNEUROSCI.6348-09.2010

Mandala, S., Hajdu, R., Bergstrom, J., Quackenbush, E., Xie, J., Milligan, J., et al. (2002). Alteration of lymphocyte trafficking by sphingosine-1-phosphate receptor agonists. *Science* 296, 346–349. doi: 10.1126/science.1070238

Mannaioni, G., Orr, A. G., Hamill, C. E., Yuan, H., Pedone, K. H., McCoy, K. L., et al. (2008). Plasmin potentiates synaptic N-methyl-D-aspartate receptor function in hippocampal neurons through activation of protease-activated receptor-1. *J. Biol. Chem.* 283, 20600–20611. doi: 10.1074/jbc.M803015200

Mansoor, M., and Melendez, A. J. (2008). Recent trials for FTY720 (fingolimod): a new generation of immunomodulators structurally similar to sphingosine. *Rev. Recent Clin. Trials* 3, 62–69. doi: 10.2174/157488708783330486

Maroso, M., Balosso, S., Ravizza, T., Iori, V., Wright, C. I., French, J., et al. (2011). Interleukin-1β biosynthesis inhibition reduces acute seizures and drug resistant chronic epileptic activity in mice. *Neurotherapeutics* 8, 304–315. doi: 10.1007/s13311-011-0039-z

Masopust, D., Vezys, V., Marzo, A. L., and Lefrançois, L. (2001). Preferential localization of effector memory cells in nonlymphoid tissue. *Science* 291, 2413–2417. doi: 10.1126/science.1058867

Matloubian, M., Lo, C. G., Cinamon, G., Lesneski, M. J., Xu, Y., Brinkmann, V., et al. (2004). Lymphocyte egress from thymus and peripheral lymphoid organs is dependent on S1P receptor 1. *Nature* 427, 355–360. doi: 10.1038/nature02284

Mehling, M., Brinkmann, V., Antel, J., Bar-Or, A., Goebels, N., Vedrine, C., et al. (2008). FTY720 therapy exerts differential effects on T cell subsets in multiple sclerosis. *Neurology* 71, 1261–1267. doi: 10.1212/01.wnl.0000327609.57688.ea

Meisel, C., Schwab, J. M., Prass, K., Meisel, A., and Dirnagl, U. (2005). Central nervous system injury-induced immune deficiency syndrome. *Nat. Rev. Neurosci.* 6, 775–786. doi: 10.1038/nrn1765

Mencl, S., Hennig, N., Hopp, S., Schuhmann, M. K., Albert-Weissenberger, C., Sirén, A. L., et al. (2014). FTY720 does not protect from traumatic brain injury in mice despite reducing posttraumatic inflammation. *J. Neuroimmunol.* doi: 10.1016/j.jneuroim.2014.07.010. [Epub ahead of print].

Mielke, M. M., Haughey, N. J., Bandaru, V. V. R., Zetterberg, H., Blennow, K., Andreasson, U., et al. (2014). Cerebrospinal fluid sphingolipids, β-amyloid and tau in adults at risk for Alzheimer's disease. *Neurobiol. Aging* doi: 10.1016/j.neurobiolaging.2014.05.019. [Epub ahead of print].

Miron, V. E., Hall, J. A., Kennedy, T. E., Soliven, B., and Antel, J. P. (2008). Cyclical and dose-dependent responses of adult human mature oligodendrocytes to fingolimod. *Am. J. Pathol.* 173, 1143–1152. doi: 10.2353/ajpath.2008.080478

Miron, V. E., Ludwin, S. K., Darlington, P. J., Jarjour, A. A., Soliven, B., Kennedy, T. E., et al. (2010). Fingolimod (FTY720) enhances remyelination following demyelination of organotypic cerebellar slices. *Am. J. Pathol.* 176, 2682–2694. doi: 10.2353/ajpath.2010.091234

Noda, H., Takeuchi, H., Mizuno, T., and Suzumura, A. (2013). Fingolimod phosphate promotes the neuroprotective effects of microglia. *J. Neuroimmunol.* 256, 13–18. doi: 10.1016/j.jneuroim.2012.12.005

Ntranos, A., Hall, O., Robinson, D. P., Grishkan, I. V., Schott, J. T., Tosi, D. M., et al. (2014). FTY720 impairs CD8 T-cell function independently of the sphingosine-1-phosphate pathway. *J. Neuroimmunol.* 270, 13–21. doi: 10.1016/j.jneuroim.2014.03.007

Osenkowski, P., Ye, W., Wang, R., Wolfe, M. S., and Selkoe, D. J. (2008). Direct and potent regulation of gamma-secretase by its lipid microenvironment. *J. Biol. Chem.* 283, 22529–22540. doi: 10.1074/jbc.M801925200

Papadopoulos, D., Rundle, J., Patel, R., Marshall, I., Stretton, J., Eaton, R., et al. (2010). FTY720 ameliorates MOG-induced experimental autoimmune encephalomyelitis by suppressing both cellular and humoral immune responses. *J. Neurosci. Res.* 88, 346–359. doi: 10.1002/jnr.22196

Paugh, S. W., Cassidy, M. P., He, H., Milstien, S., Sim-Selley, L. J., Spiegel, S., et al. (2006). Sphingosine and its analog, the immunosuppressant 2-amino-2-(2-[4-octylphenyl]ethyl)-1,3-propanediol, interact with the CB1 cannabinoid receptor. *Mol. Pharmacol.* 70, 41–50.

Payne, S. G., Oskeritzian, C. A., Griffiths, R., Subramanian, P., Barbour, S. E., Chalfant, C. E., et al. (2007). The immunosuppressant drug FTY720 inhibits cytosolic phospholipase A2 independently of sphingosine-1-phosphate receptors. *Blood* 109, 1077–1085. doi: 10.1182/blood-2006-03-011437

Peng, X., Hassoun, P. M., Sammani, S., McVerry, B. J., Burne, M. J., Rabb, H., et al. (2004). Protective effects of sphingosine 1-phosphate in murine endotoxin-induced inflammatory lung injury. *Am. J. Respir. Crit. Care Med.* 169, 1245–1251. doi: 10.1164/rccm.200309-1258oc

Pfeilschifter, W., Czech-Zechmeister, B., Sujak, M., Foerch, C., Wichelhaus, T. A., and Pfeilschifter, J. (2011a). Treatment with the immunomodulator FTY720 does not promote spontaneous bacterial infections after experimental stroke in mice. *Exp. Transl. Stroke Med.* 3:2. doi: 10.1186/2040-7378-3-2

Pfeilschifter, W., Czech-Zechmeister, B., Sujak, M., Mirceska, A., Koch, A., Rami, A., et al. (2011b). Activation of sphingosine kinase 2 is an endogenous protective mechanism in cerebral ischemia. *Biochem. Biophys. Res. Commun.* 413, 212–217. doi: 10.1016/j.bbrc.2011.08.070

Pham, T. H. M., Okada, T., Matloubian, M., Lo, C. G., and Cyster, J. G. (2008). S1P1 receptor signaling overrides retention mediated by G alpha i-coupled receptors to promote T cell egress. *Immunity* 28, 122–133. doi: 10.1016/j.immuni.2007.11.017

Pitman, M. R., Woodcock, J. M., Lopez, A. F., and Pitson, S. M. (2012). Molecular targets of FTY720 (fingolimod). *Curr. Mol. Med.* 12, 1207–1219. doi: 10.2174/156652412803833599

Puglielli, L., Ellis, B. C., Saunders, A. J., and Kovacs, D. M. (2003). Ceramide stabilizes beta-site amyloid precursor protein-cleaving enzyme 1 and promotes amyloid beta-peptide biogenesis. *J. Biol. Chem.* 278, 19777–19783. doi: 10.1074/jbc.m300466200

Qin, J., Berdyshev, E., Goya, J., Natarajan, V., and Dawson, G. (2010). Neurons and oligodendrocytes recycle sphingosine 1-phosphate to ceramide: significance for apoptosis and multiple sclerosis. *J. Biol. Chem.* 285, 14134–14143. doi: 10.1074/jbc.M109.076810

Rao, R. S., Medhi, B., Saikia, U. N., Arora, S. K., Toor, J. S., Khanduja, K. L., et al. (2008). Experimentally induced various inflammatory models and seizure: understanding the role of cytokine in rat. *Eur. Neuropsychopharmacol.* 18, 760–767. doi: 10.1016/j.euroneuro.2008.06.008

Rauskolb, S., Zagrebelsky, M., Dreznjak, A., Deogracias, R., Matsumoto, T., Wiese, S., et al. (2010). Global deprivation of brain-derived neurotrophic factor in the CNS reveals an area-specific requirement for dendritic growth. *J. Neurosci.* 30, 1739–1749. doi: 10.1523/JNEUROSCI.5100-09.2010

Ravizza, T., Balosso, S., and Vezzani, A. (2011). Inflammation and prevention of epileptogenesis. *Neurosci. Lett.* 497, 223–230. doi: 10.1016/j.neulet.2011.02.040

Rolland, W. B., Lekic, T., Krafft, P. R., Hasegawa, Y., Altay, O., Hartman, R., et al. (2013). Fingolimod reduces cerebral lymphocyte infiltration in experimental models of rodent intracerebral hemorrhage. *Exp. Neurol.* 241, 45–55. doi: 10.1016/j.expneurol.2012.12.009

Rolland, W. B., Manaenko, A., Lekic, T., Hasegawa, Y., Ostrowski, R., Tang, J., et al. (2011). FTY720 is neuroprotective and improves functional outcomes after intracerebral hemorrhage in mice. *Acta Neurochir. Suppl.* 111, 213–217. doi: 10.1007/978-3-7091-0693-8_36

Rossi, S., Lo Giudice, T., De Chiara, V., Musella, A., Studer, V., Motta, C., et al. (2012). Oral fingolimod rescues the functional deficits of synapses in experimental autoimmune encephalomyelitis. *Br. J. Pharmacol.* 165, 861–869. doi: 10.1111/j.1476-5381.2011.01579.x

Ruvolo, P. (2003). Intracellular signal transduction pathways activated by ceramide and its metabolites. *Pharmacol. Res.* 47, 383–392. doi: 10.1016/s1043-6618(03)00050-1

Salomon, D. S., Brandt, R., Ciardiello, F., and Normanno, N. (1995). Epidermal growth factor-related peptides and their receptors in human malignancies. *Crit. Rev. Oncol. Hematol.* 19, 183–232. doi: 10.1016/1040-8428(94)00144-i

Sandhoff, K., and Christomanou, H. (1979). Biochemistry and genetics of gangliosidoses. *Hum. Genet.* 50, 107–143. doi: 10.1007/bf00390234

Schiffmann, S., Ferreiros, N., Birod, K., Eberle, M., Schreiber, Y., Pfeilschifter, W., et al. (2012). Ceramide synthase 6 plays a critical role in the development of experimental autoimmune encephalomyelitis. *J. Immunol.* 188, 5723–5733. doi: 10.4049/jimmunol.1103109

Schmid, D. A., Yang, T., Ogier, M., Adams, I., Mirakhur, Y., Wang, Q., et al. (2012). A TrkB small molecule partial agonist rescues TrkB phosphorylation deficits and improves respiratory function in a mouse model of Rett syndrome. *J. Neurosci.* 32, 1803–1810. doi: 10.1523/JNEUROSCI.0865-11.2012

Schwalm, S., Döll, F., Römer, I., Bubnova, S., Pfeilschifter, J., and Huwiler, A. (2008). Sphingosine kinase-1 is a hypoxia-regulated gene that stimulates migration of human endothelial cells. *Biochem. Biophys. Res. Commun.* 368, 1020–1025. doi: 10.1016/j.bbrc.2008.01.132

Sharkey, J., Crawford, J. H., Butcher, S. P., and Marston, H. M. (1996). Tacrolimus (FK506) ameliorates skilled motor deficits produced by middle cerebral artery occlusion in rats. *Stroke* 27, 2282–2286. doi: 10.1161/01.str.27.12.2282

Shichita, T., Sugiyama, Y., Ooboshi, H., Sugimori, H., Nakagawa, R., Takada, I., et al. (2009). Pivotal role of cerebral interleukin-17-producing gammadeltaT cells in the delayed phase of ischemic brain injury. *Nat. Med.* 15, 946–950. doi: 10.1038/nm.1999

Skon, C. N., Lee, J.-Y., Anderson, K. G., Masopust, D., Hogquist, K. A., and Jameson, S. C. (2013). Transcriptional downregulation of S1pr1 is required for the establishment of resident memory CD8+ T cells. *Nat. Immunol.* 14, 1285–1293. doi: 10.1038/ni.2745

Sonoda, Y., Yamamoto, D., Sakurai, S., Hasegawa, M., Aizu-Yokota, E., Momoi, T., et al. (2001). FTY720, a novel immunosuppressive agent, induces apoptosis in human glioma cells. *Biochem. Biophys. Res. Commun.* 281, 282–288. doi: 10.1006/bbrc.2001.4352

Sugita, K., Kabashima, K., Sakabe, J.-I., Yoshiki, R., Tanizaki, H., and Tokura, Y. (2010). FTY720 regulates bone marrow egress of eosinophils and modulates late-phase skin reaction in mice. *Am. J. Pathol.* 177, 1881–1887. doi: 10.2353/ajpath.2010.100119

Sun, Y., Li, Q.-F., Zhang, Y., Hu, R., and Jiang, H. (2013). Isoflurane preconditioning increases survival of rat skin random-pattern flaps by induction of HIF-1α expression. *Cell. Physiol. Biochem.* 31, 579–591. doi: 10.1159/000350078

Takasugi, N., Sasaki, T., Ebinuma, I., Osawa, S., Isshiki, H., Takeo, K., et al. (2013). FTY720/fingolimod, a sphingosine analogue, reduces amyloid-β production in neurons. *PLoS One* 8:e64050. doi: 10.1371/journal.pone.0064050

Takasugi, N., Sasaki, T., Suzuki, K., Osawa, S., Isshiki, H., Hori, Y., et al. (2011). BACE1 activity is modulated by cell-associated sphingosine-1-phosphate. *J. Neurosci.* 31, 6850–6857. doi: 10.1523/JNEUROSCI.6467-10.2011

Tamboli, I. Y., Prager, K., Barth, E., Heneka, M., Sandhoff, K., and Walter, J. (2005). Inhibition of glycosphingolipid biosynthesis reduces secretion of the beta-amyloid precursor protein and amyloid beta-peptide. *J. Biol. Chem.* 280, 28110–28117. doi: 10.1074/jbc.m414525200

Thangada, S., Khanna, K. M., Blaho, V. A., Oo, M. L., Im, D.-S., Guo, C., et al. (2010). Cell-surface residence of sphingosine 1-phosphate receptor 1 on lymphocytes determines lymphocyte egress kinetics. *J. Exp. Med.* 207, 1475–1483. doi: 10.1084/jem.20091343

Thijs, V. N., Adami, A., Neumann-Haefelin, T., Moseley, M. E., and Albers, G. W. (2002). Clinical and radiological correlates of reduced cerebral blood flow measured using magnetic resonance imaging. *Arch. Neurol.* 59, 233–238. doi: 10.1001/archneur.59.2.233

Tsai, C.-F., Thomas, B., and Sudlow, C. L. M. (2013). Epidemiology of stroke and its subtypes in Chinese vs. white populations: a systematic review. *Neurology* 81, 264–272. doi: 10.1212/WNL.0b013e31829bfde3

Tzartos, J. S., Friese, M. A., Craner, M. J., Palace, J., Newcombe, J., Esiri, M. M., et al. (2008). Interleukin-17 production in central nervous system-infiltrating T cells and glial cells is associated with active disease in multiple sclerosis. *Am. J. Pathol.* 172, 146–155. doi: 10.2353/ajpath.2008.070690

Van Brocklyn, J. R., Jackson, C. A., Pearl, D. K., Kotur, M. S., Snyder, P. J., and Prior, T. W. (2005). Sphingosine kinase-1 expression correlates with poor survival of patients with glioblastoma multiforme: roles of sphingosine kinase isoforms in growth of glioblastoma cell lines. *J. Neuropathol. Exp. Neurol.* 64, 695–705. doi: 10.1097/01.jnen.0000175329.59092.2c

Van Brocklyn, J., Letterle, C., Snyder, P., and Prior, T. (2002). Sphingosine-1-phosphate stimulates human glioma cell proliferation through Gi-coupled receptors: role of ERK MAP kinase and phosphatidylinositol 3-kinase beta. *Cancer Lett.* 181, 195–204. doi: 10.1016/s0304-3835(02)00050-2

Van Brocklyn, J. R., Young, N., and Roof, R. (2003). Sphingosine-1-phosphate stimulates motility and invasiveness of human glioblastoma multiforme cells. *Cancer Lett.* 199, 53–60. doi: 10.1016/s0304-3835(03)00334-3

van Doorn, R., Nijland, P. G., Dekker, N., Witte, M. E., Lopes-Pinheiro, M. A., van het Hof, B., et al. (2012). Fingolimod attenuates ceramide-induced blood-brain barrier dysfunction in multiple sclerosis by targeting reactive astrocytes. *Acta Neuropathol.* 12, 397–410. doi: 10.1007/s00401-012-1014-4

Verderio, C., Muzio, L., Turola, E., Bergami, A., Novellino, L., Ruffini, F., et al. (2012). Myeloid microvesicles are a marker and therapeutic target for neuroinflammation. *Ann. Neurol.* 72, 610–624. doi: 10.1002/ana.23627

Vezzani, A., and Friedman, A. (2011). Brain inflammation as a biomarker in epilepsy. *Biomark. Med.* 5, 607–614. doi: 10.2217/bmm.11.61

Wacker, B. K., Park, T. S., and Gidday, J. M. (2009). Hypoxic preconditioning-induced cerebral ischemic tolerance: role of microvascular sphingosine kinase 2. *Stroke* 40, 3342–3348. doi: 10.1161/STROKEAHA.109.560714

Wacker, B. K., Perfater, J. L., and Gidday, J. M. (2012). Hypoxic preconditioning induces stroke tolerance in mice via a cascading HIF, sphingosine kinase and CCL2 signaling pathway. *J. Neurochem.* 123, 954–962. doi: 10.1111/jnc.12047

Walzer, T., Chiossone, L., Chaix, J., Calver, A., Carozzo, C., Garrigue-Antar, L., et al. (2007). Natural killer cell trafficking in vivo requires a dedicated sphingosine 1-phosphate receptor. *Nat. Immunol.* 8, 1337–1344. doi: 10.1038/ni1523

Webb, M., Tham, C.-S., Lin, F.-F., Lariosa-Willingham, K., Yu, N., Hale, J., et al. (2004). Sphingosine 1-phosphate receptor agonists attenuate relapsing-remitting experimental autoimmune encephalitis in SJL mice. *J. Neuroimmunol.* 153, 108–121. doi: 10.1016/j.jneuroim.2004.04.015

Wei, Y., Yemisci, M., Kim, H.-H., Yung, L. M., Shin, H. K., Hwang, S.-K., et al. (2011). Fingolimod provides long-term protection in rodent models of cerebral ischemia. *Ann. Neurol.* 69, 119–129. doi: 10.1002/ana.22186

Wilson, E., Olcott, M. C., Bell, R. M., Merrill, A. H., and Lambeth, J. D. (1986). Inhibition of the oxidative burst in human neutrophils by sphingoid long-chain bases. Role of protein kinase C in activation of the burst. *J. Biol. Chem.* 261, 12616–12623.

Wu, C., Leong, S. Y., Moore, C. S., Cui, Q. L., Gris, P., Bernier, L.-P., et al. (2013). Dual effects of daily FTY720 on human astrocytes in vitro: relevance for neuroinflammation. *J. Neuroinflammation* 10:41. doi: 10.1186/1742-2094-10-41

Xie, D., Yin, D., Tong, X., O'Kelly, J., Mori, A., Miller, C., et al. (2004a). Cyr61 is overexpressed in gliomas and involved in integrin-linked kinase-mediated Akt and beta-catenin-TCF/Lef signaling pathways. *Cancer Res.* 64, 1987–1996. doi: 10.1158/0008-5472.can-03-0666

Xie, D., Yin, D., Wang, H.-J., Liu, G.-T., Elashoff, R., Black, K., et al. (2004b). Levels of expression of CYR61 and CTGF are prognostic for tumor progression and survival of individuals with gliomas. *Clin. Cancer Res.* 10, 2072–2081. doi: 10.1158/1078-0432.ccr-0659-03

Xiong, Y., and Hla, T. (2014). S1P control of endothelial integrity. *Curr. Top. Microbiol. Immunol.* 378, 85–105. doi: 10.1007/978-3-319-05879-5_4

Yanagawa, Y., Sugahara, K., Kataoka, H., Kawaguchi, T., Masubuchi, Y., and Chiba, K. (1998). FTY720, a novel immunosuppressant, induces sequestration of circulating mature lymphocytes by acceleration of lymphocyte homing in rats. II. FTY720 prolongs skin allograft survival by decreasing T cell infiltration into grafts but not cytokine production in vivo. *J. Immunol.* 160, 5493–5499.

Young, N., Pearl, D. K., and Van Brocklyn, J. R. (2009). Sphingosine-1-phosphate regulates glioblastoma cell invasiveness through the urokinase plasminogen activator system and CCN1/Cyr61. *Mol. Cancer Res.* 7, 23–32. doi: 10.1158/1541-7786.mcr-08-0061

Young, N., and Van Brocklyn, J. R. (2009). Roles of sphingosine-1-phosphate (S1P) receptors in malignant behavior of glioma cells. Differential effects of S1P2 on cell migration and invasiveness. *Exp. Cell Res.* 313, 1615–1627. doi: 10.1016/j.yexcr.2007.02.009

Yuan, H., Vance, K. M., Junge, C. E., Geballe, M. T., Snyder, J. P., Hepler, J. R., et al. (2009). The serine protease plasmin cleaves the amino-terminal domain of the NR2A subunit to relieve zinc inhibition of the N-methyl-D-aspartate receptors. *J. Biol. Chem.* 284, 12862–12873. doi: 10.1074/jbc.m805123200

Yung, L. M., Wei, Y., Qin, T., Wang, Y., Smith, C. D., and Waeber, C. (2012). Sphingosine kinase 2 mediates cerebral preconditioning and protects the mouse brain against ischemic injury. *Stroke* 43, 199–204. doi: 10.1161/strokeaha.111.626911

Zhang, M., Martin, B. R., Adler, M. W., Razdan, R. J., Kong, W., Ganea, D., et al. (2009). Modulation of cannabinoid receptor activation as a neuroprotective strategy for EAE and stroke. *J. Neuroimmune Pharmacol.* 4, 249–259. doi: 10.1007/s11481-009-9148-4

Zhang, L., Wang, H.-D., Ji, X.-J., Cong, Z.-X., Zhu, J.-H., and Zhou, Y. (2013). FTY720 for cancer therapy (Review). *Oncol. Rep.* 30, 2571–2578. doi: 10.3892/or.2013.2765

Zheng, H., and Koo, E. H. (2011). Biology and pathophysiology of the amyloid precursor protein. *Mol. Neurodegener.* 6:27. doi: 10.1186/1750-1326-6-27

Zuccato, C., Ciammola, A., Rigamonti, D., Leavitt, B. R., Goffredo, D., Conti, L., et al. (2001). Loss of huntingtin-mediated BDNF gene transcription in Huntington's disease. *Science* 293, 493–498. doi: 10.1126/science.1059581

18

Fractalkine is a "find-me" signal released by neurons undergoing ethanol-induced apoptosis

Jennifer D. Sokolowski[1,2,3] **_*, Chloe N. Chabanon-Hicks_**[1]**_, Claudia Z. Han_**[4,5]**_, Daniel S. Heffron_**[1] **_and James W. Mandell_**[1,5]

[1] *Department of Pathology, School of Medicine, University of Virginia, Charlottesville, VA, USA*
[2] *Medical Scientist Training Program, School of Medicine, University of Virginia, Charlottesville, VA, USA*
[3] *Neuroscience Graduate Program, School of Medicine, University of Virginia, Charlottesville, VA, USA*
[4] *Department of Microbiology, Immunology and Cancer Biology, School of Medicine, University of Virginia, Charlottesville, VA, USA*
[5] *Center for Cell Clearance, University of Virginia, Charlottesville, VA, USA*

***Correspondence:**
Jennifer D. Sokolowski, Department of Pathology, School of Medicine, University of Virginia, 415 Lane Road, MR5 3220, Charlottesville, VA 22908, USA
e-mail: jde2z@virginia.edu

Apoptotic neurons generated during normal brain development or secondary to pathologic insults are efficiently cleared from the central nervous system. Several soluble factors, including nucleotides, cytokines, and chemokines are released from injured neurons, signaling microglia to find and clear debris. One such chemokine that serves as a neuronal–microglial communication factor is fractalkine, with roles demonstrated in several models of adult neurological disorders. Lacking, however, are studies investigating roles for fractalkine in perinatal brain injury, an important clinical problem with no effective therapies. We used a well-characterized mouse model of ethanol-induced apoptosis to assess the role of fractalkine in neuronal–microglial signaling. Quantification of apoptotic debris in fractalkine-knockout (KO) and CX3CR1-KO mice following ethanol treatment revealed increased apoptotic bodies compared to wild type mice. Ethanol-induced injury led to release of soluble, extracellular fractalkine. The extracellular media harvested from apoptotic brains induces microglial migration in a fractalkine-dependent manner that is prevented by neutralization of fractalkine with a blocking antibody or by deficiency in the receptor, CX3CR1. This suggests fractalkine acts as a "find-me" signal, recruiting microglial processes toward apoptotic cells to promote their clearance. Next, we aimed to determine whether there are downstream alterations in cytokine gene expression due to fractalkine signaling. We examined mRNA expression in fractalkine-KO and CX3CR1-KO mice after alcohol-induced apoptosis and found differences in cytokine production in the brains of these KOs by 6 h after ethanol treatment. Collectively, this suggests that fractalkine acts as a "find me" signal released by apoptotic neurons, and subsequently plays a critical role in modulating both clearance and inflammatory cytokine gene expression after ethanol-induced apoptosis.

Keywords: apoptosis, fractalkine, ethanol, cytokine, chemokine, neuron, microglia, clearance

INTRODUCTION

Clearance of apoptotic neurons is critical for normal central nervous system (CNS) development and for resolution of injury due to pathologic processes. Failure to clear apoptotic neurons leads to secondary necrosis with leakage of intracellular contents that are toxic and inflammatory. Efficient clearance is thought to be critical in order to avoid an adverse immune reaction and secondary degeneration (Ravichandran and Lorenz, 2007). However, the precise mechanisms by which apoptotic neurons are cleared have yet to be elucidated. Most of the work on apoptotic cell clearance has been done in non-neural systems or in invertebrate animal models (Truman et al., 2008; Elliott et al., 2009; Gronski et al., 2009). Elucidation of molecular mechanisms used for clearance of apoptotic cells in the developing and adult mammalian brain is an important goal.

Studies in peripheral tissues have shown that as cells undergo apoptosis, they release soluble signals that attract phagocytes and modulate their clearance (Ravichandran and Lorenz, 2007), and the chemokine fractalkine has been described as one of many "find me" signals released by apoptotic cells (Truman et al., 2008). Fractalkine is a transmembrane chemokine that is cleaved constitutively by matrix metalloprotease ADAM10 and inducibly by ADAM 17 (also known as the TNFα-converting enzyme, TACE) to release an extracellular soluble fragment. Inducible cleavage occurs following cell stress or injury, and the soluble fragment acts as a chemotactic factor for T cells, monocytes, and microglia (Bazan et al., 1997; Harrison et al., 1998). The study describing fractalkine as a "find me" signal showed that it is released following induction of apoptosis and that the fractalkine receptor, CX3CR1, modulates recruitment of phagocytes to apoptotic germinal center B cells (Truman et al., 2008). In this study we asked whether fractalkine and its receptor, CX3CR1 are important for apoptotic neuron clearance *in vivo* utilizing a mouse model of fetal alcohol syndrome.

In the CNS, fractalkine is expressed by neurons and cleaved by matrix metalloproteases to release a soluble fragment after neuronal stress. Microglia are the only CNS cell that expresses appreciable levels of the fractalkine receptor, CX3CR1 *in vivo* (Harrison et al., 1998). Studies in CNS models have largely focused on the role of fractalkine in neurotoxicity and have shown that fractalkine signaling modulates the inflammatory response of microglia (Mizuno et al., 2003; Noda et al., 2011). However, whether fractalkine signaling promotes a beneficial versus a detrimental response has been unclear, as studies have come to different conclusions depending on the injury model and the outcomes measured (Mizuno et al., 2003; Cardona et al., 2006; Fuller and Van Eldik, 2008; Staniland et al., 2010; Noda et al., 2011).

Other studies in the CNS have also shown that fractalkine signaling plays a role in developmental pruning of neurons. Mice lacking CX3CR1 have increased density of dendritic spines (Paolicelli et al., 2011), and CX3CR1 deficiency leads to delayed development of the barrel cortex (Hoshiko et al., 2012). There are corollaries between events that occur during pruning and events that occur in neuronal degeneration after apoptosis.

A well-characterized mouse model of ethanol-induced injury has proven very useful for studying developmental neuronal apoptotic mechanisms. Ethanol injection at postnatal day 7 causes robust forebrain neuronal apoptosis (as opposed to other forms of cell death such as necrosis) and the dose required and time course have been well-characterized (Ikonomidou et al., 2000). This model has been extensively used to study factors involved in the neuronal apoptotic cascade (Young et al., 2003; Ghosh et al., 2009). However, this model has not been employed to assess what factors may be involved in orchestrating clearance of apoptotic neurons or the response of neighboring glia.

Our data provide strong evidence of a role for fractalkine signaling in the response to acute alcohol neurotoxicity. We show that deficiency in fractalkine or the receptor leads to increased apoptotic debris and an altered inflammatory reaction after ethanol-induced apoptosis. Our experiments suggest that fractalkine release from apoptotic neurons may act as a "find me" signal to modulate the microglial response and promote clearance.

MATERIALS AND METHODS

MICE

All animal procedures were approved by the University of Virginia Animal Care and Use Committee. Mice used were C57/bl6 (Charles River), CX3CR1$^{eGFP/+}$ and CX3CR1$^{eGFP/eGFP}$ (Jung et al., 2000) or fractalkine-knockout (KO; Cook et al., 2001) on C57/bl6 background. CX3CR1^{eGFP} mice have green fluorescent protein (GFP) inserted into the CX3CR1 locus, therefore CX3CR1$^{eGFP/eGFP}$ animals are functional KOs.

ETHANOL INJURY

Ethanol was injected subcutaneously in postnatal day 7 pups as a 20% solution in 0.9% saline at 15.9 μL/g body weight. Control animals were injected with 0.9% saline at 15.9 μL/g body weight. It was administered twice, 2 h apart (as described by Ghosh et al., 2009).

IMMUNOSTAINING AND QUANTIFICATION OF APOPTOTIC DEBRIS

We quantified the number of apoptotic corpses in the cortex in ethanol-treated and control-treated animals. We used CX3CR1$^{eGFP/eGFP}$, fractalkine-KO, and wild type (WT) mice. We used 3–6 animals per condition. Brain tissue was harvested 4 or 6 h after the first injection and was fixed in either 4% paraformaldehyde or 70% ethanol. Anti-fractin, an antibody against caspase-cleaved actin, is a sensitive and specific marker of apoptotic neuronal debris (Suurmeijer et al., 1999; Sokolowski et al., 2014), therefore we quantified apoptosis by counting the number of fractin-stained corpses. For fractin staining, tissue was processed into paraffin by standard methods. Paraffin-embedded sections were dewaxed, rehydrated, underwent antigen retrieval (Tris-EDTA pH 9, 12 min over a boiling water bath), were quenched (15 min, 0.6% H_2O_2 in dH_2O) and blocked (1 h, 2% horse serum, 0.1% Tween in PBS) prior to incubation with primary antibody (overnight at 4°C, diluted in block), fractin (Millipore, 1:1000). Immunoperoxidase detection was performed using the ImmPress polymeric peroxidase reagents (Vector). Diaminobenzidine (Dako) 1 mg/ml plus 0.02% hydrogen peroxide was applied for 3–5 min. We quantified apoptosis by counting the number of fractin-stained corpses in the cortex and hippocampus. We averaged the number of corpses in three sections per animal, and quantified 3–6 animals per condition. Brightfield images were acquired with an Olympus BX40 upright microscope and a Scion Firewire CCD camera (Scion, Frederick, MD, USA).

BRAIN-CONDITIONED MEDIA

Brain-conditioned media (BCM) was prepared from WT mice as follows: brains harvested at 6 h after ethanol or saline treatments were hemisected and three coronal cuts were made. These tissue chunks were incubated in DMEM (no antibiotics, 1 mL per brain) in a 15 mL conical tube for 2 h on ice, on a rocker. The media was then isolated, excluding the tissue, and filtered through a 0.4 μm filter and stored at –20°C until use.

WESTERN BLOTTING

Brain-conditioned media from 2 brains was collected and a BCA protein assay (Pierce) was performed. Protein (2 mg) was precipitated in 15% TCA at 4°C for 2 h. The precipitate was spun down at 12 k rpm for 15 min at 4°C. The resulting pellet was washed three times with ice-cold acetone. The pellet was resuspended in 2X alkaline sample buffer (100 mM Tris pH 8.0, 4% SDS, 200 mM DTT, 20% glycerol). A NuPAGE gel (Life Technologies) was loaded with 50 μg of protein per lane and separated by electrophoresis using standard procedures. Gels were transferred to a PVDF membrane (Immobilon) for 90 min with a semidry transfer apparatus and treated with blocking reagent (LI-COR block; LI-COR, Lincoln NE) for 1 h and then probed with primary antibodies overnight. Antibodies used were the following: rat monoclonal anti-fractalkine (1:500, R&D systems). For visualization, blots were incubated with fluorescent secondary antibodies (1:2000, LI-COR) for 2 h and imaged on a LI-COR Odyssey infrared scanner.

CELL CULTURE

Glia were harvested from the forebrain of newborn pups (postnatal day 1–3). Briefly, meninges were removed from the brain and tissue was dissociated in 0.05% trypsin EDTA for 10 min at 37°C. Following trituration, cells were suspended in DMEM supplemented with 10% fetal bovine serum and plated into flasks. Cells were grown in an incubator at 37°C, 5% CO_2. Media was replaced twice per week for 2 weeks to obtain mixed glial culture. To harvest glia-conditioned media, media on mixed glial cultures was changed to fresh growth media (DMEM with 10% FBS), then this media was collected after 24–48 h and filtered through a 0.4 μm filter and used immediately. Microglia were isolated via the shake-off method. Briefly, flasks were shaken for 2–4 h at 37°C and the resultant detached microglia were spun down and resuspended at desired cell density.

Bone marrow-derived macrophages were prepared from mice by flushing the femurs with 1% FBS in PBS and then cultured in RPMI containing 10% L929 media for 7 days. Resident peritoneal macrophages were collected from mice by flushing the peritoneal cavity with 1% FBS in PBS and then plating collected cells in XVIVO-10 supplemented with 1% PSQ (Pen-Strep-Glut). Cells were allowed to adhere overnight and floaters were washed off; remaining cells were used in the phagocytosis assay a day later.

MIGRATION ASSAY

Chemoattractants included soluble fractalkine (sFKN; 0.1–10 nM, chemokine domain, R&D systems), CXCL12 (100 ng/mL, R&D systems), and BCM harvested from control or ethanol-treated pups. An anti-fractalkine antibody (3.5 μg/mL, rat monoclonal, R&D systems) was used in some experiments to neutralize fractalkine. Chemokines were prepared in 0.1% BSA in DMEM and BCM was used neat. Chemoattractants were added to 12-well plates at a volume of 600 μL per well and allowed to equilibrate in the incubator for 30 min prior to addition of transwell inserts (Millicell-PCF inserts, 8 um pore size, Millipore) and microglia. Microglia were isolated via the shake-off method, resuspended in 0.1% BSA in DMEM, and 5×10^4 cells were added in 400 μL to the upper chamber, according to transwell instructions. Plates were placed in the incubator for the duration of migration. After 3 h, transwells were placed in 4% PFA with DAPI for 20 min in order to fix cells and stain nuclei. The top of the inserts was wiped clean and only migrated cells remained on the membrane. The membrane was imaged (6–8 fields), and the number of cells per field was averaged for each transwell. Replicates were biological replicates, that is, each replicate data point represents microglia harvested from a different animal.

CONFOCAL IMAGING

Free-floating sections were cut to a thickness of 40 μm and stained with DAPI. Confocal imaging was performed using a Leica SP5 X. Images in stacks were 0.5 μm apart and the depth collected was 20 μm. Images were acquired from the cortex and data represents the average of 3–6 fields per animal. Microglia were visualized with endogenous GFP expression and apoptotic cells were identified via their DAPI-stained pyknotic nuclei.

PHAGOCYTOSIS

Thymocytes from 6 to 8 week old mice were incubated with 50 μM of dexamethasone for 4 h and then labeled with CypHer5E. Stained thymocytes were resuspended in glia-conditioned medium and added to phagocytes. The cells were then spun down and incubated at 37°C, 5% CO_2 for 1 h. After completion of the engulfment assay, the wells were washed three times with PBS, trypsinized, and resuspended in glia-conditioned medium and analyzed by two-color flow cytometry. The microglial cells were recognized by their GFP fluorescence. For each point, 10,000 GFP-positive events were collected and the data was analyzed using FlowJo software.

QUANTITATIVE PCR

For quantitative PCR using brain tissue, pieces of lateral cortex were isolated and stored at −80°C until RNA isolation. RNA was isolated using RNeasy Lipid Mini kit (Qiagen). Reverse transcription was performed using 1000 ng of RNA according to manufacturer's instructions (High Capacity cDNA kit, Applied Biosystems). Quantitative PCR was performed with Sybr green according to manufacturer's instructions (Platinum Sybr kit, Life Technologies) with annealing temperatures of 60°C. Primers used were: actin, forward CCCAGAGCAAGAGAGGTGTC, reverse AGAGCATAGCCCTCGTAGAT; IL-6, forward GAGGATACCACTCCCAACAGACC, reverse AAGTGCATCATCGTTGTTCATACA; TNFα, forward GGCAGGTCTACTTTGGAGTCATTGC, reverse ACATTCGAGGCTCCAGTGAATTCGG; CX3CL1, forward CTCACGAATCCCAGTGGCTT, reverse TTTCTCCTTCGGGTCAGCAC; CX3CR1, forward TGCAGAAGTTCCCTTCCCATC, reverse GGCCTCAGCAGAATCGTCATA; CXCR1eGFP, forward (same as CX3CR1) TGCAGAAGTTCCCTTCCCATC, GFP reverse CTGAACTTGTGGCCGTTTAC. Specificity of CX3CR1, CX3CR1eGFP, and CX3CL1 was confirmed by lack of amplification in respective KO tissues.

RESULTS

FRACTALKINE OR CX3CR1 DEFICIENCY LEADS TO AN INCREASE OR PERSISTENCE OF APOPTOTIC DEBRIS IN THE BRAIN AFTER ETHANOL-INDUCED APOPTOSIS

We quantified the amount of apoptotic debris 4 and 6 h after ethanol-induced apoptosis in CX3CR1-KO mice and found that at 6 h the CX3CR1-deficient mice had increased apoptotic debris in the cortex compared to WT mice (**Figures 1A,D,F**). Next, we aimed to determine whether the ligand KO mice phenocopied the receptor KO. We quantified the amount of apoptotic debris 6 h after injury in fractalkine-KO mice, and found that they also had increased apoptotic debris compared to WT animals, and the amount of apoptotic debris was similar to the amount seen in the CX3CR1-KO animals (**Figures 1B,F,H**). Of note, there was no difference between genotypes in the amount of apoptotic corpses in control, uninjured animals (**Figures 1B,C,E,G**). CX3CR1-heterozygous (HET) mice (which were used for subsequent

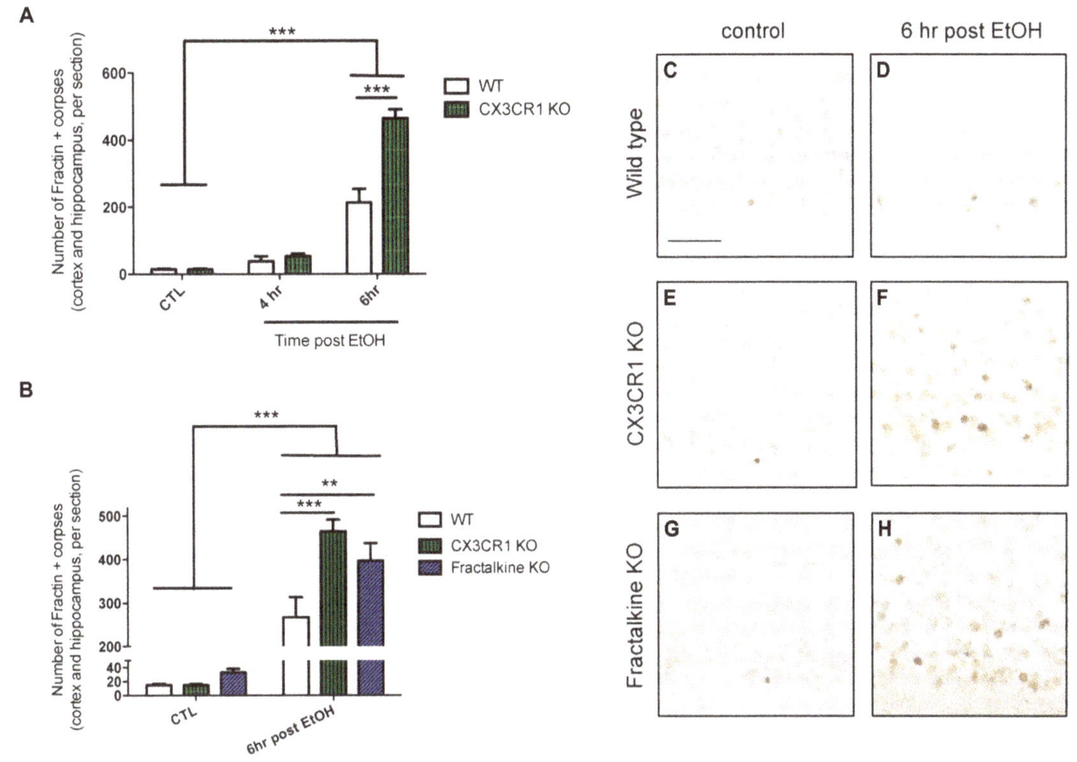

FIGURE 1 | Deficiency in fractalkine or CX3CR1 leads to increased apoptotic debris. (A) P7 mice were injected with saline as a control (CTL) or ethanol to induce neuronal apoptosis. Brain tissue was harvested at 4 or 6 h after the initial injection and the number of fractin-positive apoptotic corpses in the cortex and hippocampus was counted (three sections averaged per animal). **(A)** CX3CR1-knockout (KO) and wild type (WT) mice were compared at 4 and 6 h after injection. At 6 h after ethanol injection, the number of fractin-positive corpses was increased in CX3CR1-KO mice compared to WT mice **(B)**. Tissue from WT, CX3CR1-KO, and fractalkine-KO mice was collected 6 h after ethanol injection. CX3CR1-KO and fractalkine-KO mice had increased fractin-positive corpses compared to WT mice. Representative images from the cortex are shown in **(C–H)**. **(A,B**; $n = 3–6$) Two-way ANOVA, $**p < 0.01$, $***p < 0.005$. Scale = 50 μm.

experiments) had levels of debris comparable to WT animals (Figure S1).

IN VIVO ETHANOL-INDUCED NEURONAL APOPTOSIS LEADS TO RELEASE OF SOLUBLE FRACTALKINE

We observed increased apoptotic debris in mice that are deficient in fractalkine signaling, which suggests fractalkine plays an important role in the response to alcohol injury. We hypothesized that the cleaved fragment of fractalkine is released during ethanol-induced apoptosis. We harvested brains 6 h after ethanol-induced apoptosis and incubated them in media to isolate diffusible extracellular factors and tested whether fractalkine was present. We detected sFKN in BCM from animals treated with ethanol, but not in saline-treated controls (**Figure 2A**). This shows that fractalkine is released as a soluble fragment in response to ethanol-induced injury. Recombinant fractalkine and lysate from mixed neural cultures were used as controls for the western blot.

MICROGLIA MIGRATE TOWARD APOPTOTIC BRAIN-CONDITIONED MEDIA IN A FRACTALKINE AND CX3CR1-DEPENDENT MANNER

We hypothesized that fractalkine released during injury plays a role in the microglial reaction to apoptotic neurons. Microglia are the only cells in the brain that express appreciable levels of the fractalkine receptor, CX3CR1. Fractalkine is a known chemotactic factor, and we aimed to determine whether fractalkine released from apoptotic neural cells was necessary and sufficient to induce microglial chemotaxis.

We found that microglia migrate toward sFKN; migration toward fractalkine was dose-dependent, and as expected, CX3CR1-KO microglia did not migrate toward fractalkine (Figure S2). CX3CR1 deficiency does not lead to a general migration defect as KO microglia are still able to migrate toward another chemokine, CXCL12 (Figure S2). A fractalkine-neutralizing antibody blocks migration toward fractalkine, and this antibody is not a general inhibitor of migration, as it has no effect on migration toward CXCL12 (**Figure 2B**).

Next, we tested whether microglia respond to the fractalkine in the extracellular media from apoptotic brains. The apoptotic BCM from ethanol-treated animals was sufficient to induce migration (**Figure 2C**). Microglia did not migrate toward the BCM from the non-apoptotic control tissue. Fractalkine signaling was absolutely required to stimulate migration toward the apoptotic BCM. Neutralizing fractalkine blocked migration toward the apoptotic BCM (**Figure 2C**), and CX3CR1-deficient microglia failed to migrate toward it (**Figure 2D**). This data suggests that in the context of ethanol-induced injury, sFKN signals

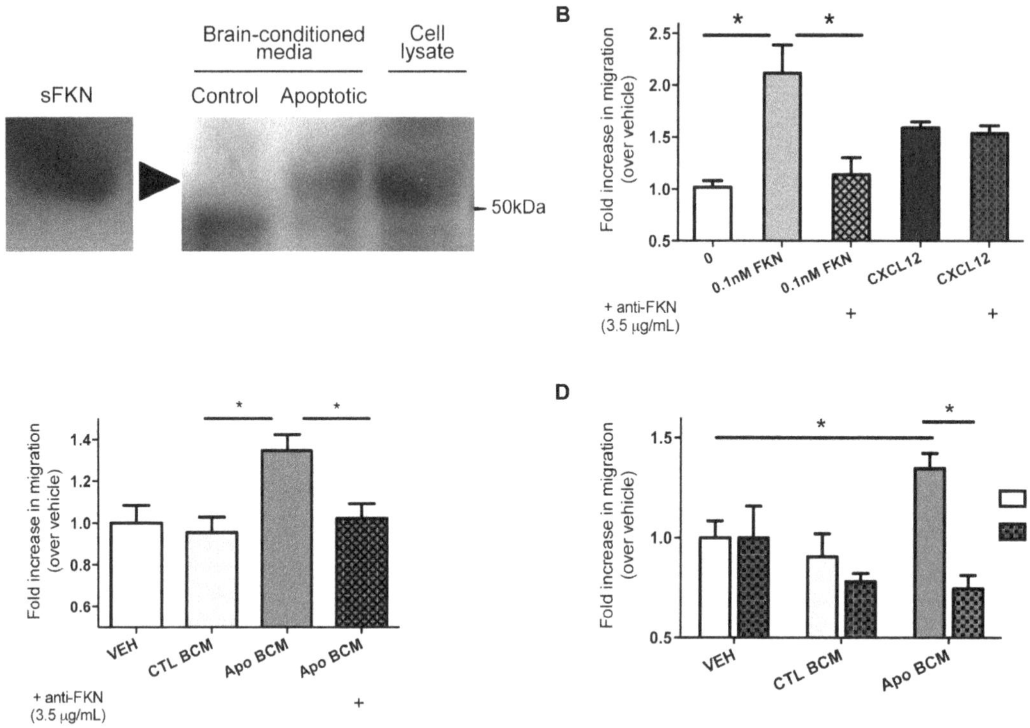

FIGURE 2 | Soluble fractalkine (sFKN) is released into the extracellular space after injury and acts as a chemotactic factor for microglia. (A) P7 mice were treated with saline (control) or ethanol to induce neuronal apoptosis (apoptotic), and the brains were incubated in DMEM on ice for 2 h to isolate brain-conditioned media (BCM). 2 mg of protein were TCA precipitated, run on a gel, and probed with anti-fractalkine via western blot. sFKN and lysate from mixed neural cultures were used for comparison. We found fractalkine in BCM from apoptotic, but not control brain (a, arrowhead points to band of interest). **(B–D)** Transwell migration assays were performed to determine whether microglia transmigrate toward fractalkine. Microglia were isolated from mixed glial cultures via the shake-off method and added to the upper chamber of a transwell insert. Attractant of interest was added to the bottom of the transwell. After 3 h of migration, the cells that had migrated to the bottom surface of the transwell were fixed, stained with DAPI, and counted. **(B)** Microglia migrate toward 0.1 nM of sFKN. A fractalkine-neutralizingantibody (3.5 μg/mL) was pre-incubated with either 0.1 nM of sFKN or CXCL12 [indicated by (+)]. This antibody specifically blocked fractalkine-induced migration, as CXCL12-induced migration was not inhibited. **(C,D)** Microglia migrate toward apoptotic BCM in a fractalkine-dependent manner. P7 mice were treated with saline as a control or ethanol to induce neuronal apoptosis. Brains were then incubated in DMEM on ice for 2 h to isolate BCM from saline-treated control (CTL BCM) or apoptotic brain (Apo BCM). BCM was used as a chemoattractant in the lower chamber for transwell migration assays. **(C)** Microglia migrate toward apoptotic BCM but not control BCM. A fractalkine-neutralizing antibody (3.5 μg/mL) was pre-incubated with apoptotic BCM [indicated by (+)] to block fractalkine-dependent migration and this prevented migration toward the apoptotic BCM. **(D)** Migration toward BCM was quantified in CX3CR1 heterozygous (HET) versus KO microglia. CX3CR1 deficient microglia fail to migrate toward apoptotic BCM. **(B–D)** Data is from repeated experiments, each replicate represents microglia harvested from a different animal ($n = 4$–6). **(B–C)** One-way ANOVA, $*p < 0.05$; **(D)** Two-way ANOVA, $*p < 0.05$.

to microglia in a CX3CR1-dependent manner. Our data suggests that this signaling helps attract microglia toward apoptotic neurons.

IN VIVO ANALYSIS OF PROXIMITY BETWEEN MICROGLIA AND APOPTOTIC NEURONS

We hypothesized that fractalkine signaling modulates microglial recruitment to apoptotic cells. Brain tissue from CX3CR1-KO or CX3CR1-HET pups was collected at 6 h after ethanol treatment and confocal stacks were acquired (orthogonal views seen in **Figures 3A,C**). Microglia were identified via endogenous GFP expression and apoptotic cells were identified via their pyknotic, DAPI-positive nuclei. We analyzed the confocal stacks and identified apoptotic cells as either untouched, touched or engulfed by microglia (**Figures 3B,D** are diagrams depicting the analysis for **Figures 3A,C**). An association index was calculated by quantifying the fraction of microglia touching apoptotic cell bodies (arrowheads in **Figure 3D** indicate microglial processes that fail to associate with nearby apoptotic corpses). CX3CR1-KO microglia had a lower association index at 6 h after injury (**Figure 3E**).

There was no difference in microglial cell density between the HET or the KO animals (**Figure 3F**). Therefore the increase in debris in the CX3CR1-KO brain is not attributable to a difference in number of microglia available to participate in clearance. Microglia are normally ubiquitous throughout brain tissue, therefore long distance migration may not be required for the microglial response. Instead, fractalkine may signal for local "recruitment" of microglia, and this could manifest as movement of just the arms or processes of the cell as opposed to the entire cell.

An increase in apoptotic debris could be due to defects in microglial recruitment, but could also be due to a defect in microglial phagocytosis and clearance. We used the same confocal images to determine whether CX3CR1-deficient microglia

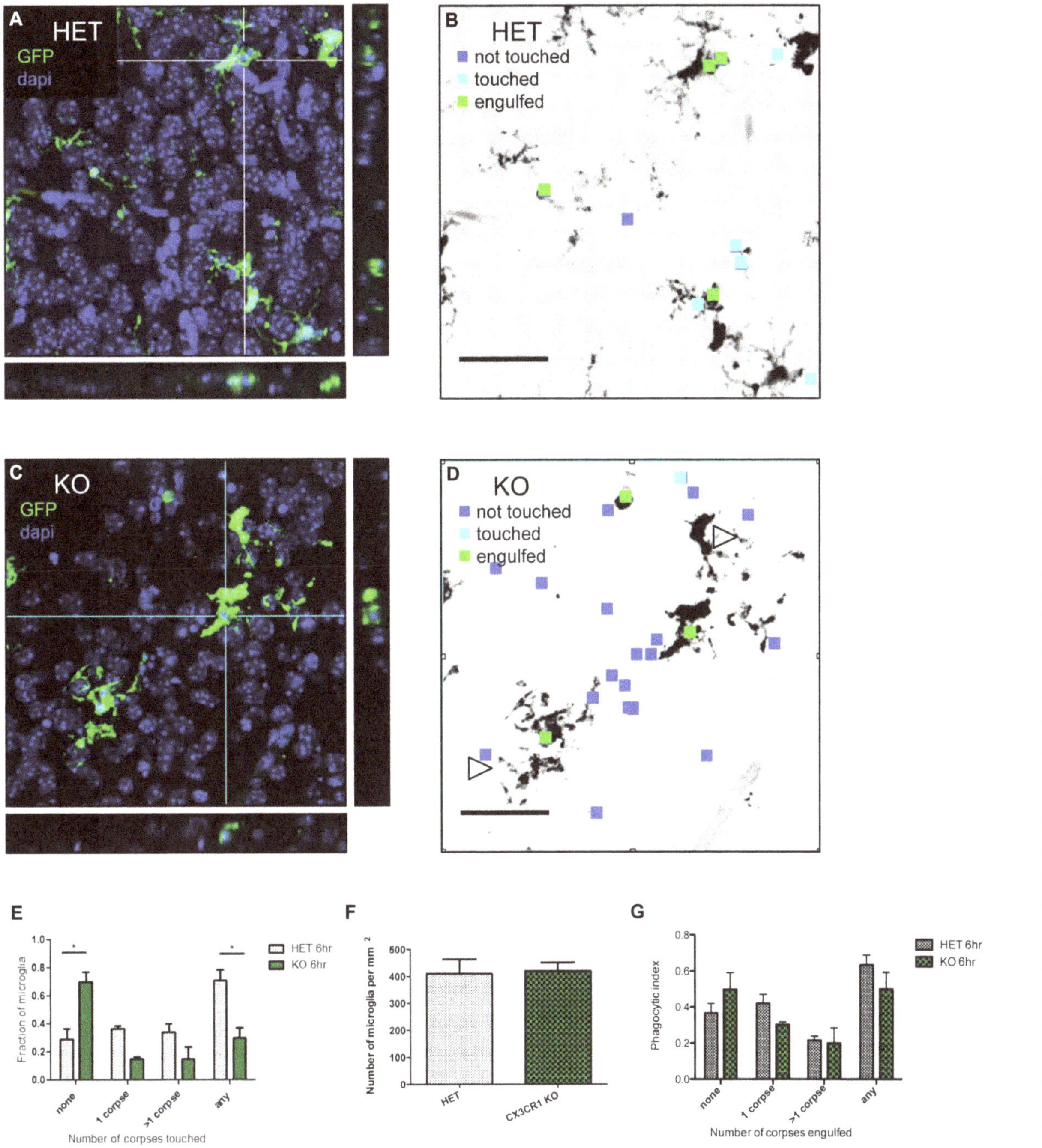

FIGURE 3 | CX3CR1-deficient microglia have a defect in association with apoptotic debris after ethanol-induced apoptosis, but no overt defect in phagocytosis. (A–D) CX3CR1-HET and CX3CR1-KO pups were injected with ethanol to induce neuronal apoptosis and tissue was harvested 6 h later. Microglia express GFP and nuclei were labeled with DAPI. 40 μm sections were cut and 20 μm thick confocal stacks were acquired from the cortex. Apoptotic corpses were identified via their pyknotic nuclei. **(A,C)** Representative images with orthogonal projections acquired from CX3CR1-HET **(A)** and CX3CR1-KO **(C)** after ethanol treatment. **(B,D)** We analyzed each confocal stack and identified apoptotic cells as either untouched (blue square), touched (cyan square) or engulfed (green square) by microglia. Open arrowheads in **(D)** indicate microglial processes that fail to associate with nearby apoptotic corpses. **(E)** An association index was determined by quantifying the fraction of microglia touching apoptotic corpses at 6 h after injury. By 6 h, fewer microglia from the CX3CR1-KO had associated with apoptotic corpses as compared to the CX3CR1-HET microglia. **(F)** The density of microglia was quantified and there was no difference between the CX3CR1-HET and CX3CR1-KO. **(G)** Confocal stacks were also used to calculate a phagocytic index, the fraction of GFP-positive microglia that contained corpses. There was no significant difference in phagocytosis measures in the brain of the CX3CR1-KO compared to the CX3CR1-HET mice. (**E–G**; $n = 3$, three fields were averaged per animal) Two-way ANOVA, $^*p < 0.05$. Scale = 50 μm.

had an *in vivo* defect in phagocytosis. The microglial phagocytic index was quantified by measuring the fraction of microglia containing engulfed apoptotic cells (**Figure 3G**). We found no change in the phagocytic index at 6 h after ethanol treatment.

We also performed *in vitro* phagocytosis assays to determine whether fractalkine signaling modulates phagocytosis. We tested whether sFKN promotes phagocytosis and whether CX3CR1-KO cells have a defect in phagocytosis. We utilized multiple approaches. We used apoptotic thymocytes as targets and tested macrophages pretreated with fractalkine or treated concurrent with addition of apoptotic cells (Figure S3). Addition of exogenous fractalkine had no effect and CX3CR1-deficient macrophages had a comparable phagocytic index. Next, we tried pure cultures of microglia isolated from CX3CR1 HET or KO glial cultures, but found no effect of fractalkine or CX3CR1 deficiency (Figure S3). Finally, we tried mixed cultures of astrocytes and microglia. We added apoptotic thymocytes to mixed glial cultures from CX3CR1 HET or KO animals treated with or without fractalkine and quantified the microglial phagocytic index and found that neither exogenous fractalkine nor CX3CR1-deficiency had an effect (Figure S3). The combination of *in vitro* and *in vivo* data suggest that fractalkine signaling does not have a prominent role in regulating the engulfment phase of phagocytosis.

We have not ruled out the possibility that CX3CR1-KO microglia have a defect in their ability to digest apoptotic cells, which could also lead to a persistence of debris after ethanol-induced apoptosis. It is also possible that CX3CR1 deficiency leads to increased apoptotic debris through a combination of decreased clearance and increased neurotoxicity.

FRACTALKINE OR CX3CR1 DEFICIENCY LEADS TO AN ALTERED INFLAMMATORY GENE EXPRESSION RESPONSE TO ETHANOL-INDUCED APOPTOSIS

Apoptotic cells and fractalkine are both known to modulate inflammatory responses. Therefore, we hypothesized that the increased apoptotic load and/or defective fractalkine signaling would lead to an altered inflammatory response in the brain after ethanol injury. We quantified mRNA expression of the cytokines IL-6 and TNFα as well as fractalkine and CX3CR1 (**Figure 4**; Figure S4). IL-6 levels were similar in control-treated animals of each genotype. In WT animals, we found increased IL-6 mRNA at 6 h after ethanol treatment. IL-6 expression was further increased in both fractalkine- and CX3CR1-KO mice compared to WT. TNFα levels were similar in control-treated WT and CX3CR1 mice, but only CX3CR1-KOs upregulated TNFα at 6 h after ethanol injury. In contrast, fractalkine-KO mice had increased TNFα expression at baseline, at levels comparable to the levels seen in ethanol-treated CX3CR1 mice, and the level did not change with ethanol treatment (**Figure 4**).

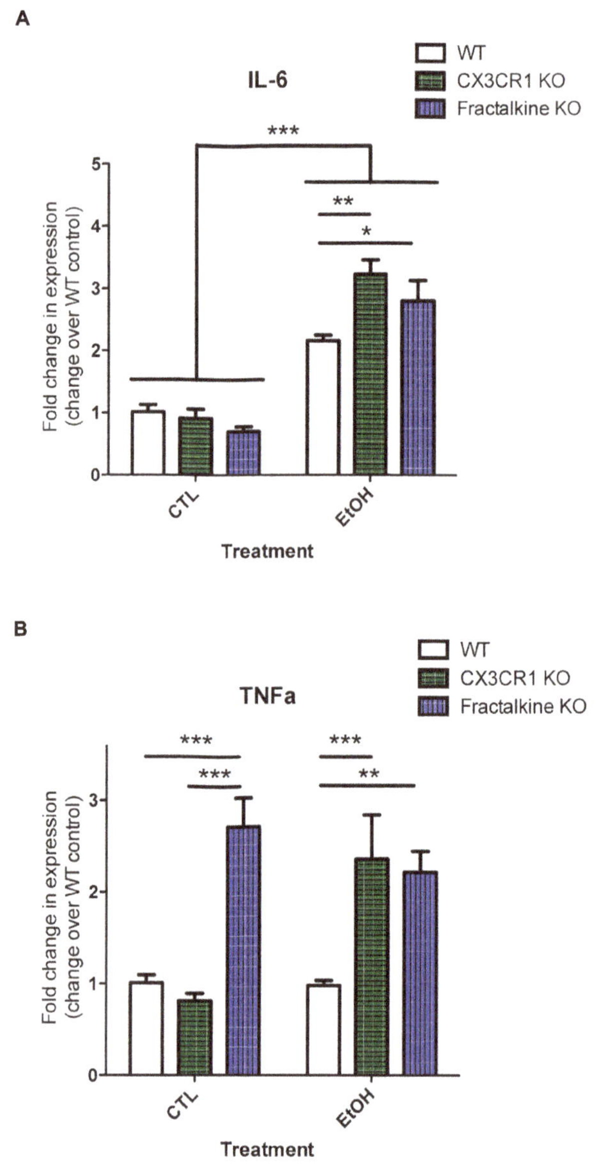

FIGURE 4 | Ethanol-induced apoptosis leads to fractalkine-dependent alteration of cytokines gene expression. P7 animals were treated with saline (CTL) or ethanol and brain tissue was harvested 6 h later. Brain tissue and RNA was harvested from WT, CX3CR1-knockout, and fractalkine-knockout mice. Quantitative PCR was used to assess mRNA expression of IL-6 **(A)** and TNAα **(B)**. IL-6 expression is elevated after ethanol treatment, and is significantly higher in the CX3CR1 knockout and the fractalkine-knockout than in the wild type brain. In fractalkine-knockout brain, TNFα expression is higher in control conditions as compared to wild type or CX3CR1 knockout. CX3CR1-knockout brain has increased TNFα compared to wild type after ethanol treatment. ($n = 3$–6; **A,B**) Two-way ANOVA, $*p < 0.05$, $**p < 0.01$, $***p < 0.001$.

We also tested whether fractalkine or CX3CR1 expression was modulated by ethanol-induced apoptosis (Figure S3). We found no difference in mRNA expression in the brain of WT animals after ethanol treatment compared to control. We also analyzed expression in the KO animals. We found an increase in fractalkine mRNA expression in the CX3CR1-KO animals after ethanol treatment. We assessed expression of transcript for the receptor and we found increased CX3CR1 in the fractalkine-KO. The CX3CR1-KO does not express functional CX3CR1, however, GFP transcript can be used as a reporter for gene expression. We used a primer set designed to amplify CX3CR1-eGFP transcript and we found increased production of this transcript in the CX3CR1-KO after ethanol treatment. This suggests that fractalkine signaling could have a role in feedback regulation of the expression of the receptor and ligand in the context of injury.

DISCUSSION

Fractalkine has been previously described as a neuron–microglia communication factor and is known to be a chemokine that can modulate migration of immune cells (Ransohoff et al., 2007). Our data additionally illuminates the role of fractalkine signaling in the response to apoptotic neuronal cells in the context of perinatal brain injury.

Only one previous study has investigated fractalkine regulation after ethanol injury. In that study, the quantity of fractalkine protein increased after prenatal ethanol injury in WT mice (Roberson et al., 2011). Using our model, we did not detect changes in fractalkine mRNA expression in WT mice after postnatal ethanol injury (Figure S3). However, when we isolated BCM, that is, the extracellular soluble components from the brain, we detected an increase in cleaved sFKN after ethanol injury (**Figure 2A**).

Cleaved fractalkine released from apoptotic neurons may create a gradient that allows microglia to hone in on apoptotic neurons. A previous study showed that fractalkine acts as a "find me" signal to guide phagocytes such as macrophages to apoptotic cells (Truman et al., 2008), and others have shown that fractalkine can modulate chemotaxis of microglia (Maciejewski-Lenoir et al., 1999). However, these studies predominantly used *in vitro* models or peripheral systems. We show that fractalkine acts as an important "find me" signal to modulate microglial recruitment in order to help clear apoptotic neurons in *in vivo* CNS injury.

Apoptosis may result in the release of many factors, and fractalkine is only one of many possible chemoattractants (Ravichandran, 2003; Ravichandran and Lorenz, 2007). However, we show that fractalkine signaling is critical for migration toward apoptotic BCM: blocking fractalkine signaling by neutralizing fractalkine or through CX3CR1 deficiency prevents migration (**Figure 2**). Does this suggest other "find me" signals are irrelevant?

Other signals such as ATP and UDP have been shown to modulate microglial movement and phagocytosis (Davalos et al., 2005; Koizumi et al., 2007). ATP and UDP are unstable in the extracellular space due to the presence of ubiquitous ATPases (Zimmermann, 2000). It seems possible that fractalkine may have a longer half-life than other potential "find-me" signals and therefore fractalkine may be the dominant chemoattractant remaining in apoptotic BCM. These other signals may still be relevant in other conditions.

Our *in vitro* data suggests that fractalkine "find me" signaling is the critical factor for recruitment of microglia; however, *in vivo*, other signals are probably also involved. Although we found that microglia from CX3CR1-KO mice did not associate with apoptotic debris as well as WT microglia (**Figure 3**), there was not a large *in vivo* defect in engulfment (Figure S2). This suggests two possibilities: (a) microglia are ubiquitous and motile enough that in the absence of fractalkine signaling they are still able to encounter apoptotic debris by chance and engulf it, or (b) perhaps there are other factors that can act to recruit microglia in the absence of fractalkine signaling. For example cell surface "eat me" signals are likely involved.

A defect in recruitment or the association of microglia with apoptotic neurons would lead to failed or slowed clearance of debris. We speculate that this explains why the fractalkine and CX3CR1-KO brains have more apoptotic debris after ethanol injury compared to WT animals (**Figure 1**).

The increased apoptotic debris could be attributable to a defect in recruitment, but could also be due to a defect in phagocytosis. A previous study showed that addition of sFKN to injured cultured neurons induces phagocytosis (Noda et al., 2011). However, we could not find any evidence for an *in vivo* defect in phagocytosis, as the microglial phagocytic index was similar in WT and CX3CR1-KO animals (**Figure 3**). In addition, we tested *in vitro* phagocytosis and found no effect of fractalkine and no defect in the CX3CR1-deficient microglia (Figure S2). Another factor that would influence the amount of debris is the rate of degradation of apoptotic material, and we have not ruled out the possibility that CX3CR1-KO microglia could have a defect in the ability to digest corpses. This could be tested by following the fate of apoptotic cells in time lapse imaging experiments both *in vitro* and perhaps *in vivo* using slice cultures of alcohol-injured brain.

We do not know if other glia also plays a role in clearance of apoptotic cells. Astrocytes are capable of engulfment (Noda et al., 2011), and it is possible that they may engulf debris after alcohol injury. However, we were unable to identify parenchymal astrocytes via conventional astrocyte markers such as glial fibrillary aidic protein (GFAP) or S100β at this age in development. Therefore, we were unable to determine whether astrocytic engulfment contributed to clearance. Astrocytes do not express appreciable levels of CX3CR1 *in vivo*; therefore they are unlikely to be responding to fractalkine in this injury.

A common dogma in the field of apoptotic cell clearance is that cells must be cleared in order to prevent an exaggerated immune response (Ravichandran and Lorenz, 2007). Interestingly, we find that in conjunction with the increased apoptotic cell load, we see an exaggerated immune response in the fractalkine and CX3CR1-KO animals. It would be interesting if this exaggerated inflammatory response were due to persistence of apoptotic debris and secondary necrosis. However, we cannot tease apart whether this altered immune response is due the persistence of apoptotic cells or due to the defect in fractalkine signaling, as both apoptotic cells and fractalkine have been shown to modulate inflammatory responses (Mizuno et al., 2003; Griffiths et al., 2009). Related to this, another possibility we have not ruled out is that the increase in apoptotic debris could be due to increased neurotoxicity because of an adverse inflammatory response. Fractalkine may be important for immunomodulation (perhaps suppression). Fractalkine has been shown to downregulate production of pro-inflammatory factors in response to LPS (Mizuno et al., 2003). Avoiding the exaggerated immune response may be critical to avoid secondary degeneration.

Another goal of this study was to determine whether there is an inflammatory response after acute ethanol injury. Our data supports previous data that showed that fetal alcohol injury leads to an increase in factors such as TNFα, and IL-6 (Vink et al., 2005).

We similarly find that ethanol injury induces an inflammatory response in the developing brain. We additionally show that this response appears to be modulated by fractalkine signaling. Ultimately, *in vivo* we cannot tease apart whether the ethanol or the apoptotic cells are signaling for the production of cytokines, and we do not know the downstream functional consequences of this inflammation.

It is interesting that the ligand and receptor KO phenocopied with respect to increased apoptotic debris after injury, but had differences in mRNA expression of TNFα. It is possible that intact fractalkine transmembrane protein has other important functions distinct from its role in CX3CR1-receptor signaling that would explain baseline (pre-injury) differences in TNFα expression in the fractalkine-KO brain. Fractalkine is known as an adhesion molecule. Perhaps it also associates with and modulates other signaling molecules or has an (as of yet unidentified) intracellular signaling component. It is also interesting that fractalkine and TNFα are both cleaved by ADAM 17 (also known as the TNFα-converting enzyme, TACE). Perhaps fractalkine deficiency somehow leads to dysregulation of TNFα due to this shared relationship with ADAM 17.

CONCLUSION

We have used a well-characterized mouse model of ethanol-induced apoptosis to assess the role of fractalkine in neuronal–microglial signaling. Our data suggests that fractalkine released after apoptosis recruits microglial processes toward apoptotic cells to promote their clearance and that defects in this signaling lead to increased apoptotic debris. Secondly, our data suggests that defects in clearance or fractalkine signaling lead to altered cytokine production after ethanol injury. Collectively, this suggests that fractalkine acts as a "find me" signal released by apoptotic neurons and subsequently plays a critical role in modulating clearance and inflammatory cytokine gene expression after ethanol-induced apoptosis.

AUTHOR CONTRIBUTIONS

Jennifer D. Sokolowski and James W. Mandell conceived and designed the project. Jennifer D. Sokolowski, Chloe N. Chabanon-Hicks, Claudia Z. Han, and Daniel S. Heffron performed the experiments. Jennifer D. Sokolowski prepared all the figures and wrote the manuscript with assistance from Chloe N. Chabanon-Hicks. All authors reviewed the manuscript.

REFERENCES

Bazan, J. F., Bacon, K. B., Hardiman, G., Wang, W., Soo, K., Rossi, D., et al. (1997). A new class of membrane-bound chemokine with a CX3C motif. *Nature* 385, 640–644. doi: 10.1038/385640a0

Cardona, A. E., Pioro, E. P., Sasse, M. E., Kostenko, V., Cardona, S. M., Dijkstra, I. M., et al. (2006). Control of microglial neurotoxicity by the fractalkine receptor. *Nat. Neurosci.* 9, 917–924. doi: 10.1038/nn1715

Cook, D. N., Chen, S. C., Sullivan, L. M., Manfra, D. J., Wiekowski, M. T., Prosser, D. M., et al. (2001). Generation and analysis of mice lacking the chemokine fractalkine. *Mol. Cell. Biol.* 21, 3159–3165. doi: 10.1128/MCB.21.9.3159-3165.2001

Davalos, D., Grutzendler, J., Yang, G., Kim, J. V., Zuo, Y., Jung, S., et al. (2005). ATP mediates rapid microglial response to local brain injury *in vivo. Nat. Neurosci.* 8, 752–758. doi: 10.1038/nn1472

Elliott, M. R., Chekeni, F. B., Trampont, P. C., Lazarowski, E. R., Kadl, A., Walk, S. F., et al. (2009). Nucleotides released by apoptotic cells act as a find-me signal to promote phagocytic clearance. *Nature* 461, 282–286. doi: 10.1038/nature08296

Fuller, A. D., and Van Eldik, L. J. (2008). MFG-E8 regulates microglial phagocytosis of apoptotic neurons. *J. Neuroimmune Pharmacol.* 3, 246–256. doi: 10.1007/s11481-008-9118-2

Ghosh, A. P., Walls, K. C., Klocke, B. J., Toms, R., Strasser, A., and Roth, K. A. (2009). The proapoptotic BH3-only, Bcl-2 family member, Puma is critical for acute ethanol-induced neuronal apoptosis. *J. Neuropathol. Exp. Neurol.* 68, 747–756. doi: 10.1097/NEN.0b013e3181a9d524

Griffiths, M. R., Gasque, P., and Neal, J. W. (2009). The multiple roles of the innate immune system in the regulation of apoptosis and inflammation in the brain. *J. Neuropathol. Exp. Neurol.* 68, 217–226. doi: 10.1097/NEN.0b013e3181996688

Gronski, M. A., Kinchen, J. M., Juncadella, I. J., Franc, N. C., and Ravichandran, K. S. (2009). An essential role for calcium flux in phagocytes for apoptotic cell engulfment and the anti-inflammatory response. *Cell Death Differ.* 16, 1323–1331. doi: 10.1038/cdd.2009.55

Harrison, J. K., Jiang, Y., Chen, S., Xia, Y., Maciejewski, D., McNamara, R. K., et al. (1998). Role for neuronally derived fractalkine in mediating interactions between neurons and CX3CR1-expressing microglia. *Proc. Natl. Acad. Sci. U.S.A.* 95, 10896–10901. doi: 10.1073/pnas.95.18.10896

Hoshiko, M., Arnoux, I., Avignone, E., Yamamoto, N., and Audinat, E. (2012). Deficiency of the microglial receptor CX3CR1 impairs postnatal functional development of thalamocortical synapses in the barrel cortex. *J. Neurosci.* 32, 15106–15111. doi: 10.1523/JNEUROSCI.1167-12.2012

Ikonomidou, C., Bittigau, P., Ishimaru, M. J., Wozniak, D. F., Koch, C., Genz, K., et al. (2000). Ethanol-induced apoptotic neurodegeneration and fetal alcohol syndrome. *Science* 287, 1056–1060. doi: 10.1126/science.287.5455.1056

Jung, S., Aliberti, J., Graemmel, P., Sunshine, M. J., Kreutzberg, G. W., Sher, A., et al. (2000). Analysis of fractalkine receptor CX3CR1 function by targeted deletion and green fluorescent protein reporter gene insertion. *Mol. Cell. Biol.* 20, 4106–4114. doi: 10.1128/MCB.20.11.4106-4114.2000

Koizumi, S., Shigemoto-Mogami, Y., Nasu-Tada, K., Shinozaki, Y., Ohsawa, K., Tsuda, M., et al. (2007). UDP acting at P2Y6 receptors is a mediator of microglial phagocytosis. *Nature* 446, 1091–1095. doi: 10.1038/nature05704

Maciejewski-Lenoir, D., Chen, S., Feng, L., Maki, R., and Bacon, K. B. (1999). Characterization of fractalkine in rat brain cells: migratory and activation signals for CX3CR-1-expressing microglia. *J. Immunol.* 163, 1628–1635.

Mizuno, T., Kawanokuchi, J., Numata, K., and Suzumura, A. (2003). Production and neuroprotective functions of fractalkine in the central nervous system. *Brain Res.* 979, 65–70. doi: 10.1016/S0006-8993(03)02867-1

Noda, M., Doi, Y., Liang, J., Kawanokuchi, J., Sonobe, Y., Takeuchi, H., et al. (2011). Fractalkine attenuates excito-neurotoxicity via microglial clearance of damaged neurons and antioxidant enzyme heme oxygenase-1 expression. *J. Biol. Chem.* 286, 2308–2319. doi: 10.1074/jbc.M110.169839

Paolicelli, R. C., Bolasco, G., Pagani, F., Maggi, L., Scianni, M., Panzanelli, P., et al. (2011). Synaptic pruning by microglia is necessary for normal brain development. *Science* 333, 1456–1458. doi: 10.1126/science.1202529

Ransohoff, R. M., Liu, L., and Cardona, A. E. (2007). Chemokines and chemokine receptors: multipurpose players in neuroinflammation. *Int. Rev. Neurobiol.* 82, 187–204. doi: 10.1016/S0074-7742(07)82010-1

Ravichandran, K. S. (2003). "Recruitment signals" from apoptotic cells: invitation to a quiet meal. *Cell* 113, 817–820. doi: 10.1016/S0092-8674(03)00471-9

Ravichandran, K. S., and Lorenz, U. (2007). Engulfment of apoptotic cells: signals for a good meal. *Nat. Rev. Immunol.* 7, 964–974. doi: 10.1038/nri2214

Roberson, R., Kuddo, T., Benassou, I., Abebe, D., and Spong, C. (2011). Neuroprotective fractalkine in fetal alcohol syndrome. *Am. J. Obstet. Gynecol.* 204, 400.e1–400.e3. doi: 10.1016/j.ajog.2011.03.034

Sokolowski, J. D., Gamage, K. K., Heffron, D. S., Leblanc, A. C., Deppmann, C. D., and Mandell, J. W. (2014). Caspase-mediated cleavage of actin and tubulin is a common feature and sensitive marker of axonal degeneration in neural development and injury. *Acta Neuropathol. Commun.* 2:16. doi: 10.1186/2051-5960-2-16

Staniland, A. A., Clark, A. K., Wodarski, R., Sasso, O., Maione, F., D'Acquisto, F., et al. (2010). Reduced inflammatory and neuropathic pain and decreased spinal microglial response in fractalkine receptor (CX3CR1) knockout mice. *J. Neurochem.* 114, 1143–1157. doi: 10.1111/j.1471-4159.2010.06837.x

Suurmeijer, A. J., van der Wijk, J., van Veldhuisen, D. J., Yang, F., and Cole, G. M. (1999). Fractin immunostaining for the detection of apoptotic cells and apoptotic bodies in formalin-fixed and paraffin-embedded tissue. *Lab. Invest.* 79, 619–620.

Truman, L. A., Ford, C. A., Pasikowska, M., Pound, J. D., Wilkinson, S. J., Dumitriu, I. E., et al. (2008). CX3CL1/fractalkine is released from apoptotic lymphocytes to stimulate macrophage chemotaxis. *Blood* 112, 5026–5036. doi: 10.1182/blood-2008-06-162404

Vink, J., Auth, J., Abebe, D. T., Brenneman, D. E., and Spong, C. Y. (2005). Novel peptides prevent alcohol-induced spatial learning deficits and proinflammatory cytokine release in a mouse model of fetal alcohol syndrome. *Am. J. Obstet. Gynecol.* 193, 825–829. doi: 10.1016/j.ajog.2005.02.101

Young, C., Klocke, B. J., Tenkova, T., Choi, J., Labruyere, J., Qin, Y. Q., et al. (2003). Ethanol-induced neuronal apoptosis *in vivo* requires BAX in the developing mouse brain. *Cell Death Differ.* 10, 1148–1155. doi: 10.1038/sj.cdd.4401277

Zimmermann, H. (2000). Extracellular metabolism of ATP and other nucleotides. *Naunyn Schmiedebergs Arch. Pharmacol.* 362, 299–309. doi: 10.1007/s002100000309

Permissions

All chapters in this book were first published by Frontiers; hereby published with permission under the Creative Commons Attribution License or equivalent. Every chapter published in this book has been scrutinized by our experts. Their significance has been extensively debated. The topics covered herein carry significant findings which will fuel the growth of the discipline. They may even be implemented as practical applications or may be referred to as a beginning point for another development.

The contributors of this book come from diverse backgrounds, making this book a truly international effort. This book will bring forth new frontiers with its revolutionizing research information and detailed analysis of the nascent developments around the world.

We would like to thank all the contributing authors for lending their expertise to make the book truly unique. They have played a crucial role in the development of this book. Without their invaluable contributions this book wouldn't have been possible. They have made vital efforts to compile up to date information on the varied aspects of this subject to make this book a valuable addition to the collection of many professionals and students.

This book was conceptualized with the vision of imparting up-to-date information and advanced data in this field. To ensure the same, a matchless editorial board was set up. Every individual on the board went through rigorous rounds of assessment to prove their worth. After which they invested a large part of their time researching and compiling the most relevant data for our readers.

The editorial board has been involved in producing this book since its inception. They have spent rigorous hours researching and exploring the diverse topics which have resulted in the successful publishing of this book. They have passed on their knowledge of decades through this book. To expedite this challenging task, the publisher supported the team at every step. A small team of assistant editors was also appointed to further simplify the editing procedure and attain best results for the readers.

Apart from the editorial board, the designing team has also invested a significant amount of their time in understanding the subject and creating the most relevant covers. They scrutinized every image to scout for the most suitable representation of the subject and create an appropriate cover for the book.

The publishing team has been an ardent support to the editorial, designing and production team. Their endless efforts to recruit the best for this project, has resulted in the accomplishment of this book. They are a veteran in the field of academics and their pool of knowledge is as vast as their experience in printing. Their expertise and guidance has proved useful at every step. Their uncompromising quality standards have made this book an exceptional effort. Their encouragement from time to time has been an inspiration for everyone.

The publisher and the editorial board hope that this book will prove to be a valuable piece of knowledge for researchers, students, practitioners and scholars across the globe.

List of Contributors

Maxime Gauberti, Axel Montagne, Aurélien Quenault and Denis Vivien
Inserm, Inserm UMR-S U919, Serine Proteases and Pathophysiology of the Neurovascular Unit, Université de Caen Basse-Normandie – GIP Cyceron, Caen, France

Susanne M. Schwarzmaier
Department of Anesthesiology, University of Munich Medical Center, Munich, Germany
Institute for Stroke and Dementia Research (ISD), University of Munich Medical Center, Munich, Germany

Nikolaus Plesnila
Institute for Stroke and Dementia Research (ISD), University of Munich Medical Center, Munich, Germany
Munich Cluster of Systems Neurology, Munich, Germany

Eva Mracsko
Department of Neurology, University Heidelberg, Heidelberg, Germany

Roland Veltkamp
Department of Neurology, University Heidelberg, Heidelberg, Germany
Division of Brain Sciences, Imperial College, London, UK

Francesca Gullo, Giulia Donvito, Marzia Lecchi, Barbara Costa and Enzo Wanke
Department of Biotechnologies and Biosciences, University of Milano-Bicocca, Milan, Italy

Alida Amadeo
Department of Biomolecular Sciences and Biotechnology, University of Milan, Milan, Italy

Andrew Constanti
UCL School of Pharmacy, University of London, London, UK

Katie N. Murray and Stuart M. Allan
Faculty of Life Sciences, University of Manchester, Manchester, UK

Adrian R. Parry-Jones
Salford Royal NHS Foundation Trust, Salford, UK

Corinne Benakis, Lidia Garcia-Bonilla, Costantino Iadecola and Josef Anrather
Feil Family Brain and Mind Research Institute, Weill Cornell Medical College, New York, NY, USA

Franca Orsini, Elisa R. Zanier and Maria-Grazia De Simoni
Department of Neuroscience, IRCCS – Istituto di Ricerche Farmacologiche Mario Negri, Milan, Italy

Daiana De Blasio
Department of Neuroscience, IRCCS – Istituto di Ricerche Farmacologiche Mario Negri, Milan, Italy
Department of Experimental and Clinical Sciences, University of Chieti, Pescara, Italy

Rosalia Zangari
Department of Neuroscience, IRCCS – Istituto di Ricerche Farmacologiche Mario Negri, Milan, Italy
Department of Anesthesia and Critical Care Medicine, Fondazione IRCCS Ca' Granda Ospedale Maggiore Policlinico, University of Milan, Milan, Italy

Abby L. Dotson
Neuroimmunology Research, VA Medical Center, Portland, OR, USA
Department of Neurology, Oregon Health and Science University, Portland, OR, USA

Wenbin Zhu and Nicole Libal
Department of Anesthesiology and Perioperative Medicine, Oregon Health and Science University, Portland, OR, USA

Nabil J. Alkayed
Department of Neurology, Oregon Health and Science University, Portland, OR, USA
Department of Anesthesiology and Perioperative Medicine, Oregon Health and Science University, Portland, OR, USA
Knight Cardiovascular Institute, Oregon Health and Science University, Portland, OR, USA

Halina Offner
Neuroimmunology Research, VA Medical Center, Portland, OR, USA
Department of Neurology, Oregon Health and Science University, Portland, OR, USA
Department of Anesthesiology and Perioperative Medicine, Oregon Health and Science University, Portland, OR, USA

Silvia Alfonso-Loeches, Juan R. Ureña-Peralta, Maria José Morillo-Bargues, Jorge Oliver-De La Cruz and Consuelo Guerri
Molecular and Cellular Pathology of Alcohol Laboratory, Prince Felipe Research Center, Valencia, Spain

Friedrich Koch-Nolte
Department of Immunology, University Medical Center Hamburg-Eppendorf, Hamburg, Germany

Xabier Urra and Angel Chamorro
Functional Unit of Cerebrovascular Diseases, Hospital Clínic, Barcelona, Spain
August Pi i Sunyer Biomedical Research Institute (IDIBAPS), Barcelona, Spain

Anna M. Planas
August Pi i Sunyer Biomedical Research Institute (IDIBAPS), Barcelona, Spain
Department of Brain Ischemia and Neurodegeneration, Instituto de Investigaciones Biomédicas de Barcelona (IIBB), Consejo Superior de Investigaciones Científicas (CSIC), Barcelona, Spain

Robert Brunkhorst and Waltraud Pfeilschifter
Cerebrovascular Research Group, Department of Neurology, Frankfurt University Hospital, Frankfurt am Main, Germany

Athanasios Lourbopoulos and Farida Hellal
Laboratory of Experimental Stroke Research, Institute for Stroke and Dementia Research (ISD), University of Munich Medical School, Munich, Germany

Ali Ertürk
Laboratory of Acute Brain Injury, Institute for Stroke and Dementia Research (ISD), University of Munich Medical School, Munich, Germany

Hyun Ah Kim, Stephanie C. Whittle, Seyoung Lee, Hannah X. Chu, Shenpeng R. Zhang, Zihui Wei and Anthony Vinh
Department of Pharmacology, Monash University, Clayton, VIC, Australia

Thiruma V. Arumugam
Department of Physiology, Yong Loo Lin School of Medicine, National University of Singapore, Singapore, Singapore
School of Pharmacy, Sungkyunkwan University, Suwon, South Korea
School of Biomedical Sciences, The University of Queensland, St Lucia, QLD, Australia

Grant R. Drummond and Christopher G. Sobey
Department of Pharmacology, Monash University, Clayton, VIC, Australia
Department of Surgery, Monash Medical Centre, Southern Clinical School, Monash University, Clayton, VIC, Australia

Christiane Albert-Weissenberger, Stine Mencl, Sarah Hopp and Christoph Kleinschnitz
Department of Neurology, University Hospital of Würzburg, Würzburg, Germany

Anna-Leena Sirén
Department of Neurosurgery, University Hospital of Würzburg, Würzburg, Germany

Takashi Shichita
Department of Microbiology and Immunology, School of Medicine, Keio University, Tokyo, Japan
Precursory Research for Embryonic Science and Technology, Japan Science and Technology Agency, Tokyo, Japan

Minako Ito and Akihiko Yoshimura
Department of Microbiology and Immunology, School of Medicine, Keio University, Tokyo, Japan

Mathias Gelderblom, Priyadharshini Arunachalam, Björn Rissiek and Tim Magnus
Department of Neurology, University Medical Center Hamburg-Eppendorf, Hamburg, Germany

Francesc Miró
August Pi i Sunyer Biomedical Research Institute (IDIBAPS), Barcelona, Spain

Rajkumar Vutukuri
Institute of General Pharmacology and Toxicology, pharmazentrum frankfurt, Goethe University Frankfurt, Frankfurt am Main, Germany

Jennifer D. Sokolowski
Department of Pathology, School of Medicine, University of Virginia, Charlottesville, VA, USA
Medical Scientist Training Program, School of Medicine, University of Virginia, Charlottesville, VA, USA
Neuroscience Graduate Program, School of Medicine, University of Virginia, Charlottesville, VA, USA

Chloe N. Chabanon-Hicks and Daniel S. Heffron
Department of Pathology, School of Medicine, University of Virginia, Charlottesville, VA, USA

Claudia Z. Han
Department of Microbiology, Immunology and Cancer Biology, School of Medicine, University of Virginia, Charlottesville, VA, USA
Center for Cell Clearance, University of Virginia, Charlottesville, VA, USA

James W. Mandell
Department of Pathology, School of Medicine, University of Virginia, Charlottesville, VA, USA
Center for Cell Clearance, University of Virginia, Charlottesville, VA, USA

Index

L

M

N

O

P

R

S

T

V